# Essentials of
# GYNECOLOGIC PATHOLOGY

# Essentials of
# GYNECOLOGIC PATHOLOGY

**Pranab Dey**
MBBS MD MIAC FRCPath
Professor
Department of Cytology and Gynecologic Pathology
Postgraduate Institute of Medical Education and Research
Chandigarh, India

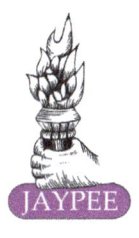

The Health Sciences Publisher
New Delhi | London | Panama

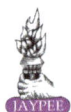 **Jaypee Brothers Medical Publishers (P) Ltd**

#### Headquarters

Jaypee Brothers Medical Publishers (P) Ltd
4838/24, Ansari Road, Daryaganj
New Delhi 110 002, India
Phone: +91-11-43574357
Fax: +91-11-43574314
Email: jaypee@jaypeebrothers.com

#### Overseas Offices

J.P. Medical Ltd
83 Victoria Street, London
SW1H 0HW (UK)
Phone: +44 20 3170 8910
Fax: +44 (0)20 3008 6180
Email: info@jpmedpub.com

Jaypee-Highlights Medical Publishers Inc
City of Knowledge, Bld. 235, 2nd Floor, Clayton
Panama City, Panama
Phone: +1 507-301-0496
Fax: +1 507-301-0499
Email: cservice@jphmedical.com

Jaypee Brothers Medical Publishers (P) Ltd
17/1-B Babar Road, Block-B, Shaymali
Mohammadpur, Dhaka-1207
Bangladesh
Mobile: +08801912003485
Email: jaypeedhaka@gmail.com

Jaypee Brothers Medical Publishers (P) Ltd
Bhotahity, Kathmandu, Nepal
Phone: +977-9741283608
Email: kathmandu@jaypeebrothers.com

Website: www.jaypeebrothers.com
Website: www.jaypeedigital.com

© 2017, Jaypee Brothers Medical Publishers

The views and opinions expressed in this book are solely those of the original contributor(s)/author(s) and do not necessarily represent those of editor(s) of the book.

All rights reserved. No part of this publication may be reproduced, stored or transmitted in any form or by any means, electronic, mechanical, photocopying, recording or otherwise, without the prior permission in writing of the publishers.

All brand names and product names used in this book are trade names, service marks, trademarks or registered trademarks of their respective owners. The publisher is not associated with any product or vendor mentioned in this book.

Medical knowledge and practice change constantly. This book is designed to provide accurate, authoritative information about the subject matter in question. However, readers are advised to check the most current information available on procedures included and check information from the manufacturer of each product to be administered, to verify the recommended dose, formula, method and duration of administration, adverse effects and contraindications. It is the responsibility of the practitioner to take all appropriate safety precautions. Neither the publisher nor the author(s)/editor(s) assume any liability for any injury and/or damage to persons or property arising from or related to use of material in this book.

This book is sold on the understanding that the publisher is not engaged in providing professional medical services. If such advice or services are required, the services of a competent medical professional should be sought.

Every effort has been made where necessary to contact holders of copyright to obtain permission to reproduce copyright material. If any have been inadvertently overlooked, the publisher will be pleased to make the necessary arrangements at the first opportunity.

**Inquiries for bulk sales may be solicited at:** jaypee@jaypeebrothers.com

*Essentials of Gynecologic Pathology*

*First Edition*: **2017**

ISBN: 978-93-86261-20-5

**Dedicated to**

*Shree Shree Satyananda Giri, Rini and Madhumanti*

# Preface

Gynecological pathology is a major component of histopathology. It is essential to have practical knowledge in this subject. In this book I have discussed various lesions in Gynecology and Obstetrics. The etiology, clinical features, macroscopy, histopathology, immunohistochemistry, molecular pathology and treatment of gynecological lesions have been discussed. Multiple tables, boxes and microscopical figures have been provided to illustrate the lesions. I strongly believe that this book will be very helpful to both the students and practicing pathologists who are interested in gynecologic pathology. I also hope that the book will also be helpful to Gynecologists.

**Pranab Dey**

# Acknowledgments

Idea flies in the world to take shape and materialize. My wife Rini helped me to catch the idea of writing my three decades experience in this book. She really deserves the major credit of the book.

I wish to express my special thanks to Dr Suvradeep Mitra. He helped me in every aspect during the preparation of the manuscript by giving his valuable suggestions and also active cooperation.

Subrata Adhikari of Jaypee Brothers Medical Publishers provided me active encouragement and assistance in writing and publishing the book. I also express my gratitude to the full team of the publishing company who helped me from beginning to end.

I am thankful to Late Professor Subhash Kumari Gupta, Professor Arvind Rajwanshi and Professor Raje Nijhawan for sharing their knowledge with me in last three decades.

Lastly, I express my gratitude to God Almighty because without His blessings no work can be done.

# Contents

### Chapter 1: Embryology and Developmental Defects in Female Genital Tract  1–7
- Gonadal Development  1
- Primordial Germ Cells  2
- Reproductive Tract Development  3
- Molecular Genetics in the Development of the Gonads and Reproductive Tract  4
- External Genitalia Development  4
- Disorders of Gonadal and Genital Tract Development  4

### Chapter 2: Inflammatory and Benign Neoplastic Lesions of Vulva  8–23
- Anatomy  8
- Infectious Diseases of Vulva  8
- Non-infectious Inflammatory Diseases of Vulva  12
- Bullous Lesions of Vulva  16
- Vulvodynia  17
- Benign Diseases of Vulva  17
- Miscellaneous Conditions of Vulva  22

### Chapter 3: Premalignant and Malignant Tumors of Vulva  24–36
- World Health Organization Classification of Tumors of Vulva 2014  24
- Squamous Tumors  24
- Squamous Cell Carcinoma of Vulva  27
- Paget Disease of Vulva  31
- Malignant Melanoma of Vulva  33
- Other Uncommon Malignant Tumors of Vulva  34

### Chapter 4: Benign and Malignant Diseases of Vagina  37–49
- WHO Classification of Tumors of Vagina (2014)  37
- Developmental Disorders of Vagina  37
- Infectious Inflammatory Disorders  38
- Noninfectious Inflammatory Diseases of Vagina  40
- Traumatic, Surgery and Radiation-induced Lesions  40
- Postoperative Spindle Cell Nodule  41
- Vaginal Cysts  41
- Müllerian Cyst  41
- Vaginal Adenosis  42
- Vaginal Intraepithelial Neoplasia  43
- Neoplasms of Vagina  44

### Chapter 5: Benign Diseases of Cervix  50–60
- Anatomy  50
- Histology  50
- Squamous Epithelium  50
- Columnar Epithelium  51
- Stroma  51

- Squamocolumnar Junction and Transformation Zone 51
- Changes in Normal Menstrual Cycle 53
- Pregnancy-induced Changes 53
- Arias-Stella Reaction 53
- Squamous Metaplasia 53
- Immature Squamous Metaplasia 54
- Tubal Metaplasia 54
- Transitional Cell Metaplasia 54
- Inflammation of Cervix 55
- Hyperplasia of Cervix 56
- Deep Endocervical Glands and Cysts 59
- Endocervical Polyp 59
- Cervical Cysts 59
- Tunnel Clusters 59

## Chapter 6: Preneoplastic and Neoplastic Lesions of Cervix    61–77
- WHO Classification of Tumors of the Uterus Cervix 61
- The Human Papilloma Virus 62
- Terminology of Preneoplastic Lesions of Cervix 64
- Cervical Intraepithelial Neoplasm Grade 1 or Low Grade Squamous Intraepithelial Lesion 65
- High Grade Squamous Intraepithelial Lesions 66
- Squamous Cell Carcinoma 71
- Variants of Squamous Cell Carcinoma 74

## Chapter 7: Glandular and Miscellaneous Lesions of Cervix    78–95
- Preneoplastic Lesion of Cervical Adenocarcinoma 78
- Early Invasive Adenocarcinoma (Microinvasive Adenocarcinoma) 80
- Adenocarcinoma 81
- Endometrioid Adenocarcinoma 84
- Clear Cell Carcinoma 85
- Serous Adenocarcinoma 85
- Mesonephric Carcinoma 85
- Adenosquamous Carcinoma 86
- Glassy Cell Carcinoma 86
- Adenoid Cystic Carcinoma (ADC) 87
- Adenoid Basal Cell Carcinoma (ABC) 88
- Neuroendocrine Carcinoma 88
- Small Cell Carcinoma of Cervix 88
- Carcinoid and Atypical Carcinoid of Cervix 89
- Large Cell Neuroendocrine Carcinoma 89
- Metastatic Carcinoma in Cervix 89
- Mesenchymal Tumors 90
- Lymphoma of Cervix 92
- Mixed Mesodermal Tumor 92
- Adenomyoma 94

## Chapter 8: Endometrium: Benign Lesions    96–115
- Anatomy and Histology of the Uterus 96
- Cyclic Endometrium 97
- Endometrial Dating and Biopsy 102
- Postmenopausal Endometrium 102
- Pregnancy-induced Changes 103
- Artifacts in Endometrium 104

- Dysfunctional Uterine Bleeding   105
- Hormone-induced Changes   107
- Endometritis   108
- Endometrial Polyp   109
- Adenomyomatous Polyp   110
- Atypical Polypoid Adenomyoma (APAM)   110
- Endometrial Metaplastic and Reactive Changes   111
- Asherman's Syndrome   113
- Endometriosis   113

## Chapter 9: Uterus: Preneoplastic Lesions and Carcinoma          116–139
- WHO Classification of the Tumors of the Uterine Corpus   116
- Endometrial Hyperplasia   117
- Endometrial Intraepithelial Neoplasia   119
- Endometrial Carcinoma   120
- Variants of Endometrioid Carcinoma   125
- Serous Carcinoma   129
- Clear Cell Adenocarcinoma   131
- Mixed Types of Carcinoma   133
- Squamous Cell Carcinoma   133
- Transitional Cell Carcinoma   133
- Small Cell Carcinoma   133
- Ovarian Carcinoma along with Uterine Carcinoma   133
- Tumors of the Epithelial and Mesenchymal Component (Mixed Müllerian Tumor)   135

## Chapter 10: Mesenchymal Tumor of Uterus          140–156
- Endometrial Stromal Tumors   140
- Smooth Muscle Tumors   144
- Leiomyosarcoma   149
- Myxoid Variant   151
- Epithelioid Leiomyosarcomas   151
- Uterine Smooth Muscle Tumors of Uncertain Malignant Potential   152
- Perivascular Epithelioid Cell Tumors   153
- Adenomatoid Tumor   153
- Adenomyosis and Adenomyoma   154
- Uterine Tumors Resembling Ovarian Sex Cord-like Elements   155

## Chapter 11: Anatomy, Histology and Non-neoplastic Lesions of Ovary          157–168
- Anatomy of the Ovary   157
- Histology   157
- Follicle and Derivatives   157
- Infections of Ovary   160
- Non-neoplastic Lesions of the Follicular and Stromal Elements   161
- Polycystic Ovarian Syndrome (PCOS)   163
- Stromal Hyperplasia and Stromal Hyperthecosis   165
- Hilus Cell Hyperplasia   165
- Massive Stromal Edema and Fibromatosis   165
- Pregnancy Luteoma   166
- Ovarian Decidua (Ectopic Decidua)   166
- Ovarian Torsion and Infarction   166
- Ovarian Failure   167
- Congenital Lesions of Ovary   167

### Chapter 12: Ovarian Tumor: General Aspect — 169–178
- Classification of Ovarian Tumors   169
- Classification   171
- Clinical Features   171
- Etiology and Risk Factors   171
- Pathogenesis and Precursor Lesions of Ovarian Carcinoma with Molecular Pathology   171
- Diagnosis and Screening   175
- Staging   176
- Prognostic Factors   176
- Treatment   177

### Chapter 13: Epithelial Carcinoma of Ovary — 179–208
- Serous Tumor   179
- Serous Carcinoma   184
- Mucinous Tumor of Ovary   186
- Endometrioid Carcinoma of Ovary   192
- Malignant Müllerian Mixed Tumor (Carcinosarcoma)   195
- Endometrioid Stromal Sarcoma   197
- Clear Cell Tumors of Ovary   198
- Transitional Cell Tumor   201
- Mixed Epithelial Tumor   204
- Squamous Cell Carcinoma   205
- Undifferentiated Carcinoma   205
- Neuroendocrine Carcinoma of the Ovary   205

### Chapter 14: Sex Cord Tumors of Ovary — 209–227
- Granulosa Cell Tumor   209
- Sertoli–Leydig Cell Tumor   219
- Sertoli Cell Tumor   224
- Gynandroblastoma   225
- Sex Cord Tumor with Annular Tubules   225
- Steroid Cell Tumors   225

### Chapter 15: Germ Cell Tumor of Ovary — 228–244
- Dysgerminoma   228
- Yolk Sac Tumors   230
- Embryonal Carcinoma   234
- Polyembryoma   235
- Choriocarcinoma   235
- Teratoma   236
- Mixed Malignant Germ Cell Tumors   243
- Gonadoblastoma   243

### Chapter 16: Metastatic and Miscellaneous Tumors of Ovary — 245–250
- Metastatic Tumors of Ovary   245
- Miscellaneous Tumors of Ovary   248

### Chapter 17: Fallopian Tube — 251–261
- Anatomy   251
- Histology   251
- Blood Supply and Lymphatics   252
- Non-neoplastic Lesions of Fallopian Tube   252
- Salpingitis Isthmica Nodosa   253
- Tubal Pregnancy   254

- Infections  254
- Torsion  256
- Tumors of the Fallopian Tube  256
- Cysts  259
- Female Adnexal Tumor of Probable Wolffian Origin  260

## Chapter 18: Pathology of Placenta                                                                              262–277
- Normal Development  262
- Microscopy  263
- Placenta Gross  264
- Indications of Placental Examination  264
- Abnormalities of the Shape of Placenta  264
- Abnormal Adherence of Placenta  265
- Multiple Gestations  266
- Placental Inflammation and Intrauterine Infections  268
- Circulatory Disorders of Placenta: Maternal Circulatory Disorder  271
- Chorangiosis  274
- Placenta in Maternal and Fetal Disorders  274
- Pathology of Membranes  275
- Non-trophoblastic Tumors  275
- Umbilical Cord Pathology  276

## Chapter 19: Gestational Trophoblastic Disease                                                                   278–287
- Hydatidiform Mole  278
- Invasive Hydatidiform Mole  280
- Choriocarcinoma  280
- Placental Site Trophoblastic Tumor  283
- Epithelioid Trophoblastic Tumor  285
- Exaggerated Placental Site Reaction  286
- Placental Site Nodule  286

## Chapter 20: Gross Examination of the Samples and Synoptic Reporting Format                                      288-295
- Essential Things Required before Grossing  288
- Grossing Room  288
- Individual Specimen  288
- Vulvectomy Specimen  292
- Salpingectomy Specimen  292
- Oophorectomy  293
- Examination of the Placenta  293
- Synoptic Reporting of Gynecological Lesions  294

*Index*                                                                                                           297

# Embryology and Developmental Defects in Female Genital Tract

The complete knowledge of the development of the female genital tract is essential to understand various congenital anomalies of this area. The essential components of the female genital tract are ovaries, reproductive tract and external genitalia. These organs differentiate within the utero before the end of the first trimester. Human fetus has the capability to develop in either sex till first 7 weeks after conception. As the early genital tract development is similar in both female and male so this period is called as indifferent gonadal phase. The exact phenotype of human fetus is determined by the presence of sex chromosome XX or XY. In absence of Y chromosome the fetus differentiates as female. Under the influence of Y chromosome the testis develops and fetus develops as male (Figure 1.1). Key outline of female genital tract is shown in the Box 1.1.

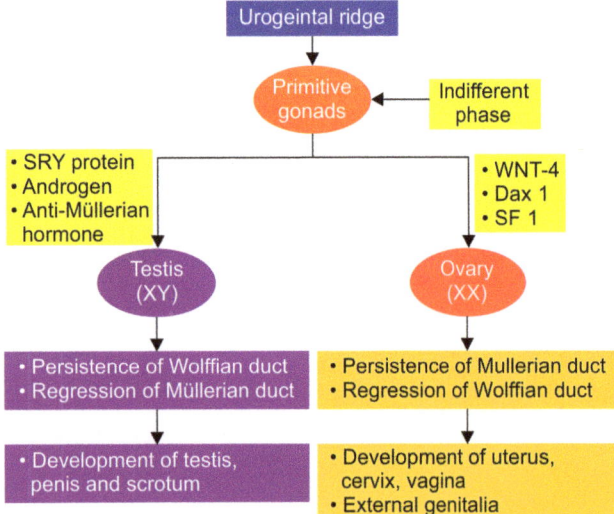

Figure 1.1: Schematic diagram of overall development of ovary and testis in relation to sex chromosome

**Box 1.1:** Key chronology of female genital tract development
- 4th to 6th week:
  - Migration of germ cells towards genital ridge
  - Paramesonephric (Müllerian) duct formation
- 7th to 8th week:
  - Gonadal differentiated phase. Cortical cords formation
  - Müllerian duct fusion starts from the cephalic part and fallopian tubes, uterus, cervix form
- 10th to 12th week:
  - External genitalia develops
- 4th to 5th month
  - Primordial follicles formation in ovary complete
  - Lower vaginal canal fuses with upper vaginal canal

## GONADAL DEVELOPMENT

The development of the gonads starts from the 5th week. The gonads develop in two phases:
1. Initial indifferent phase and
2. Later differentiated phase.

In the initial indifferent phase, the gonads are bipotential to develop male or female as the cells in the gonads can differentiate in either direction. Later phase of gonadal development is more differentiated and this is solely influenced by genes in the Y chromosome. The initial gonads develop from the gonadal ridges. The gonadal ridge develops in the medial side of the mesonephros as a bulge due to proliferation of the epithelial lining along with the underlying mesoderm (Figure 1.2). The epithelial cells invaginate within the mesoderm as multiple cords like structures known as primary sex cord. The primitive germ cells are noted in the yolk sac during the 4th week. During 6th week the primitive germ cells migrate by amoeboid movement and travels from original source of the yolk sac along the pathway of the dorsal mesentery of the hind gut to the ultimate destination of the gonadal ridge. At this time the epithelial cells of the genital ridge proliferate and invaginate into the mesenchymal

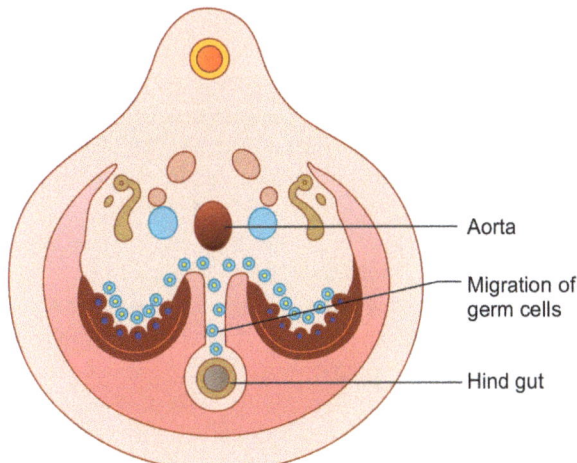

**Figure 1.2:** Schematic diagram shows development of genital ridge and migration of the germ cells from the yolk sac to the genital ridge

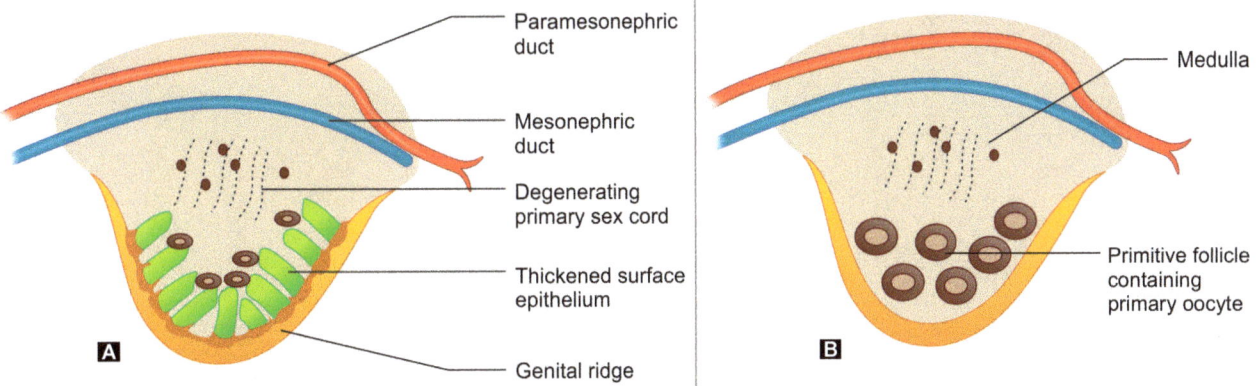

**Figures 1.3A and B:** (A) At first primary sex cord develops that regress in course of time; (B) the surface epithelium of the genital ridge proliferates and invaginates in the mesoderm to form primordial follicles

tissue underneath it to form primary sex cord. The germ cells are incorporated into the primary sex cord. As the Y chromosome is absent so the primary sex cords in the female embryo break down as small clusters in 8th week and remain as rudimentary structure with the primitive germ cells within the medullary part of ovary (Figure 1.3). Later part these cords disappear and are replaced by blood vessels. Under the influence of X chromosome the secondary generation of cortical epithelial cells develop and invaginate within the mesoderm of the ovary to form secondary sex cords. These cortical cords increase in size and then break down in multiple small fragments. The single layer of cortical epithelial cells encircles the primordial germ cells to form primordial follicle.

## PRIMORDIAL GERM CELLS

The primitive germ cells (PGC) do not develop from the genital ridge. Their source of origin is totally different. PGCs develop in the yolk sac and travels to the genital ridge by the influence of stella, fragilis and BMP-4 genes. The PGCs characteristically express a special transcription factor OCT4. The PGC survives during migration by the complex interaction of its surface receptors c-kit and the stem cell factors liberated by the surrounding mesoderm.[1] Once the PGCs arrive in the genital ridge, they become static and aggregates in the stroma of the genital ridge. These PGCs in the genital ridge proliferate by mitotic division into several million cells. The germ cells are encircled by cortical epithelial cells and form primordial follicles. The germ cell in the center of the follicle is known as oocyte. Once meiotic division of the oocyte starts the further mitosis is not possible. The oocytes remain frozen in the first phase of meiosis till the time of ovulation. In course of time the large number of the oocytes undergoes apoptosis and degenerate. At the time of menarche near about four lakhs primordial follicles remain in the ovary.

## REPRODUCTIVE TRACT DEVELOPMENT

The embryonic genitourinary tract is composed of three things: pronephros, mesonephros and metanephros. The pronephros and mesonephros both are transient structures and disappear in course of time. The mesonephric duct also known as Wolffian duct takes important role in the development of male reproductive system. However, the Wolffian duct slowly disappears in the female during embryonic development. The mesonephros and mesonephric duct remain as vestigial structures such as Gartner duct cyst, epoophoron and paraoophoron. The paramesonephric duct is also known as Müllerian duct. It generates from the longitudinal invagination of coelomic epithelium lateral to the Wolffian duct. It starts cranially from the abdominal cavity and extends caudally up to the pelvis. At first it runs laterally parallel to the Wolffian duct and then this duct crosses the Wolffian duct caudo-medially to meet with opposite paramesonephric duct (Figure 1.4). Uterus, cervix and vagina (upper 2/3rd) develops from the Müllerian ducts due to the fusion of the caudal end of the Müllerian ducts. The fusion of two Müllerian ducts occurs between 7th to 9th weeks. In this time fusion of the vertical parts of the two ducts may be incomplete and a midline septum remains (Figure 1.5). This midline septum of the uterus disappears around 20th week (Figure 1.6). The terminal caudal end of the fused Müllerian ducts comes in contact with the posterior part of urogenital sinus and induces the formation of the sinovaginal bulb. The sinovaginal bulb later on canalizes to generate lower 1/3rd of vagina (Figure 1.7). The proximal or cranial part of the Müllerian ducts does not fuse together and form the two fallopian tubes that open in the peritoneal cavity.

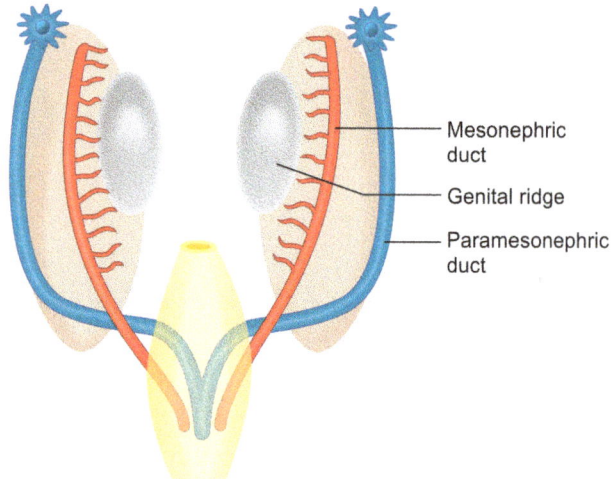

**Figure 1.4:** Schematic diagram of mesonephric duct along with paramesonephric duct. The paramesonephric duct runs parallel to the mesonephric duct

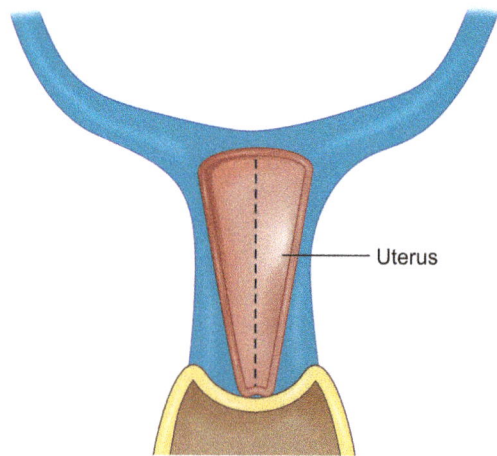

**Figure 1.6:** Midline septum separating the two paramesonephric ducts also slowly dissolves and single uterine, cervix and vaginal cavity develops

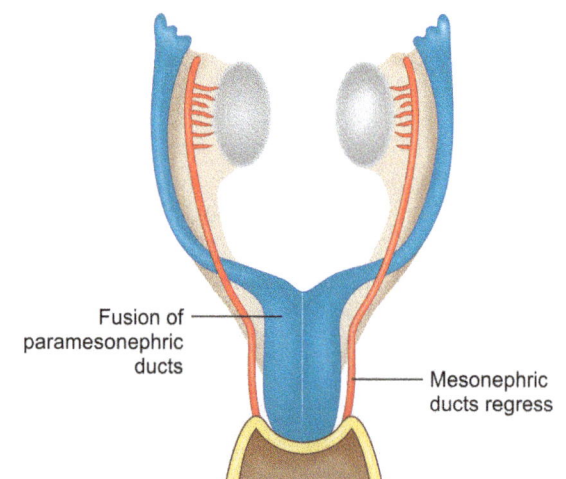

**Figure 1.5:** Mesonephric ducts regress and two paramesonephric duct fuse to form uterus, cervix and upper part of vagina

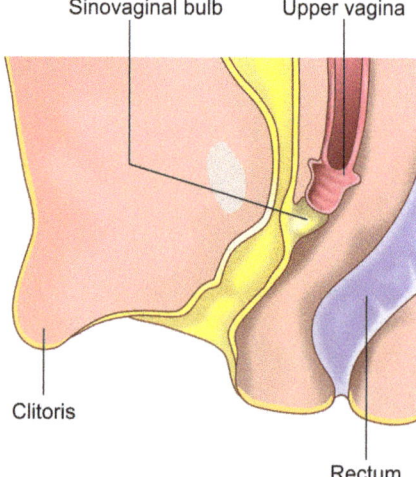

**Figure 1.7:** A protrusion known as sinovaginal bulb arises from the urogenital sinus and projects towards the vagina. Later on the upper 1/3rd of vagina and sinovaginal bulb fuses to form a complete vagina

During the fusion of the Müllerian ducts the peritoneal fold is brought together that later on forms the broad ligament. Successively, the rectouterine and vesicouterine pouch form. The proliferation and differentiation of surrounding mesenchymal tissue around the uterus form parametrium.

## MOLECULAR GENETICS IN THE DEVELOPMENT OF THE GONADS AND REPRODUCTIVE TRACT

The sex of the human fetus is determined by the presence of XX for female and XY for male. It was assumed long back that Y chromosome contains a gene known as testis determining factor (TDF). Later on, the gene of the TDF was isolated and identified from the short arm of Y chromosome. This part is labeled as sex determining region gene in the Y chromosome (SRY).[2,3] The presence of SRY gene induces the development of male fetus. The SRY gene is situated in the short arm of chromosome Y. The SRY gene produces several nuclear proteins that specifically binds with DNA. This DNA-binding protein acts as a transcriptional activation factor of many other genes. The exact target gene of SRY is not known, however SRY gene products possibly act on SOX9 gene. By the influence of SRY gene the somatic cell populations of the gonads develop pre-sertoli cells followed by sertoli cells. This is an important event that stimulates the subsequent cascade of development of male fetus. As mentioned before, the female reproductive tract is produced in default and in the absence of SRY gene in the Y chromosome female reproductive system develops. In absence of SRY gene the primary germ cells proliferate and are surrounded by cortical epithelial cells to form primordial follicles. It has been proposed that several other genes are also responsible for the initial development of female genital tract such as LIM homeobox gene 9 (Lhx9), steroidogenic factor 1 (SF1), empty-spiracles homeobox gene 2(Emx2), paired-box gene 2(Pax2), Pax8 and Wnt7a.[4-8] These genes are mainly responsible for Müllerian tract development and they act by an unknown complex interaction.

## EXTERNAL GENITALIA DEVELOPMENT

In the initial period up to 7th week the external genitalia of both sexes are similar and indifferent as like gonads. This period is known as indifferent period of external genitalia. The distinct sexual characteristics of the external genitalia start from 9th week. At first the genital tubercle arises at the proximal end of the cloacal membrane due to proliferation of the mesenchyme. This occurs in the 4th week in both female and male fetus. This genital tubercle enlarges and forms the primordial phallus. On each side of the cloaca two folds develop: medially urogenital fold and laterally labioscrotal

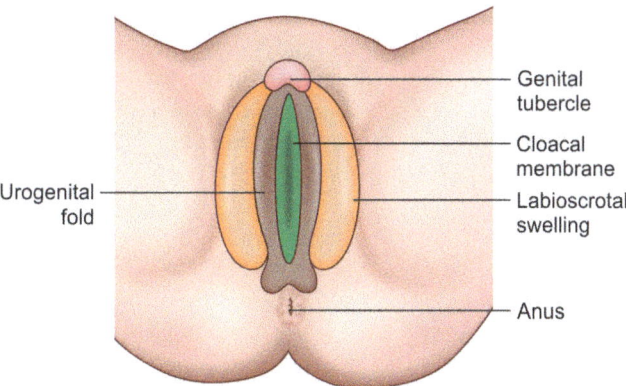

**Figure 1.8:** Schematic diagram showing the development of external genitalia. Labia minora develop from the urogenital folds and labia majora develop from the labioscrotal swelling

fold (Figure 1.8). The anterior fusion of labioscrotal fold is known as anterior labial commissure and the posterior fusion of the labioscrotal fold is labeled as posterior labial commissure. A ridge of mesenchyme (urorectal septum) develops in between the cloacal membrane and rectum that separates the genitourinary system from the rectum. The clitoris develops from the primordial phallus in case of female. The inner urogenital folds give rise to labia minora and the outer labioscrotal folds develop as labia minora.

## DISORDERS OF GONADAL AND GENITAL TRACT DEVELOPMENT

The common causes of congenital abnormalities of female genital tract are:
1. **Environmental:** Viral infections, ionizing radiations, etc.
2. **Genetic:** Chromosomal disorders such as 45X in Turner syndrome, 47XXY in Klinefelter's syndrome, etc.

### Gonadal Abnormalities

*Ovarian Dysgenesis or Agenesis*

The patients are 46XX and karyotypically normal. However, the primordial germ cells (PGC) do not develop or migrate from the yolk sac and so gonads are free of any PGC. The ovaries fail to develop in such cases. On histopathology, the ovaries show streak gonads.

*Ovarian Hypoplasia*

This is typically occurs in Turner syndrome with karyotypically 45X chromosome. In majority of the cases, the X chromosome is derived from the mother. These patients do not show any Barr bodies in buccal smear. In Turner syndrome, the PGC develops and migrates to the genital ridge to form gonads. Due to the absence of other extra X chromosome the PGCs do not sustain and fail to develop any primordial follicle. The ovaries do not develop and no ovarian sex hormones are produced. As there is no Y chromosome so SRY gene is absent and the Müllerian tract persists to form internal genitalia. Lack of ovarian sex hormone causes failure of development of female external genitalia. In some cases, the patients may show 45X/46XY karyotyping. Unlike classic 45X Turner syndrome, these patients are in higher risk of gonadoblastoma and dysgerminoma.

*Histopathology:* The ovaries are small and streak like. The outer cortex of the ovary is thin and composed of spindle shaped cells. The oocytes are characteristically absent. The hilum of the ovary may contain rete ovarii and hilar cells.

### Testicular Feminization

The patients are genotypically male and show 46XY karyotyping. This disease is an X-linked recessive disorder. In this disease, there is lack of testosterone sensitivity in the receptor. The incidence of testicular feminization is about one in 60,000 male births.[9] In this disease, SRY gene in the Y chromosome is retained. Due to the presence of SRY gene the Müllerian duct development is suppressed. Uterus and cervix are absent and the vagina terminates in a blind pouch. However, at puberty there is estradiol secretion from the testis because of lack of any negative feedback control. Therefore, the patients are phenotypically female and they show scanty pubic hair with normal breast development. The patients usually present with amenorrhea. The testes are cryptorchid and remains either in abdomen or in inguinal canal. The chances of malignancies are increased in higher age group and seminoma is the commonest malignant tumor.

*Biology:* Testosterone is synthesized in the testis under the influence of luteinizing hormone liberated from the pituitary gland. Dihydrotestosterone is formed by the enzymatic modification of testosterone in the target tissue with the help of 5 α reductase. Both the testosterone and dihydrotestosterone bind with their respective receptors on the nuclear membrane and the receptor-hormone complex enters into the nucleus and acts on the gene to produce necessary substances (Figure 1.9). Dihydrotestosterone, the metabolite of testosterone is more potent than testosterone and is responsible for the formation of various external male organ such as external genitalia, prostate and also urethra. In testicular feminization syndrome the following defects may happen: (1) Absence of

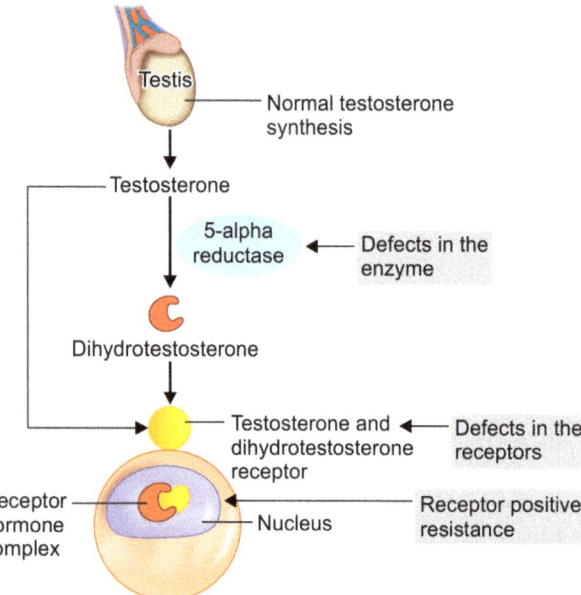

**Figure 1.9:** The schematic diagram showing the causes of androgen insensitivity in testicular feminization

5 α reductase enzyme, (2) Defects of androgen receptors, (3) Receptor positive resistance.

*Histopathology:* Microscopically, the testis show immature seminiferous tubules without any sign of spermatogenesis. The empty sertoli tubules may form nodule like structure. There is abundant interstitial stroma along with large sheet of Leydig cells.

## Hermaphrodites
## (Intersex or Disorders of Sex Differentiation)

Hermaphrodite may be two types: True hermaphrodite and pseudo hermaphrodite.

*True Hermaphrodite:* The patient shows both male and female gonads and external genitalia.

*Pseudohermaphrodite:* The patient shows internal genitalia of the same genotype and external genitalia opposite to the genotype. The terminologies such as intersex, hermaphrodite, pseudohermaphrodite, etc. are often confusing and therefore, LWPES1/ESPEW2 consensus groups suggested the terminology as "disorder of sex development" (DSD).[10] Chicago Consensus Conference,[10] 2005 also propsed to replace the term male pseudohermaphrodite as 46,XY DSD, female pseudohermaphrodite as 46, XX DSD, true hermaphrodite as ovotesticular DSD and XX male or XX reversal as 46, XX testicular DSD. The classification of the DSD was based primarily on the pathogenesis of DSD[10] (Table 1.1).

## Essentials of Gynecologic Pathology

Table 1.1: Disorder of sex development[10]

| Sex chromosome | 46,XY DSD | 46,XX DSD |
|---|---|---|
| • 45,X (Turner syndrome and variants)<br>• 47,XXY (Klinefelter syndrome and variants)<br>• 45,X/46,XY (Mixed gonadal dysgenesis, ovotesticular DSD)<br>• 46,XX/46,XY (Chimeric, ovotesticular DSD) | • Disorder of gonadal (testicular) development: Complete gonadal dysgenesis, pure gonadal dysgenesis, gonadal regression and ovotesticular DSD<br>• Disorder in androgen synthesis or action<br>• Other: Severe hypospadias, cloacal extrophy | • Disorder of gonadal (ovarian) development: Ovotesticular DSD, testicular DSD, gonadal dysgenesis<br>• Androgen excess: Fetal, fetoplacental, maternal<br>• Other: Müllerian agenesis or hypoplasia, vaginal atresia |

**DSD:** Disorder of sex development

### Developmental Anomalies of Uterus and Cervix

The developmental anomalies of uterus and cervix may be due to:
a. Complete or partial failure of the development of Müllerian duct
b. Failure of fusion of two Müllerian ducts
c. Incomplete removal of the septum of the fused Müllerian duct.

#### Complete Failure of the Development of Müllerian Duct

The complete agenesis of the Müllerian ducts may cause total failure of the development of fallopian tube to upper part of vagina. This is also known as Mayer-Rokitansky-Küster–Hauser (MRKH) syndrome. Skeletal and cardiac malformation may also be seen in MRKH syndrome. Till date no specific genetic abnormality is detected in this syndrome.

#### Failure of Fusion or Incomplete Removal of Septum (Figure 1.10)

The defective fusion of the two Müllerian ducts may be the cause of various abnormalities in the uterus, cervix and upper 1/3rd of vagina. Majority of the women with Müllerian duct anomalies do not experience any significant problem of conception or abnormality in menstruation. However, there are higher rates of spontaneous abortion, premature delivery or abnormal placement of fetus in uterus in Müllerian anomalies.[11] The prevalence of Müllerian anomalies varies from 0.16 to 10%.[11] The wide variation of incidence is due to the variability of the detection rate of such anomalies as many such Müllerian anomalies remain silent for long time till the specific investigations are carried out. According to American Fertility Society the Müllerian duct anomalies have been classified into six type depending on the degree of failure of fusion or regression of the septum.[12] In addition the defects caused by diethylstilbestrol exposure in utero has been also included.

**Class I: Segmental agenesis**—Complete or partial agenesis of uterus, cervix, vagina.

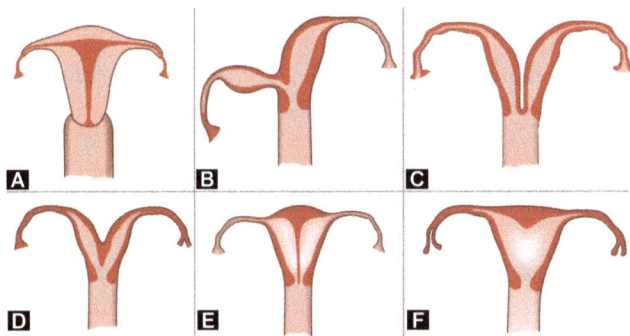

Figure 1.10: The schematic diagram of various anomalies of the development of uterus; (A) Normal uterus; (B) Unicornuate uterus; (C) Didelphus uterus; (D) Bicornuate uterus; (E) Septate uterus; (F) Arcuate uterus

**Class II: Unicornuate uterus**—One rudimentray horn is present. This horn may or may not communicate with main uterine cavity.

**Class III: Uterine didelphys**—There is partial or complete failure of fusion of the Müllerian ducts resulting in double uterus, cervix or vagina.

**Class IV: Bicornuate uterus**—In this condition, the uterus has two horns. Bicornuate uterus is the commonest abnormality of the uterine malformation. This is caused by the failure of fusion of Müllerian duct at the apex of the uterus. The degree of the defect of fusion may vary and there may be two horns of uterus at the fundus or the fusion defect may be more extensive and may reach upto cervical canal.

**Class V: Sepatate uterus**—Uterine cavity is separated longitudinally by a septum. In case of septate uterus, the uterovaginal septum fails to dissolve after the fusion of the two Müllerian ducts. This is one of the commonest Müllerian duct anomalies. The septate uterus is frequently associated with spontaneous abortion. In case of Uterus subseptus, the uterine septum is partial or incomplete and does not reach up to the cervix.

**Class VI: Arcuate uterus**—Here the uterus is almost normal except a small notch in the fundus. This type of uterine anomaly is not related with any clinical side effect.

**Class VII: Diethylstilbestrol exposure related anomalies.**

## Anomalies of Vaginal Development

**Vaginal agenesis:** Here the vagina does not develop at all due to absence of Müllerian duct. In addition, the uterus and cervix also do not develop. This is the part of MRKH syndrome as described before.

**Disorders of longitudinal fusion of vagina:** This develops due to incomplete fusion of the two Müllerian ducts in the caudal end. The patient usually complains of dyspareunia or disorders in menstrual flow.

**Disorders of transverse fusion of the vagina:** This is due to the incomplete canalization of the vagina at the junction of Müllerian duct and sinovaginal bulb resulting in transverse vaginal septum or imperforate hymen. The patient complains of primary amenorrhea. Retention of menstrual blood may cause hematocolpos and urinary retention.

## REFERENCES

1. Bendel-Stenzel M, Anderson R, Heasman J, Wylie C. The origin and migration of primordial germ cells in the mouse. Semin Cell Dev Biol. 1998;9:393-400.
2. Palmer MS, Sinclair AH, Berta P, Ellis NA, Goodfellow PN, Abbas NE, et al. Genetic evidence that ZFY is not the testis-determining factor. Nature. 1989;342:937-9.
3. Sinclair AH, Berta P, Palmer MS, Hawkins JR, Griffiths BL, Smith MJ, et al. A gene from the human sex-determining region encodes a protein with homology to a conserved DNA-binding motif. Nature. 1990;346:240-4.
4. Hammes A, Guo JK, Lutsch G, Leheste JR, Landrock D, Ziegler U, et al. Two splice variants of the Wilms' tumor 1 gene have distinct functions during sex determination and nephron formation. Cell. 2001;106:319-29.
5. Luo X, Ikeda Y, Parker KL. A cell-specific nuclear receptor is essential for adrenal and gonadal development and sexual differentiation. Cell. 1994;77:481-90.
6. Miyamoto N, Yoshida M, Kuratani S, Matsuo I, Aizawa S. Defects of urogenital development in mice lacking Emx2. Development. 1997;124:1653-64.
7. Katoh-Fukui Y, Tsuchiya R, Shiroishi T, Nakahara Y, Hashimoto N, Noguchi K, et al. Male-to-female sex reversal in M33 mutant mice. Nature. 1998;393:688-92.
8. Birk O, Casiano D, Wassif C, Cogliati T, Zhao L, Zhao Y, et al. The LIM homeobox gene Lhx9 is essential for mouse gonad formation. Nature. 2000;403:909-13.
9. Schweikert HU. The androgen resistance syndromes: clinical and biochemical aspects. Eur J Pediatr. 1993; 152: S50-7.
10. Houk CP, Hughes IA, Ahmed SF, Lee PA; Writing Committee for the International Intersex Consensus Conference Participants. Summary of consensus statement on intersex disorders and their management. International Intersex Consensus Conference. Pediatrics. 2006;118(2):753-7.
11. Troiano RN, McCarthy SM. Müllerian duct anomalies: imaging and clinical issues. Radiology. 2004;233:19-34.
12. The American Fertility Society classifications of adnexal adhesions, distal tubal occlusion, tubal occlusion secondary to tubal ligation, tubal pregnancies, müllerian anomalies and intrauterine adhesions. [No authors listed] Fertil Steril. 1988;49(6):944-55.

# Inflammatory and Benign Neoplastic Lesions of Vulva

## ANATOMY

The female external genitalia consists of: mons pubis labia majora, labia minora, clitoris, prepuce and vestibule (Figure 2.1).

### Mons Pubis

It is the fibrofatty tissue over the pubic bone and pubic symphysis. This is covered with the skin containing hair.

### Labia Majora

Labia majora represents two longitudinal folds of skin situated lateral to the pudendal cleft. They extend from the mons pubis to the perineum and is covered with skin containing loose connective tissue, smooth muscles, fat, glands and blood vessels. Many sweat glands and sebaceous glands open into the labia majora.

### Labia Minora

Labia minora are present medial to the labia majora. They extend from the clitoris to downwards encircling the vaginal orifice. Anteriorly each labia minus divides around the clitoris. The upper part of the labia minus joins to the other labia minus and forms the prepuce of the clitoris and lower art forms the frenulum. Labia minora are rich in elastic fibers and abundant sebaceous follicles. They are devoid of any smooth muscle, fat and any glandular elements.

### Vestibule

The vestibule is the cleft-like space that is situated in between the two labia minora. The glands of Bartholin and many minor vestibular glands open into the vestibule. Two orifices open in the vestibular space: anteriorly urethral orifice and the posteriorly vaginal orifice. The vaginal orifice is partially narrowed by thin layer of fibrofatty tissue known as hymen.

### Clitoris

This is situated anteriorly in between the two folds of labia minora. This is the homologous of male penis and contains root, body and a glans. The glans of the clitoris is a round spongy erectile structure and is very much touch sensitive. The clitoris is rich in blood vessels and nerves and is covered by thin layer of stratified squamous epithelium.

Mons pubis, labia majora and minora are covered by keratinized stratified squamous epithelium. Unlike mons pubis and labia majora, the labia minora are devoid of fat and adnexal glands. The vestibule is lined by squamous epithelium.

### Lymphatic Drainage

Vulval lymphatics drain into the femoral and inguinal lymph node. The lymphatic from the deep inguinal lymph node drains into the pelvic lymph node via femoral canal.

## INFECTIOUS DISEASES OF VULVA

Vulva is infected by a large number of organisms consisting of bacterial, fungal and viral infections (Table 2.1). Many

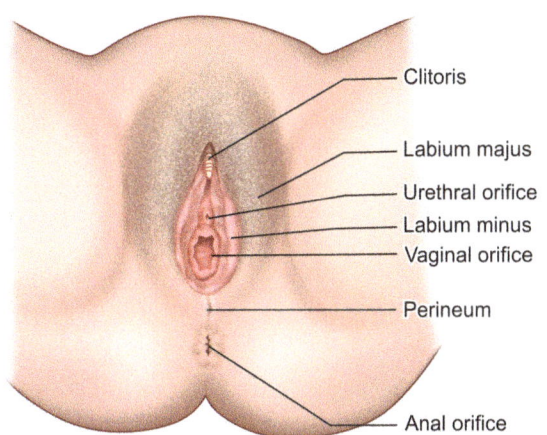

**Figure 2.1:** Schematic diagram showing anatomy of vulva

**Table 2.1:** Infections of vulva

| Bacterial | Fungal | Parasitic | Viral |
|---|---|---|---|
| • Syphilis<br>• Tuberculosis<br>• Granuolma ingunale<br>• Lymphogranuloma venereum<br>• Malakoplakia | • Candida<br>• Pityriasis versicolor<br>• Actinomycosis<br>• Chromoblastomycosis | • Scabies<br>• Pubic lice | • Herpes virus<br>• Human papilloma virus<br>• Molluscum contagiosum |

such infections are diagnosed by the clinical examination alone and pathologists play little role.

## Bacterial Infections

### Syphilis

Syphilis is caused by the spirochetes *Treponema pallidum*. If untreated, the disease undergoes through three phases: primary, secondary and tertiary. This natural phase of the disease is rare because of the intervention by antibiotic penicillin.

**Primary syphilis (10 days to 3 months after the infection):** It is characterized by the chancre. This is a round to oval painless, indurated, shallow ulcer. In addition to the vulva, it may occur in anal mucosa, oral mucosa and cervix. The large numbers of treponema are shed from the chancre and the patient is highly infective at his stage. In untreated case the lesion slowly heals without any scar and the patient undergoes in the secondary stage.

*Histopathology:* In chancre there is beach of surface epithelium. The dermis shows infiltration by lymphocytes, polymorphs and plasma cells. Perivascular infiltration of lymphocytes and plasma cells are noted. The features are non-specific for syphilis.

**Secondary syphilis (few weeks to several months):** In untreated patient the secondary syphilis develops. The patient develops systemic manifestations like fever and arthralgia. Macules and maculopapular lesions in the skin are seen involving mucosa and the skin of the sole of foot or hand.

*Histopathology:* The histopathology of condyloma lata shows hyperkeratosis and acanthosis of the epidermis. The dermis shows lymphocytes and marked plasma cells infiltration. The smaller arteries show inflammation and obliteration of the lumen.

**Tertiary syphilis:** Tertiary syphilis is uncommon in vulva. It may show nodular soft lesions known as gumma. The lesion shows central necrosis along with epithelioid cell granulomas.

**Diagnostic tests of syphilis:** In the initial period: the special stain such as Warthin –Starry stain shows the spirochetes in the dermis.

**Serological test of syphilis:** Venereal disease laboratory test (VDRL), fluorescent treponemal antibody absorption test (FTA-ABS) and rapid plasma regain (RPR). VDRL and RPR tests have almost equal specificity and become positive one month after the infection.[1,2]

**Differential diagnosis:** Condyloma lata, plasma cell vulvitis.

**Treatment:** Penicillin is the treatment of choice in case of syphilis. Serological tests are helpful to assess the success of the treatment and also to exclude any reinfection.

### Chancroid

*Haemophilus ducreyi*, a gram negative bacillus, is the causative organism. The patient develops multiple small 1 to 2 mm painful genital ulcers after 4/5 days of initial exposure of the infection that may coalesce to form large confluent ulcer and if untreated may develop fistulas.

**Histopathology:** The histopathological features of chancre are non-specific and biopsy is done to exclude the other lesions. The ulcer bed presents with necrosis and infiltration by polymorphs. The deeper tissue shows lymphocytes, plasma cells and granulomas. The diagnosis of chancroid is usually confirmed by PCR.[3]

**Differential diagnosis:** Herpes simplex virus (HSV) and syphilis.

### Granuloma Inguinale

Gram negative rod *Klebsiella granulomatis*, is the causative organism. The incubation period of the disease is a week to few months. The patient presents with painless erythematous papules in the vulva, vagina and cervix.

**Histopathology:** The biopsy of the ulcer shows extensive mixed inflammatory cells consisting of polymorphs, lymphocytes, plasma cells and macrophages. There may be pseudoepitheliomatous hyperplasia in the adjacent surface epithelium of the ulcer. The diagnosis of granulomas inguinale is confirmed by the demonstration of rod-shaped Donovan bodies within the vacuoles of the macrophages in the hematoxylin and eosin stain or Giemsa stain.[4]

**Differential diagnosis:** Different ulcerative lesions of the vulva are considered in the differential diagnosis of granuloma inguinale (Table 2.2). Demonstration of

**Table 2.2:** Vulval ulcerative lesions

| Disease | Causative agent | Incubation period | STD | Clinical feature | Histopathology | Diagnostic test | Treatment |
|---|---|---|---|---|---|---|---|
| Herpes simplex | HSV-2, HSV-1 (15% cases) (DNA virus) | 4 days–14 days | Yes | Papule, vesicle followed by ulcer. Painful, multiple ulcer | Ground glass nuclear chromatin, multinucleate giant cells, intranuclear inclusion | Cytological scraping smear, HSV serology, immunohistochemistry, PCR, culture | Antiviral agent (Acyclovir) |
| Molluscum contagiosum | MSV (DNA pox virus) | 2–6 weeks | Yes | Multiple, flesh colored papules with central-dome shaped notch | Basophilic intracytoplasmic molluscum body | Cytological scraping, histopathology | Self-limited, cryotherapy, tropical agent |
| Granuloma inguinale | *Klebsiella granulomatis* | Weeks to months | Yes | Painless erythematous ulcer bleeds on touch | Polymorphs, lymphocytes, plasma cells and macrophages. Rod-shaped organism within the macrophages | Giemsa and silver stain | Antibiotic |
| Lymphogranuloma venerum | *Chlamydia trachomatis* | 3 days–6 weeks | Yes | Nontender ulcer | Lymphocytes, polymorphs, giant cells | Complement fixation test, immunofluorescence test, intradermal skin test | Antibiotic |
| Chancroid | *Haemophilus ducreyi* | 4–5 days | Yes | Small 1–2 mm multiple painful ulcer | Lymphocytes, plasma cells granulomas | PCR | Antibiotic |
| Syphilitic chancre | *Treponema pallidum* | 10 days–3 months | Yes | Painless, indurated shallow ulcer | Lymphocytes, plasma cells, vasculitis | VDRL, FTA-ABS, RPR, Silver stain | Penicillin |
| Tuberculosis | *Mycobacterium tuberculosis* | 3–4 weeks | No | Painless ulcer | Lymphocytes, plasma cells, epithelioid granulomas, giant cells, necrosis | AFB stain, culture | Anti-tubercular therapy |

*Abbreviations:* PCR, Polymerase chain reaction
VDRL, Venereal Disease Research Laboratory
FTA-ABS, Fluorescent treponemal antibody-absorption
RPR, Rapid plasma regain
AFB, Acid-fast Bacilli

intracellular rod shaped Donovan bodies is diagnostic of granulomas inguinale.

**Treatment:** Antibiotic therapy.

### Lymphogranuloma Venereum (LGV)

*Chlamydia trachomatis* is the causative organism.

**Clinical feature:** The disease passes through three stages: (1) Initial phase of ulcer formation, (2) lymphadenitis: The inguinal lymph node becomes enlarged, painful and purulent, (3) anorectal and genital involvement with fibrosis and stricture formation.[4]

**Histopathology:** Non-specific changes: (1) Dense lymphocytic and plasma cell infiltration along with multinucleated giant cells and granulomas. (2) The lymph node biopsy shows stellate abscess along with granulomas and chronic inflammation.

**Diagnosis:** The diagnosis of LGV is confirmed by complement fixation test (CFT), microimmunofluorescence (MIF) test, and intradermal skin test.

**Treatment:** Tetracycline or doxycycline is the drug of choice for LGV.

### Tuberculosis

Tuberculosis of vulva is rare.[5] The vulval tuberculosis may be primary or secondary. The primary tuberculosis of vulva occurs due to direct inoculation of the bacteria in the skin. The secondary tuberculosis of vulva occurs as an association of tuberculosis in other parts of female genital system.

## Viral Infections

### Herpes Simplex Infection

Herpes simplex infection is caused by: (a) HSV-2 subtype (majority) (b) HSV-1 causes only 15% of genital herpes simplex infection.

**Incubation period:** 2 weeks.

**Clinical features:** The vulva becomes reddish and swollen. A large number of vesicles appear and they undergo sequential change of pustules to ulcer. The ulcer is painful and is often secondarily infected. The ulcer spontaneously heals without any scarring within 3–4 weeks. The recurrent infection of HSV is less extensive and heals within a week. HSV-2 is mainly responsible for the recurrent infection.

**Histopathology:** The ulcer of HSV is usually superficial. The ulcer bed shows necrosis. The nuclei of the epithelial cells show homogenization of chromatin resulting in typical ground glass appearance. As the disease progresses many multinucleated giant cells appear. The cells show typical intranuclear inclusion. The viral inclusions within the nuclei are usually more evident in the peripheral part of the ulcer. The dermis may show neutrophilic infiltration.

**Diagnostic tests:** (a) Cytological scrapping: (b) HSV serology: Type specific HSV-2 antibody (IgG type) is helpful in diagnosis. (c) Others: Immunohistochemistry on paraffin embedded histopathology section with the help of HSV-antibody. Polymerase chain reaction may be done with the help of HSV specific primer.[6] The viral culture may take 1 week to 1 month time.

**Differential diagnosis:** Various ulcerative lesions of vulva will come in the differential diagnosis (Table 2.2).

**Treatment:** The patients are treated by antiviral therapy such as acyclovir. However antiviral therapy fails to eradicate the latent virus.

### Cytomegalovirus

The histopathology section shows typical intracytoplasmic and intranuclear viral inclusions in the epithelial and vascular endothelial cells. The further confirmation can be done by immunohistochemistry (antibody against CMV) or by PCR.

### Molluscum Contagiosum

Molluscum contagiosum is caused by Molluscum contagiosum virus, a DNA poxvirus. The incubation period is 2–6 weeks. The patient develops multiple small 5–6 mm flesh colored papules with central dome-shaped notch that are mainly self-limited and regress spontaneously.

**Histopathology:** Properly oriented lesion shows dome-shaped depression. The section shows marked acanthosis. The epithelial cells show characteristic eosinophilic oval-shaped viral inclusions popularly known as molluscum bodies or Henderson-Patterson bodies[7] (Figures 2.2 and 2.3). In later stage, the cytoplasmic inclusion takes bluish color. The

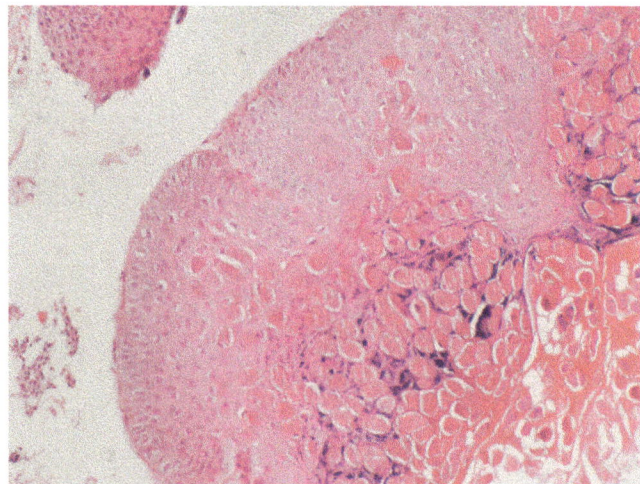

**Figure 2.2:** Molluscum contagiosum of vulva showing molluscum bodies

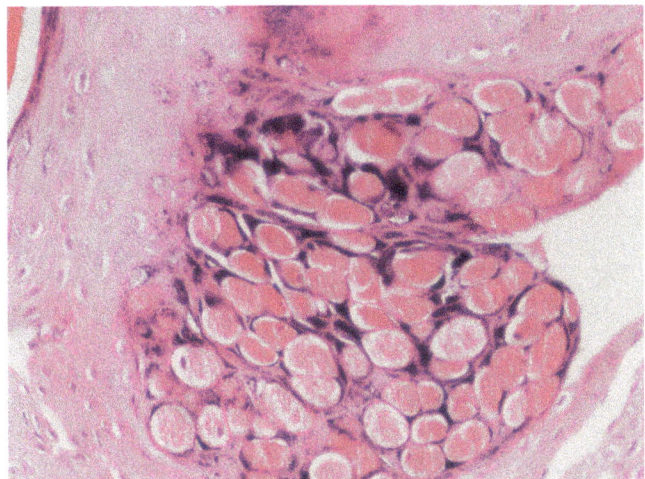

Figure 2.3: Higher magnification showing eosinophilic oval shaped viral inclusions

inclusion totally occupies the cytoplasmic area and pushes the nucleus in the periphery. Deeper dermis may show vascular proliferation along with chronic inflammation.

**Diagnosis:** Clinical examination and cytological scrapping.

## Fungal Infections

Candida infection is the commonest fungal infection that may, occur in the immunocompromised patients more frequently.

## NON-INFECTIOUS INFLAMMATORY DISEASES OF VULVA

In 1986, the revised International Society for the Study of Vulvar Disease (ISSVD) classification of non-neoplastic vulval epithelial diseases was proposed as:[8] (1) lichen sclerosis, (2) squamous cell hyperplasia (formerly hyperplastic dystrophy), (3) other dermatoses.

In 2006, this classification was revised again[9] and the newer revised classification was proposed as mentioned in Box 2.1.

## Lichen Planus

Vulval lichen planus (LP) is an uncommon chronic inflammatory dermatosis that usually affects the woman of more than 40 years age and the age range varies from 30–60 years. LP occurs in oral mucosa, genital mucous membranes, skin, of scalp and nails. The exact etiology of LP is not known. However, it is postulated that LP is a T-cell mediated immune disease.[10] The patient may have pruritus, burning pain and dyspareunia. There are three types of vulval LPs: classical, hypertrophic and erosive forms. In the classical type the patient shows multiple purple polygonal papules with thin

**Box 2.1:** ISSVD classification of vulvar non-neoplastic non-infective lesions[9]

- **Spongiotic pattern**
  - Atopic dermatitis
  - Contact dermatitis
  - Irritant contact dermatitis
- **Acanthotic pattern (previously squamous hyperplasia)**
  - Psoriasis
  - Lichen simplex chronicus
- **Lichenoid pattern**
  - Lichen sclerosus
  - Lichen planus
- **Dermal homogenization**
  - Lichen sclerosis
- **Vesiculobullous pattern**
  - Pemphigoid, cicatricial type
  - Linear IgA disease
- **Acantholitic pattern**
  - Hailey-Hailey disease
  - Darier's disease
- **Granulomatous disease**
  - Crohn's disease
- **Vasculopathic pattern**
  - Aphthous ulcer
  - Behcet's disease
  - Plasma cell vulvitis

white lines known as Wickham's striae. The hypertrophic form of LP, affects the vulval along with perianal mucosa. In case of erosive LP, there is desquamation of the epithelial cells with erosion and involvement of vagina.

The vaginal orifice may be distorted or completely obliterated causing dyspareunia. The vulval LP is often associated with extra vulvar lesions and recognition of such lesions is helpful in diagnosis. LP typically presents Koebner phenomenon that means the occurrence of the disease at the sites of prior trauma.

### Histopathology (Figures 2.4 and 2.5)

The characteristic histopathological features of LP include:[11]
1. Band-like infiltration of lymphocytes admixed with few macrophages in the papillary dermis. The lymphocytes are mainly T-cells and occasionally B-cells.
2. Degenerated keratinocytes forming eosinophilic colloid bodies (Civatte bodies) in the upper papillary dermis.
3. Vacuolar changes in the basal cells of epidermis,
4. Compact orthokeratosis in the cornified layer characterized by the absence of any parakeratotic cells.
5. The granular cells enlarge and proliferate to form characteristic wedge-shaped hypergranulosis. In addition, there may be hyperkeratosis, and acanthosis. Elongation

- Lichenoid drug eruption: Eosinophils are significant in number in case of lichenoid drug eruptions.
- Bullous lesions: Unlike bullous lesions, LP shows band like lymphocytic infiltration.

*Prognosis and Treatment*

Majority of the cases of LP undergo spontaneous remission within one to two year. The erosive form of LP is usually difficult to treat. The use of tropical corticosteroid such as clobetasol propionate ointment is the first line of treatment in LP. Systemic corticosteroid is applied in case of extensive involvement. The patient needs regular follow up to evaluate the lesion for any significant changes.

## Lichen Sclerosis (Lichen Sclerosis Atrophicus)

It is a common chronic inflammatory fibrosing lesion and commonly occurs in perimenopausal and postmenopausal patients. The exact etiology of LS is unknown. Possibly the lesion is an autoimmune diseases. The patients usually present with porcelain white thinned out epithelium which is often symmetrical in appearance. The lesion may extend to the perineum and may give rise to "figure of eight" appearance (hour glass pattern). At times LS involves the labia minora and fuse them together causing stenosis and dyspareunia. Anal stenosis may also occur in LS and the patient may have painful defecation.

*Histopathology*

The histopathological features of LS depend on the age of the lesion.[12] In early stage LS shows mild lymphocytic infiltration in epidermo-dermal junction, occasional degenerated keratinocytes along with mild sclerosis. In established cases of LS shows following characteristic features (Figures 2.6 and 2.7):

1. Homogenization and loss of collagen: Edema occurs in the upper dermis along with homogenization and loss of collagen. The fibrillary appearance of collagen is lost and it looks like amorphous eosinophilic material.
2. The epidermis shows thinning and loss of rete pegs: The stratum Malpighii becomes thinned out and atrophic. Basal layer cells show hydropic degeneration and melanin pigment incontinence is seen.
3. Marked hyperkeratosis: Marked hyperkeratosis occurs and the horny layer is remarkably more pronounced than the stratum Malpighi.
4. Inflammation in the mid-dermis: Chronic inflammatory cell infiltration is seen below the sclerosis zone.

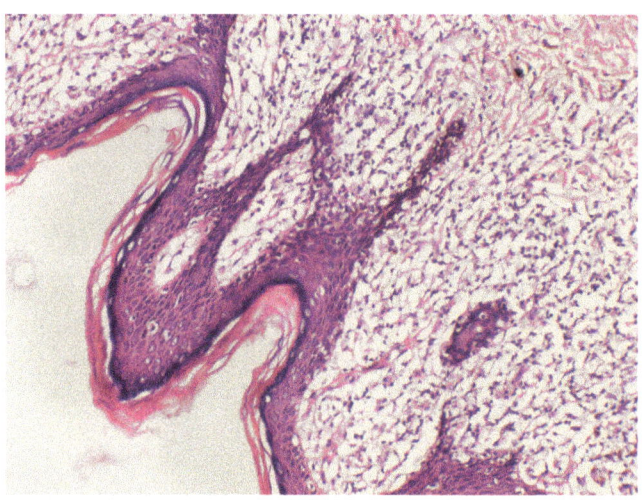

**Figure 2.4:** Wedge-shaped hypergranulosis of epidermal layer along with band-like lymphocytic infiltrate in the upper dermis in lichen planus

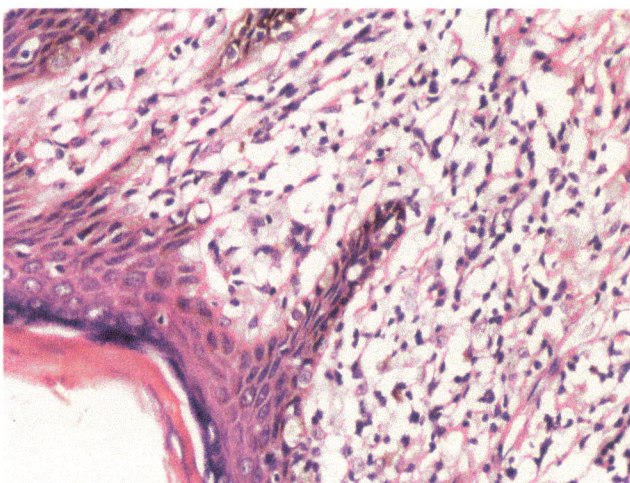

**Figure 2.5:** Thinned out papillary epidermis and vacuolar degeneration in lichen planus

of rete pegs may produce saw tooth-like appearance. There may be melanin incontinence due to the destruction of the basal layer of epidermis.

*Immunofluorescence*

Direct immunofluorescent stain shows shaggy deposits of fibrinogen in epidermo-dermal junction. Occasionally IgM, IgG and C3 are seen in the band-like infiltrate of the epidermo-dermal junction. Necrotic keratinocytes are stained mainly by IgM and occasionally IgG, C3 and IgA.[11]

*Differential Diagnosis*

- Lichen sclerosis: LS shows absence of dense band like lymphocytes

*Differential Diagnosis*

1. Lichen planus: Early lesions of LS may often be confused with LP (Table 2.3).

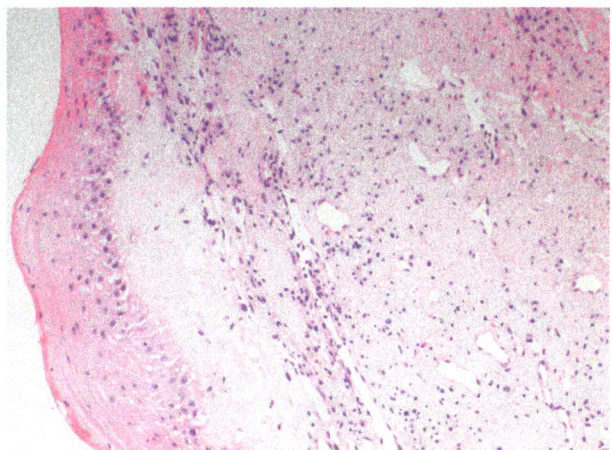

Figure 2.6: Eosinophilic homogenization of collagen in the upper dermis in lichen sclerosis

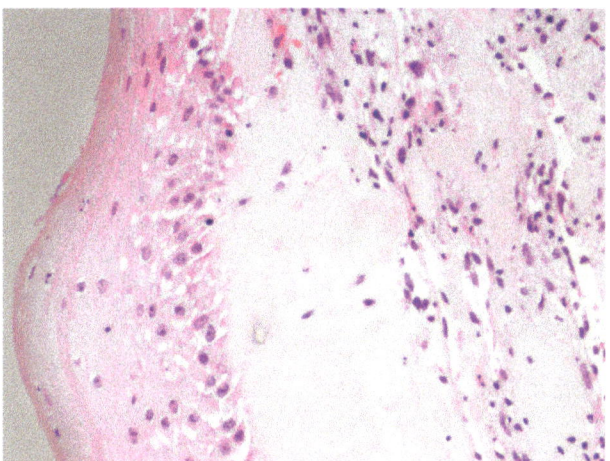

Figure 2.7: Thinned out epidermis, homogenized collagen band and mild inflammation in the upper dermis in lichen sclerosis

2. Morphea: No basal cell degeneration or hyperkeratosis is seen in morphea.
3. Radiation-induced fibrosis: Many thick walled blood vessels and large atypical cells are frequently seen in radiation changes.

Table 2.3: Lichen sclerosis versus lichen planus

| Features | Lichen sclerosis | Lichen planus |
| --- | --- | --- |
| Lymphocytic infiltration | In mid-dermis. In early stage upper dermis | Band-like dense infiltration in epidermo-dermal junction |
| Hyperkeratosis with follicular plugging | Absent | Present |
| Basal cell hydropic degeneration | Present | Absent |
| Homogenization and loss of collagen | Present | Absent |
| Colloid bodies | Absent | Present |

*Treatment*

Long-term tropical corticosteroid such as ultrapotent clobetasol propionate is the treatment of choice. The patient should be advised to wear cotton gloves at night to prevent injury due to scratching. Many cases of LS resolve spontaneously. Surgical treatment may be needed to prevent stricture. Cancer risk: About 5% of LS may develop squamous cell carcinoma.

## Lichen Simplex Chronicus (Squamous Hyperplasia)

Lichen simplex chronicus (LSC) is not a distinctive disease and is considered as a non-specific inflammatory disease of skin. The patients experience repeated itching in the perianal and genital region particularly labia majora. The lesion presents as thickened reddish scaly area. Chronic itching may cause hyperpigmentation. Excoriation and fissure formation may also occur due to the extensive itching.

*Histopathology*

Histology section shows non-specific changes such as epidermal hyperplasia with thickened rete ridges, dermal fibrosis and chronic inflammation in the dermis (Figure 2.8). The epidermis is thickened and shows hyperkeratosis and parakeratosis. The squamous epithelial cells do not show any atypia. The superficial dermis shows thick eosinophilic vertical strands of collagen bundles.

*Differential Diagnosis*

- Infection: Chronic infection due to candida and tinea cruris.
- Psoriasis: The presence of plaque-like parkeratosis and narrow deep rete ridges are distinctive features of psoriasis.

*Treatment*

It is important to protect the skin from severe itching. Local corticosteroid application helps to prevent itching.

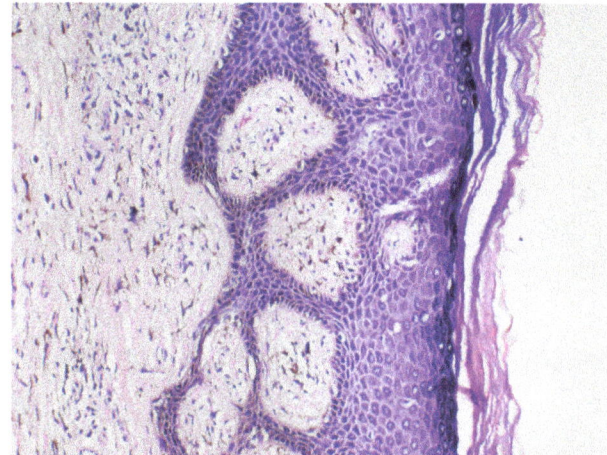

Figure 2.8: Hyperplastic epidermal layer along with chronic inflammation in the upper dermis

Emollients, antipruritic agents and barrier occlusion such as wearing cotton gloves in the night may break the itch-scratch cycle.

## Psoriasis

Psoriasis is a chronic relapsing hyperproliferative disease of skin with an inherent autosomal dominant trait. In the genital region it usually affects in the lateral part of the labia majora. The patient classically presents well-circumscribed erythematous plaque with a silvery top. The removal of the silvery scale produces pin point bleeding point (Auspitz sign).

*Histopathology*

Psoriasis is characterized by following features (Figures 2.9 and 2.10):
1. Epidermal hyperplasia with elongation of the rete ridges: The epidermis shows acanthosis and thickening. The tip of the rete ridges is widened and club-shaped.
2. Parakeratosis.
3. The thinned out supra-papillary epidermis and spongiosis with polymorphs collection.
4. Loss of granular layer.
5. The collection of neutrophils within the epidermis termed as Munro's micro abscess.
6. Edema and vascular congestion of the dermis. Mild perivascular lymphocytic infiltration may be seen in the dermis.

*Differential Diagnosis*

Chronic fungal infection, Psorasiform drug reaction and seborrheic dermatitis.

*Treatment*

Psoriasis is a chronic disease and treatment is often frustrating. Mild form of the disease is treated by local application of steroids, emollients and vitamin D analogs. In severe disease, systemic therapy is done by the use of methotrexate, retinoid or phototherapy.

## Atopic Dermatitis

Atopic dermatitis (AD) is a chronic pruritic skin lesion caused by hypersensitivity reaction.[13] AD is probably an IgE mediated hypersensitivity reaction. The patients have history of allergy. The patient complains of burning pain and itching. The physical findings include thickening and scaling of skin. The histopathology section shows epidermal hyperplasia and lymphocytes, eosinophils and mast cells infiltrate in the upper dermis. Epidermis also shows intercellular edema or spongiosis and exocytosis of lymphocytes. In chronic condition, the lesions show variable epidermal hyperplasia, lymphocytic exocytosis and parakeratosis.

*Immunofluorescent*

It shows IgE on epidermal Langerhans cells.

*Treatment*

The treatment include avoidance of allergens and using antipruritic agents.

## Contact Dermatitis

Contact dermatitis (CD) may be irritant type due to irritation by physical and chemical reagents or it may be allergic type due to exposure to allergens.

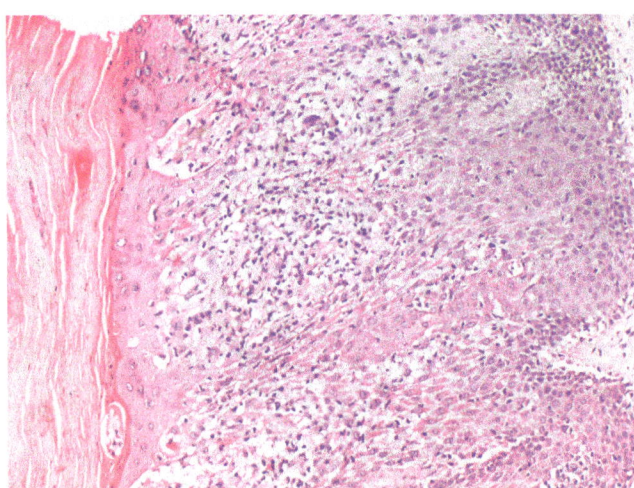

**Figure 2.9:** Epidermal hyperplasia with elongation of the rete ridges in psoriasis

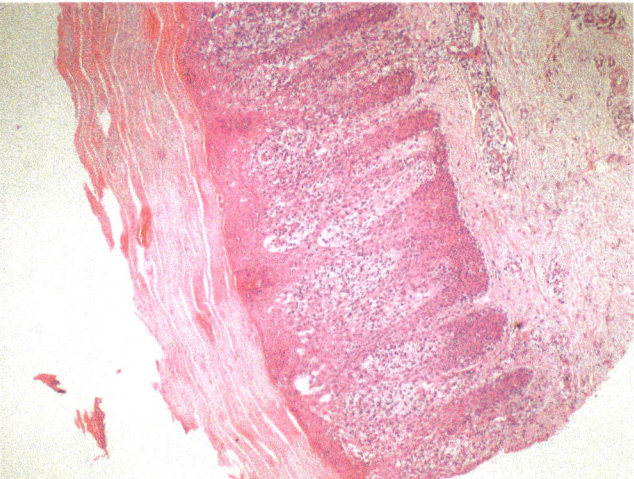

**Figure 2.10:** The collection of neutrophils within the epidermis in psoriasis

### Irritant Contact Dermatitis

The irritant contact dermatitis is more common and shows erythema, eczematous changes along with vesiculobullous lesions. In vulval region urine is the most common cause of CD in cases of urinary incontinence.

### Allergic Contact Dermatitis

Allergic CD is a type IV hypersensitivity reaction. It commonly occurs within 2 days of the exposure with the allergens. The common allergens are cosmetics, dyes, chemicals and metallic substances.

**Histopathology:** Histology section shows epidermal spongiosis. There is formation of spongiotic microvesicles within the epidermis. Upper dermis shows nonspecific perivascular chronic inflammation consisting of lymphocytes, histiocytes and eosinophils.

## BULLOUS LESIONS OF VULVA

### Bullous Pemphigoid and Cicatrical Pemphigoid

Bullous pemphigoid (BP) and cicatrical pemphigoid (CP) are autoimmune diseases and caused by autoantibodies against plakin. BP is the commonest bullous disease and the patient presents with multiple tense fluid filled vesicles in the labia majora, minora, perianal region, groin, lower abdomen, arms and legs. The bullae rupture and produce ulcers. CP is relatively more common in vulva than BP. In CP the vesicles ruptures followed by the desquamation and scarring of the tissue. Progressive scarring may cause severe distortion of the vulva.

### Histopathology

Pemphigoid lesion is characterized by subepidermal bullae. There is cleavage of the tissue between the epidermis and superficial dermis. The bullae contain serum, fibrin and also polymorphs in case of associated inflammation.

### Immunofluorescence

Direct immunofluorescence: Linear deposition of IgG and C3 in the basement membrane.

### Treatment

Pemphigoid is treated by using systemic and also tropical corticosteroid.

### Pemphigus Vulgaris

Pemphigus vulgaris (PV) is autoimmune in origin and is caused due to autoantibody against desmoglein. The patient presents with recurrent painful bullae in the anorectal and vulval region. If the pressure is given to the border of the bullae the margin of the vesicle is extended. This is known as positive Nikolsky's sign.

### Histology

Microscopy of the lesion shows acantholysis and suprabasal separation of cells. The basal keratinocytes are separated from each other but remain attached to the dermis. These viable rows of basal cells appear as "row of tombstones" (Figures 2.11 and 2.12). This intra-epidermal separation of the cells is the characteristic of PV. The bullae contain acantholytic keratinocytes and sparse eosinophils. The cytology smear of Tzanck preparation of the blister shows acantholytic cells which is diagnostic of intraepidermal bullae of PV.

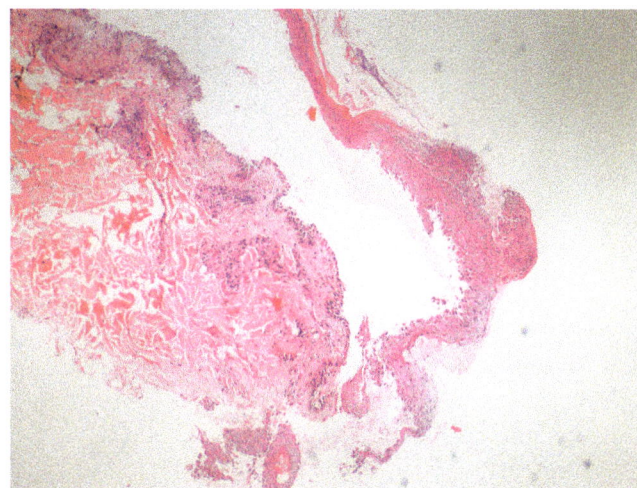

Figure 2.11: Suprabasal and intraepidermal bullae in pemphigus vulgaris

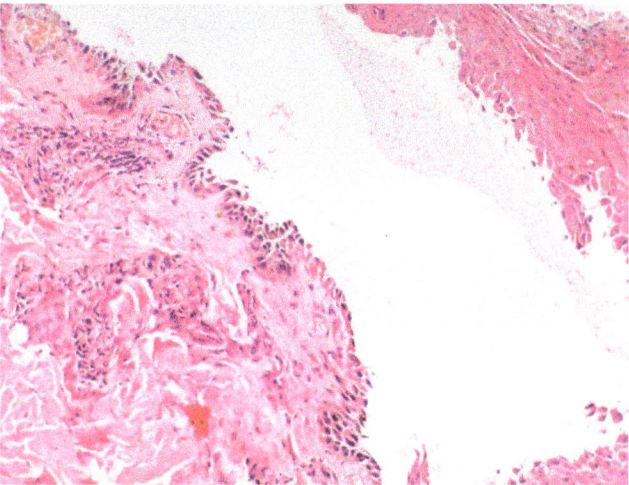

Figure 2.12: Pemphigus vulgaris: Higher magnification showing "row of tombstones" of basal cells bullae in pemphigus vulgaris

## Immunofluorescence

Immunofluorescence of the lesion shows IgG deposition at the intercellular junction of the epidermis.

## Differential Diagnosis

The differential diagnosis of PV is BP and other causes of bullae. The cleavage point of BP is subepidermal whereas it is intraepidermal in PV. Immunofluorescence studies show linear IgG and C3 deposition in BP. In contrast, PV shows this deposition in intercellular junction of the epidermis (Table 2.4).

Table 2.4: Distinguishing features between pemphigus vulgaris and bullous pemphigoid

| Features | Pemphigus vulgaris | Bullous pemphigoid |
|---|---|---|
| Location of bullae | Intraepidermal | Subepidermal |
| Acantholysis of suprabasal cells | Present | Absent |
| Immunofluorescence | IgG deposition in the intercellular junction of the epidermis | Linear IgG and C3 deposition on the basement membrane |
| Tzanck preparation of the blister | Acantholytic cells present | Absent |

## Treatment

Pemphigus vulgaris is treated by systemic corticosteroid. Rarely cytotoxic drug such as methotrexate is used.

## VULVODYNIA

The term vulvodynia indicates vulval pain without any specific disorder and vulval does not show much change except mild erythema. The vulval pain may be generalized or in a specific area. ISSVD classified vulval pain in two broad categories[14,15] (Box 2.2):
1. Vulval pain due to specific disorder and
2. Vulvodynia: Vulval pain without any apparent cause in a normal looking vulva.

Box 2.2: ISSVD terminology of vulval pain (2003)

→ Vulval pain related to specific disorder
- Infection: Herpes, candida
- Inflammation: Lichen sclerosis, bullous disease
- Neoplastic: Squamous cell carcinoma, Paget's disease
- Neurologic: Herpes neuralgia

→ Vulvodynia
- Generalized
  - Provoked: Sexual, nonsexual or both
  - Unprovoked
  - Mixed
- Localized
  - Provoked: Sexual, nonsexual or both
  - Unprovoked
  - Mixed

## Histopathology

Histopathology section of vulvodynia is essentially normal. Histopathological features of vulval pain due to infection depend on the specific cause. Vulval pain due to infection shows mild to moderate infiltration of lymphocytes, histiocytes and occasional plasma cells.

## Treatment

The therapy of vulvodynia is variable. The local care of vulva, tropical application of anesthetic ointment, interferon therapy and biofeedback of pelvic floor muscle training, and acupuncture are the main ways of management of vulvodynia.

## BENIGN DISEASES OF VULVA

### Vulval Cyst

The various types of cysts are seen in vulva derived from different source of origin and are lined by different types of epithelium (Table 2.5).

### Bartholin Duct Cyst

Two major vestibular glands, known as Bartholin gland, are located in the vulvar vestibules and open through a duct

Table 2.5: Cysts of vulva

| Cyst | Source of origin | Lining epithelium |
|---|---|---|
| Bartholin duct cyst | Bartholin duct | Squamous epithelium, transitional epithelium or columnar epithelium surrounded by dense fibrous tissue |
| Epithelial inclusion cyst | Skin adnexal gland | Stratified squamous epithelium including granular layer |
| Mucinous cyst | Lesser vestibular glands | Mucous secreting cuboidal to columnar epithelium |
| Wolffian duct cyst or cysts of Gartner duct | Wolffian duct remnant | Nonciliated cuboidal to tall columnar epithelium |
| Cysts of the canal of nuck | Peritoneal lining | Single layer of flattened epithelium similar to the peritoneal lining |

in the posterior introitus. The Bartholin gland is lined by columnar mucus secreting cells and the duct is lined mainly by transitional epithelium except its tip that is lined by squamous epithelium. Bartholin duct cyst is found in the posterior introitus around the opening of the Bartholin duct.

The obstruction of the Bartholin duct causes accumulation of fluid and formation of cyst.[16] The obstruction may occur due to either inspissated secretion or inflammation due to bacterial infection.

**Histopathology:** Bartholin cyst is lined by lined by squamous epithelium, or transitional epithelium or columnar epithelium surrounded by dense fibrous tissue (Figures 2.13 and 2.14). The nature of the lining epithelium depends on the part of the duct affected. At times the epithelial lining may be totally flattened and the nature of the cyst is difficult to ascertain.

**Management:** The Bartholin cyst is treated by word catheter placement or marsupialization.

### Epithelial Inclusion Cyst

Epithelial inclusion cysts are single or multiple, and commonly seen on the labia majora. The cysts are less than 5 mm in size and contain cheesy or yellowish material.

**Histology:** The cyst is lined by stratified squamous epithelium including granular layer. The cyst wall may show foreign body reaction with many multinucleated giant cells. Calcification on the cyst wall may also be seen.

### Mucinous Cyst

Mucinous cyst probably develops from the lesser vestibular glands.[17] These cysts are commonly seen in multiparous woman. The cysts are usually single and 1 to 2 cm in diameter.

**Histopathology:** The cyst wall is lined by mucous secreting cuboidal to columnar epithelium similar to the cells of endocervical canal (Figure 2.15). Squamous metaplasia may also occur in the lining epithelium.

### Cysts of Gartner Duct (Wolffian Duct Cyst)

These cysts are originated from the Wolffian ducts that are vestigial mesonephric duct. The cysts are usually situated in the lateral wall of the vagina and lateral aspect of vulva. The Gartner duct cyst. Wolffian duct cyst is lined by non-ciliated cuboidal to tall columnar epithelium (Figure 2.16). Subepithelium shows smooth muscle fibers.

### Cysts of the Canal of Nuck

The cyst is developed from the processus vaginalis which is an extension of the peritoneal membrane with the round

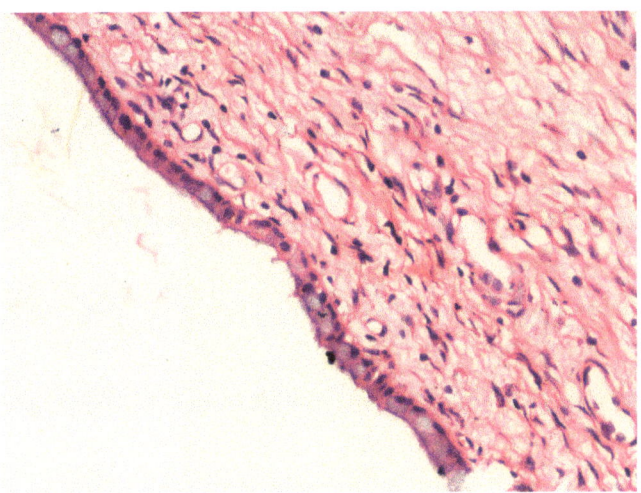

Figure 2.13: Columnar lining of cells in Bartholin cyst

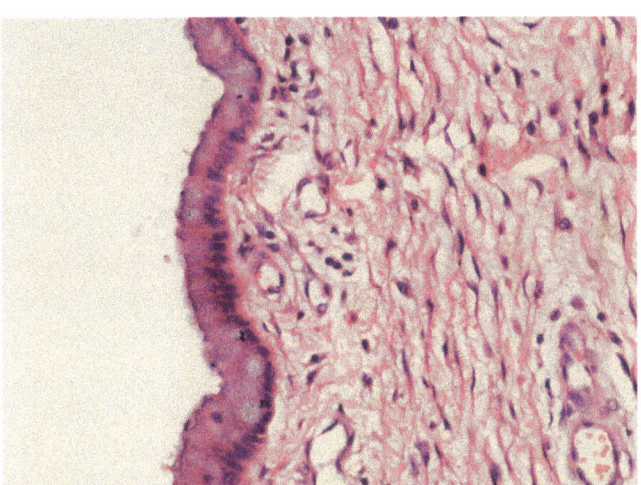

Figure 2.14: Bartholin cyst: Higher magnification showing tall columnar cells with basally placed nuclei and underlying fibrous tissue

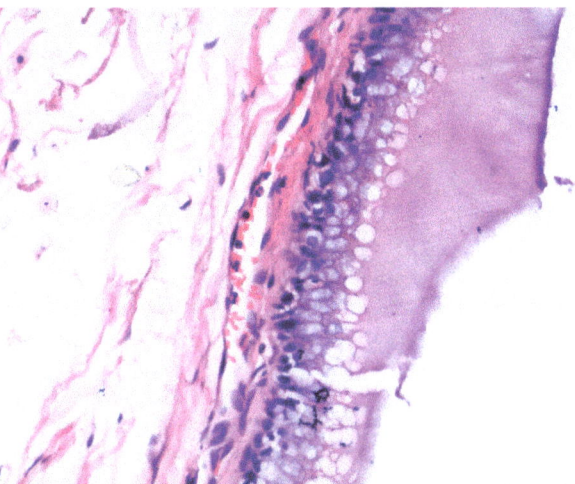

Figure 2.15: Mucinous cyst: The wall of the cyst is lined by mucus secreting columnar epithelium

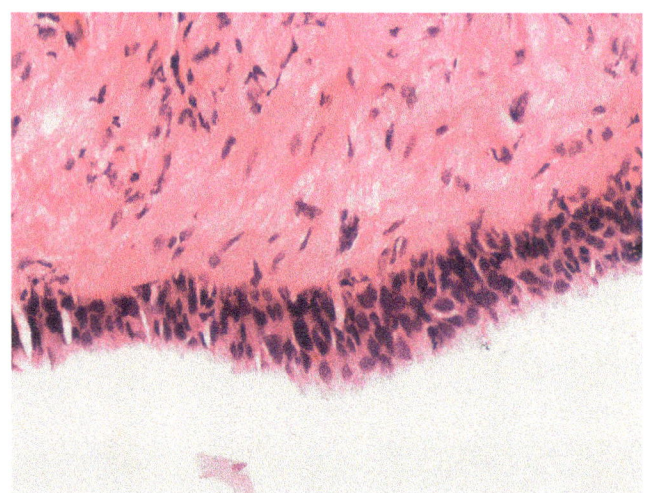

Figure 2.16: Gartner duct cyst: The cyst wall lined by multilayered cuboidal epithelium

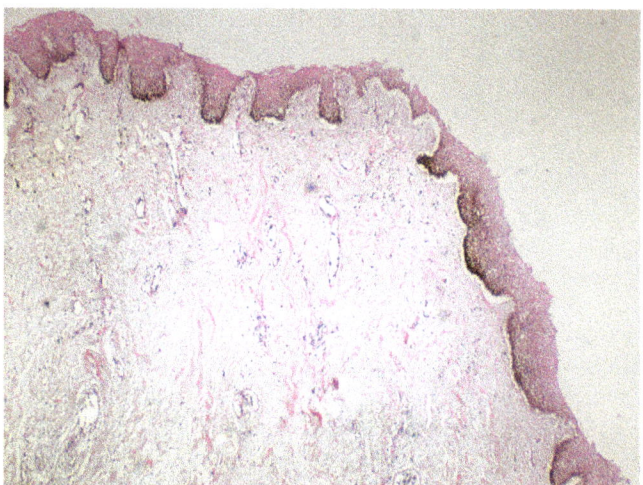

Figure 2.17: Fibroepithelial polyp covered with squamous epithelium and underlying mesenchymal tissue

ligament. The cysts commonly present as small mass on the labia majus. They may also present as indirect inguinal hernia.

**Histopathology:** The cyst is lined by single layer of flattened epithelium similar to the peritoneal lining. The epithelium is surrounded by smooth muscle and fibrous tissue.

## Benign Squamous Tumor of Vulva

The common benign squamous tumors of vulva are fibro-epithelial polyp, seborrheic keratosis and keratoacanthoma.

## Adnexal Tumor of Vulva

The various adnexal tumors in this region include hidradenoma papilliferum, syringoma and nodular hidradenoma.

## Mesenchymal Lesions of Vulva

### Fibroepithelial Stromal Polyp

It is a benign a slow growing painless tumor. The lesion is usually solitary, polypoid and less than 5 cm in diameter.

**Histopathology:** The polyp is covered with squamous epithelium that may show hyperkeratosis and papillomatosis. The underlying stroma is composed of stellate shaped stromal cells and good number of vascular channels (Figures 2.17 and 2.18). The stromal cells are often multinucleated and moderately pleomorphic. Brisk mitotic activities (more than 10/10 high power field) may also be seen.[18]

**Immunocytochemistry:** The tumor cells are positive for vimentin, desmin and receptors for estrogen and progesterone.

**Differential diagnosis:** (a) Sarcoma. (b) Botryoid rhabdomyosarcoma.

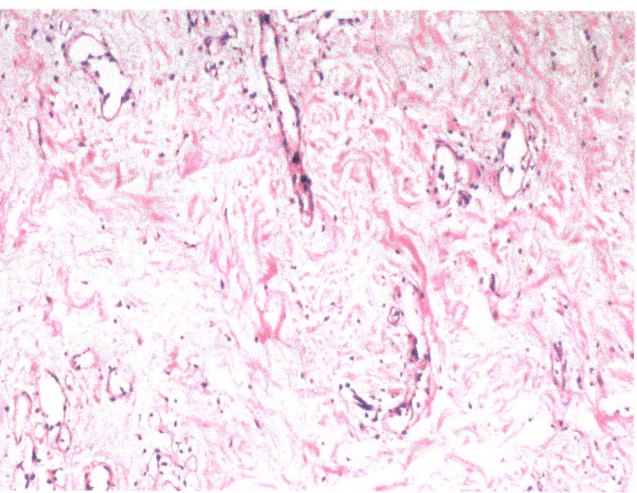

Figure 2.18: Higher magnification showing sparse elongated stromal cells in fibroepithelial polyp

**Prognosis and treatment:** Complete surgical excision of the polyp is required. The polyp is prone to recur due to incomplete removal.

### Superficial Angiomyxoma

It is a benign soft tissue tumor and occurs in 4th to 5th decade. The patient presents with a painless, slow growing mass in the vulva about 2.5–5 cm diameter in size.

**Histopathology:** The tumor is soft and lobulated mass with gelatinous appearance in the cut section. The lesion is well-demarcated within the dermis and subcutaneous tissue. The tumor shows scanty to moderate number of stellate-shaped cells with elongated nuclei having eosinophilic cytoplasm. The cells have bland monomorphic nuclei. Mitotic activities are absent to scanty. The stellate cells are embedded in myxoid stroma. Variable amount of thin and thick walled blood vessels are also noted.

**Immunocytochemistry:** The tumor cells are positive for CD 34 and vimentin. The cells are negative for smooth muscle actin, desmin, S-100 protein, estrogen and progesterone receptors.

**Differential diagnosis:** Superficial angiomyxoma should always be differentiated from deep angiomyxoma (Table 2.6).

**Treatment:** Complete surgical resection of the tumor is recommended for superficial angiomyxoma. Near about 33% of the tumor recurs after surgical resection.

### Aggressive (Deep) Angiomyxoma

Aggressive angiomyxoma (AA) is also known as deep angiomyxoma. This is a locally invasive and non-metastasizing tumor. AA commonly occurs in the reproductive age period particularly in adult female of 4th decade. Other than vulvovaginal region the tumor is also seen in the deep pelvis and perineum. The patient presents with an asymptomatic slow growing mass in the vulva. The tumor is infiltrative in the deeper tissue but does not metastasize. The tumor is usually large with more than 10 cm diameter at the time of discovery. The mass is lobulated and poorly circumscribed from the surrounding fat and stromal tissue. The cut section of the tumor is soft rubbery, myxoid or gelatinous consistency. Foci of cystic changes may also be seen.

**Histopathology:** The tumor shows sparse cellularity. The cells are predominantly spindle to stellate-shaped with bland nuclei and scanty cytoplasm (Figures 2.19 to 2.21). The nuclei show minimal atypia. In general mitotic figures are absent. The spindle cells are embedded in a myxoid stroma. Tumor with predominant fibrous stroma is usually seen in recurrent tumors. The tumor also shows numerous stromal blood vessels of variable sized ranging from thin walled vessels to large thick walled hyalinized vessel. The tumor characteristically shows perivascular small bundles of oval to spindle-shaped smooth muscle cells and collagen fibers around the thick walled blood vessels. In addition smooth muscles are also noted in the stroma. Occasionally multinucleated tumor giant cells, mast cells and extravasated RBCs are seen. This tumor is unencapsulated and shows an infiltrative margin within the adipose tissue and adjacent skeletal muscle.

**Immunocytochemistry:** AA lacks any specific immunological marker/s. The tumor cells are positive for vimentin, desmin, alpha smooth muscle actin, and CD34. The cells are also positive for estrogen and progesterone receptors. HMGA2, the architectural transcription factor, is often mutated in AA. The demonstration of nuclear expression of HMGA2 in AA may be helpful to distinguish this tumor from the surrounding blood vessels and connective tissue of vulva.[19]

**Differential diagnosis**
- Fibroepithelial stromal polyp: See Table 2.6.

Table 2.6: Differential diagnosis of vulval mesenchymal tumors

| Lesions | Age | Location | Margin | Cellular homogeneity | Blood vessels | Immunohistochemistry | Behavior |
|---|---|---|---|---|---|---|---|
| Fibroepithelial stromal polyp | Reproductive | Superficial | Not well-demarcated | Central cellularity | Scanty vessels | Positive for vimentin, desmin and receptors for estrogen and progesterone | Benign |
| Superficial angiomyxoma | Reproductive | Superficial | Well-circumscribed | Hypocellular | Many delicate blood vessels | • Positive for CD 34 and vimentin<br>• Negative for SMA, desmin, S-100 protein, estrogen and progesterone receptors | Benign but Local recurrence may occur |
| Aggressive angiomyxoma | Reproductive | Deep | Infiltrative | Hypocellular | Thick walled hyalinized blood vessels | • Positive for desmin, vimentin, estrogen and progesterone receptors<br>• Positive for CD 34 | Local recurrence |
| Angiomyo-fibroblastoma | Early post-menopausal | Superficial | Well-circumscribed | Heterogeneous cellularity | Thin walled blood vessels | Positive for vimentin and desmin, and estrogen and progesterone receptors | Benign but Local recurrence may occur |
| Cellular angiofibroma | Middle aged women | Superficial | Well-circumscribed | Cellular | Small to medium sized blood vessels | • Positive for vimentin and CD 34<br>• Variable expression SMA, desmin | Benign |

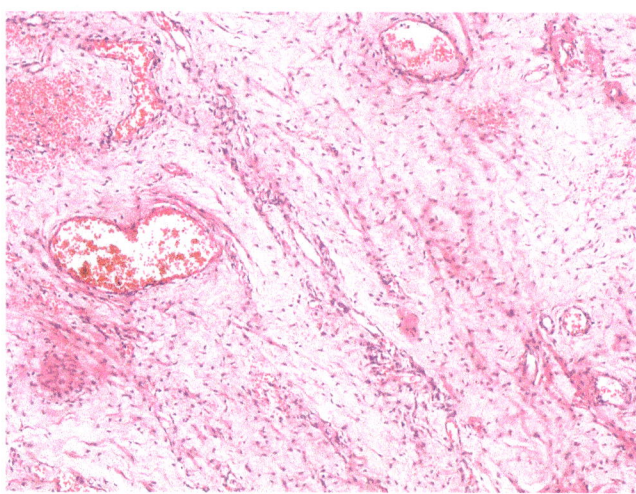

**Figure 2.19:** Spindle cells in a myxoid stroma in deep angiomyxoma

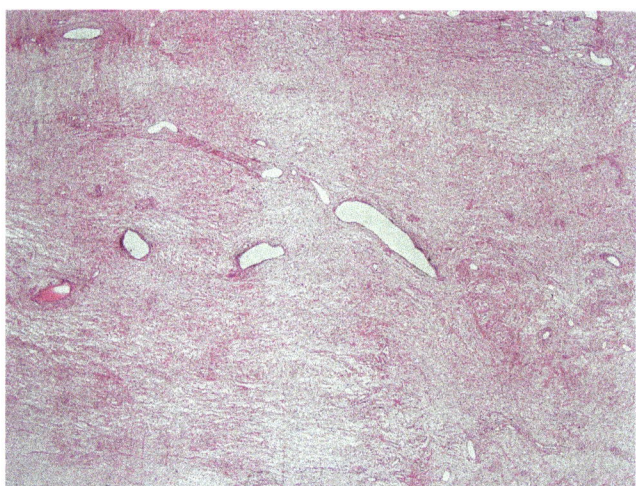

**Figure 2.20:** Numerous stromal blood vessels and blunt looking spindle cells in deep angiomyxoma

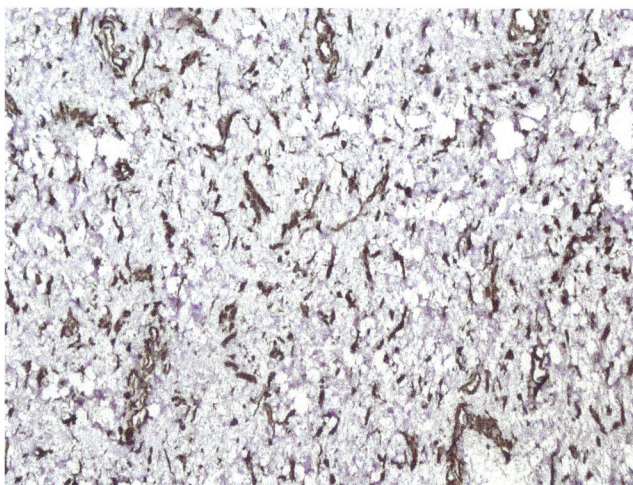

**Figure 2.21:** Strong vimentin positive cells in deep angiomyxoma. (Immunostaining X 240)

- Angiomyofibroblastoma: Aggressive angiomyxoma is distinguished from Angiomyofibroblastoma by these following features:
  - Deep location
  - Infiltration in deeper tissue
  - Thick walled hyalinized blood vessels.
- Superficial angiomyxoma: Discussed previously (see Table 2.6).
- Other myxoid neoplasms: myxoid fibrosarcoma and myxoid fibrous histiocytoma may also pose diagnostic difficulties. Nuclear pleomorphism and high mitotic activities help in differentiating between sarcomas and aggressive angiomyxoma.

**Prognosis and treatment:** Near about 35–40% cases of aggressive angiomyxoma recurs locally.[20] This tumor never metastasizes. Complete local excision with 1 cm free lateral margin and free deep resection plane is the treatment of choice. Due to high chances of local recurrence, frequent follow up is needed.

### Angiomyofibroblastoma

Angiomyofibroblastoma is a benign nonrecurring mesenchymal tumor of vulva. The tumor occurs in adult female in the reproductive age as painless slow growing small mass.

**Gross features:** Angiomyofibroblastoma is usually less than 5 cm in size. The tumor is soft and well-circumscribed. Cut section of the tumor is myxomatous to rubbery.

**Histopathology:** Angiomyofibroblastoma is well-circumscribed but un-encapsulated swelling. The tumor typically shows simultaneous presence of hypocellular and hypercellular areas. The tumor is composed of numerous thin walled capillary like blood vessels in myxomatous stroma. The individual cells are oval to spindle shaped. However, in the cellular areas the cells are epithelioid or plasmacytoid. The epithelioid cells have moderate to abundant cytoplasm with oval shaped nuclei in central to eccentric position. The cells are usually aggregated around the vascular channels and are also seen as small groups or cords. Mitotic activity is infrequent to nil. Mast cells and lymphocytes are also seen in the stroma. In the periphery of tumor adipocytes are found.

**Immunohistochemistry:** The tumor cells are positive for vimentin and desmin, and estrogen and progesterone receptors. The cells are usually negative for smooth muscle actin and variably express CD 34.

**Differential diagnosis**

- Aggressive angiomyxoma: Discussed before
- Cellular angiofibroma: Cellular angioma shows less blood vessels, thick walled hyalinized vessels, relatively homogenous cellularity and lack of cell aggregation

around vessels. The tumor cells are negative for desmin and positive for CD34.

**Treatment:** Local excision of the tumor is adequate. The tumor does not recur after excision. The chance of malignancy from this tumor is exceedingly rare.

### Cellular Angiofibroma

Cellular angiofibroma is an uncommon benign soft tissue tumor and that occurs in the middle aged female. The tumor appears as small well-circumscribed painless lesion. Gross appearance: The tumor is well-circumscribed. Cut section is grey white rubbery in appearance.

**Histopathology:** The tumor is unencapsulated. It is cellular and composed of numerous small to medium sized blood vessels along with monomorphic spindle cells. The spindle cells are arranged in short interlacing fascicles in a fibrous stroma. Vague nuclear palisading arrangement is also seen. The individual spindle cells show scanty cytoplasm and ovoid nuclei. Mitotic activity is usually less, however, high mitotic activities (more than 10/10 high power fields) have also been described. The blood vessels are small to medium in size. They often have hyalinization in the wall. There may be degenerative changes in the tumor such as hemorrhage or cyst formation. The tumor often shows many mast cells around collagen fibers.

**Immunocytochemistry:** The tumor cells are positive for vimentin and CD 34 (nearly 50% cases). The cells are negative for of smooth muscle actin (SMA), desmin and h-caldesmon.[21] The tumor is persistently negative for S-100. Most of the tumor cells are positive for estrogen and progesterone receptors.

**Differential diagnosis:**
- Angiomyofibroblastoma: Discussed before.
- Leiomyoma: Cellular angiofibroma is distinguished from leiomyoma with the help of numerous vessels and short fascicles.

**Behavior and treatment:** This is a benign tumor and does not show any recurrence. Complete local excision of the tumor with tumor free margin is adequate treatment.

## MISCELLANEOUS CONDITIONS OF VULVA

### Mixed Tumor of Vulva

This is a rare benign neoplasm and occurs near the Bartholin gland. The tumor is composed of tubules of epithelial cells admixed with chondromyxoid and osseous stroma.

### Ectopic Breast Tissue

Ectopic breast tissue may be seen any site along the milk line from the nipple to groin. Ectopic breast tissue in the vulva is rare.[22] Histology of the lesion shows ducts and lobules of breast simulating normal breast tissue. Rare cases of fibroadnoma, lactational changes and duct papilloma have been described in vulva.[22]

The ectopic breast tissue in this region should not be mistaken as adenocarcinoma and careful observation is needed.

### Endometriosis

Endometriosis may occur in vulva particularly after surgery. The lesion presents as painful bluish nodule. The lesion may bleed at the time of menstruation. Histopathology section shows the characteristic endometrial glands, stroma and hemosiderin laden histiocytes. In longstanding cases, the lesion may show fibrosis and the classical features may be obscured.

## REFERENCES

1. Young H. Syphilis. Serology. Dermatol Clin. 1998;16(4):691-8.
2. Jaffe HW. The laboratory diagnosis of syphilis. New concepts. Ann Intern Med. 1975;83(6):846-50.
3. Orle KA, Gates CA, Martin DH, Body BA, Weiss JB. Simultaneous PCR detection of Haemophilus ducreyi, Treponema pallidum, and herpes simplex virus types 1 and 2 from genital ulcers. J Clin Microbiol. 1996;34(1):49-54.
4. Brown TJ, Yen-Moore A, Tyring SK. An overview of sexually transmitted diseases. Part I. J Am Acad Dermatol. 1999;41(4):511-32.
5. Millar JW, Holt S, Gilmour HM, Robertson DH. Vulval tuberculosis. Tubercle. 1979;60(3):173-6.
6. Thomas CA, Smith SE, Morgan TM, White WL, Feldman SR. Clinical application of polymerase chain reaction amplification to diagnosis of herpes virus infection. Am J Dermatopathol. 1994;16(3):268-74.
7. Epstein WL Molluscum contagiosum. Semin Dermatol. 1992;11:184-9
8. Ridley CM. International Society for the Study of Vulvar Disease—Progress Report British Journal of Dermatology. 1988; 118;732-3.
9. Lynch PJ, Moyal-Barracco M, Bogliatto F, Micheletti L, Scurry JJ. 2006 ISSVD classification of vulvar dermatoses: pathologic subsets and their clinical correlates. Reprod Med. 2007;52(1):3-9.
10. Shiohara T. The lichenoid reaction. An immunological perspective. Am J Dermatopathol. 1988;10:252-6.
11. Toussaint S, Kamino H. Noninfectious erythemotous, papular and squamous diseases. In: Elder D (ed) Lever's histopathology of the skin, 8th edn. 1997. Lippincott-Raven, Philadelphia, pp 151-84.

12. Mullins DL, Wilkinson EJ. Pathology of the vulva and vagina. Curr Opin Obstet Gynecol. 1994;6:351-8.
13. Pincus SH. Vulvar dermatoses and pruritus vulva. Dermatol Clin. 1992;10:297-308.
14. Haefner HK. Report of the International Society for the Study of Vulvovaginal Disease terminology and classification of vulvodynia. J Low Genit Tract Dis. 2007;11(1):48-9.
15. Moyal-Barracco M, Lynch PJ. 2003 ISSVD terminology and classification of vulvodynia: a historical perspective. J Reprod Med. 2004;49(10):772-7.
16. Sarrel PM, Steege JF, Maltzer M, Bolinsky D. Pain during sex response due to occlusion of the Bartholin gland duct. Obstet Gynecol. 1983;62:261-4.
17. Friedrich EG Jr, Wilkinson EJ. Mucous cysts of the vulvar vestibule. Obstet Gynecol. 1973;42:407-14.
18. Carter J, Elliott P, Russell P. Bilateral fibroepithelial polyp of labium minus with atypical stromal cells. Pathology. 1992;24:37-9.
19. Rabban JT, Dal Cin P, Oliva E. HMGA2 rearrangement in a case of vulvar aggressive angiomyxoma. Int. J. Gynecol. Pathol. 2006;25:403-7.
20. Fetsch JF, Laskin WB, Lefkowitz M et al. Aggressive angiomyxoma: a clinicopathologic study of 29 female patients. Cancer. 1996;78:79-90.
21. McCluggage WG, Ganesan R, Hirschowitz L, et al. Cellular angiofibroma and related fibromatous lesions of the vulva: Report of a series with a morphological spectrum wider than previously described. Histopathology. 2004;45:360-8.
22. van der Putte SCJ. Mammary-like glands of the vulva and their disorders. Int J Gynecol. 1994;13:150-60.

# Premalignant and Malignant Tumors of Vulva

## 3

## WORLD HEALTH ORGANIZATION CLASSIFICATION OF TUMORS OF VULVA 2014[1]

**Epithelial tumors**
Squamous cell tumors and its precursors
- Squamous intraepithelial lesions
  - Low grade squamous intraepithelial lesion
  - High grade squamous intraepithelial lesions
  - Differentiated-type vulvar intraepithelial lesions
- Squamous cell carcinoma
  - Keratinizing
  - Non-keratinizing
  - Basaloid
  - Warty
  - Verrucous
- Basal cell carcinoma
- Benign squamous lesions
  - Condyloma accuminatum
  - Vestibular papilloma
  - Seborrheic keratosis
  - Keratoacanthoma
- Glandular tumors
  - Paget disease
  - Tumors arising from Bartholin and other specialized anogenital glands
    - Adenocarcinoma
    - Squamous cell carcinoma
    - Adenosquamous cell carcinoma
    - Adenoid cystic carcinoma
    - Transitional cell carcinoma
  - Adenocarcinoma of other types
  - Benign tumors and cysts
- Neuroendocrine tumors
  - High grade neuroendocrine carcinoma
  - Markel cell tumor

**Neuroectodermal tumors**
*Soft tissue tumors:*
- Benign tumors
  - Lipoma
  - Fibroepithelial stromal polyp
  - Superficial angiomyxoma
  - Superficial myofibroblastoma
  - Aggressive angiomyxoma
  - Leiomyoma
- Malignant tumors
  - Rhabdomyosarcoma
  - Leiomyosarcoma
  - Epithelioid sarcoma
  - Alveolar soft part sarcoma

**Melanocytic tumors**
- Melanocytic naevi
- Malignant melanoma
- Germ cell tumors
- Lymphoid and myeloid tumors
- Secondary tumors.

## SQUAMOUS TUMORS

### Condyloma Accuminata

Condyloma accuminata (CA), a preneoplastic condition, is related with HPV 6 and HPV 11.[2] CA is usually multifocal and affects vulva, perineal region, vagina and cervix. The lesion in the vulva appears as white maculopapular lesion, papillary or verrucous type. CA is associated with sexual promiscuity, immunosuppression and diabetes mellitus.

*Histopathology (Figures 3.1 to 3.3)*

The lesion shows multiple papillae like structures that are lined by squamous cells. The lining epithelium shows hyperkeratosis, acanthosis, and parakeratosis along with basal cell hyperplasia. The characteristic finding in CA is koilocytotic changes in the superficial epithelium. Koilocytosis is characterized by perinuclear halo with central pyknotic or enlarged nucleus. The superficial cells may show mild nuclear atypia and binucleation.

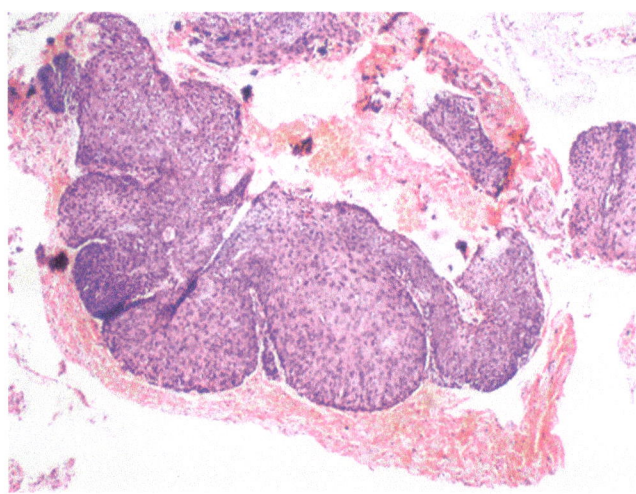

Figure 3.1: Condyloma: Papillary projections

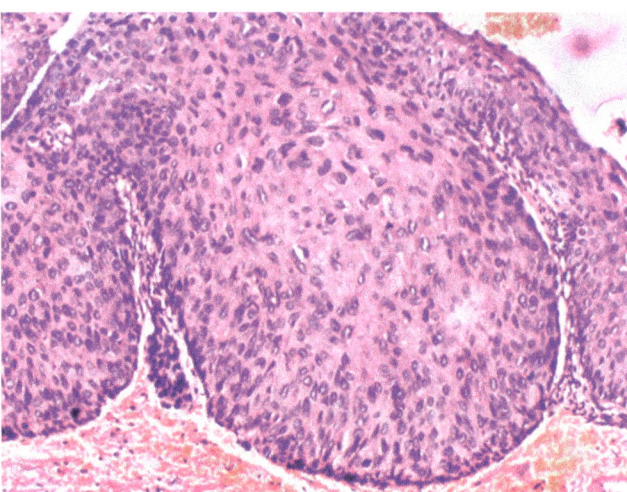

Figure 3.2: Condyloma: High power view showing papillary structure

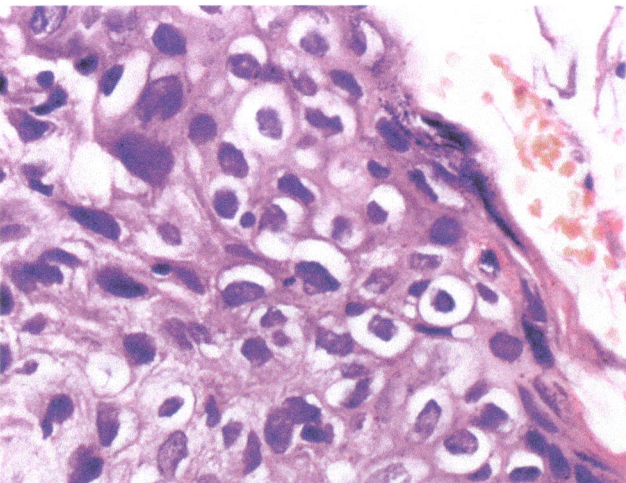

Figure 3.3: Condyloma: Koilocytic cells show central nucleus surrounded by clear halo

*Differential Diagnosis*

- *Vulval intraepithelial neoplasia (VIN)*: Condyloma accuminata is differentiated from VIN by the presence of parabasal hyperplasia, koilocytosis and absence of mitosis.
- *Fibroepithelial mucosal polyp*: Fibroepithelial mucosal polyp lack any koilocytotic change.

*Natural History and Management*

Majority of the CA regresses slowly and in a minority of cases the lesions persist. Occasional cases of CA may progress to VIN to squamous cell carcinoma.[3] Small lesions can be treated with topical application of Podophylin and the larger lesions are treated by surgical resection, laser ablation, electrocauterization, etc.[4]

## Vulval Intraepithelial Neoplasia

The term vulval intraepithelial neoplasia (VIN) is often noted along with cervical intraepithelial neoplasia (CIN). Strong correlation is observed with cigarette smoking, immunosuppression, sexually transmitted disease and VIN.[5] HPV 16 is isolated in nearly 70% of VIN cases.[6]

*Clinical Features*

Vulval intraepithelial neoplasia is usually seen in older patient and the mean age is about 40 years. The patient complains of pruritus and irritation. However, most of them are asymptomatic. The lesions are usually multifocal (2/3rd) and commonly appear as white or pigmented maculopapular raised lesion in the labia minora and perineum.

*Terminology*

In 2014, World Health Organization (WHO) classified vulval precursor lesion in three categories LSIL, HSIL, and differentiated type vulvar intraepithelial lesion (Table 3.1).[1] ISSVD, in 2004, classified VIN as usual VIN (u-VIN) and differentiated VIN (d-VIN) (Table 3.2).[7] u-VIN is also known as classic VIN. It includes both VIN-2 and VIN-3 (high grade lesions). These lesions are more common, multifocal; HPV associated and occur in relatively younger patient than d-VIN group. The other group d-VIN is already considered as high grade lesion and is HPV-independent.

**Histopathology:** VIN shows nuclear enlargement, hyperchromasia, and pleomorphism of the epithelial cells (Figures 3.4 and 3.5). Nuclear chromatin is coarse. Mitotic activity is noted in all layers of epithelium. Abnormal mitotic figures are also seen.

## Classic or Usual Type of VIN

There are two histological types of u-VIN:
1. Warty type and
2. Basaloid type.

Table 3.1: WHO classification of vulval intraepithelial neoplasia

| Low-grade squamous intraepithelial lesion | High-grade squamous intraepithelial lesion | Differentiated-type vulvar intraepithelial lesion |
|---|---|---|
| • It is a synonym of vulval intraepithelial neoplasia (VIN) grade 1<br>• It shows the features of productive HPV infection | It is a synonym of Vulval intraepithelial neoplasia (VIN) grade 2 and 3. The lesion involves lower third to full thickness of epithelium. It includes basaloid and warty type of lesion | • The lesion is HPV negative.<br>• It shows atypia of the basal cells and abnormal differentiation of keratinocytes |

Table 3.2: ISSVD terminology

| VIN-1 | VIN-2 and VIN-3 | |
|---|---|---|
| This terminology is omitted | ISSVD Terminology | |
| • Flat condyloma accuminatum<br>• Or HPV effect | Usual VIN (u-VIN) | Differentiated VIN as (d-VIN) |
| | • Includes both VIN-2 and VIN-3<br>• Warty, basaloid or mixed type<br>• Multifocal<br>• More common<br>• Lower age group<br>• HPV dependent | • High grade differentiated lesion<br>• Unifocal<br>• Less common<br>• Post-menopausal<br>• HPV independent |

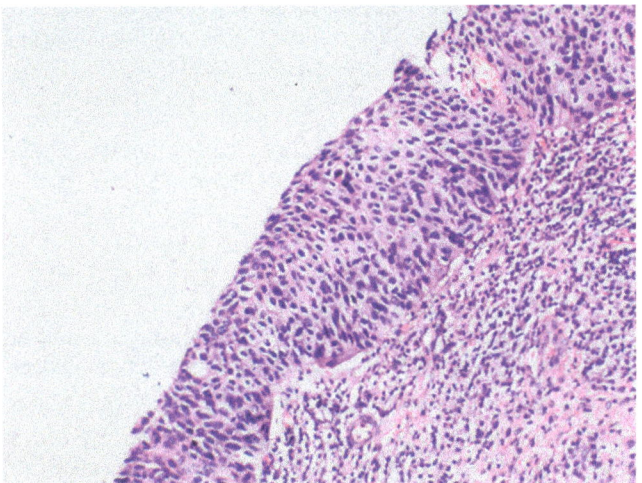

Figure 3.4: Vulval intraepithelial neoplasia 3: Full thickness involvement in usual type of VIN

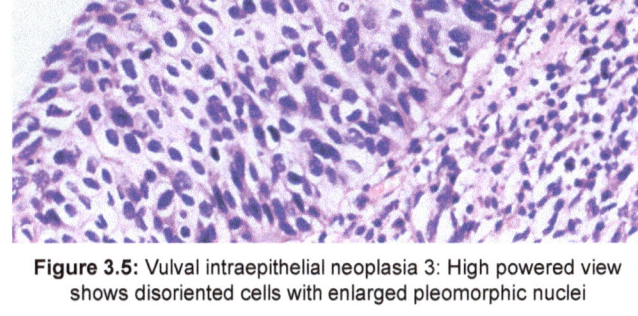

Figure 3.5: Vulval intraepithelial neoplasia 3: High powered view shows disoriented cells with enlarged pleomorphic nuclei

*Warty type*: In low power examination warty type of VIN gives a striking papillary appearance. The epithelium shows hyperkeratosis, parakeratosis along with prominent acanthosis. The rete ridges are wide and extend deep in the dermis. Individual cell keratinization is also noted. The epithelial cells show koilocytotic changes characterized by hyperchromatic nuclei and perinuclear halo.

*Basaloid type*: It presents as flat type of lesion. The epithelial cells are relatively small, uniform with high nucleo-cytoplasmic ratio and coarse chromatin. The cells resemble basal cells. Koilocytes are uncommon in this type of lesion.

## Differentiated (Simplex) Type of VIN

Abnormalities of d-VIN are subtle and may be missed by routine pathological examination. d-VIN is characterized by epithelial thickening with elongated anastomosing rete pegs and parakeratosis.

The basal and parabasal cells show marked nuclear atypia. The nuclei are large, moderately pleomorphic having vesicular chromatin and prominent nucleoli. The upper part of the epithelium shows normal appearing differentiated cells. Dyskeratotic cells are seen in the whole thickness of the epithelium. These cells are parabasal cells with premature maturation characterized by increased eosinophilia of the cells. Mitotic activities are more frequent in the parabasal and basal cells.

*Differential Diagnosis (Table 3.3)*

- *Reactive nonspecific atypia*: P-16 immunostain is always negative in reactive atypia whereas VIN cases are positive for p-16.[8]

Table 3.3: Differential diagnosis of vulval intraepithelial neoplasia

| Lesions | Histopathology | Immunocytochemistry | | | | |
|---|---|---|---|---|---|---|
| | | CK7 | CEA | CAM5.2 | HMB 45 | Melan A |
| VIN | Atypical epithelial cells | – | – | – | – | – |
| Paget's disease | Large cell with pale cytoplasm | + | + | + | | |
| Melanoma | Melanin containing cells | – | – | – | + | + |

Table 3.4: Ancillary studies in different types of vulval intraepithelial neoplasia

| Lesions | HPV infection | p16 | p53 | Ki 67 index |
|---|---|---|---|---|
| Usual (classical) VIN | HPV 6 and 11 | Intense nuclear p-16 | Negative | High |
| Differentiated (simplex) VIN | Independent of HPV | Usually negative | Strongly positive in immature basal and parabasal cells | High |

- *Paget's disease of vulva*: Paget cells are positive for CK 7, CEA, CAM 5.2 and GDFP-15.[9]
- *Superficial spreading malignant melanoma*: Melanomas are positive for HMB-45, Melan A and S-100 protein.
- *Multinucleated atypia of vulva*: This entity does not show any nuclear atypia.

The differential diagnoses of differentiated VIN (d-VIN) are:
- *Squamous hyperplasia*: Orderly maturation of the hyperplastic epithelial cells in squamous hyperplasia helps to distinguish it from d-VIN.
- *Lichen sclerosis*: Lack of nuclear atypia helps in distinguishing LS from u-VIN.

### Ancillary Studies (Table 3.4)

- HPV: HPV virus (HPV 16) is demonstrated in majority of the cases of u-VIN by molecular studies and rarely seen in d-VIN.[10]
- p-16: Intense nuclear p-16 is seen in the entire paraneoplastic epithelium of u-VIN. In contrast, p-16 immunostain is negative in d-VIN cases[11]
- Ki 67: Ki 67 index is a reliable proliferation marker and its expression is increased in VIN.[12] However, Ki 67 is more useful in grading of VIN than its diagnosis.
- p53: p53 staining is strongly positive in immature basal and parabasal cells of d-VIN.

### Prognosis and Treatment

There is substantial risk if VIN 3 cases are not treated as they may develop invasive carcinoma within 8 years after the primary diagnosis.[13] Small proportion of high grade VIN regresses spontaneously. The following treatment protocol is available for VIN lesions:

**Surgery:** Complete local excision is the treatment of choice. The resection margins should be free of any tumor.

**Laser excision, laser vaporization and loop electrosurgical excision procedure (LEEP):** Laser excision helps in the removal of the lesion along with histopathological examination, whereas, laser vaporization destroys the tissue. LEEP is an alternative technique of laser vaporization.

**Medical treatment:** Local application of 5-flurouracil may eradicate the lesion. However, the occult invasion may be missed as no histopathological study could be done.

## SQUAMOUS CELL CARCINOMA OF VULVA

Carcinoma of vulva accounts for 5–8% of all gynecological malignancies worldwide.[14] Approximately 90% of vulval cancers are squamous cell carcinoma. The mean age of vulval carcinoma is 65 years. The risk factors for vulval carcinoma include HPV infection, sexual promiscuity, cigarette smoking, immunodeficiency, and vulval dermatosis such as lichen sclerosis, squamous hyperplasia, etc.[15] HPV 16 is commonly related with vulval squamous cell carcinoma (VSCC) and less commonly other HPV types (HPV 18, 31, 33, 45) are related with VSCC.[16] Most of the vulval carcinomas develop from VIN lesion. Probably, there are two distinct groups of vulval carcinoma cases (Figure 3.6):
- *HPV associated*: The patients are associated with HPV and VIN lesions (30% of vulval carcinoma cases).
- *HPV independent*: The large majority of the patients has various vulval dermatosis and are not related with HPV.

### Clinical Features

The patient presents with ulcer, black macule, nodule or pedunculated mass. The patient may complaints of pruritus, bleeding, dyspareunia, or foul smell. The tumor is usually solitary and is located in the labia majus or minus (Figure 3.7). Less than 10% of VSCCs are multifocal in origin.

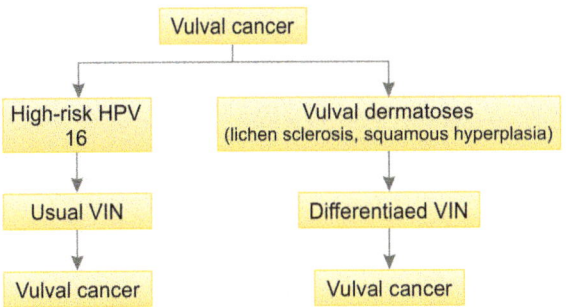

Figure 3.6: Two distinct etiological origin of vulval cancer

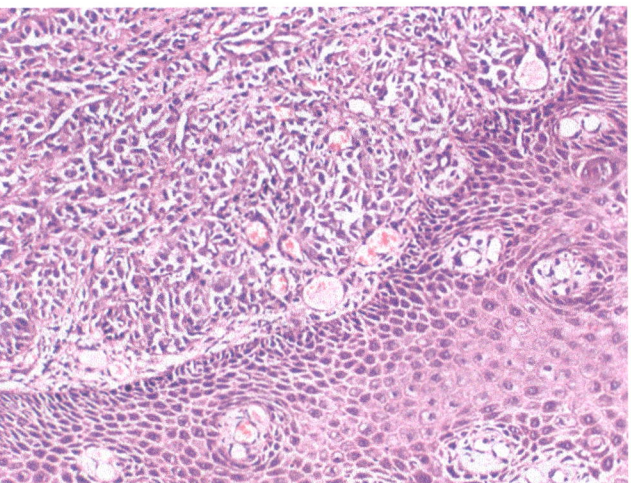

Figure 3.8: Nonkeratinizing squamous cell carcinoma: Diffuse sheet of cells

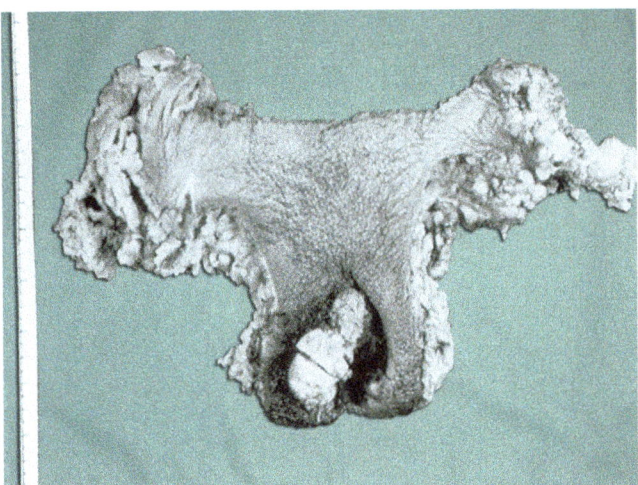

Figure 3.7: Squamous cell carcinoma: Large ulcerated swelling over the right labia major of vulva

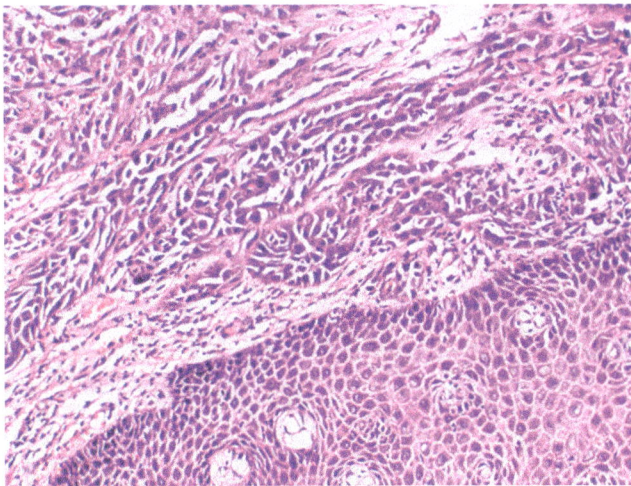

Figure 3.9: Nonkeratinizing squamous cell carcinoma: Nest and diffuse sheets of cells

## Histology of Squamous Cell Carcinoma of Vulva

### Nonkeratinizing Squamous Cell Carcinoma

Here the individual cells show keratinization but the tumor lacks squamous pearl (Figures 3.8 to 3.10).

### Keratinizing Squamous Cell Carcinoma

This is the most common variety of squamous cell carcinoma. The tumor shows multiple squamous pearls (Figures 3.11 and 3.12). The tumor cells infiltrate in the deeper stromal tissue with desmoplastic reaction. The malignant cells are large and contain abundant eosinophilic cytoplasm having moderate nuclear enlargement and pleomorphism.

### Basaloid Carcinoma

It consists of nests of small monomorphic cells having scanty cytoplasm. The nuclei show granular chromatin. The cells resemble basal cells (Figure 3.13). Keratin pearls are not usually not seen in this carcinoma, however focal keratinization may be seen. Basaloid carcinoma usually shows HPV 16 DNA.

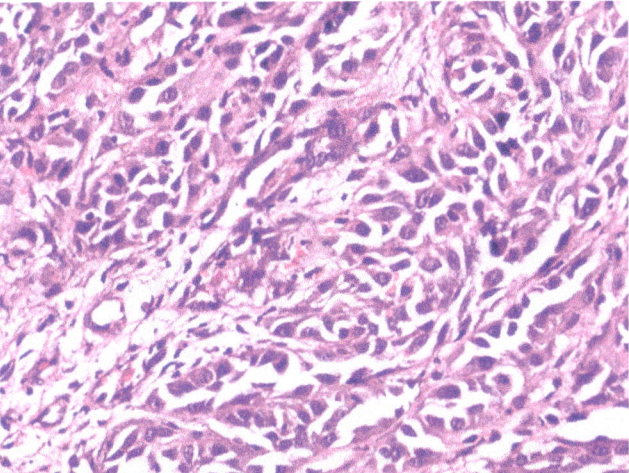

Figure 3.10: Non keratinizing squamous cell carcinoma: Oval to polyhedral cells with intracellular keratinization

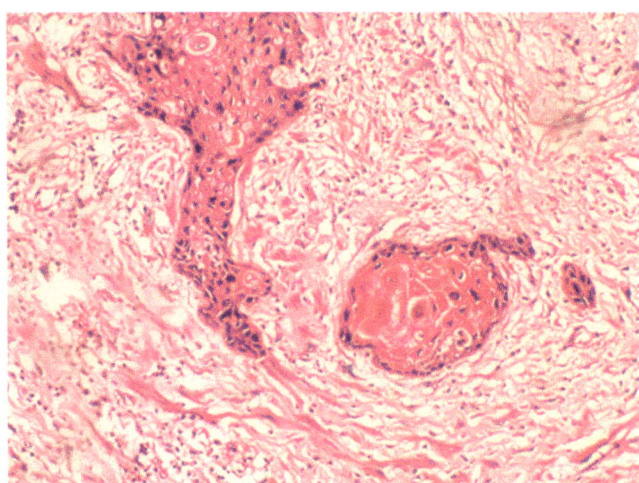

**Figure 3.11:** Keratinizing squamous cell carcinoma: Squamous pearl

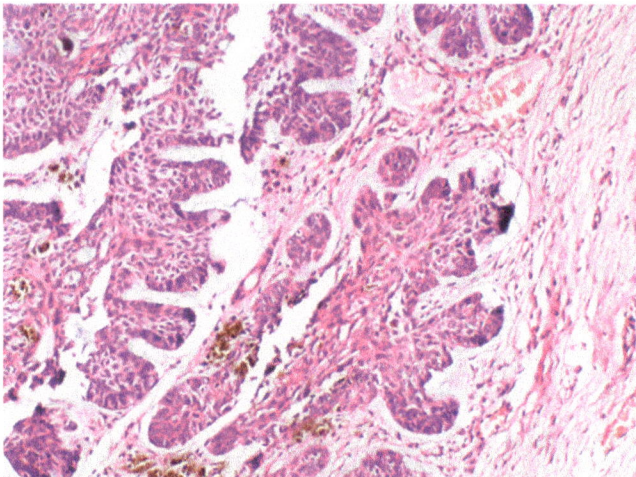

**Figure 3.13:** Basaloid squamous cell carcinoma: Basaloid arrangement of cells in the periphery of cell cluster

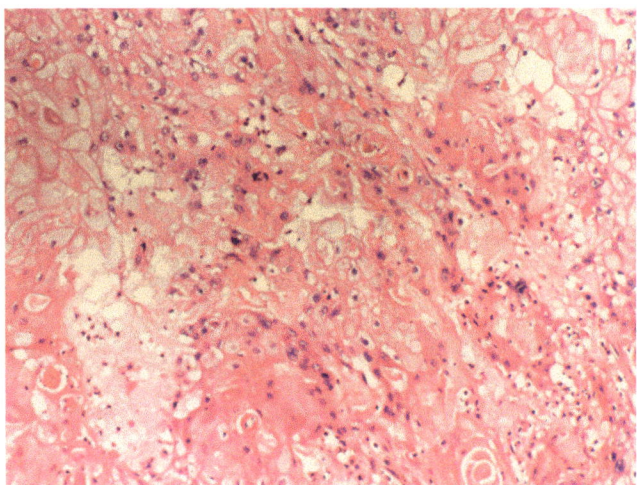

**Figure 3.12:** Keratinizing squamous cell carcinoma: Intracellular keratinization

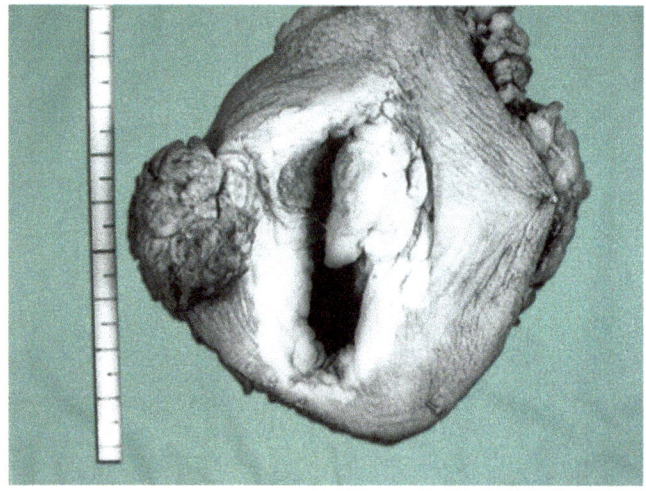

**Figure 3.14:** Verrucous carcinoma: Papillary exophytic growth in the right labia majora of vulva

### Warty Carcinoma

The tumor shows warty surface consists of multiple papillary projections with fibrovascular core. The papillae are lined by squamous cells. The individual tumor cells show nuclear enlargement and pleomorphism along with increased mitotic activity. Many cells show koilocytoctic changes. Warty carcinoma also frequently associated with HPV 16 infection.

### Verrucous Carcinoma (Figures 3.14 to 3.17)

It is a well-differentiated type of squamous cell carcinoma characterized by broad based papillary growth that pushes the stroma downwards by bulldozer like pattern. This broad pushing margin of the malignant cells is difficult to recognize as invasion. Hyperkeratosis and parakertosis are seen. The individual cells have abundant cytoplasm. Nuclear atypia and mitotic activity are nil to absent.

The tumor may recur after local excision however metastasis in the regional lymph node is extremely uncommon and re-evaluation of the tumor should be done in such cases.

### Keratoacanthoma Like Carcinoma

The tumor resembles keratoacanthoma and is included in VSCC by WHO. The tumor is characterized by central crater filled with proliferating squamous cells and keratin. The tumor is self-limiting and complete remission of the tumor may occur spontaneously due to unknown immune mechanism.

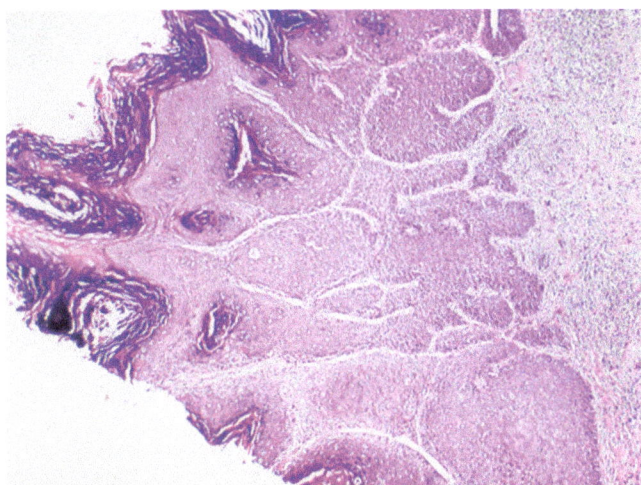

Figure 3.15: Verrucous carcinoma: Broad based bulbous growth of tumor cells

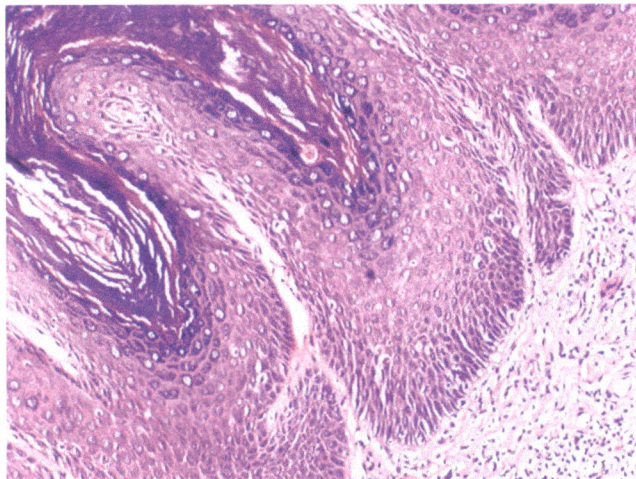

Figure 3.16: Verrucous carcinoma: Broad based bulbous growth of tumor cells with pushing margin

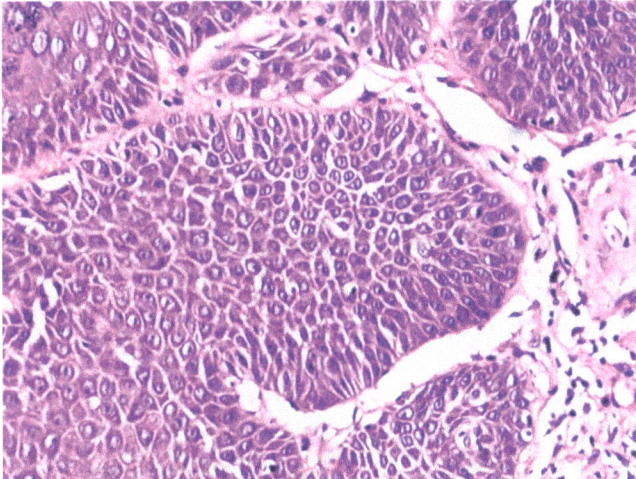

Figure 3.17: Verrucous carcinoma: The tumor cells show minimal nuclear atypia and scanty mitotic activity

## Differential Diagnosis (Table 3.5)

- **Verrucous carcinoma versus other lesions:**
  - Keratinizing squamous cell carcinoma
  - Warty carcinoma, condyloma accuminatum
- **Amelanotic melanoma versus squamous cell carcinoma (SCC) with multinucleated giant cells:** The presence of adjacent VIN or focal squamous differentiation may be helpful morphological features of SCC. In case of difficulty immunostaining such as HMB 45 and Melan A may be helpful to confirm the diagnosis of melanoma.
- **Basaloid squamous cell carcinoma versus small cell carcinoma, Merkel cell carcinoma, and basal cell carcinoma:** Frequent molding and the absence of any squamoid differentiation help in identification of small cell carcinoma. The cells of Merkel cell carcinoma is small round monomorphic and arranged in diffuse sheet or in trabecular pattern. The cells show NSE, chromogranin and CK20 positivity. The cells of basal cell carcinoma are monomorphic, bland and show characteristic peripheral palisading pattern.

## Tumor Spread and Staging

The staging of vulvar carcinoma is recommended by Federation of Gynecology and Obstetrics (FIGO) in 2014 (Table 3.6).[17]

The depth of invasion is defined as the measurement of the tumor from the epithelialstromal junction of the adjacent most superficial dermal papilla to the deepest point of invasion.

It is important to provide necessary information in the surgical pathology report of vulva as recommended by college of American Pathologist and Royal College of Australian Pathologist[18] (Box 3.1) (Figure 3.18).

## Prognosis

Prognosis of VSCC is dependent on the FIGO stage of the tumor (Box 3.2). The overall 5 year survival of Stage 1 tumor is as high as 98% in comparison to 29% in case of stage IV tumors.[19] The various other factors related with prognosis are tumor size, depth of invasion, lymph node involvement, lymphovascular invasion and the presence of high grade VIN along the margin of the tumor.

## Treatment

The main treatment of vulvar carcinoma is surgical resection. The operative procedure may be partial vulvectomy or radical vulvectomy. In case of partial vulvectomy a part of vulva is removed. In case of total vulvectomy, the whole vulva along with appropriate integument is removed.

Table 3.5: Differential diagnosis of verrucous carcinoma

| Features | Verrucous carcinoma | Keratinizing squamous cell carcinoma | Warty carcinoma | Condyloma accuminatum |
|---|---|---|---|---|
| Growth pattern | Broad based papillary growth pushing the stroma | Small islands or isolated cells | Irregular and exophytic growth | Vascular papillary growth |
| Nuclear atypia | Absent | Present: Moderate to marked | Present: Moderate | Mild atypia |
| Mitosis | Absent | Present: | Present | Absent |
| Koilocytosis | Absent | Absent | Present | Present |

Table 3.6: FIGO staging of carcinoma of vulva

| Stage | Description |
|---|---|
| Sage I | • Tumor confined to the vulva<br>• IA Lesions ≤ 2 cm in size, confined to the vulva or perineum and with stromal invasion, ≤1.0 mm[a], no nodal metastasis<br>• IB Lesions > 2 cm in size or with stromal invasion >1.0 mm[a], confined to the vulva or perineum, with negative nodes |
| Stage II | Tumor of any size with extension to adjacent perineal structures (lower third of urethra, lower third of vagina, anus) with negative nodes |
| Stage III | Tumor of any size with or without extension to adjacent perineal structures (lower third of urethra, lower third of vagina, anus) with positive inguinofemoral nodes<br>• IIIA (i) with 1 lymph node metastasis (≥5 mm), or (ii) with 1–2 lymph node metastasis(es) (<5 mm)<br>• IIIB (i) with 2 or more lymph node metastases (≥5 m), or (ii) with 3 or more lymph node metastases (<5 mm)<br>• IIIC with positive nodes with extracapsular spread |
| Stage IV | Tumor invades other regional (upper 2/3 urethra, upper 2/3 vagina), or distant structures<br>• IVA tumor invades any of the following:<br>  - (i) upper urethral and/or vaginal mucosa, bladder mucosa, rectal mucosa, or fixed to pelvic bone, or<br>  - (ii) fixed or ulcerated inguinofemoral lymph nodes<br>• IVB Any distant metastasis including pelvic lymph nodes |

Box 3.1: Microscopy report of vulval carcinoma

- The gross diameter of the tumor in surgical specimen
- The number of primary tumors
- The exact depth of invasion of the tumor and the method of measurement
- The diameter of tumor on histopathology section
- The presence of vascular invasion
- The presence of any perineural invasion
- The status of tumor margins and deep resection plane
- Associated VIN, if any
- Total number of lymph nodes and their involvement with location
- The size of metastatic lymph node

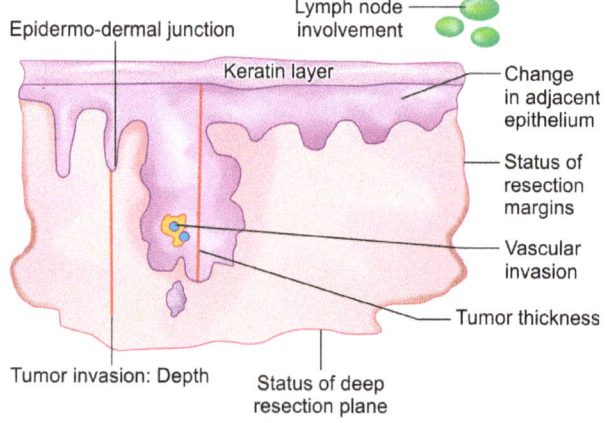

Figure 3.18: Vulval carcinoma: Reporting the various microscopic features

Box 3.2: Prognostic factor of vulval carcinoma

- Main prognostic factor (by multivariate analysis)
  • FIGO staging
- Other prognostic factors (by univariate analysis)
  • Tumor size
  • Depth of invasion
  • Lymph node involvement
  • Lymphovascular invasion

## PAGET DISEASE OF VULVA

Paget disease is an intraepithelial adenocarcinoma of vulva with eccrine or apocrine differentiation. This represents only 1% of vulval carcinoma. The lesion occurs in postmenopausal woman. Approximately 10–20% vulval Paget disease is accompanied by invasive adenocarcinoma. The patients usually complain of pruritus or pain along with red to pink eczematous plaque-like lesion.

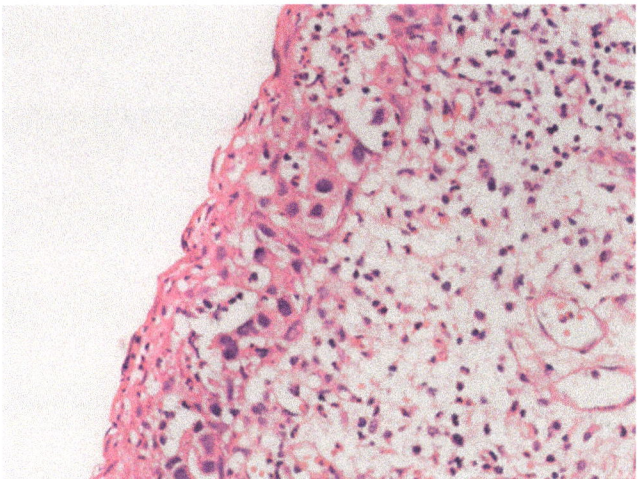

Figure 3.19: Paget's disease: The epidermis shows many Paget's cells

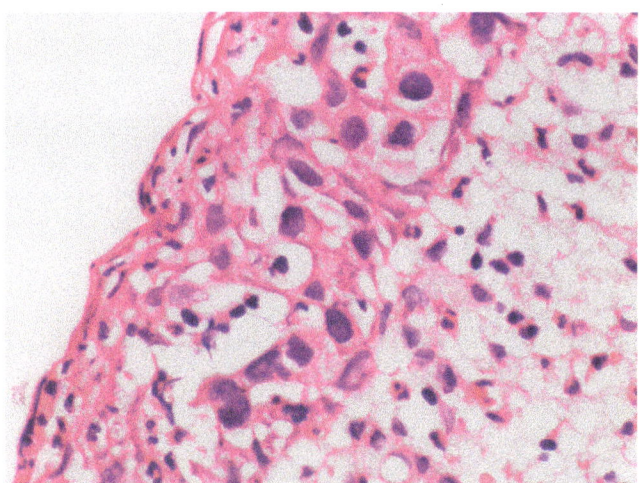

Figure 3.20: Paget's disease: Paget's cells show large hyperchromatic nuclei with clear cytoplasm

Table 3.7: Differential diagnosis of Paget disease

| Lesion | Simulating features | Distinguishing features |
| --- | --- | --- |
| In situ and invasive squamous cell carcinoma (pagetoid Bowen disease) | • Single dispersed tumor cells in the epidermis | • Tumor cells are located in the suprabasal region of the epidermis with intact keratinocytes<br>• Intracellular mucin<br>• Signet ring cells<br>• Glandular structures |
| Superficial spreading malignant melanoma | • Single dispersed cells in the epidermis<br>• Occasional cases show melanin within the Paget cell | • Cells of melanoma are collected as a nest in dermoepidermal junction<br>• Intracellular mucin and acini<br>• HMB 45 and Melan A positivity |
| Mycosis fungoides | • Single large cells in the epidermis | • Large convoluted cerebriform cells<br>• Intraepidermal collection of lymphoid cells<br>• T-cell marker (CD 3) positive |

## Histopathology

The tumor shows single or nests of Paget cells in the epidermis predominantly located in the basal or parabasal region. The individual Paget cells are large and contain abundant pale vacuolated cytoplasm (Figures 3.19 and 3.20). The nuclei of the cells are central in position and large with vesicular having prominent nucleoli. Uncommonly glands or acini like structures are seen. Infrequent mitotic activity may also be noted. Occasionally, the Paget cells may contain melanin pigment due to transfer of melanin from melanocytes to Paget cell.

## Special Stains

Paget cells are positive for Periodic acid Schiff (PAS) stain and resistant to diastase. The cells contain mucin and therefore positive for Alcian blue and mucicarmine. The cells are also positive for mucin core protein (MUC) 1 and MUC 5. On immunohistochemistry, Paget cells are positive for CEA, epithelial membrane antigen (EMA), low-molecular weight cytokeratin and gross cystic disease fluid protein 15 (GCDFP-15). Immunocytochemistry is particularly helpful in distinguishing primary intraepidermal Paget's disease and Paget's disease that developed from an associated internal adenocarcinoma.

## Differential Diagnosis

The differential diagnosis and detailed immunohistochemistry of Paget's disease have been mentioned in Tables 3.7 and 3.8 respectively.
- In situ and invasive squamous cell carcinoma (pagetoid Bowen disease).
- Superficial spreading malignant melanoma.
- Mycosis fungoides and Paget's disease.

## Prognosis and Treatment

The prognosis of Paget disease depends on the extent of the lesion. The prognosis of totally intraepithelial Paget disease without any invasion is much better than invasive Paget

Table 3.8: Immunohistochemistry of extra-mammary Paget disease

| Lesion | Immunohistochemistry | | | | |
|---|---|---|---|---|---|
| | CK7 | CK20 | GCDFP15 | Uroplakin | CEA |
| Primary Paget | + | – | + | – | + |
| Paget due to underlying anorectal carcinoma | – | + | – | – | + |
| Paget due to underlying urothelial carcinoma | + | + | – | + | – |

Gross cystic disease fluid protein (GCDFP-15)

disease. The primary intraepithelial Paget progresses slowly and has an indolent course. The disease is often multifocal and the normal appearing skin around the Paget disease may also show involvement. Therefore, the recurrence of Paget is common even after successful resection margin free tumor removal.

The treatment of Paget disease of vulva is surgical resection of the tumor. There should be at least 1 cm tumor free margin of the skin.[20] In case of invasive Paget disease ipsilateral inguinal–femoral lymphadenectomy is recommended.

## MALIGNANT MELANOMA OF VULVA

Malignant melanoma represents 10% of all malignant tumors of vulva.[21] The disease predominantly occurs in elderly white woman and rarely seen under 30 year of age.

**Clinical features:** The patients complain vulval bleeding, pruritus and dysuria. They usually present with pigmented nodule or polypoid mass and rarely as ulcerated lesion. Approximate one-third of vulval melanoma may be amelanotic. The vulval melanomas are often multifocal with satellite nodules around the main tumor (20%).

### Histopathology (Figures 3.21 and 3.22)

There are three histological pattern of malignant melanoma of vulva:
1. **Mucosallentiginous melanoma:** Mucosal lentiginous melanoma is the commonest type in the vulval region. The tumor may show both radial and vertical growth pattern. The large atypical melanocytes are spread singly or nest-like pattern in the epidermis. The cells in the invasive epidermo-dermal zone are elongated spindle-shaped and invade the dermis in small fascicles or nests. The atypical cells in the intra-epidermal region are large. The tumor cells contain abundant cytoplasm with round nuclei and prominent nucleoli.
2. **Nodular melanoma:** Nodular melanoma usually does not show any radial growth pattern. The neoplastic cells may be present within the epidermis with an invasive component. The tumor cells are large polygonal with

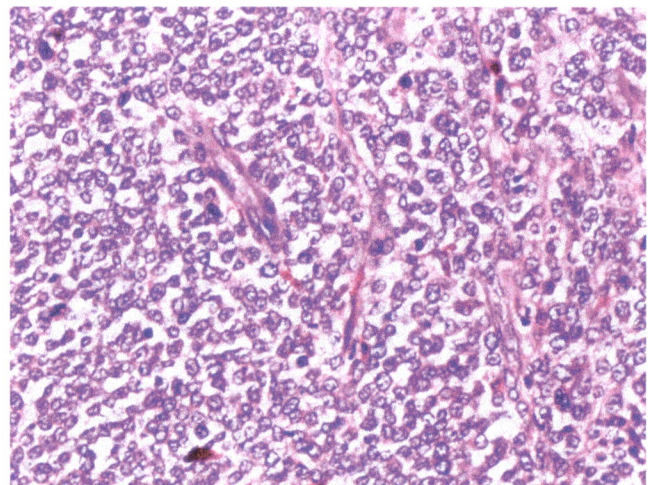

Figure 3.21: Melanoma of vulva: Diffuse sheets of cells with malignant cells

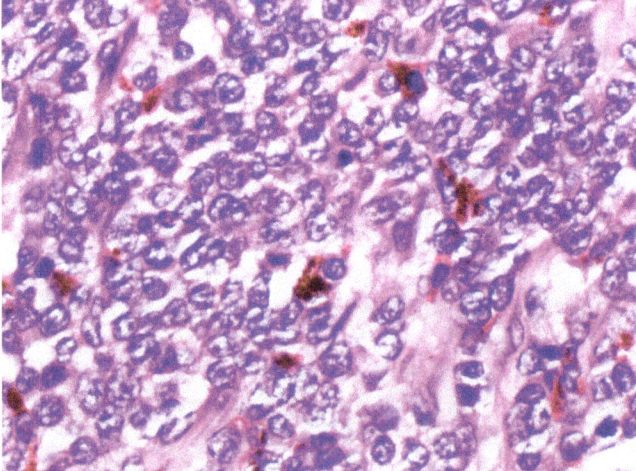

Figure 3.22: Melanoma of vulva: Higher magnification shows cells with enlarged nuclei and prominent nucleoli. The cells contain brownish melanin pigment

abundant cytoplasm having enlarged nuclei with prominent nucleoli. The other cell types are spindle-shaped and dendritic cells with oval to elongated nuclei. The cells are arranged in small fascicles. The dendritic cells contain elongated cytoplasmic process simulating nerve cells. The cells show moderate nuclear pleomorphism.

3. **Superficial spreading melanoma:** Superficial spreading melanoma predominantly shows radial pattern of growth. There is evidence of invasion. The malignant cells are large polygonal with abundant cytoplasm having centrally placed nuclei. Nuclei are relatively monomorphic with prominent nucleoli.

## Differential Diagnosis

The differential diagnoses of malignant melanoma of vulva are:
- Vulval Paget disease: Discussed before
- VIN: Discussed before
- Poorly differentiated squamous cell carcinoma: Poorly differentiated squamous cell carcinoma with spindle cell component may be mistaken as malignant melanoma.
- Spindle cell tumor of soft tissue origin: The presence of melanin in the spindle cells and immunocytochemistry (HMB 45 and Melan A) may be helpful in confirmation of melanoma.

## Prognosis

The main prognostic factors of melanoma are: (1) depth of tumor invasion, (2) tumor thickness.

**Tumor thickness:** The tumor thickness is measured by Breslow's thickness measurement. The tumor thickness is measured from the lower border of the granular layer of the epithelium to the deepest point of tumor invasion.[22] According to the depth of invasion the tumor is classified from T1 to T4 (Table 3.9). The 5 year survival rate in T1 Breslow's grade of invasion (less than 1 mm) is much higher (near about 90%).

**Tumor invasion:** Clark classified melanoma in five levels depending on the involvement of the various anatomic compartments of the skin[23] (Table 3.10). Prognosis of melanoma is excellent when melanoma is less than Clark 2 level.

**Other prognostic factors:** The other adverse prognostic factors of melanoma are: (1) surface ulceration, (2) lymphovascular invasion, (3) tumor necrosis and, (4) high dermal mitotic activities.

## Treatment

The treatment of melanoma of vulva is complete surgical excision of the lesion. There should be at least 2 cm free margins and 1-2 cm free deep resection plane. Melanoma with more than 4 mm invasion needs wide resection with removal of deep fascia and inguinal lymph nodal dissection.

Table 3.9: Breslow's classification of melanoma invasion

| Classification | Depth of tumor invasion |
|---|---|
| T1 | Less than 1 mm |
| T2 | 1–2 mm |
| T3 | 2–4 mm |
| T4 | More than 4 mm |

Table 3.10: Clark's classification

| Classification | Tumor invasion into the different anatomic subdivision |
|---|---|
| Level 1 | Intraepithelial involvement of melanoma or in situ melanoma |
| Level 2 | Involvement into the superficial papillary dermis |
| Level 3 | Melanoma extensively involves the papillary dermis |
| Level 4 | Reticular dermis is involved |
| Level 5 | Tumor invasion into the subcutaneous tissue and fat |

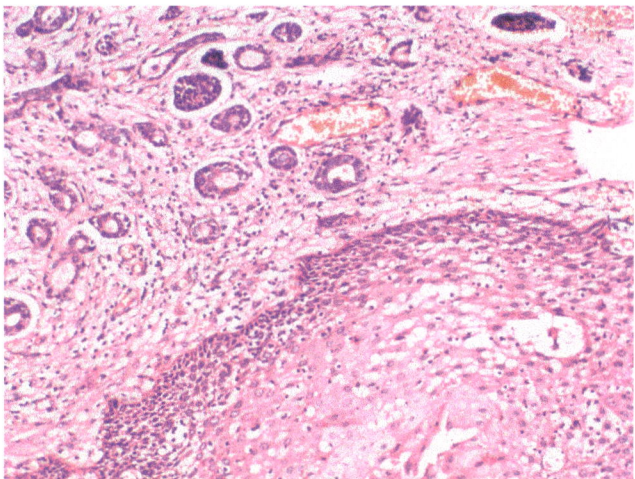

Figure 3.23: Adenoid cystic carcinoma: Tumor underneath the epidermis

## OTHER UNCOMMON MALIGNANT TUMORS OF VULVA

Vulva is rarely involved by various other malignant tumors such as adenoid cystic carcinoma (Figures 3.23 to 3.25), Markel cell carcinoma, endodermal sinus tumor and non-Hodgkin lymphoma.

## Metastatic Tumors of Vulva

Metastatic tumor comprises of 8% of vulval tumors. The common primary sources of metastasis are cervix, uterus and ovary. The other uncommon primary sites are breast, kidney and gastrointestinal tract.

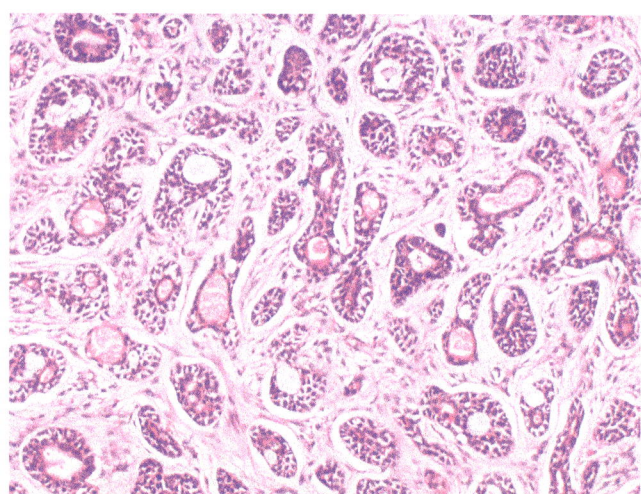

**Figure 3.24:** Adenoid cystic carcinoma: Typical pattern of adenoid cystic carcinoma

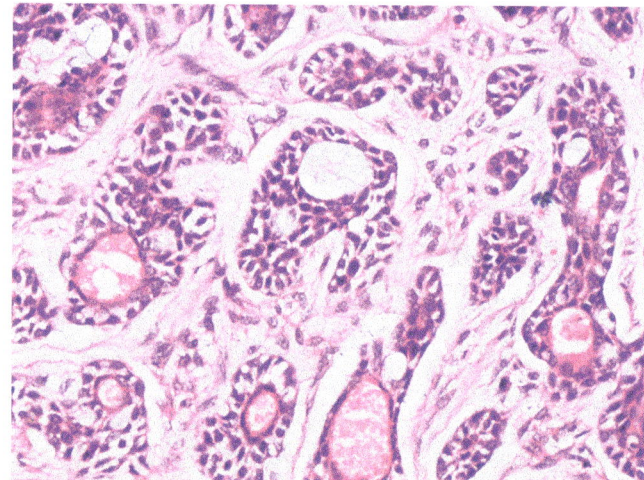

**Figure 3.25:** Adenoid cystic carcinoma: Higher magnification shows gland-like arrangement of cells around central luminal structure

## REFERENCES

1. Kurman RJ, Carcangiu ML, Herrington S, Young RH. Tumors of vulva. WHO classification of tumors of female genital reproductive organs. 4th Edition, International Agency for Research on Cancer, Lyon; 2014.
2. Kondi-Paphitis A, Deligeorgi-Politi H, Liapis A, Plemenou-Frangou M. Human papilloma virus in verrucus carcinoma of the vulva: an immunopathological study of the cases. Eur J Gynaecol Oncol. 1998; 19:319-20.
3. Traiman P, Bacchi CE, De Luca LA, Uemura G, Nahas Neto J, Nahas EA, et al. Vulvar carcinoma in young patients and its relationship with genital warts. Eur J Gynaecol Oncol. 1999; 20: 191-4.
4. Congilosi SM, Madoff RD. Current therapy for recurrent and extensive anal warts. Dis Colon Rectum. 1995;38:1101-7.
5. Mabuchi K, Bross DS, Kessler, II. Epidemiology of cancer of the vulva. A case-control study. Cancer. 1985;55(8):1843-8.
6. Haefner HK, Tate JE, McLachlin CM, Crum CP. Vulvar intraepithelial neoplasia: age, morphological phenotype, papillomavirus DNA, and coexisting invasive carcinoma. Hum Pathol. 1995;26(2):147-54.
7. Sideri M, Jones RW, Wilkinson EJ, et al. Squamous vulvar intraepithelial neoplasia:2004 modified terminology, ISSVD. Vulvar Oncology Subcommittee. J Reprod Med. 2005;50:807-10.
8. Rufforny I, Wilkinson EJ, Liu C, Zhu H, Buteral M, Massoll NA. Human papillomavirus infection and p16(INK4a) protein expression in vulvar intraepithelial neoplasia and invasive squamous cell carcinoma. J Low Genit Tract Dis. 2005;9(2):108-13.
9. McCluggage WG. Recent advances in immunohistochemistry in gynaecological pathology. Histopathology. 2002;40(4):309-26.
10. Skapa P, Zamecnik J, Hamsikova E, Salakova M, Smahelova J, Jandova K, et al. Human papillomavirus (HPV) profiles of vulvar lesions: possible implications for the classification of vulvar squamous cell carcinoma precursors and for the efficacy of prophylactic HPV vaccination. Am J Surg Pathol. 2007;31(12):1834-43.
11. Santos M, Montagut C, Mellado B, Garcia A, Ramon y Cajal S, Cardesa A, et al. Immunohistochemical staining for p16 and p53 in premalignant and malignant epithelial lesions of the vulva. Int J Gynecol Pathol. 2004;23(3):206-14.
12. Brustmann H, Naude S. Expression of topoisomerase IIalpha, Ki-67, proliferating cell nuclear antigen, p53, and argyrophilic nucleolar organizer regions in vulvar squamous lesions. Gynecol Oncol. 2002;86(2):192-9.
13. Jones RW, Rowan DM. Vulvar intraepithelial neoplasia III: a clinical study of the outcome in 113 cases with relation to the later development of invasive vulvar carcinoma. Obstet Gynecol. 1994;84(5):741-5.
14. Parkin DM, Whelan SL, Ferlay J, et al. Cancer incidence in five continents VII. Lyon, France, IARC, 1997.
15. Moore TO, Moore AY, Carrasco D, Vander Straten M, Arany I, Au W, Tyring SK. Human papillomavirus, smoking, and cancer. J Cutan Med Surg. 2001;5(4):323-8.
16. Bonvicini F, Venturoli S, Ambretti S, Paterini P, Santini D, Ceccarelli C, et al. Presence and type of oncogenic human papillomavirus in classic and in differentiated vulvar intraepithelial neoplasia and keratinizing vulvar squamous cell carcinoma. J Med Virol. 2005;77(1):102-6.
17. FIGO staging for carcinoma of the vulva, cervix, and corpus uteri. FIGO Committee on Gynecologic Oncology. Int J Gynaecol Obstet. 2014;125 (2):97-8. Epub 2014 Feb 22.
18. Wilkinson EJ. Protocol for the examination of specimens from patients with carcinomas and malignant melanomas of the vulva: a basis for checklists. Cancer Committee of the College of American Pathologists. Arch Pathol Lab Med. 2000;124:51-56: Revised 2005.

19. Homesley HD, Bundy BN, Sedlis A, et al. Assessment of current international federation of gynecology and obstetrics staging of vulvar carcinoma relative to prognostic factors for survival (a gynecologic oncology group study). Am J Obstet Gynecol. 1991;164:997-1004.
20. DeVita VT, Jr, Hellman S, Rosenberg SA. Cancers of the skin. Cancer, principles and practice of oncology. New York: Lippincott Raven, 1997:1565-6.
21. Irvin PW, Legallo RL, Stoler MH, Rice LW, Taylor PT Jr, Andersen WA. Vulvar melanoma: a retrospective analysis and literature review. Gynecol Oncol. 2001;83:457-65.
22. Breslow A. Tumor thickness, level of invasion and node dissection in stage I cutaneous melanoma. Ann Surg. 1975;182:572-5.
23. Clark WH Jr, Elder DE, Guerry D 4th, et al. Model predicting survival in stage I melanoma based on tumor progression. J Natl Cancer Inst. 1989;81:1893-904.

# Benign and Malignant Diseases of Vagina

## 4

## WHO CLASSIFICATION OF TUMORS OF VAGINA (2014)[1]

**Epithelial tumors**
Squamous cell tumors and precursors
- Low grade squamous intraepithelial lesion
- High grade squamous intraepithelial lesion

Squamous cell carcinoma
- Keratinizing
- Nonkeratinizing
- Papillary
- Basaloid
- Warty
- Verrucous

Benign squamous lesions
- Condyloma acuminatum
- Squamous papilloma
- Fibroepithelial polyp
- Tubulosquamous polyp
- Transitional cell metaplasia

**Glandular tumors**
Adenocarcinomas
- Endometrioid carcinoma
- Clear cell carcinoma
- Mucinous carcinoma
- Mesonephric carcinoma

Benign glandular lesions
- Tubulovillous adenoma
- Villous adenoma
- Müllerian papilloma
- Adenosis
- Endometriosis
- Endocervicosis
- Cyst

High grade neuroendocrine carcinoma
- Small cell neuroendocrine carcinoma
- Large cell neuroendocrine carcinoma

Other epithelial tumors
- Mixed tumor
- Adenosquamous carcinoma
- Adenoid basal carcinoma

**Mesenchymal tumors**
- Leiomyoma
- Rhabdomyoma
- Leiomyosarcoma
- Rhabdomyosarcoma
- Aggressive angiomyxoma

**Tumor-like lesions**
**Mixed epithelial and mesenchymal tumors**
**Lymphoid and myeloid tumors**
**Melanotic tumors**
**Miscellaneous tumors**
Germ cell tumors
- Mature teratoma
- Yolk sac tumors

Others
- Ewing sarcoma
- Paraganglioma

**Secondary tumors**

## DEVELOPMENTAL DISORDERS OF VAGINA

### Vaginal Agenesis

This is a rare developmental disorder that affects 1 in 5,000 female birth.[2] The vagina is not developed due to the imperfect caudal development and fusion of the distal part of Müllerian ducts. The patient has normal uterus and normally appearing external genitalia. The vaginal orifice is ended by a blind pouch. The patient usually complains of the consequences of retrograde menstruation. In Mayer–Rokitansky–Küster–Hauser syndrome, the vaginal agenesis is associated with absence of uterus, fallopian tubes and skeletal abnormalities. The patient has normal 44XX chromosomal pattern with normal ovaries.[3]

*Treatment*

Artificial reconstruction of vagina is the treatment of vaginal agenesis.

## Imperforate Hymen

This is the most common significant congenital abnormalities of vagina and represents 0.1–0.2% of female birth. The patient usually remains asymptomatic till puberty. They complain of back pain or abdominal pain, constipation or amenorrhea. If not treated in time then the patient may develop endometriosis and pelvic adhesion due to retrograde menstruation.[4] On gross examination hymen appears as shiny white tissue. Hymen consists of fibrocollagenous tissue lined by squamous epithelial cells.

*Treatment*

The treatment involves central cruciate incision of the membrane.

## Transverse Vaginal Septum

It is an uncommon congenital anomaly that represents only 0.002% of female birth. The patient has a transverse septum in the vagina. If the septum is complete then the patient presents with the same symptoms as that of imperforate hymen. Partial vaginal septum presents with dyspareunia. The septum is composed of fibrocollagenous tissue covered by squamous epithelium in caudal side and glandular epithelium in cranial side.

## INFECTIOUS INFLAMMATORY DISORDERS

## Bacterial Vaginosis

*Gardnerella vaginalis* is the main causative organism however other bacteria such as *Prevotella bivia*, *Mycoplasma hominis*, *Mobiluncus mulieris*, and *Mobiluncus curtisii* are also responsible for bacterial vaginosis.

*Clinical Features*

The presence of combination of any three features among the following features confirms the clinical diagnosis of bacterial vaginosis:[5]
1. Vaginal pH 4.5 or less,
2. Fishy smelling thin discharge,
3. The peculiar unique smell after the addition of 10% potassium hydroxide solution on the drops of vaginal secretion on slide, and
4. Large number of clue cells in either wet preparation or Papanicolaou's stained vaginal smear.

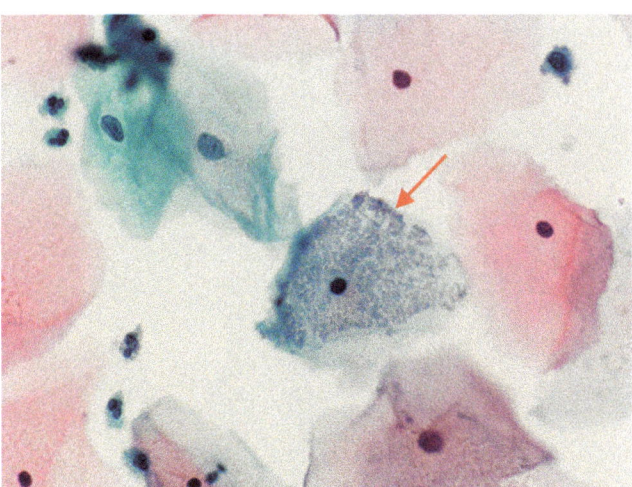

**Figure 4.1:** Bacterial vaginosis: Clue cells with granular dots in the cytoplasm

*Pathology*

Vaginal smears show alteration of normal flora of lactobacilli. Multiple "clue cells" are seen characterized by squamous cells with attached coccobacilli (Figure 4.1). In addition, inflammatory cells and background cocci and bacilli are also seen.

*Treatment*

The treatment of bacterial vaginosis may be:
1. Oral metronidazole for 7 days,
2. Tropical application of clindamycin or
3. Tropical application of metronidazole.

## Candida Infection

Near about one-third of acute vaginitis cases are caused by candidal infection, most commonly *Candida albicans*. The other candidal species are *C. tropicalis* or *C. glabrata*.

*Clinical Features*

The patient presents with thick curdy white discharge along with pruritus and burning sensation. The vagina becomes erythematous with superficial erosion. The risk factors of candida infection are nulliparity, use of broad spectrum antibiotic, spermicide, etc.

*Pathology*

The vaginal smear shows yeast and pseudohyphae of candida on Papanicolaou's stain (Figure 4.2). Tissue biopsy is rarely obtained and the section shows abundant acute inflammatory cells, congested vessels and fungal profile in the superficial epithelial layer.

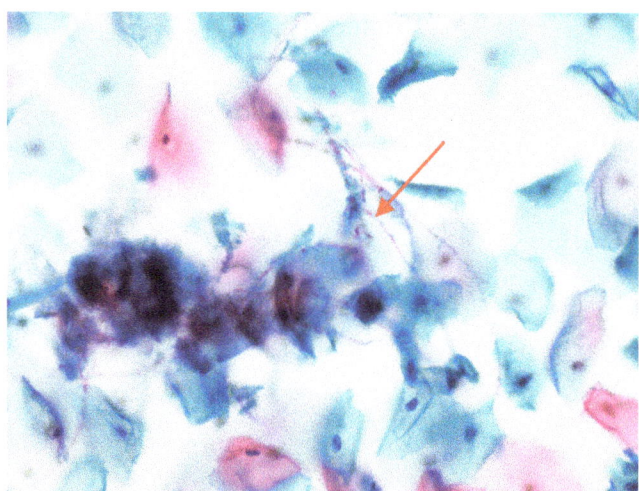

Figure 4.2: Candidal hyphae: Multiple candida pseudo hyphae

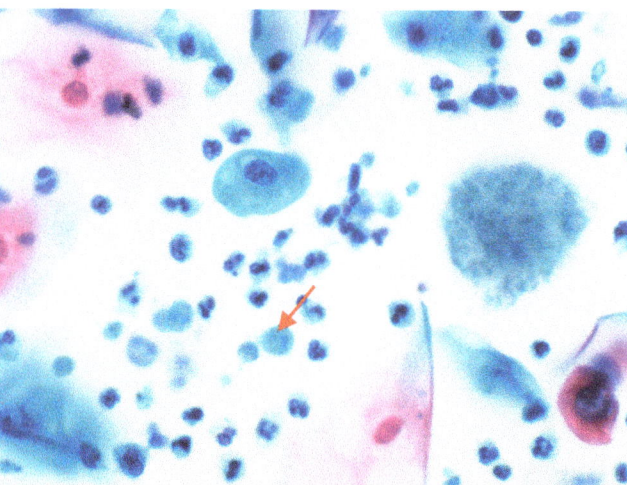

Figure 4.3: Trichomonas vaginalis: Round pear-shaped trichomonas vaginalis

*Treatment*

A single dose of oral fluconazole therapy or tropical antifungal for 7 days is used.

### Trichomonas Vaginalis

It is one of the common causes of acute vaginitis. The infection is always caused by sexual transmission.

*Clinical Feature*

The patient usually complaints of thin yellowish vaginal discharge, pruritus and dysuria. The vagina appears erythematous with many small hemorrhagic points.

*Pathology*

Cervical smear shows dirty inflammatory background along with 10–20 micron diameter pear-shaped cyanophilic organism in Papanicolaou's stain (Figure 4.3). Histopathology is rarely obtained in trichomonas vaginalis infection. Tissue section shows dense lymphocytes and plasma cells along with stromal vascular congestion.

*Treatment*

Treatment includes oral metronidazole. The treatment of male partner is also recommended to prevent recurrence.

### Actinomycosis

Actinomycosis is a Gram positive acid fast organism. The organism infects vagina in case of intrauterine contraceptive device or the presence of any other foreign objects. The patient usually complains of malodorous discharge, pruritus and postcoital bleeding. Vaginal smear shows aggregation of fine filamentous bacteria that radiate from a central core (Figure 4.4). Background of the smear shows evidences of inflammation.

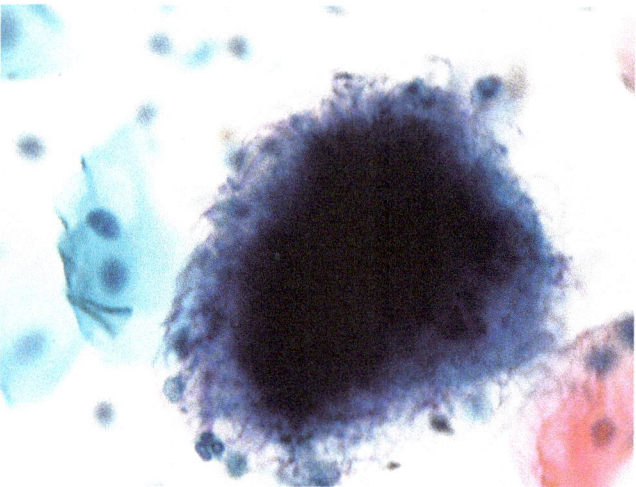

Figure 4.4: Actinomycosis: Filamentous organism in ball-like cluster

*Treatment*

Penicillin is the treatment of choice. Removal of foreign bodies is also recommended.

### Parasitic Vaginitis

Parasitic vaginitis is rare. *Entamoeba histolytica* causes vaginal amoebiasis. The patients complain with bloody vaginal discharge. Vagina becomes ulcerated simulating carcinoma. Histopathology section shows ulcerated lining epithelium with fibrinopurulent exudates. Many trophozoites of Entamoeba histolytica are also seen.

Patients with *Schistosoma mansoni* and *Schistosoma haematobium* infection present with pruritus, vaginal discharge and dyspareunia. The mucosa shows polypoidal lesion or ulceration. Histopathology section reveals many eggs of Schistosoma along with inflammation.

Vagina may be infected by fecal contamination of ova of *Enterobius vermicularis* or *Trichuris trichiura*. The parasitic ova evoke granulomatous reaction with central necrosis.

## Toxic Shock Syndrome

Toxic shock syndrome (TSS) is a systemic fatal disease. The patient shows fever, myalgia, confusion and hypotension. The disease is caused by the use of vaginal tampon that may cause proliferation of *Staphylococcus aureus*. The organisms produce toxic shock syndrome toxin-1 (TSST-1). The absorption of such TSST-1 in the systemic circulation causes TSS. TSS is mostly related with menstruation and tampon use, however, non-menstrual TSS has also been described in 10% cases.[6]

### Histopathology

Microscopical examination shows desquamated lining epithelium and inflammatory cell infiltrate predominantly around the capillaries. Vasculitis is also seen.

### Treatment

The disease may be trivial to fatal. The treatment of choice is the administration of beta-lactamase resistant anti-staphylococcal antibiotics. The patient should be provided other supportive measures of shock.

## Emphysematous Vaginitis

Emphysematous vaginitis is a rare condition.[7] The patients usually complaints of cracking rupture of gas filled cystic spaces during intercourse and vaginal discharge. The disease is probably caused by organisms like trichomonas vaginalis and *Gardnerella vaginalis*. On histology, the cyst shows inflammatory cells and multinucleated giant cells. The gas in the cyst is composed of oxygen, hydrogen sulfide, ammonia, nitrogen, etc. The disease is non-fatal and self-limited.

# NONINFECTIOUS INFLAMMATORY DISEASES OF VAGINA

## Desquamative Inflammatory Vaginitis

Exact etiology of this disease is not known and no causative organism is identified. There is exfoliation of the normal vaginal mucosa along with mucopurulent discharge. The woman is in premenopausal age and presents with purulent vaginal discharge, dyspareunia, vulvar pruritus and malodorous smell. The vaginal discharge shows large number of polymorphs. No bacterial organism is identified in the discharge. Histopathology is rarely available in this lesion. The section shows desquamated lining epithelium with underlying acute inflammatory cells. Treatment includes tropical clindamycin in vagina.

## Ligneous Vaginitis

Ligneous vaginitis is a rare systemic disease that causes pseudomembrane formation. The disease affects in oral, respiratory, middle ear and vagina. It is suggested that severe type 1 plasminogen (PLG) deficiency due to mutations in the PLG gene is the cause of ligneous vaginitis.[8] The patient usually presents with dysmenorrhea, vaginal discharge, and postcoital bleeding.

### Histopathology

The section of the lesion shows amorphous eosinophilic membrane composed of fibrin and collagen along with chronic inflammatory cells. The pseudomembrane is negative for Congo red stain.

### Treatment

Surgery, antibiotics and anti-inflammatory agents are used for treatment. The treatment has partial success.

## Reaction to Seminal Fluid

Uncommonly vagina may show allergic reaction to seminal fluid in the form of localized or systemic urticarial reaction.[9]

## Other Conditions

Rarely vagina may be affected by malakoplakia, a chronic inflammatory condition of unknown pathology. Gram negative bacilli mainly *Escherichia coli* is isolated in malakoplakia. The patients present with tumor-like lesion in the vagina.[10] Histology shows abundant histiocytes and plasma cells along with 5–10 micron diameter spherical concentrically laminated intra and extracellular inclusions known as Michaelis–Gutmann bodies.

# TRAUMATIC, SURGERY AND RADIATION-INDUCED LESIONS

## Traumatic Injury

Vagina may undergo injury due to various causes such as sexual assault, accidental fall, automobile accidents, etc.

## Tampon Ulcer

Use of tampon may cause micro ulcerations of vaginal mucosa. The patient may have abnormal vaginal discharge or intermenstrual bleeding. The ulcers are shallow with smooth margins and clean floor made up of granulation tissue. Discontinuation of tampon helps in healing of the ulcers.

## Granulation Tissue

After hysterectomy operation, granulation tissue is often seen in the vaginal vault. This is a common cause of post-surgical bleeding.

## Radiation-induced Changes

Radiation therapy in the malignancy of female genital tract may induce atrophy in vaginal mucosal membrane. The mucus membrane of the vagina becomes thin and friable.[11] The vaginal vault shows mass-like lesion. The histopathology of such lesion exhibits plasma cells, stromal cell proliferation and vascular endothelial cell proliferation. The atypical stromal cells may simulate malignancy because of nuclear enlargement and pleomorphism. However, the nucleo-cytoplasmic ratio of these cells is not altered and the nuclear chromatin is smudged.

## Prolapse of Vagina

Due to loss of support of the ligaments the vagina may prolapse. This is particularly seen in multiple pregnancies.

## Prolapse of Fallopian Tube

This uncommon complication is seen after hysterectomy. The patient complains of vaginal discharge and bleeding. Red nodular mass is seen in the apex of the vagina. The histology section shows multiple branching tubules lined by bland looking tubal epithelium. At times the lesion may show considerable vascular and stromal proliferation and may be mistaken as mesenchymal tumors such as aggressive angiomyxoma or angiomyofibroblastoma.[12] The presence of tubal epithelium is the indicator of fallopian tube prolapse in such cases.

## POSTOPERATIVE SPINDLE CELL NODULE

This nodule typically appears 2 to 3 months after surgery. Vagina is the commonest site. However, the other parts of the genital tract such as cervix and endometrium may also be involved.[13] The lesion is usually polypoid mass. Histopathology section shows fascicles of spindle cells with elongated nuclei and vesicular chromatin. Pleomorphism is strikingly absent. The mitosis activity is high. The cells are positive for desmin.

## Differential Diagnosis

As the lesion is not well-circumscribed with high mitotic activities so it may be mistaken as sarcoma particularly leiomyosarcoma. However, the history of prior surgery and absence of nuclear atypia are the helpful features to exclude malignancy.

## Prognosis and Treatment

Prognosis of such lesion is good. Treatment includes complete local surgical resection.

## VAGINAL CYSTS

Vaginal cysts are commonly seen and are of two types: acquired and congenital.

## Mesonephric Cyst (Gartner's Duct Cyst)

These cysts are commonly seen in the anterolateral or lateral vaginal wall. Most of the patients are asymptomatic until the cyst becomes large enough to produce urinary incontinence. The cyst is developed from the mesonephric or paramesonephric duct. The Gartner's cyst is lined by low cuboidal cells (Figure 4.5).

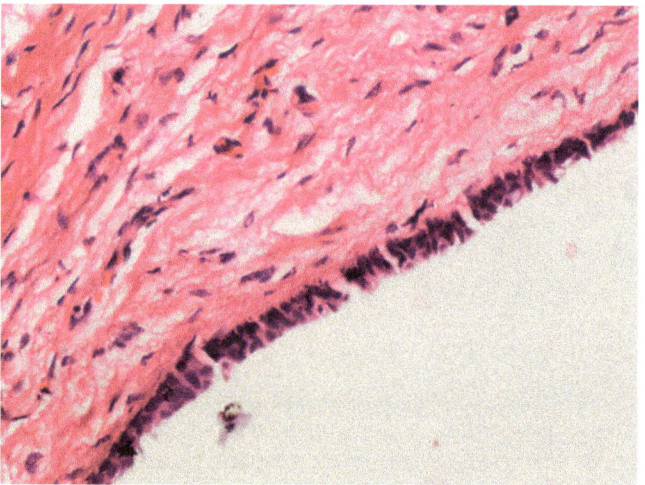

**Figure 4.5:** Mesonephric cyst (Gartner's duct cyst): The cyst is lined by low cuboidal epithelium

## MÜLLERIAN CYST

This is the commonest cyst in vagina and is located anywhere in vaginal wall. The cyst is usually small (less than 2.5 cm in diameter). The Müllerian cyst is lined by the epithelium of the Müllerian duct derivative such as mucinous endocervical, endometrial or ciliated columnar epithelium of fallopian tube (Figures 4.6 and 4.7).

## Bartholin Gland Cysts

This cyst is located around the opening of the Bartholin gland near the vestibule. The cyst is lined by squamous epithelium, transitional epithelium or columnar epithelium surrounded by dense fibrous tissue (Figures 4.8 to 4.10). The details of Bartholin gland cysts have been described in earlier chapter.

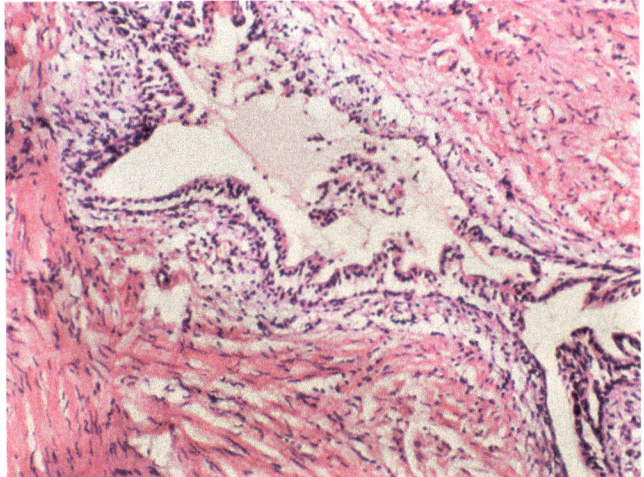

**Figure 4.6:** Müllerian cyst: The cyst is lined by mucinous epithelium

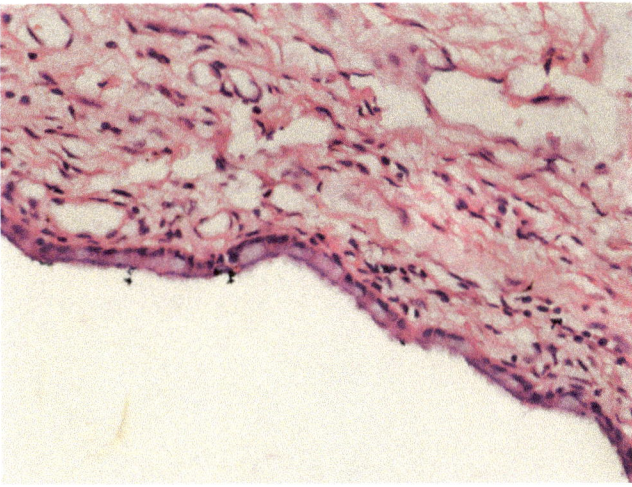

**Figure 4.9:** Bartholin cyst: Higher magnification shows tall columnar lining cells of the cyst

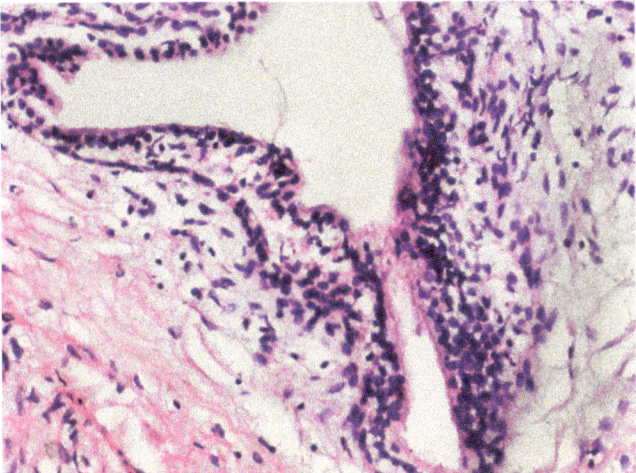

**Figure 4.7:** Müllerian cyst: Higher magnification shows tall columnar mucus secreting cells in the lining of the cyst

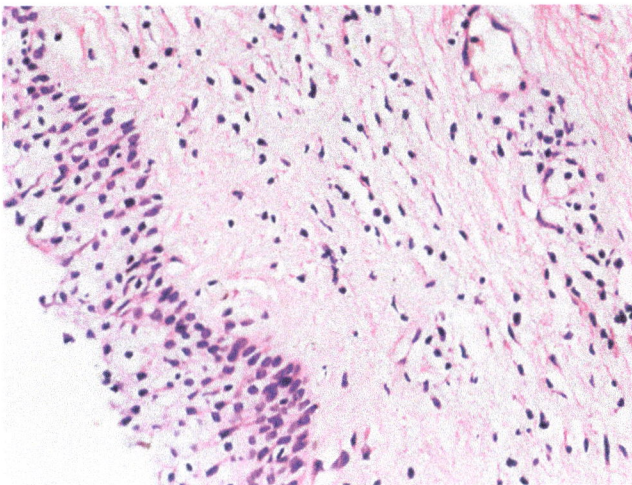

**Figure 4.10:** Bartholin cyst: The cyst is lined by transitional cells

### Epithelial Inclusion Cyst

This is the commonest vaginal cyst. The dimension of the cyst varies from few mm to few cm. The cyst is lined by stratified squamous epithelium. The granular layer is seen in the lining. The cyst wall may show foreign body reaction with many multinucleated giant cells.

*Treatment*

Most of the vaginal wall cysts are asymptomatic and do not require any treatment. However, the large symptomatic cyst should be removed.

## VAGINAL ADENOSIS

It is commonly associated with Diethylstilbestrol (DES) in utero. However, rarely vaginal adenosis may be unrelated

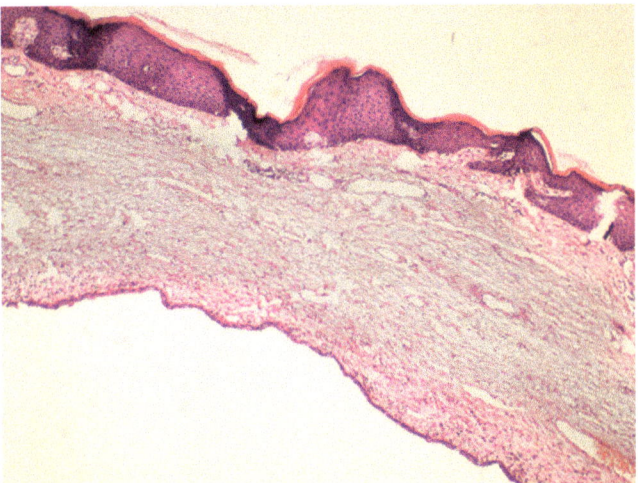

**Figure 4.8:** Bartholin cyst: The cyst is lined by single layer of columnar cells

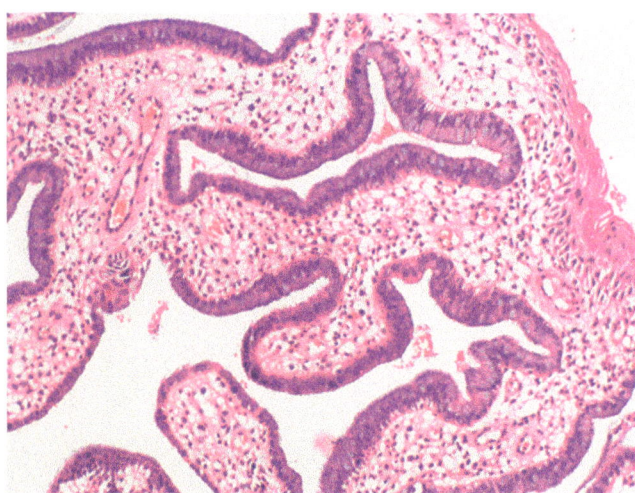

Figure 4.11: Vaginal adenosis: Multiple glands under the squamous epithelium of vagina

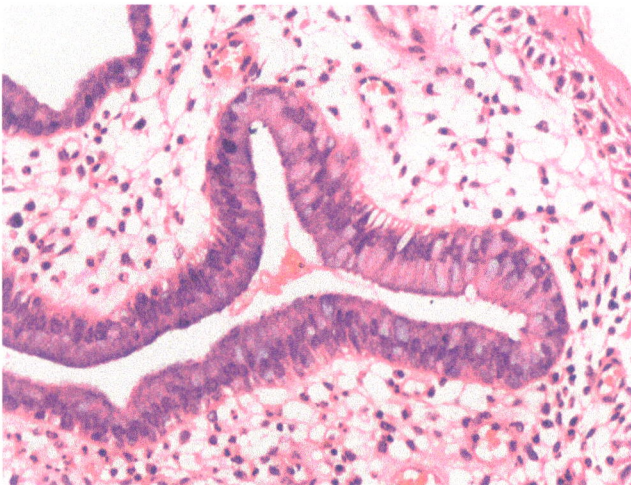

Figure 4.12: Vaginal adenosis: Higher magnification shows endocervical mucus lining of the glands

with DES exposure. The lesion usually involves the upper one-third of the vagina.

## Histopathology

Histopathology of the lesion shows multiple glands underneath the squamous lining epithelium. The glands are lined by endocervical mucin secreting epithelium (Figures 4.11 and 4.12) or endometrioid cells with tubal metaplasia. Endocervical epithelium may show squamous metaplasia. The endometrioid cells also often show tubal metaplasia with ciliated lining.

## VAGINAL INTRAEPITHELIAL NEOPLASIA

Vaginal intraepithelial neoplasia (VAIN) is relatively uncommon in comparison to cervical intraepithelial neoplasia (CIN). About 65% of VAIN is associated with CIN. The

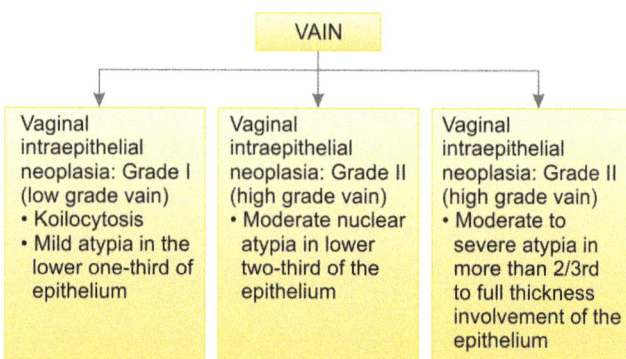

Figure 4.13: Schematic diagram of vaginal intraepithelial neoplasia (VAIN)

age of the patients varies from 18 to 72 years, with a mean age of 49 years which is almost 10 years less than CIN. The common risk factors of VAIN are immunosuppression, history of CIN, HPV infection, history of Diethylstilbestrol exposure and irradiation. VAIN is related with HPV infection (most common type HPV[16]). Mixed HPV infections are also noted in multifocal VAIN cases.[14]

## Clinical Features

The patients are mostly asymptomatic. VAINs are usually multifocal (50%). The solitary lesion is usually seen in upper third of vagina and is mostly detected by Papanicolaou's stain, colposcopic examination, or histopathological examination of upper part of vagina after hysterectomy.

## Histology

The histopathological features of VAIN are similar to CIN (Figure 4.13). VAIN I shows mild nuclear atypia of the squamous cells restricted to lower one-third of the epithelium. The superficial layer shows koilocytotic changes. VAIN 1 includes both exophytic and flat condyloma. Exophytic condyloma shows exophytic verucopapillary growth pattern whereas flat condyloma shows flat surface. These lesions are frequently related with HPV 6 and 11 infections.

VAIN II shows moderate nuclear atypia in lower 2/3rd of the surface epithelium. VAIN III exhibits more than 2/3rd to total thickness involvement of the epithelium by moderately atypical cells (Figures 4.14 and 4.15). Both VAIN II and VAIN III may show koilocytotic cells.

## Ancillary Studies

Ki 67 may be helpful in the diagnostic confirmation of VAIN. In case of normal epithelium Ki 67 is positive only in the basal and parabasal epithelium. However in VAIN I, it is positive in scattered cells of superficial epithelium and in VAIN II and III, Ki 67 positive cells are seen throughout the entire epithelium.

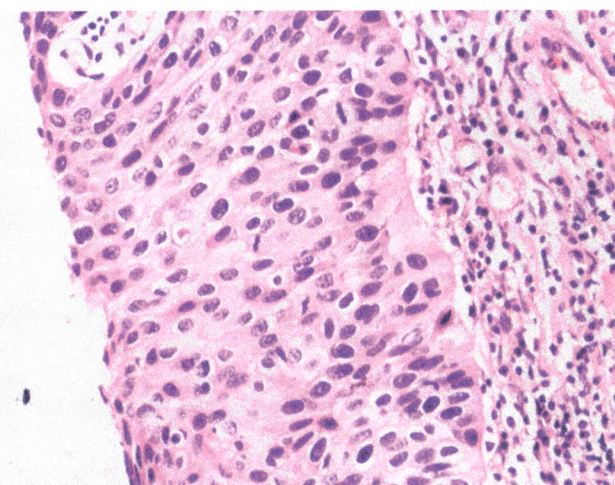

**Figure 4.14:** VAIN III: Full thickness involvement by atypical cells

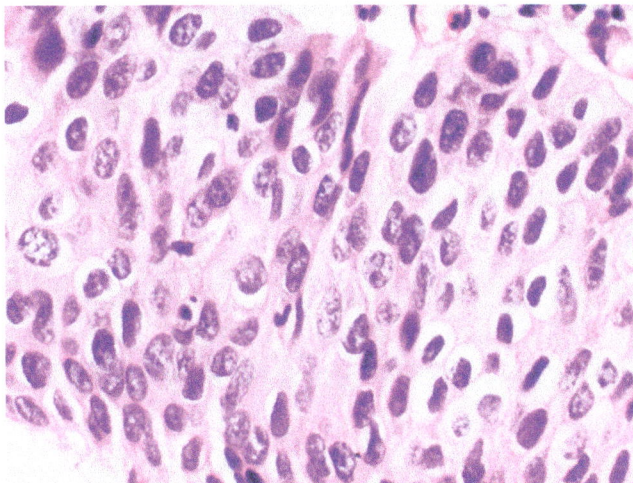

**Figure 4.15:** VAIN III: Higher magnification shows cells with nuclear enlargement and pleomorphism

## Prognosis and Management

A large follow-up study of untreated VAIN cases showed that near about 78% cases of VAIN regress over the course of time, 13% cases it may remain static, and only 9% cases may progress to carcinoma.[15] Patients with VAIN I can be followed up because the chance of progression is rare. VAIN II and VAIN III are treated by surgical excision, laser vaporization, cryosurgery, topical 5-fluorouracil.[16]

In small localized lesion, surgical excision of the lesion is the management of choice. Topical 5-fluorouracil may cause extensive desquamation of the vaginal mucosal lining and therefore its use is limited nowadays. Loop electroexcision may cause surrounding tissue damage. Laser is particularly helpful in extensive and persistent lesion.

## NEOPLASMS OF VAGINA

### Squamous Cell Carcinoma

Vaginal malignancies represent only 1–4% all gynecological cancer and out of which squamous cell carcinoma occupies the main bulk (80% of all vaginal cancer). To label a primary vaginal carcinoma the following factors should be considered: (1) No involvement of cervix or vulva. (2) Vaginal carcinoma within 5 years of cervical carcinoma is not considered as primary vaginal carcinoma.

*Risk Factors*

The risk factors of vaginal squamous cell carcinoma are HPV infection, low social economic status, immunosuppression, smoking, and prior pelvic radiation.[17]

*Clinical Features*

Vaginal squamous cell carcinoma may involve in patients of any age. The mean age of the patient is 64 year. The patients usually present with vaginal discharge and painless bleeding and occasionally may have postcoital bleeding or dyspareunia.

*Gross*

Grossly, the tumor may be exophytic, fungating, ulcerated, annular or constrictive. The size of the tumor may vary from small to several cm.

*Histopathology*

The vaginal squamous cell carcinoma shows same histopathological features as noted in other areas. The tumor may be keratinizing or non-keratinizing squamous cell carcinoma (Figures 4.16 and 4.17). The invasive carcinoma should

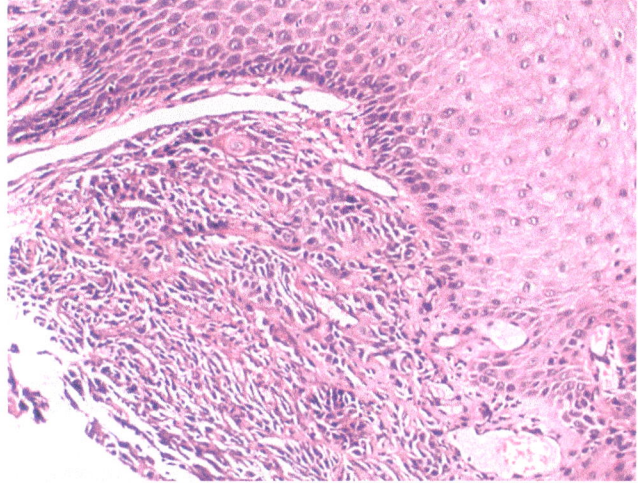

**Figure 4.16:** Vaginal squamous cell carcinoma: The tumor cells infiltrating into deeper tissue

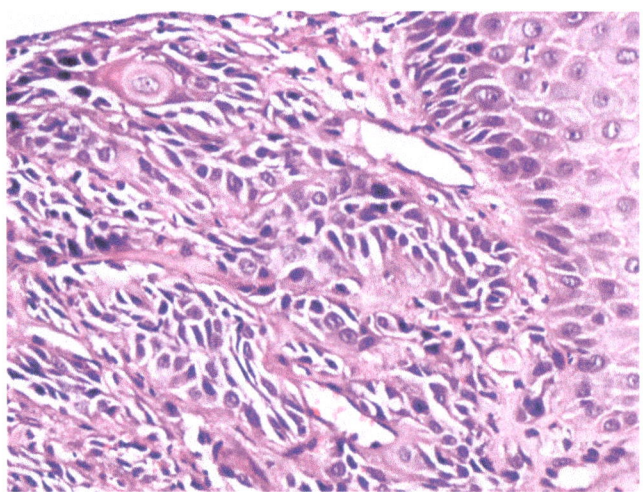

Figure 4.17: Vaginal squamous cell carcinoma: Nonkeratinizing squamous cell carcinoma of vagina. Polyhedral cells with intracytoplasmic keratinization

be differentiated from VAIN. Narrow rows of tumor cells invasion in the stroma, stromal desmoplasia and inflammatory response are helpful features to distinguish invasive squamous cell carcinoma from carcinoma in situ (VAIN III).

*Management and Prognosis*

The prognosis depends on FIGO staging (Table 4.1).
Five year survival rates for different stages vaginal carcinoma are:[18]
Stage I: 73–75%, Stage II: 50–60%, Stage III: 30–43%, Stage IV: 20–36%.

Table 4.1: FIGO staging of carcinoma of vagina[19]

| Stage | Clinical description |
| --- | --- |
| Stage 0 | Intraepithelial: Carcinoma in situ |
| Stage I | Carcinoma limited to vaginal wall |
| Stage II | Carcinoma extends to subvaginal tissue but not to pelvic wall |
| Stage III | Carcinoma extends to pelvic side wall |
| Stage IV | Carcinoma extends beyond the true pelvis or involves mucosa of the bladder or rectum. Bullous edema as such does not permit a case to be allotted to stage IV |
| Stage IV a | Adjacent organ such as bladder and/or rectal mucosa involved and/or direct extension beyond the true pelvis |
| Stage IV b | Distant spread |

Radiotherapy is the treatment of choice of squamous cell carcinoma of vulva. Both brachytherapy and external beam radiation are included in radiation therapy. Surgery is advocated only in selective cases. Carcinoma in upper part of vagina is treated by radical hysterectomy and vaginectomy.

## Verrucous Carcinoma

This is a rare tumor with indolent course. The tumor presents as slow growing exophytic fungating growth. Microscopy of the tumor shows hyperkeratosis and acanthosis of the surface epithelium. The tumor consists of relatively monomorphic squamous cells. The broad based tumor margin pushes the stroma in a bulldozer-like fashion. Surgical resection is the treatment of choice and incomplete resection may cause recurrence. Radiation is not recommended in verrucous carcinoma as radiation may transform this tumor into squamous cell carcinoma.[20]

## Squamotransitional Cell Carcinoma

This is a rare type of carcinoma and known as various names such as, transitional cell carcinoma, mixed squamous and transitional cell carcinoma and papillary squamous carcinoma. The tumor shows multiple papillae lined by cells simulating transitional cells. The tumor cells are positive for CK 7 and negative for CK 20.[21]

## Clear Cell Adenocarcinoma

This tumor is mainly associated with the use of DES, a synthetic nonsteroidal estrogen, during pregnancy of the victim's mother.[22] The patient with history of DES exposure mother develops clear cell adenocarcinoma in earlier age and the peak incidence is 19 years. The patients without any DES exposure develop clear cell adenocarcinoma in the age 45–65 year.

*Clinical Features*

The patient complaints of vaginal bleeding, discharge or dyspareunia. The tumor is usually situated in the anterior aspect of upper one-third of vagina. Primary vaginal growth may also involve cervix. Near about 2/3rd of DES exposed cases develop growth in vagina and 1/3rd in cervix.[23] The growth is polypoidal, papillary and often ulcerated. Occasional tumors may be very small and invisible in naked eye or by colposcopic examination.

*Histopathology*

The tumor shows various architectural pattern: tubulocystic, papillary, solid and mixed (Figure 4.18). The malignant cells are of two types: clear cell and hobnail cells. The clear cells contain abundant clear cytoplasm. The nuclei are pleomorphic, central in position with round prominent nuclei (Figure 4.19). The hobnail cells show bulbous nuclei protruding out from the cell surface to lumen (Figure 4.20).

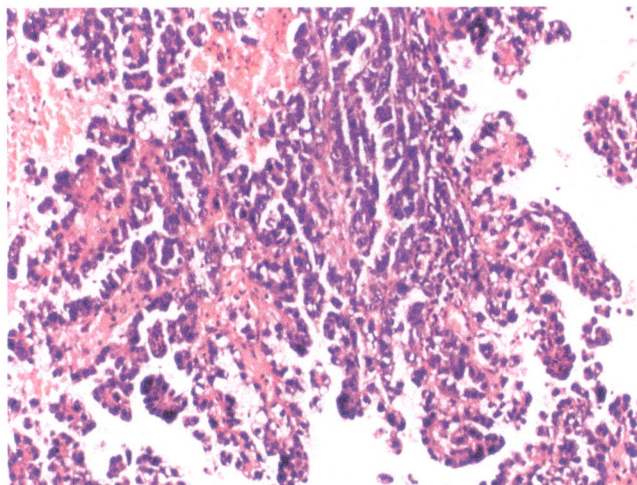

Figure 4.18: Clear cell carcinoma: Multiple papillary structures

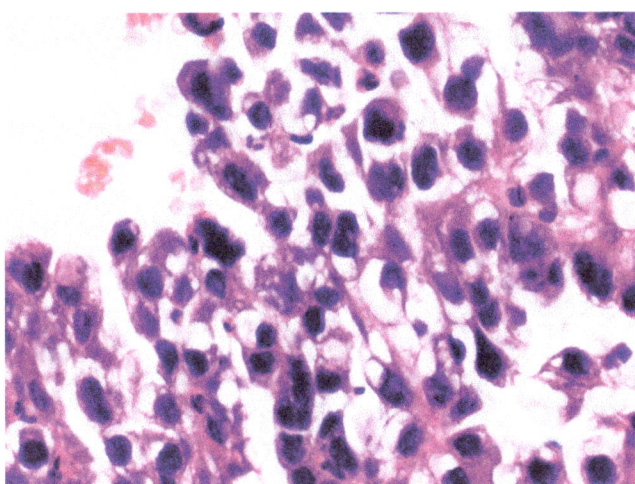

Figure 4.19: Clear cell carcinoma: Higher magnification shows cells with clear cytoplasm

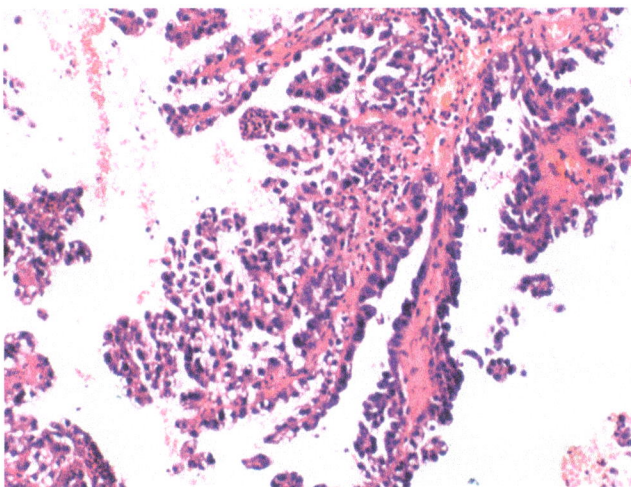

Figure 4.20: Clear cell carcinoma: Hobnail appearance is seen

Mitotic count is usually brisk. Occasionally, psammoma bodies and intracellular hyaline bodies may be noted.

*Immunocytochemistry*

The tumor is positive for CK 7 and Leu M1 (CD 15) and is negative for ER and PR.

*Differential Diagnosis*

1. Metastatic adenocarcinoma from other part of female genital tract and colon,
2. Microglandular hyperplasia of the cervix,
3. Arias–Stella reaction.

*Prognosis*

The good prognostic factors of this tumor are low stage and small tumor size and low mitotic count. Overall prognosis of stage I clear cell adenocarcinoma is good and 5 year survival rate is almost 100%.[24]

*Treatment*

Clear cell adenocarcinoma is treated by either surgery or by external beam radiation or by local radiotherapy.

## Embryonal Rhabdomyosarcoma (sarcoma botryoides)

Embryonal rhabdomyosarcoma is also known as sarcoma botryoides. This is the commonest vaginal malignancy in infant and children. Majority of embryonal rhabdomyosarcoma cases occur below 5 years age and the mean age of the patient is 2 year.[25] The patient usually presents with vaginal bleeding or mass in vagina. The tumor may be small to large nodular or polypoidal mass and often looks like bunch of grapes in the vagina.

*Histopathology*

The presence of "cambium layer" is the hallmark of this tumor. The cambium layer is defined as the thick dense aggregates of tumor cells under the subepithelium with an intervening space containing loose connective tissue. At least one microscopic field containing cambium layer should be present to diagnose sarcoma botryoides.[26] The tumor shows both hypocellular and hypercellular areas. The cells are round to oval with scanty cytoplasm. Nuclear chromatin is open with inconspicuous nucleoli. The cells with spindle-shaped nuclei are also seen. Mitotic activity is high. Occasionally cells with cytoplasmic cross striations indicating rhabdomyoblastic differentiation are noted.

*Immunohistochemistry*

The tumor cells are positive for muscle-specific actin, Myo D1, desmin, and myoglobin.

*Differential Diagnosis*

1. Fibroepithelial polyp: Lacking typical cambium layer and rhabdomyoblast and
2. Rhabdomyomas: Lack of cambium layer.

*Prognosis*

The prognosis of embryonal rhabdomyosarcoma depends on:
1. Extent of the tumor,
2. Age of the patient,
3. Histological type, and
4. Cellular atypia.

Overall 5 year survival of embryonal rhabdomyosarcoma is more than 90%.

*Treatment*

The treatment includes surgery along with chemotherapy and radiotherapy.

## Leiomyosarcoma

Leiomyosarcoma is the commonest vaginal sarcoma in adult female. The average age of the patient is 47 year. The patient commonly complains of vaginal bleeding and pain. The tumor may be exophytic or intramural with variable sized. Presently, it is recommended that vaginal smooth muscle tumor with following features should be considered as leiomyosarcoma (Figure 4.21):

1. More than 3 cm in diameter,
2. Infiltrating margin of the tumor,
3. More than 5 mitotic figures per ten high power fields,
4. Moderate nuclear atypia.[27]

*Immunohistochemistry*

The tumor cells are positive for desmin, and/or smooth muscle actin and h-caldesmon.

*Prognosis and Treatment*

The overall 5 year survival rate of leiomyosarcoma is 35 to 43% only. Surgery is the treatment of choice along with radiation therapy.

## Melanoma of Vagina

This is rare and accounts for less than 3% of all vaginal tumor. The tumor is seen in any age group. The mean age of the patient is 60 year.

*Clinical Features*

The patient usually presents with vaginal bleeding and mass. The lower 1/3rd of vagina is the common location of melanoma.

*Gross Features*

The mass is polypoidal and ulcerated and often in blackish discoloration. The lesion may be less than 1 cm to very large (several cm).

*Histopathology*

The tumor shows sold sheets, nests, trabeculae or mixed pattern of arrangement. The cells are epithelioid or spindle shaped. The nuclei are enlarged pleomorphic having prominent nucleoli. Cytoplasmic melanin pigment is seen (Figure 4.22).

*Immunocytochemistry*

Malignant melanoma cells are positive for HMB 45, melan A and S-100 protein.

*Prognosis and Treatment*

Prognosis is poor and 5 year survival rate is only 21%.[28] The median survival is only 21 months.

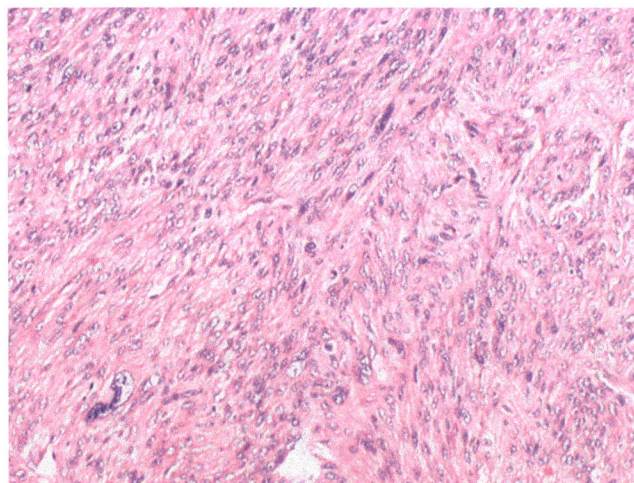

**Figure 4.21:** Leiomyosarcoma: Fascicular arrangement of spindle cells with moderate nuclear atypia and high mitotic activity

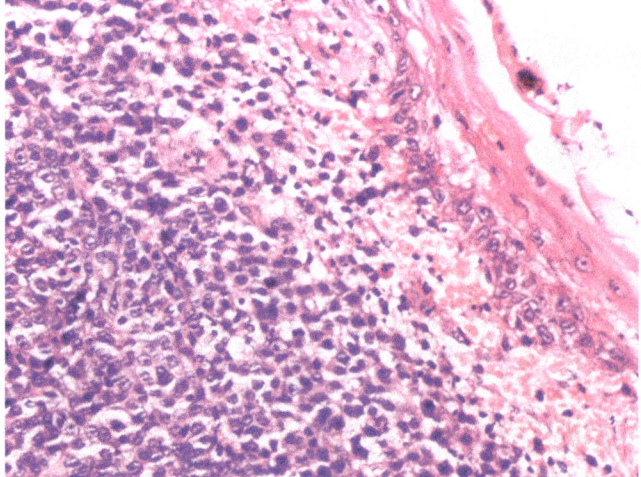

**Figure 4.22:** Melanoma vagina: Diffuse sheets of tumor cells

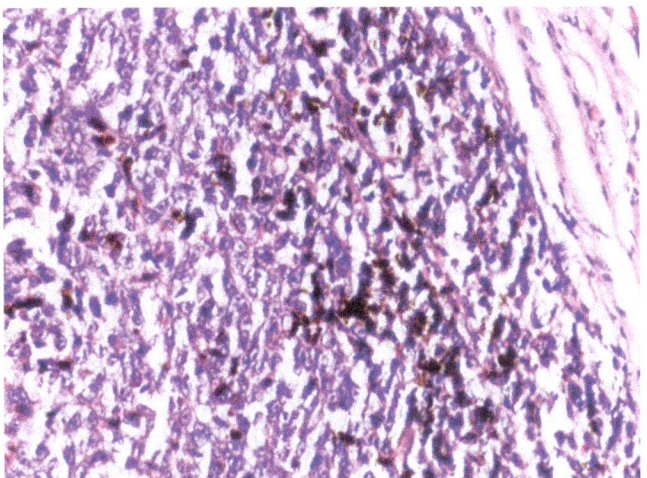

Figure 4.23: Melanoma vagina: Large cells with prominent nucleoli having cytoplasmic blotchy melanin pigment

Treatment of malignant melanoma includes radical local excision. Radiation therapy is given in non–resectable tumor. Chemotherapy is not effective in melanoma.

## Metastatic Tumors

A large variety of tumors can be metastasized to vagina. Metastatic tumors in vagina are more common than primary vaginal tumors. Metastasis may occur either by (1) direct extension or (2) by vascular spread. The commonest primary site of metastatic carcinoma of vagina from female genital tract is endometrial carcinoma.[29] The other primary sites are cervical, ovarian, and tubal carcinoma. The various primary sites other than female genital tract are colon, pancreas, stomach and urinary bladder.

### REFERENCES

1. Kurman RJ, Carcangiu ML, Herrington S, Young RH. Tumors of vulva. WHO classification of tumors of female genital reproductive organs. 4th Edition, International Agency for Research on Cancer, Lyon 2014.
2. Fujimoto V, Miller J, Klein N, Soules M. Congenital cervical atresia: report of seven cases and review of the literature. Am J Obstet Gynecol. 1997;177(6):1419-25.
3. Fliegner JR. Congenital atresia of the vagina. Surg Gynecol Obstet. 1987;165:387-91.
4. Polasek P, Erickson L, Stanhope C. Transverse vaginal septum associated with tubal atresia. Mayo Clin Proc. 1995; 70(10):965-8.
5. Davis JD, Connor EE, Clark P, Wilkinson EJ, Duff P. Correlation between cervical cytologic results and Gram stain as diagnostic tests for bacterial vaginosis. Am J Obstet Gynecol. 1997;177(3):532-5.
6. Resnick SD. Toxic shock syndrome: recent developments in pathogenesis. J Pediatr. 1990;116:321-8.
7. Christensen EF, Curry TS. 3rd. Emphysematous vaginitis. JAMA. 1967;200(11):1001-2.
8. The Working Group on Severe Streptococcal Infections (1993) Defining the Group A streptococcal toxic shock syndrome. Rationale and consensus definition. JAMA. 269:390-1.
9. Levine BB, Sriaganian RP, Schenkein I. Allergy to human seminal plasma. N Engl J Med. 1973;288:894.
10. Fishman A, Ortega E, Girtanner RE, Kaplan AL. Malacoplakia of the vagina presenting as a pelvic mass. Gynecol Oncol. 1993;49(3):380-2.
11. Roberts WS, Hoffman MS, LaPolla JP, et al. Management of radionecrosis of the vulva and distal vagina. Am J Obstet Gynecol. 1991;164:1235-8.
12. Michal M, Rokyta Z, Mejchar B, Pelikan K, Kummel M, Mukensnabl P. Prolapse of the fallopian tube after hysterectomy associated with exuberant angiomyofibroblastic stroma response: a diagnostic pitfall. Virchows Arch. 2000;437(4):436-9.
13. Clement PB. Postoperative spindle-cell nodule of the endometrium. Arch Pathol Lab Med. 1988;112(5):566-8.
14. Bergeron C, Ferenczy A, Shah KV, Naghashfar Z. Multicentric human papillomavirus infections of the female genital tract: correlation of viral types with abnormal mitotic figures, colposcopic presentation, and location. Obstet Gynecol. 1987;69(5):736-42.
15. Aho M, Vesterinen E, Meyer B, Purola E, Paavonen J. Natural history of vaginal intraepithelial neoplasia. Cancer. 1991;68(1):195-7.
16. Stuart GCE, Flagler EA, Nation JG, et al. Laser vaporization of vaginal intraepithelial neoplasia. Am J Obstet Gynecol. 1988;158:240-3.
17. Boice JD Jr, Engholm G, Kleinerman RA, Blettner M, Stovall M, Lisco H, et al. Radiation dose and second cancer risk in patients treated for cancer of the cervix. Radiat Res. 1988;116(1):3-55.
18. Tjalma WA, Monaghan JM, de Barros Lopes A, Naik R, Nordin AJ, Weyler JJ. The role of surgery in invasive squamous carcinoma of the vagina. Gynecol Oncol. 2001; 81(3):360-5.
19. Current FIGO staging for cancer of the vagina, fallopian tube, ovary, and gestational trophoblastic neoplasia. Int J Gynaecol Obstet. 2009;105(1):3-4.
20. Crowther ME, Lowe DG, Shepherd JH. Verrucous carcinoma of the female genital tract: a review. Obstet Gynecol Surv. 1988;43:263-80.
21. Niederle B, Rauthe S, Engel JB, Krockenberger M, Dietl J, Honig AJ. Papillary squamotransitional cell carcinoma of the vagina. Obstet Gynaecol Res. 2011;37(12):1851-5.
22. Palmer JR, Anderson D, Helmrich SP, Herbst AL. Risk factors for diethylstilbestrol-associated clear cell adenocarcinoma. Obstet Gynecol. 2000;95(6 Pt 1):814-20.
23. Hanselaar A, van Loosbroek M, Schuurbiers O, Helmerhorst T, Bulten J, Bernhelm J. Clear cell adenocarcinoma of the vagina and cervix. An update of the central Netherlands registry showing twin age incidence peaks. Cancer. 1997;79(11):2229-36.
24. Herbst AL. Vaginal clear cell cancer: incidence, survival and screening. In: Long-term effects of exposure to diethylstilbestrol

(DES) (NIH Workshop), 1992.23–24. Falls Church, VA, pp 19–20.
25. NewtonWA, Soule EH, Hamoudi AB, et al. Histopathology of childhood sarcomas, intergroup rhabdomyosarcoma studies I and II: clinicopathologic correlation. J Clin Oncol. 1988;6:67-75.
26. Qualman S, Coffin C, Newton W, et al. Intergroup rhabdomyosarcoma study: update for pathologists. Pediatr Dev Pathol. 1998;1:550-61.
27. Tazvassoli FA, Norris HJ. Smooth muscle tumors of the vagina. Obstet Gynecol. 1979;53:689-93.
28. Weinstock MA. Malignant melanoma of the vulva and vagina in the United States: patterns of incidence and population-based estimates of survival. Am J Obstet Gynecol. 1994;171(5):1225-30.
29. Metastases to the female genital tract. Analysis of 325 cases. Mazur MT, Hsueh S, Gersell DJ. Cancer. 1984;53(9):1978-84.

# Benign Diseases of Cervix 5

## ANATOMY

The uterus is divided into three parts: body, isthmus and cervix. Cervix is the lower most part of uterus (Figure 5.1). The cervix is attached with the lower part of the body of uterus by fibromuscular tube known as isthmus. The upper part of cervical canal opens into the body of uterus by canal through internal os. The lower part of cervix is projected into vagina. The vaginal wall is attached with cervix circumferentially and is divided cervix into two parts: upper supravaginal and a lower vaginal (Figure 5.1). The free space in between the cervix and vagina forms vaginal fornix. The portion of the cervix within the vagina is also known as exocervix or portio vaginalis. The portio vaginalis opens into the vaginal cavity through external os. The portio vaginalis has two lips anterior and posterior. The cervix is cylindrical structure with 3 cm in length and 2.5 cm in diameter in adult nulligravida. The endocervical canal is fusiform in appearance and 3 cm long. It connects with the uterus through internal os and vagina through external os. A layer of connective tissue (parametrium) separates the supravaginal part of the cervix and the urinary bladder. Posteriorly the pelvic peritoneum is reflected over the cervix, vagina and back to anterior surface of rectum and thus forming a blind pouch known as Pouch of Douglas or rectouterine pouch.

**Cervix is kept in position by two ligaments:** Lateral ligament and uterosacral ligament. The lateral ligament, also known as cardinal ligament of Mackenrodt, extends superiorly from the base of the broad ligament and inferiorly to the supravaginal part of cervix. The uterosacral ligament extends from the suparvaginal part of cervix to the sacral vertebrae (2nd, 3rd and 4th).

The descending branches of uterine arteries supplies blood to the cervix and venous system runs parallel to the arterial drainage.

The predominant lymphatic drainage of the cervix is to the external iliac, hypogastric, obturator, and common iliac lymph nodes.

## HISTOLOGY

The cervical wall is composed of mainly collagenous tissue. This is admixed with small component (15%) of smooth muscle. The exocervix is lined by stratified squamous epithelium and endocervix is lined by columnar lining epithelium.

## SQUAMOUS EPITHELIUM

The squamous epithelium of cervix is situated on the basement membrane. Cervical glands are absent in the subepithelial tissue in exocervix.

The squamous layer may be subdivided into three zones from basement membrane to luminal zone (Figures 5.2 and 5.3):
- **Lower zone (Basal/parabasal cell layer):** The basal cells are situated over the basement membrane. These

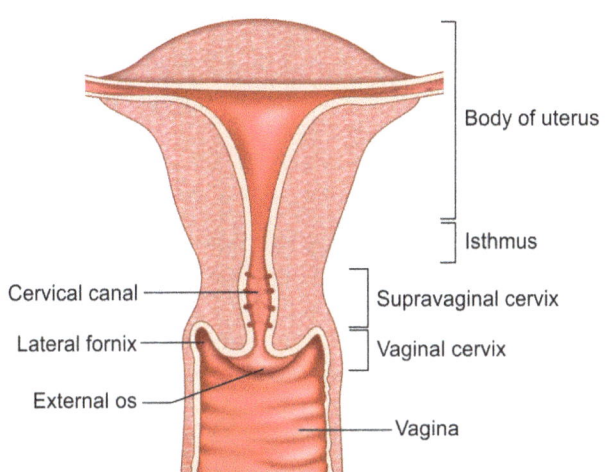

**Figure 5.1:** Cervix: Detailed anatomy of cervix

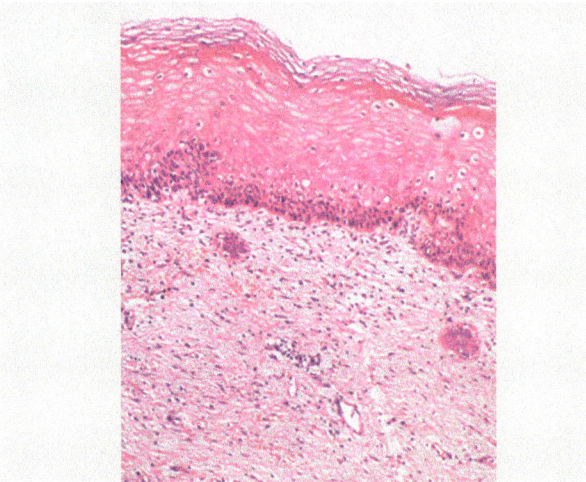

**Figure 5.2:** Benign squamous lining of cervix: Multilayered squamous epithelial cells with underlying fibroconnective tissue

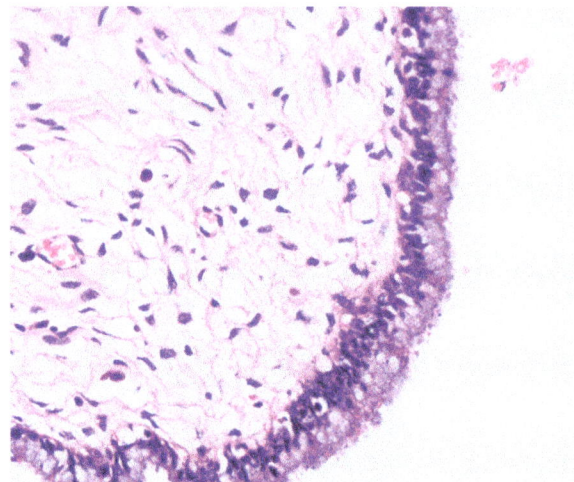

**Figure 5.4:** Endocervix: It is lined by tall mucus secreting columnar cells

## COLUMNAR EPITHELIUM

Endocervix is lined mucus secreting columnar epithelium (Figure 5.4). The cells are closely packed and give a "cobblestone pattern". In another angle they may appear as "picket fence". The individual cells are tall with abundant granular cytoplasm and basally placed round monomorphic nuclei. Occasional ciliated columnar cells are also seen. In addition isolated rare neuroendocrine cells may also be noted. Endocervical columnar cells contain mucin which is positive for Alcian blue stain. The cells are positive for CK 7, 8, 18, and 19.

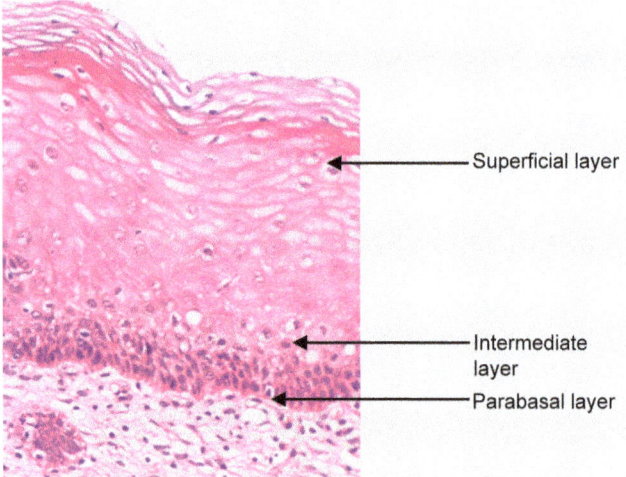

**Figure 5.3:** Benign squamous lining: Different layer of epithelium is highlighted

cells are small and contain scanty cytoplasm and round nuclei. The basal cell appears to behave as stem cells and they take active participation in regenerating the epithelial cells. Parabasal cells are situated over the basal cells and are mildly bigger than basal cells.
- **Mid zone (Intermediate cell layer):** This layer is formed by intermediate cells. The cells are larger than parabasal cells and polyhedral in shape with abundant cytoplasm. Nuclei are central with vesicular chromatin. The intermediate cell contains abundant glycogen and is positive for Periodic acid-Schiff (PAS) stain.
- **Superficial zone (Superficial cell layer):** This zone is only 2 to 3 layer thick and contains polyhedral to flattened cells with abundant cytoplasm and central pyknotic nuclei. The cells contain keratin and are orangeophilic in Papanicolaou's stained smear.

## STROMA

The stroma is composed of bundles of collagen fibers along with scanty smooth muscle fiber. Occasional lymphoid follicles may also be noted in the subepithelial tissue (Figure 5.5). The cervical stroma contains multiple mucus secreting glands that are lined by tall columnar epithelium (Figure 5.6). The glands open into the endocervical canal.

## SQUAMOCOLUMNAR JUNCTION AND TRANSFORMATION ZONE (FIGURES 5.7 to 5.10)

Squamocolumnar junction (SCJ) is the junction between the original squamous epithelium of exocervix and endocervical columnar epithelium. At birth this SCJ remains in the exocervix. During the later part of life the cervix elongates and the SCJ shifts more towards the exocervix. The columnar epithelium of the endocervix also migrates away towards the exocervix. This migration of SCJ towards the exocervix is known as cervical eversion or ectropion. In course of time the migrated endocervical cells forming cervical erosion is replaced by metaplastic squamous cells and the new SCJ at

**52** Essentials of Gynecologic Pathology

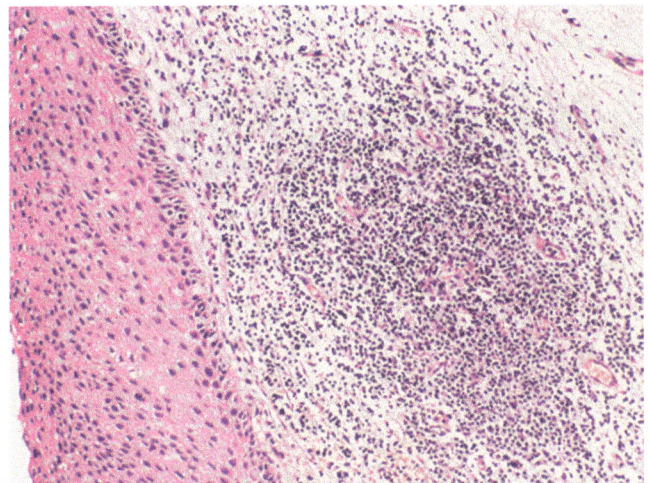

**Figure 5.5:** Lymphoid follicle in cervix: Lymphoid follicles in the subepithelium

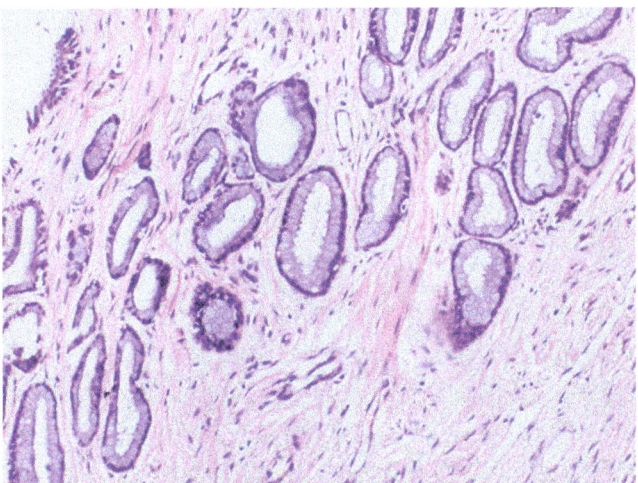

**Figure 5.6:** Benign endocervical gland: The glands are lined by tall mucus secreting columnar cells

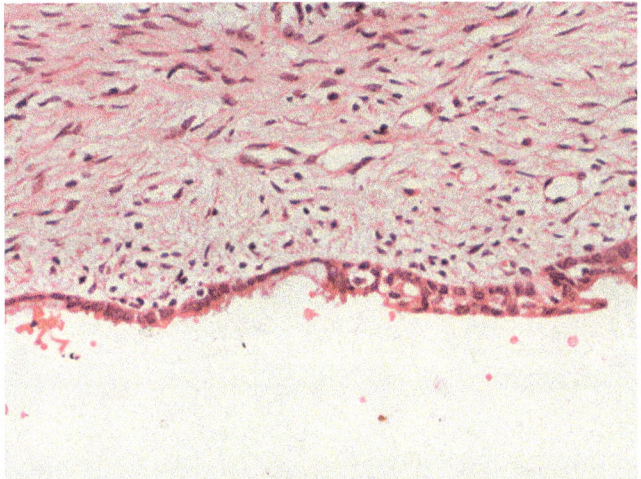

**Figure 5.7:** Squamocolumnar junction: The transition from columnar to squamous epithelium

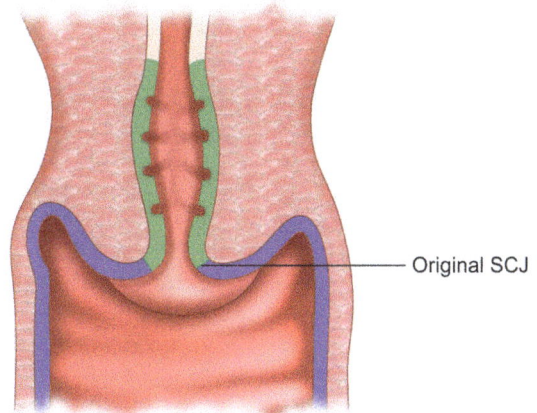

**Figure 5.8:** Original squamocolumnar junction: The junction between endocervical columnar epithelium and squamous epithelium of exocervix

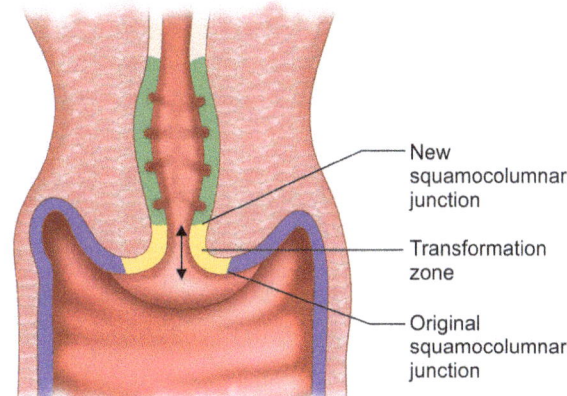

**Figure 5.9:** Transitional zone: Details of squamocolumnar junction is highlighted

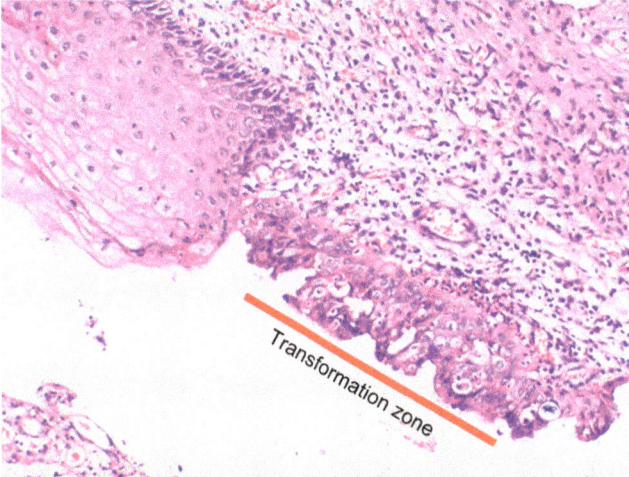

**Figure 5.10:** Squamous metaplasia in the squamocolumnar junction: The endocervical columnar cells are replaced by metaplastic cells

the junction of metaplastic squamous cells and endocervical cells known as functional or physiological SCJ. Now the area between the newly formed SCJ and original SCJ is known as transformation zone.

## Significance of Transformation Zone

The transformation zone (TZ) is a highly significant area because of:
1. TZ has higher susceptibility of HPV infection.
2. All cases of squamous cell carcinoma of cervix arise from TZ.
3. As this is the source of pre-neoplastic lesion so surveillance of this area by cervical smear may detect early cases of CIN.
4. TZ is a highly dynamic area and changes under the influence of hormone or environmental factors.

## CHANGES IN NORMAL MENSTRUAL CYCLE

The cervix undergoes changes due to the effect of estrogen hormone. Under the influence of estrogen the overall content, water and also salt content of cervical mucus increases. No demonstrable histopathological changes are seen during menstruation.

## PREGNANCY-INDUCED CHANGES

During the period of pregnancy, the cervix is enlarged due to enhanced vascularity and edema. The endocervical glands become tortuous with multilayering and papillary projections of the glandular epithelium. The stroma shows diffuse chronic inflammation. The cervical mucus becomes thick and makes a barrier between the vagina and endometrium to protect ascending infection from vagina. In addition, decidual cells may be seen in cervical stroma.

## ARIAS-STELLA REACTION

Arias-Stella reaction in cervix is not uncommon in pregnant patient.[1] The lesion is focal and is located the in proximal part of endocervix. Both superficial and deep endocervical glands may be involved. The glands show pseudostratification and papillary projections of the lining epithelium. The glandular columnar cells are enlarged with hyperchromatic nuclei. Frequent hobnail changes of the cell are also seen.

## Differential Diagnosis

Clear cell adenocarcinoma: The following features are helpful to distinguish it from clear cell adenocarcinoma:[1]
1. Lack of any mass lesion,
2. No desmoplastic response,
3. No mitotic activity and,
4. Low nucleo-cytoplasmic ratio.

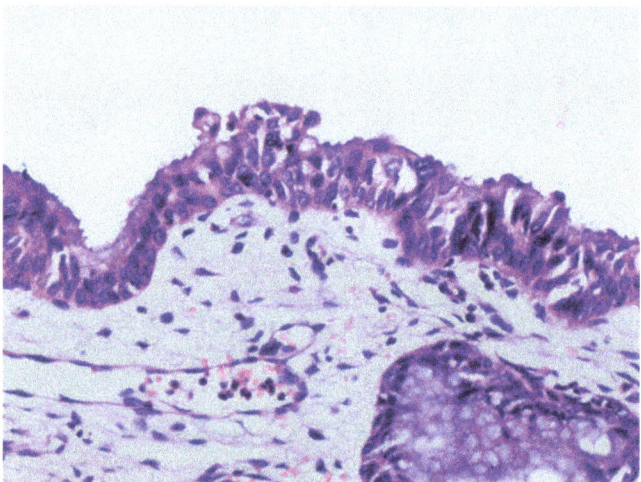

**Figure 5.11:** Squamous metaplasia of the endocervical lining epithelium. The squamous cells are in between columnar cells and basement membrane

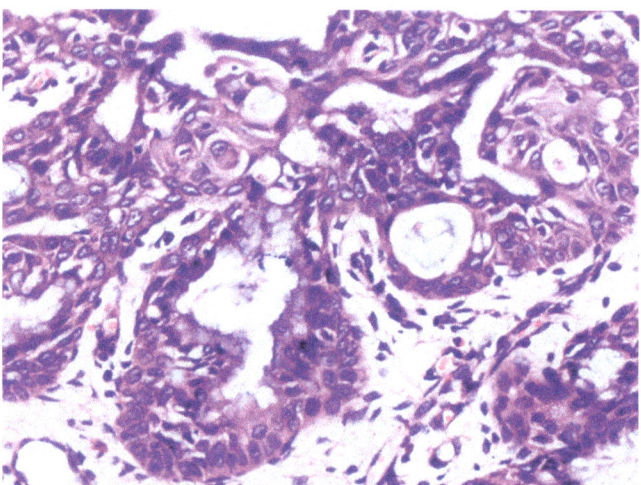

**Figure 5.12:** Endocervical glands showing squamous metaplasia

## SQUAMOUS METAPLASIA

Metaplasia means replacement of a particular type of mature tissue by other type of mature tissue. In cervix squamous metaplasia is defined as replacement of endocervical columnar epithelium by stratified squamous epithelium (Figures 5.11 and 5.12). Sites: Area of transformation zone is the site of squamous metaplasia. The endocervical epithelium is shifted towards the exocervix from its original native position and is replaced by metaplastic squamous epithelium.

## Mechanism

The two possible mechanisms may be suggested for squamous metaplasia of the endocervical epithelium:
1. **Direct extension of the mature squamous epithelium:** The mature squamous epithelium of the exocervix may

extend towards the endocervical canal underneath the endocervical epithelium. Later on as the squamous cells grow and mature the endocervical epithelium is pushed upwards. The endocervical epithelium is ultimately shredded out completely and is replaced by squamous epithelium which is also known as ''squamous epithelialization''.

2. **Reserve cells proliferation and maturation to squamous cells:** In this process, the reserve cells proliferate. These cells are located beneath the endocervical lining epithelium and usually are not recognizable. However under certain stimulus the reserve cell proliferates. These cells undergo squamous cell differentiation and later on replace the overlying endocervical cell.

## Causative Factors

Infections, local trauma, chronic irritation, surgical intervention such as electrocautery and cryosurgery.

## IMMATURE SQUAMOUS METAPLASIA (FIGURE 5.13)

Immature squamous metaplasia shows lack of surface maturation. The cells show minimal glycogen in the cytoplasm. The immature squamous metaplasia shows sharp demarcation from the normal squamous epithelium.

## Differential Diagnosis

Squamous intraepithelial lesion (SIL): Features favoring immature squamous metaplasia include:
1. Maintenance of cellular organization,
2. Absence of nuclear atypia,
3. Single rows of overlying endocervical cells may be present and
4. Absence of mitotic activities.

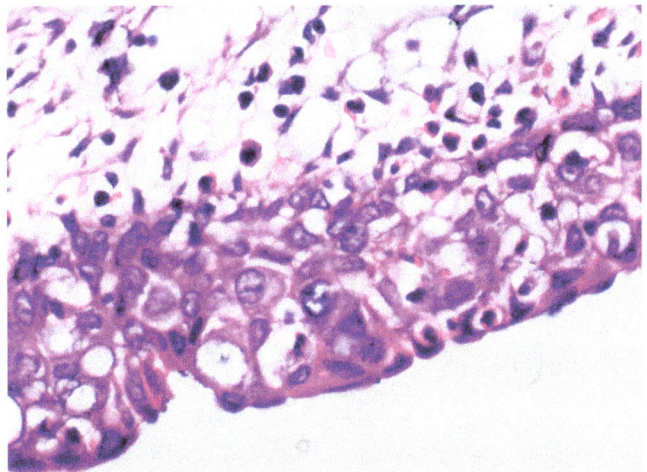

**Figure 5.13:** Immature squamous metaplasia of the lining epithelium

## TUBAL METAPLASIA

### Definition

Tubal metaplasia is defined by replacement of normal endocervical glandular epithelial cells by Müllerian type of epithelium.

### Site

Tubal metaplasia commonly occurs in the upper part of the cervix adjacent to internal os. However, it may also be seen in lower part of the cervical canal.

### Histology (Figure 5.14)

The glandular columnar cells are replaced by cells resembling tubal epithelial cells. The cells are tall columnar and they contain cilia. Tubal metaplasia of the cervix is not associated with SIL or inflammation.[2]

### Differential Diagnosis

Adenocarcinoma: The following features confirm the diagnosis of tubal metaplasia over adenocarcinoma:[3]
1. Preserved shape of the gland.
2. Absence of desmoplastic stroma.
3. Bland monomorphic nuclei.
4. Lack of mitosis.

## TRANSITIONAL CELL METAPLASIA

This metaplasia is defined as replacement of the endocervical lining epithelium by transitional cells resembling urothelial lining of urinary bladder. This is predominantly occurs in the postmenopausal patients.

### Site

Transitional cell metaplasia is seen in the transformation zone. In addition, exocervix and vagina may also be involved.

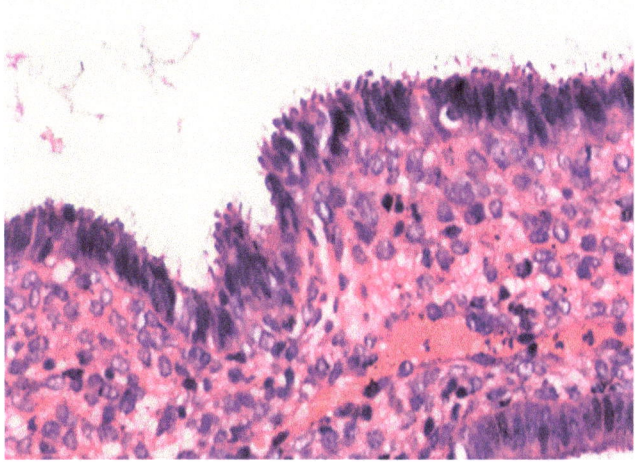

**Figure 5.14:** Tubal metaplasia: The columnar cells are replaced by ciliated tubal lining cells

## Histology

The transitional metaplastic cells are several layers thick. The cells are oval to spindle in shape and are arranged perpendicularly over the basement membrane. In the mid layer the nuclei are arranged horizontally with a streaming pattern. The superficial cell resembles umbrella cells. In addition, nests of transitional cells are also seen within the cervical stroma.[4] The individual cells have oval to spindle-shaped nuclei with tapered ends. The cells have low nucleo-cytoplasmic ratio. Perinuclear halo and deep longitudinal nuclear grooves are often seen.

## Immunohistochemistry

The transitional metaplastic cells are positive for CK 13, CK 17, CK 18 resembling urothelium of the bladder. However, unlike urothelial cell that are positive for CK 20, the metaplastic transitional cells never express CK 20.[5]

## Differential Diagnosis

High grade squamous intraepithelial lesion: The following features help to confirm transitional metaplasia
1. The presence of streaming pattern of cells,
2. Organized pattern of cells,
3. Low nucleo-cytoplasmic ratio,
4. Regular nuclear contour, and
5. Low to absent mitosis.

## INFLAMMATION OF CERVIX

### Acute Cervicitis

Acute cervicitis may be caused by physical causes such as trauma, abortion, etc. or chemical causes such as intrauterine contraceptive devices, infections, etc. Cervix becomes enlarged, edematous and red.

*Histopathology*

There is transmucosal infiltration of polymorph. Acute inflammatory cells also infiltrate in the cervical stroma. In severe condition abscess may be formed.

### Chronic Cervicitis

Chronic cervicitis occurs in women of reproductive age period. Chronic infection is the main cause of chronic cervicitis.

*Histology (Figure 5.15)*

The cervix shows infiltration of lymphocytes, plasma cells and histiocytes underneath the surface epithelium. The epithelium may be ulcerated. Vascular congestion is seen in the subepithelial tissue. There may be blockage of the endocervical crypt causing accumulation of mucus and formation of Nabothian cyst. Lymphoid follicles may also be seen.

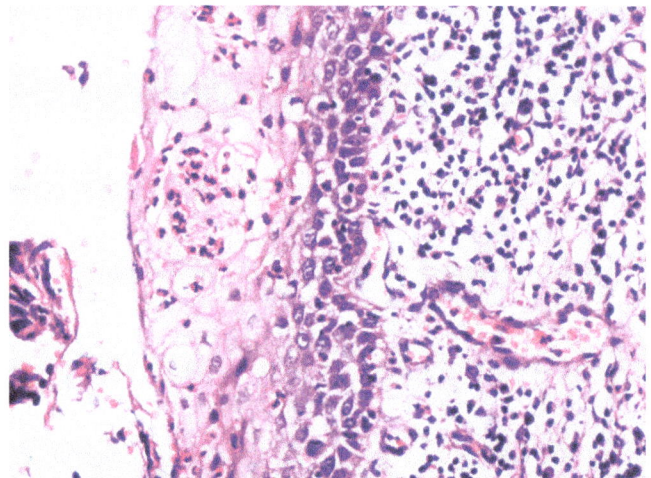

**Figure 5.15:** Chronic cervicitis: The subepithelium shows dense lymphocytic infiltration

### Specific Infections

Cervix may be affected by specific bacterial, fungal and viral infective agents.

*Tuberculosis*

Tuberculosis of cervix represents 24% of genital tract tuberculosis. Almost all cases of cervical tuberculosis are secondary to either endometrial or fallopian tube tuberculosis. Histology section of cervical tuberculosis shows granulomatous inflammation consisting of multiple epithelioid cell granulomas, multinucleated giant cells, lymphocytes and necrosis. Ziehl Neelsen stain for acid fast bacilli or bacterial culture is needed for the confirmation of tuberculosis.

**Differential diagnosis:** Rarely other causes of granulomatous inflammation such as sarcoidosis, lymphogranuloma venerum, schistosomiasis, etc. may also form granulomatous inflammation.

*Actinomycosis*

Actinomycosis is caused by *Actinomycosis israelii* infection. The infection affects the cervix either by hematogenous route or by local infection due to the use of intrauterine contraceptive devices. The presence of actinomycosis in asymptomatic patient does not bear any significance. The organism causes mild nonspecific inflammation. The bacterial colonies show radiating branching fine filaments from a central point.

## Other Bacterial Infections

Other bacterial agents such as *Chlamydia trachomatis* and *Neisseria gonorrhoeae* may also cause endocervicitis.

## Fungal Infection

*Candida* is the most common fungal infection of cervix. This has been described in previous Chapter.

## Parasitic Infection

Trichomonas vaginalis is a common parasitic infection of the cervix and is described in the section of vagina.

## Viral Infections

### Herpes Simplex Infection

Herpes simplex infection is caused by herpes simplex virus (HSV). HSV-2 subtype of HSV is responsible for 90% of the genital herpes simplex infection. HSV-1 causes only 10–15% of genital herpes simplex infection. This is a sexually transmitted disease and is mainly seen in young female. The patient becomes symptomatic about a few days to 2 weeks after initial exposure of the herpes simplex infection. Patients may have systemic symptoms such as malaise, fever, pruritus, dysuria along with inguinal lymphadenopathy. The cervical involvement of HSV is seen in majority of the cases of genital herpes infection. The cervix shows ulceration of the lining epithelium. The endocervical cells and the parabasal squamous cells show earliest changes of viral infection. The following cellular changes are noted:
1. Nuclear enlargement,
2. Margination of chromatin resulting in typical ground glass appearance,
3. Intranuclear owl eye like inclusion,
4. Multinucleation, and
5. Nuclear molding in the multinucleated cells.

### Human Papilloma Viral Infection

Discussed later.

## HYPERPLASIA OF CERVIX

### Microglandular Hyperplasia

Microglandular hyperplasia (MGH) is described long before by Taylor et al. in 1967.[6] Subsequently, the lesion was labeled as microglandular hyperplasia by Kyriakos et al.[7] MGH is important to recognize because there is a potential risk to misinterpret microglandular hyperplasia as adenocarcinoma.

### Clinical Features

Microglandular hyperplasia commonly occurs in reproductive age period. However, a small number of cases (6%) may occur in postmenopausal patients. The patient usually complains of postcoital bleeding or spotting. The cases of microglandular hyperplasia are often associated with pregnancy or oral contraceptive use. Studies also have shown the presence of microglandular hyperplasia without any such history.[8]

### Gross

Macroscopically, the microglandular hyperplasia (MGH) may be polypoidal or raised friable lesion about 1–2 cm in size. Grossly, the lining epithelium may be ulcerated and the lesion may be mistaken as carcinoma.

### Histology (Figures 5.16 to 5.18)

Microglandular hyperplasia may be unifocal or multifocal lesions. It is composed of multiple glands of varying shape and size. Many of the glands are cystically dilated. The glands are closely packed with minimal intervening fibrous stroma. Acute or chronic inflammatory cell infiltration may also be seen within the stroma. The glands are lined by cuboidal to columnar mucus secreting cells. The tip of the cells often contains mucus vacuoles. The nuclei of the cells are monomorphic. In general, the mitotic activity is low and less than 1 per 10 high power fields. Occasional cases may show signet ring cells and squamous metaplasia. The presence of focal moderate nuclear atypia, signet ring cells, hobnail appearance, solid growth pattern and stromal hyalinization in MGH may mislead to the diagnosis of carcinoma.[9]

### Differential Diagnosis

A. **Clear cell carcinoma:** The MGH shows mucin instead of glycogen, focal nuclear atypia, lack of papillary growth and true infiltration in the stroma (Table 5.1).

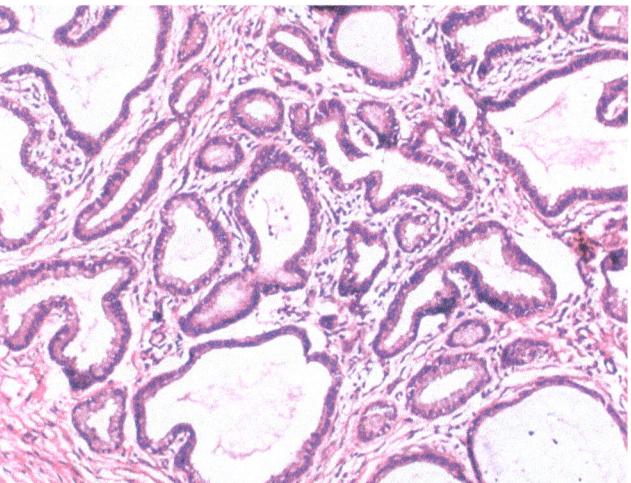

**Figure 5.16:** Microglandular hyperplasia: Multiple closely packed glands

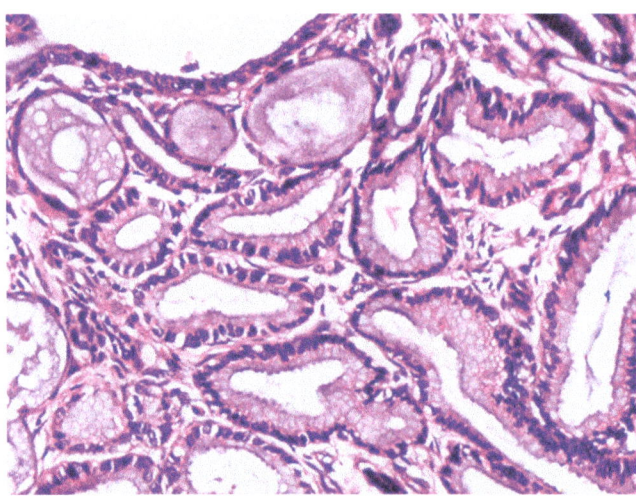

Figure 5.17: Microglandular hyperplasia: Crowded glands

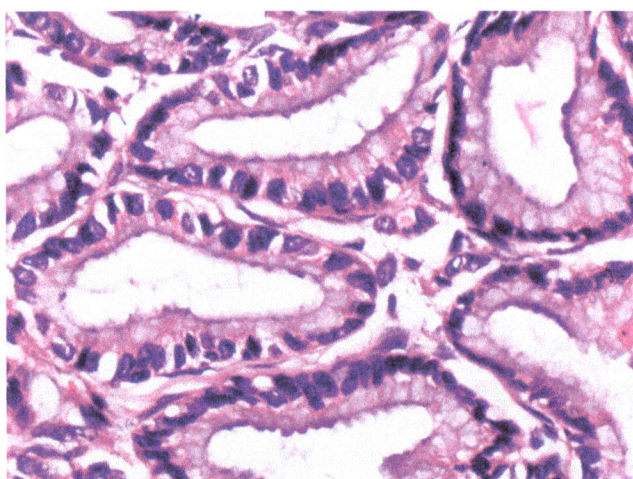

Figure 5.18: Microglandular hyperplasia: The glands are lined by tall columnar mucus secreting cells

Table 5.1: Distinguishing features of microglandular hyperplasia and clear cell carcinoma

| Features | Microglandular hyperplasia | Clear cell carcinoma |
|---|---|---|
| Glycogen | Absent | Present |
| Mucin | Present | Absent |
| Nuclear atypia | Less and focal | Greater and more diffuse |
| True infiltration | Absent | Present |
| Papillary growth pattern | Absent | Usually present |
| P16 | Negative | Strong positive |

B. **Endometrioid adenocarcinoma**: The features favoring MGH over endometrioid carcinoma are the continuity

Box 5.1: Distinction of MGH and endometrioid adenocarcinoma

**Features favoring MGH**
- Continuity of the MGH with the endocervical stroma
- The presence of sub and supranuclear vacuoles
- Reserve cell hyperplasia
- Lobulated smooth margin of MGH

**Features favoring endometrioid adenocarcinoma**
- The presence of endometrial stroma attached with the lesion
- The separate fragments of tissue showing features of atypical hyperplasia

of the MGH with the endocervical stroma, sub and supranuclear vacuoles and reserve cell hyperplasia (Box 5.1).

## Mesonephric Remnants and Hyperplasia

Mesonephric remnants represent the vestigial structures of Wolffian duct. They are commonly present in the broad ligament and lateral wall of cervix, vagina and ovarian hilum. The presence of mesonephric remnants has been described in 22% of cone biopsy sample of cervix.[10] The mesonephric duct is manly located in the lateral wall of cervix and therefore, the exact frequency of mesonephric remnants is underestimated in routine biopsy of cervix which are usually taken from anterior and posterior wall.

*Microscopy*

The mesonephric remnants are seen as multiple tubules or small cysts lined by low columnar or cuboidal cells. The cells show clear cytoplasm with bland monomorphic round nuclei. Cytoplasm of the cells does not show any demonstrable glycogen or mucin.

## Mesonephric Hyperplasia

Mesonephric remnants may show hyperplasia. This is an incidental finding and the patients are symptomatic. The mesonephric hyperplasia is usually detected in the cone biopsy or hysterectomy specimen. There are no definite criteria to distinguish mesonephric hyperplasia and mesonephric remnants. However, the lesion with more than 6 mm diameter is considered as mesonephric hyperplasia.[10]

*Histopathology*

Three histological patterns of mesonephric hyperplasia are seen: lobular, diffuse and ductal. These patterns of mesonephric hyperplasia have no clinical relevance. In lobular mesonephric hyperplasia the mesonephric tubules are arranged in lobules and in the diffuse form the tubules are arranged in diffuse pattern. The tubules may be present in the deeper stromal tissue mimicking infiltration by carcinoma. Ductal pattern is rarest type that lacks the tubules. The lesion shows multiple ducts lined by hyperplastic epithelium. Prominent papillary tufts of the epithelium is also seen.

*Differential Diagnosis*

A. **Clear cell carcinoma:** The following features are helpful in the confirmation of mesonephric hyperplasia:
   1. Lack of glycogen in the cells,
   2. No nuclear atypia
   3. No hobnail cells and
   4. No areas of solid growth.
B. **Endocervical adenocarcinoma:** Mesonephric hyperplasia is distinguished from the endocervical adenocarcinoma by the following features:
   1. Irregular shape and size of the glands are lacking,
   2. Absence of mucinous epithelium,
   3. Lack of nuclear atypia,
   4. No mitotic activity,
   5. Absence of stromal desmoplastic response.
C. **Mesonephric carcinoma:** This is a very rare tumor and may be present along with mesonephric hyperplasia.[11] The following features are helpful in the diagnosis of mesonephric carcinoma:
   1. Visible gross abnormality,
   2. Significant crowding of the glands showing back to back appearance,
   3. Irregular contour of the glands,
   4. More nuclear atypia,
   5. Stromal reaction.

## Endocervical Hyperplasia

There are two main types of endocervical hyperplasia: Lobular endocervical glandular hyperplasia (LEGH) and diffuse laminar endocervical glandular hyperplasia (DLEGH).

*Lobular Endocervical Glandular Hyperplasia (LEGH)*

The lesion is commonly seen as an incidental finding. LEGH is located in the inner wall of cervix.[12]

**Histology:** LEGH shows lobular proliferation of endocervical glands (Figures 5.19 and 5.20). The adjacent stroma is unremarkable. The glands are small to medium sized with tall mucus secreting columnar lining epithelium. The cells lack any nuclear atypia or mitotic activities.

*Diffuse Laminar Endocervical Glandular Hyperplasia*

Diffuse laminar endocervical glandular hyperplasia (DLEGH) is an incidental finding and mainly located in the inner one third of the wall of cervix. It is commonly seen in patient of reproductive age group. The lesion is shows diffuse

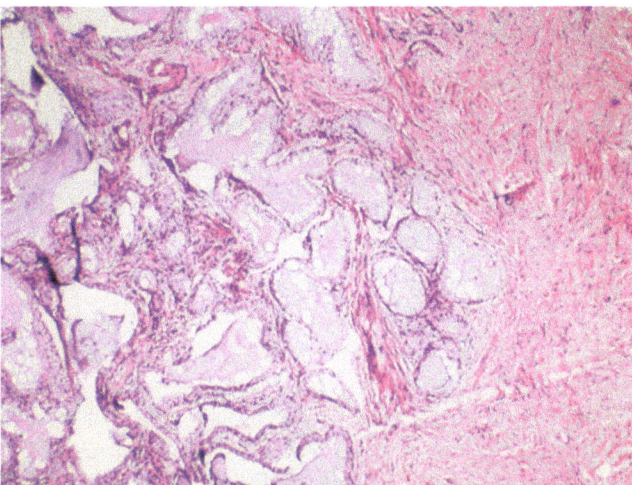

**Figure 5.19:** Endocervical glandular hyperplasia: Lobular hyperplasia of the endocervical glands

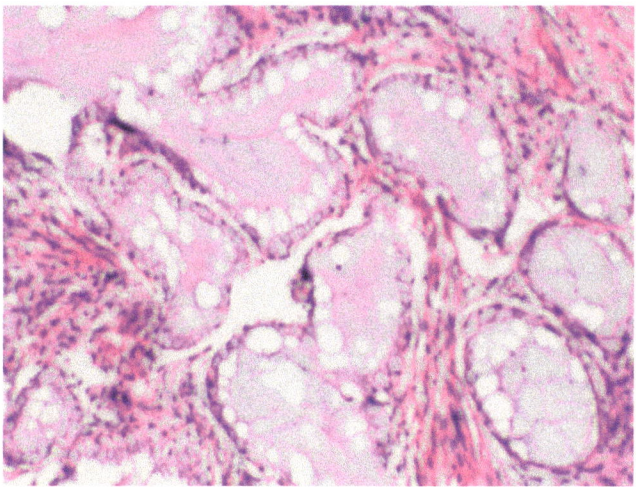

**Figure 5.20:** Higher magnification of endocervical glandular hyperplasia

proliferation of endocervical glands. The glands are closely packed of moderate in size and are well circumscribed from the surrounding stroma. The glandular lining epithelium is mucus secreting columnar cells with bland look. Mitosis is absent. Occasionally, epithelial cells may show reactive atypia. No desmoplastic stromal reaction is noted.

**Differential diagnosis of LEGH and DLEGH:** Well-differentiated adenocarcinoma: It is important to distinguish well-differentiated adenocarcinoma from LEGH and DLEGH. The following features favor endocervical hyperplasia:
1. Absence of desmoplastic stromal reaction,
2. Absent of irregular shape of the gland,
3. No stromal infiltration, and
4. No nuclear atypia or mitosis.

## DEEP ENDOCERVICAL GLANDS AND CYSTS

Uncommonly, the endocervical glands and cysts may be seen in the deeper cervical stroma and may be confused with well-differentiated adenocarcinoma. However, the lack of desmoplastic reaction, lack of architectural distortion or complexity and absent nuclear atypia exclude the possibility of malignancy.

## ENDOCERVICAL POLYP

Endocervical polyps are very common. They are commonly located in the endocervical canal. They commonly occur in the 4th and 5th decade of life. The presenting symptoms are profuse mucus secretion or bleeding per vagina from the ulceration of the surface lining epithelium.

### Gross

The polyp is smooth round or lobulated mass and may be of variable sized small to large. They may be sessile or pedunculated with a small stalk.

### Histology (Figure 5.21)

The polyp is lined by columnar epithelium. The sub-epithelium shows variable sized glands and many of which are cystically dilated. Occasionally, focal squamous metaplasia of the surface epithelium or glandular lining is seen. The stroma of the polyp is usually loose and may show inflammatory cells. Fibrosis or exuberant proliferation of blood vessels within the stroma may be seen. Polyp in the isthmic location may show lining of both endocervical and endometrial epithelium.

Ectocervical polyp is uncommon and the lining epithelium of the polyp is stratified squamous epithelium. The stroma consists of dense fibrocollagenous tissue.

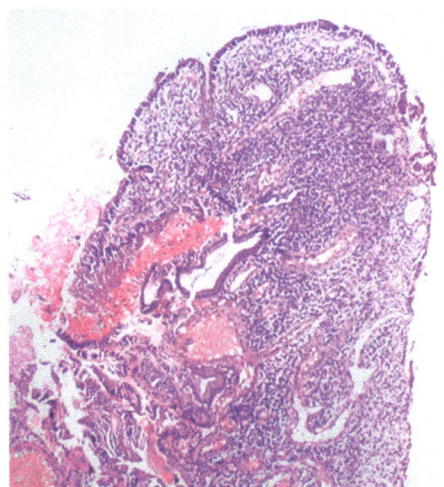

Figure 5.21: Endocervical polyp: Benign endocervical polyp with marked stromal inflammation

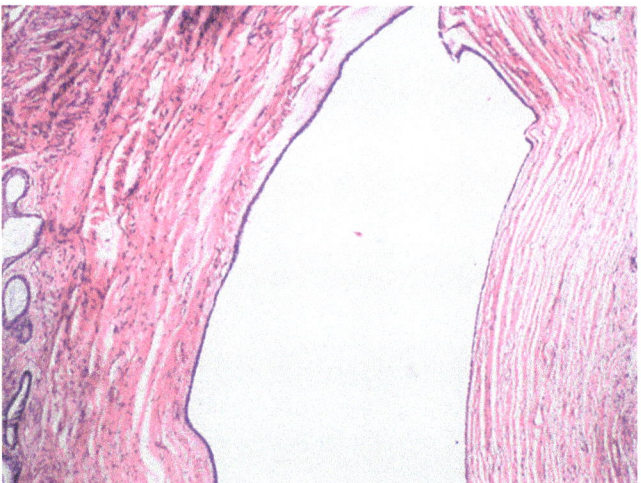

Figure 5.22: Nabothian cyst: Cystically dilated gland lined by endocervical cuboidal to flat cells

## CERVICAL CYSTS

The cysts in the cervix may be congenital or acquired.

### Congenital Cyst

The congenital cysts are mesonephric duct cyst and Müllerian duct cyst. Mesonephric duct cyst is developed from the dilatation of mesonephric duct remnants. The cyst is lined by low cuboidal cells. The Müllerian duct cyst is commonly seen in posterior cervical wall. The cyst is lined by endometrial or tubal lining epithelium.

### Acquired Cysts

The commonest acquired cyst is nabothian cyst. This is a type of retention cyst formed due to blockage of the glandular drainage pathway. The neck of the crypt is blocked due to fibrosis or squamous metaplasia. Microscopically, there is cystic dilatation of the glands (Figure 5.22). The glands are lined by tall columnar epithelium. Foci of squamous metaplasia may also be noted.

The other acquired cysts are endometriotic cyst, cystic degeneration of leiomyoma, hydatid cyst, etc.

## TUNNEL CLUSTERS

The term "tunnel cluster" was first used by Fluhmann in 1961.[13] Tunnel cluster (TC) is a relatively common lesion in the cervix and is usually located near the surface epithelium of cervix. TC was originally classified by Fluhmann in two types: type A and type B.

### Type A tunnel Cluster

The type A TC is seen in the superficial part of the cervical wall. On histology, the lesion shows multiple small closely packed glands in lobulated manner. The glands are well-circumscribed and the lining shows bland looking cuboidal to columnar cells.

*Differential Diagnosis*

Well-differentiated adenocarcinoma: Type A TC should be differentiated from well-differentiated adenocarcinoma of cervix. The following features are helpful to distinguish TC from carcinoma:
1. Lobular architecture,
2. Lack of desmoplastic reaction,
3. Absence of infiltration.

## Type B Tunnel Cluster

Type B tunnel cluster is characterized by cystically dilated glands arranged in lobular pattern. The glands are lined by small cuboidal to almost flattened epithelium. This lesion is easier to identify because of the cystic dilation of the gland. The cystic dilatation is possibly due to blockage of the neck of the crypt.

## REFERENCES

1. Nucci MR, Young RH. Arias-Stella reaction of the endocervix: a report of 18 cases with emphasis on its varied histology and differential diagnosis. Am J Surg Pathol. 2004;28(5): 608-12.
2. Jonasson JG, Wang HH, Antonioli DA, et al. Tubal metaplasia of the uterine cervix: a prevalence study in patients with gynecologic pathologic findings. Int J Gynecol Pathol. 1992; 11(2):89-95.
3. Suh KS, Silverberg SG. Tubal metaplasia of the uterine cervix. Int J Gynecol Pathol. 1990;9(2):122-28.
4. Weir MM, Bell DA, Young RH. Transitional cell metaplasia of the uterine cervix and vagina: an underrecognized lesion that may be confused with high-grade dysplasia. A report of 59 cases. Am J Surg Pathol. 1997;21(5):510-7.
5. Harnden P, Kennedy W, Andrew AC, et al. Immunophenotype of transitional metaplasia of the uterine cervix. Int J Gynecol Pathol. 1999;18(2):125-29.
6. Taylor HB, Irey NS, Norris HJ. Atypical endocervical hyperplasia in women taking oral contraceptives. JAMA. 1967;202:637-9.
7. Kyriakos M, Kempson RL, Konikov NF. A clinical and pathologic study of endocervical lesions associated with oral contraceptives. Cancer. 1968;22:99-110.
8. Greeley C, Schroeder S, Silverberg SG. Microglandular hyperplasia of the cervix: a true "pill" lesion? Int J Gynecol Pathol. 1995;14:50-54.
9. Nucci MR. Symposium part III: tumor-like glandular lesions of the uterine cervix. Int J Gynecol Pathol. 2002;21(4):347-59.
10. Ferry JA, Scully RE. Mesonephric remnants, hyperplasia, and neoplasia in the uterine cervix. A study of 49 cases. Am J Surg Pathol. 1990;14:1100-11.
11. Bague S, Rodriquez IM, Prat J. Malignant mesonephric tumors of the female genital tract: a clinicopathologic study of 9 cases. Am J Surg Pathol. 2004;28:601-7.
12. Nucci MR, Clement PB, Young RH. Lobular endocervical glandular hyperplasia, not otherwise specified: a clinico-pathologic analysis of thirteen cases of a distinctive pseudoneoplastic lesion and comparison with fourteen cases of adenoma malignum. Am J Surg Pathol. 1999;23:886-91.
13. Fluhmann CF. Focal hyperplasia (tunnel clusters) of the cervix uteri. Obstet Gynecol. 1961;17:206-14.

# Preneoplastic and Neoplastic Lesions of Cervix

## 6

### WHO CLASSIFICATION OF TUMORS OF THE UTERINE CERVIX:[1]

- Epithelial tumors
- Squamous cell tumors and its precursors
  - Squamous intraepithelial lesions
    - Low grade squamous intraepithelial lesions
    - High grade squamous intraepithelial lesions
  - Squamous cell carcinoma, NOS
    - Keratinizing
    - Non-keratinizing
    - Papillary
    - Basaloid
    - Warty
    - Verrucous
    - Sqaumotransitional
    - Lymphoepithelioma like
  - Benign squamous cell lesions
    - Squamous metaplasia
    - Condyloma acuminatum
    - Squamous papilloma
    - Transitional metaplasia
- Glandular tumors and precursors
  - Adenocarcinoma in situ
  - Adenocarcinoma
    - Endocervical adenocarcinoma, usual type
    - Mucinous carcinoma
      - ◊ Gastric type
      - ◊ Intestinal type
      - ◊ Signet-ring cell type
    - Villoglandular carcinoma
    - Endometrioid carcinoma
    - Clear cell carcinoma
    - Serous carcinoma
    - Mesonephric carcinoma
    - Adenocarcinoma admixed with neuroendocrine carcinoma
- Benign glandular tumors and tumor-like lesions
  - Endocervical polyp
  - Müllerian papilloma
  - Nabothian cyst
  - Tunnel clusters
  - Microglandular hyperplasia
  - Lobular endocervical glandular hyperplasia
  - Diffuse laminar endocervical hyperplasia
  - Arias Stella reaction
- Other epithelial tumors
  - Adenosquamous carcinoma
  - Glassy cell carcinoma
  - Adenoid basal carcinoma
  - Undifferentiated carcinoma
- Neuroendocrine tumors
  - Low grade neuroendocrine tumors
    - Carcinoid tumors
    - Atypical carcinoid
  - High grade neuroendocrine carcinoma
    - Small cell neuroendocrine carcinoma
    - Large cell neuroendocrine carcinoma
- Mesenchymal tumors and tumors-like lesions
  - Benign
    - Leiomyoma
    - Rhabdomyoma
  - Malignant
    - Leiomyosarcoma
    - Rhabdomyosarcoma
    - Alveolar soft part sarcoma
    - Angiosarcoma
    - Malignant peripheral nerve sheath tumor
    - Others
- Mixed epithelial and mesenchymal tumors
  - Adenomyoma
  - Adenosarcoma
  - Carcinosarcoma
- Melanocytic tumors
- Germ cell tumors
- Lymphoid and myeloid tumors
- Secondary tumors

Cervical carcinoma is considered as the 5th commonest cancer in the world and the incidence of new cases is 500000 women worldwide.[2] In the developing countries cervical cancer accounts for 12% of all cancers of female. The molecular studies have demonstrated HPV DNA in every cases of cervical carcinoma and preneoplastic conditions.[3] The cervical cancer undergoes four important steps in its evolution:
1. Infection by HPV
2. Persistent viral infection
3. A clone of infected cells progress to pre-neoplastic lesions
4. Invasion.

The steps are not always progressive because the viral load may be cleared and the patient may regress to normal.

## THE HUMAN PAPILLOMA VIRUS

### Subtypes of HPV

Human papilloma virus (HPV) is a double stranded non-enveloped DNA virus. Presently about 200 subtypes of HPV have been identified on the basis of genotypic character. The virus is epitheliotropic and absolutely species specific virus that infect only human species. HPV subtypes are of two types: low-risk and high-risk depending on their oncogenic potential[4] (Table 6.1).

Table 6.1: Risk potential and HPV subtypes

| Risk classification | HPV types |
|---|---|
| Low-risk | 6, 11, 42, 43, 44, 54, 61, 70, 72, 81 |
| High-risk | 16, 18, 31, 33, 35, 39, 45, 51, 52, 56, 58, 59, 61, 66, 68, 73 |
| Probably high-risk type | 26, 53, 66, 73, and 82 |

It has been noted that HPV 16, 18, 45, 31, 33, 52, 58, and 35 are responsible for major bulk (95%) of cervical squamous-cell carcinomas. HPV 16 is the most common type (55%) followed by HPV 18 (13 to 22%).[5]

### Viral Genomic Organization

HPV (55 nm in diameter) contains an inner circular genome and an outer protein capsid layer. The inner circular genome is a double-stranded circular DNA that contains 8000 nucleotides and encodes 8 viral proteins. The outer capsid layer of the virus is a non-lipid membrane and is mainly formed by L1 protein. In addition the viral capsid also contains small amount of L2 protein.

### Viral Genome

The 8 kb viral genomic DNA is divided mainly in 3 major regions: early, late, and a long control region (LCR) and

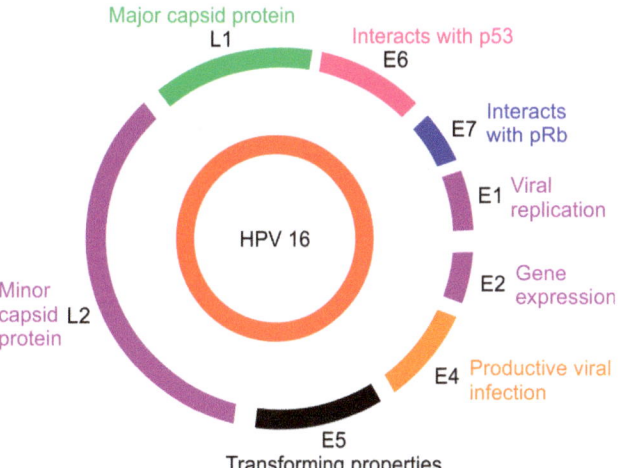

Figure 6.1: HPV: Schematic diagram of HPV genome

these regions are separated by two polyadenylation (pA) sites (Figure 6.1):

1. **An early region:** Early (E) region consists of about 50% of the virus genome and encodes a total of six open reading frames (ORF) nonstructural proteins such as E1, E2, E4, E5, E6 and E7 which are involved in viral replication, transcription and transformation. They also help in viral adaptation in changing environment.
2. **A late (L) region:** L region occupies almost 40% of the virus genome and encodes viral capsid proteins L1 and L2. These proteins are expressed late in viral life. The capsid proteins form the structure of the virus and facilitate in DNA maturation and packaging.
3. **The long control region (non-coding region):** The long control region (LCR) of HPV has a size of 850 bp and occupies 12% of viral genome. This genetic segment of HPV does not contain any open reading frame. LCR is located in between the end of the L1, and the beginning of the E6 gene. It contains the viral promoters that control regulates transcription and replication of the viral DNA.

### Viral Protein Interaction and Oncogenic Transformation

In benign proliferative lesions of cervix HPV DNA is present as extra chromosomal or episomal. During persistent infection HPV DNA integrates within the host DNA.

#### E1 and E2

E1 and E2 protein take active participation in viral replication. E2 protein binds with the promoter site of E1 gene and activates the replication of E1 to produce E1 protein. E2 protein controls the expression of E6 and E7 protein. It has been noted that at the time of viral integration and carcinogenesis, E2 expression is typically lost. Therefore, E6 and E7 are released from the control of E2 and excessive E6 and E7 proteins are produced leading to carcinogenesis.

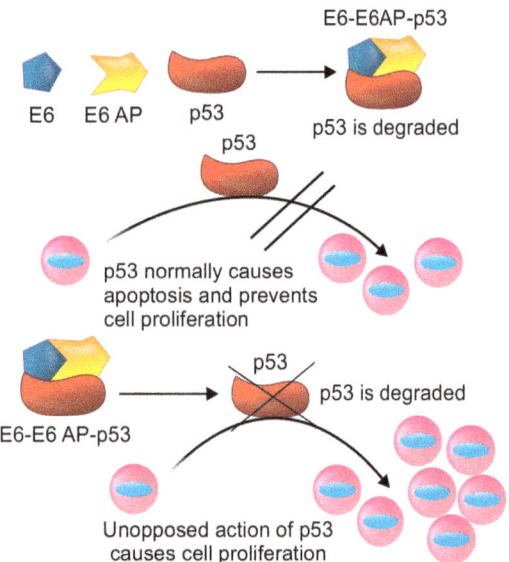

**Figure 6.2:** E6 and p53 action is shown in the schematic diagram

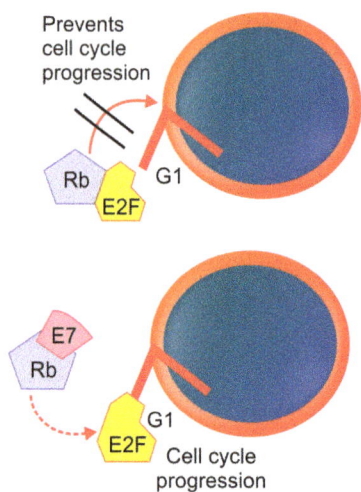

**Figure 6.3:** Schematic diagram shows E6 and pRb interaction

## E6 Protein

HPV E6 protein particularly binds with tumor suppressor protein p53 and inhibits the function of p53. High-risk HPV E6 binds to E6 associated protein (E6AP). This E6-E6AP complex functions as an ubiquitin protein ligase and degrades p53 6 (Figure 6.2). As p53 normally acts as genomic safe guard and prevents cell proliferation, so loss of p53 causes genomic instability and uncontrolled cell proliferation leading to carcinogenesis. The low-risk HPV E6 does not bind with the core region of p53.

## E7 Protein

E7 proteins are small, acidic polypeptides and contains only 100 amino acids. This protein has no intrinsic enzymatic activity. E7 of both low and high-risk HPV types combine with pRb. Compared to high-risk HPV, E7 of low-risk HPV has much lower affinity with pRb. E7 protein binds with pRb and causes proteasomal degradation and subsequently releases transcription factor E2F. Released E2F facilitates cell cycle progression by helping the cell to enter into G1/S phase (Figure 6.3). E7 also directly binds with E2F and promotes transcriptional activity. E7 deregulates the centriole synthesis and produces aberrant number of centrioles. It also causes missegregation of chromosome. This may lead to the formation of extrachromosomal material and aneuploidy. In addition E7 protein also binds with E2F cyclin A complex, histone H1 kinase, cyclin E and TATA box binding protein.[7]

## E4 Protein

E4 protein interacts with the cytoskeletal structure of the host epithelial cells and permits HPV to leave the cell. E4 and cytoskeleton interaction is responsible for koilocytotic changes. E4 protein interacts with the mitotic spindle formation and cytokinesis and therefore causes multinucleation.[8]

## E5 Protein

E5 protein interacts with growth factor receptors and ligands of the cell and enhances cellular growth. This protein also inhibits apoptosis and helps in continuous replication of epithelial cells.

**Table 6.2:** Functions of HPV proteins

| Viral protein | Function |
|---|---|
| E6 | **Main: Degradation of p53 function**<br>• Cell proliferation<br>• Prevents apoptosis<br>• Genomic instability |
| E7 | **Main: Degradation of pRb function**<br>• Cell cycle progression (G1 to S)<br>• Cell death deregulation<br>• Genomic instability<br>• Deranged gene transcription<br>• Deranged cell metabolism<br>• Epigenetic reprogramming |
| E5 | • Enhance cell proliferation<br>• Prevents apoptosis |
| E4 | • Interacts with the cytoskeletal structure of host<br>• Interacts with the mitotic spindle formation and cytokinesis<br>• Facilitates release of viral particle |
| E2 | E2 protein controls viral transcription and replication. |
| E1 | Viral DNA replication |

## Viral Life Cycle and Natural History

HPV infection is a sexually transmitted disease. The primary route of infection of HPV is through vagina or anal canal

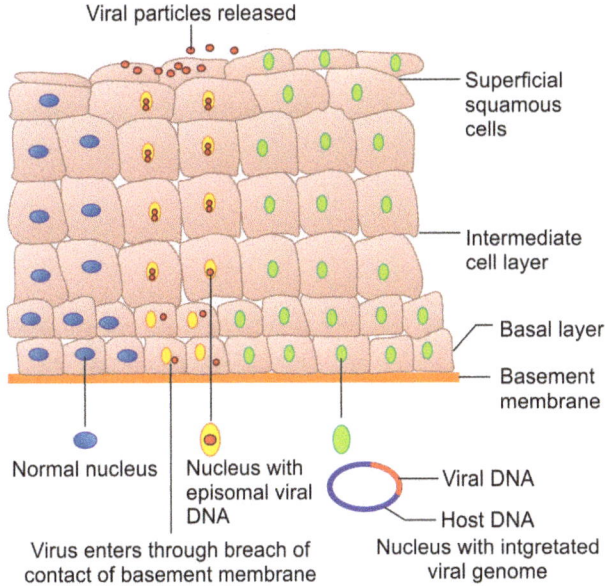

Figure 6.4: HPV life cycle within the cervical epithelium

and the virus is transmitted to the body by skin or mucosal contact. During sexual intercourse, HPV enters into the female genital tract by small superficial abrasions. The virus particles are attached within the basement membrane by a primary receptor in L1 and possibly virus enters into the basal cell at that point of time. The metaplastic epithelium is more thin and fragile and therefore much more susceptive to HPV infection.

The viral particle may remain in the cells as:

a. **Latent or dormant phase:** HPVs remain in the nucleus in low number as a circular DNA and stay free and independent to host DNA. No cytological abnormalities are demonstrable in this stage (Figure 6.4).
b. **Productive phase:** The virus proliferates within the epithelial cells irrespective of epithelial cell cycle and infect the adjacent epithelium. Viral related cytomorphological changes such as koilocytosis, nucleomegaly, and binucleation are seen.

At first, the viral replication occurs in the basal layer of the epithelium. The viral DNA is amplified at low copy number and each basal cell is infected only by 50 to 100 copies of the virus. In course of time the infected basal cells proliferate and the viral particle remains as episome in the nucleus. In this phase, the expression of viral gene is minimal. Both E6 and E7 gene is in tight regulation in this time. No cytological abnormality is noted in this stage. Once the epithelial cell stop proliferation and differentiates then the virus starts DNA replication in huge number. There is also massive upregulation of viral oncoprotein E6 and E7. The virus also express L1 and L2 protein and viral particle is assembled in the superficial epithelial cells. Ultimately, the virus is released from the epithelial cells and re-infect the adjacent epithelial cells. This whole process takes usually three weeks that corresponds to the maturation time of basal cells to squamous cells. Uncommonly HPV infection persists and viral DNA integrates within the host DNA (Figure 6.4). The circular E2 becomes linear and is incorporated within host DNA. Loss of the function of E2 permits over expression of oncoproteins E6 and E7.

Majority of the cases of HPV infection is subclinical and transient and clears within 1 to 2 year. More than 90% of infected women becomes disease free by cell-mediated immunity. The infection persists only in a small fraction of women (10–15%). The viral DNA remains within the cell and the viral replication may be ongoing in this group of women. This small group of the women with high-risk HPV infection is at increased risk for high grade intraepithelial neoplasia and progression to carcinoma.

## TERMINOLOGY OF PRENEOPLASTIC LESIONS OF CERVIX

Earlier to late 1960, the intraepithelial lesions of cervix were classified in four categories: mild dysplasia, moderate dysplasia, severe dysplasia and carcinoma in situ.[9] Richart RM[10] introduced the concept that various intraepithelial lesions of cervix are actually a single disease entity and he labeled them together as "cervical intraepithelial neoplasm" (CIN). The CIN terminology divided the preneoplastic lesions into three categories, CIN 1, CIN 2, and CIN 3, with carcinoma in situ being incorporated into the CIN 3 category. This new terminology of CIN replaced arbitrary differentiation between severe dysplasia and carcinoma in situ. It was shown that 60%, 40% and 33% of CIN 1, CIN 2 and CIN 3 spontaneously regress respectively. Only 1%, 5% and near about 12% of CIN 1, CIN 2 and CIN 3 progress to invasion[11] (Table 6.3).

Table 6.3: Natural history of CIN cases[11]

|       | Regression | Persist | Progression CIN 3 | Progression to invasion |
|-------|------------|---------|-------------------|------------------------|
| CIN 1 | 60%        | 30%     | 10%               | 1%                     |
| CIN 2 | 40%        | 40%     | 20%               | 5%                     |
| CIN 3 | 33%        | 56%     |                   | 12%                    |

Therefore CIN 1 may not be a true neoplastic lesion and just reflects the changes due to HPV infection that resolves spontaneously. There are two distinct biological entities of HPV related cervical lesions:

1. Lesions with productive viral infections that are self-limited and regress spontaneously. These lesions are histologically referred as "low grade" lesions.
2. Lesions that are really neoplastic and have the potential to develop invasive carcinoma in course of time, if not treated. On histology, these lesions are labeled as "high grade".

Table 6.4: Nomenclature of cervical preneoplastic lesions

|  | Grades | | | | |
| --- | --- | --- | --- | --- | --- |
| Older classifications | Mild dysplasia | Moderate dysplasia | Severe dysplasia | Carcinoma in situ | Carcinoma |
| CIN terminology | CIN 1 | CIN 2 | CIN 3 | | Carcinoma |
| Bethesda | LSIL | HSIL | | | Carcinoma |
| Modified CIN terminology | Low grade CIN | High grade CIN | | | Carcinoma |

The Bethesda system classified cervical preneoplastic lesions as two tiered system:[12]

1. **Low grade squamous intraepithelial lesions (LSIL):** LSIL includes both HPV induced changes and cervical intraepithelial neoplasm grade 1.
2. **High grade intraepithelial lesions (HSIL):** HSIL includes cervical intraepithelial neoplasm grade 2, grade 3 and also carcinoma in situ.

Bethesda system closely reflects the biology of cervical preneoplastic lesions and unifies the cervical cytology and histology reporting. Table 6.4 shows the comparison of different classification of cervical preneoplastic lesions.

In histopathology section, the cervical intraepithelial neoplasm may be classified as two tiered Bethesda system: low grade SIL and high grade SIL. Alternatively, these lesions may be reported as CIN 1 as low grade CIN, and CIN 2 and CIN 3 as high grade CIN.

## CERVICAL INTRAEPITHELIAL NEOPLASM GRADE 1 OR LOW GRADE SQUAMOUS INTRAEPITHELIAL LESION

### General Features

Low grade squamous intraepithelial lesion (LSIL) is caused by both low and high-risk HPV. However, the majority of LSIL is caused by low-risk HPV 6 and 11.

### Clinical Features

Cervical intraepithelial neoplasm 1 (CIN1) is mainly seen in young population. It uncommonly occurs in postmenopausal women. The patient is usually asymptomatic. The lesions are mostly detected by routine cervical smear examination.

### Colposcopic Examination

The lesions of CIN 1 appears as aceto-white area in colposcopic examination. The condylomata accuminata appears as papillary raised area.

### Histology

The CIN 1 lesion includes flat condyloma (CIN 1), condyloma accuminata and papillary immature metaplasia. Overall CIN 1 lesions show atypical squamous cells in lower

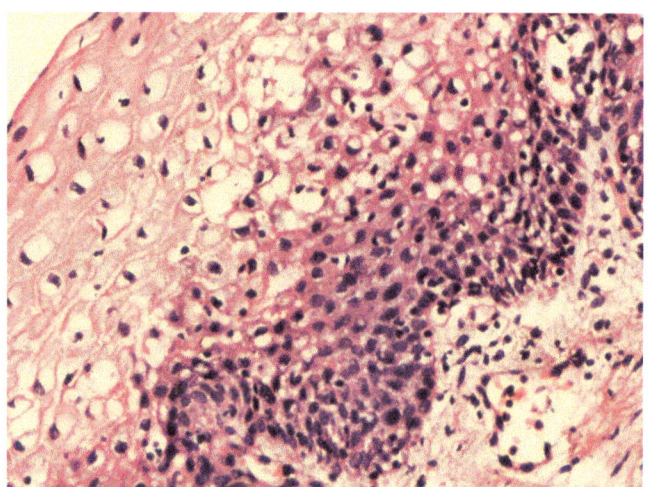

Figure 6.5: CIN 1: Dysplastic cells involving less than 1/3rd of the epithelium

third of the squamous epithelium (Figure 6.5). The upper 2/3rd of the epithelium shows normal squamous maturation. The epithelial layer is usually thickened with increased cells in the lower third zone. The nucleus of the cells shows mild atypia and koilocytotic changes. Nuclei also show mild enlargement, pleomorphism, hyperchromasia and irregular membrane. Bi and multinucleated cells are also seen. The cells show koilocytotic changes characterized by enlarged nuclei surrounded by perinuclear cytoplasmic vacuoles with sharp condensed thick cytoplasmic margin. Mitotic activities are seen only in the basal –parabasal cell layers.

### Flat Condyloma

Here the surface of the lesion is flat. The cells show mild degree nuclear atypia and koilocytosis. Majority of flat condyloma (approximately 60-70%) are associated with high-risk HPV types.

### Exophytic Condyloma

The lesions are commonly associated with HPV 6 and 11. These lesions are less common and show exophytic papillary projections. The papillae are broad based and blunt type. The cells show nuclear enlargement, binucleation and hyperchromasia. Characteristic koilocytotic changes are also seen.

*Immature Condyloma (Papillary Immature Metaplasia)*

It is also mainly associated with HPV 6 or 11. The infected cells do not mature and resemble immature metaplastic cells. The lesion often shows filiform papillae lined by the immature looking squamous cells with scanty cytoplasm, mild nuclear atypia and regular nuclear margin. The mature keratinocytes are minimal to absent. Koilocytotic changes are also minimal.

## Cytology of LSIL

Smears show abnormality of superficial and intermediate squamous cells. The cells show mild nuclear enlargement and hyperchromasia with inconspicuous nucleoli. The nucleus occupies 1/3rd of the cytoplasmic area (Figures 6.6 and 6.7). Chromatin is finely granular. Koilocytosis are frequently seen in LSIL cases.

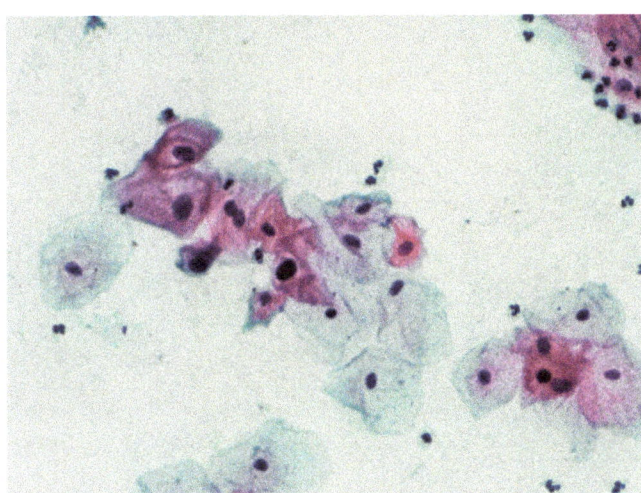

**Figure 6.6:** LSIL: Smears show discrete cells with mild nuclear enlargement and pleomorphism

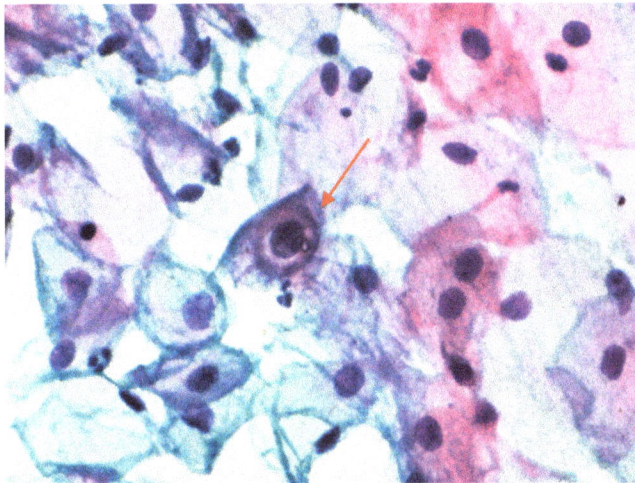

**Figure 6.7:** LSIL: Higher magnification shows enlarged hyperchromatic nuclei and koilocytic cell

## Differential Diagnosis of LSIL

- Reactive inflammatory changes in squamous epithelial cells: The metaplasia cells do not show any nuclear pleomorphism and nuclear margin irregularity. Typical koilocytotic cell is absent in the metaplastic cells.
- Nonspecific perinuclear halos: This may be seen in inflammation or trichomonas infection. Prominent cytoplasmic haloes in the glycogenated epithelial cells may be mistaken as koilocytosis. No nuclear atypia is seen in these conditions.
- HSIL: Discussed later.

## Prognosis and Management

Almost 60% LSIL cases regress within 2 year period, 30% persists and 10% progress to HSIL. Once LSIL is diagnosed on Pap smear then the management of such cases is:
- Colposcopy.
- If there is no lesion in colposcopy, unsatisfactory colposcopy then endocervical sampling is preferred.
- If colposcopy does not show CIN 2 or 3 then HPV DNA testing or repeat cervical cytology should be done.
- In postmenopausal or adolescent patients repeat cytology testing at 6 monthly intervals can be done.

## HIGH GRADE SQUAMOUS INTRAEPITHELIAL LESIONS

High grade squamous intraepithelial lesion (HSIL) cases are usually seen in relatively older patient than LSIL. Incidence of HSIL cases is 31 per 100,000 women. The patients of HSIL are usually asymptomatic and are detected by routine cervical cancer screening.

## Colposcopy

Colposcopy of HSIL cases show acetowhite area and leukoplakia. The margin of the acetowhite area is well-defined and sharp along with irregular uneven surface. The intensity of the color of the acetowhite area may be variable in different areas. In addition considerable changes are seen in the superficial vessels in the form of punctuation and mosaicism (Box 6.1). Punctuation in the colposcopy is the

**Box 6.1:** Colposcopy of HSIL

- Acetowhite area:
  - Well-defined and sharp
  - Irregular uneven surface
  - Variable color intensity
- Coarse punctuation
- Coarse mosaicism
- Umbilication

result of hairpin like turn of the small vessels from the surface to stroma. The anatomizing complex branching pattern of the vessels is reflected as "mosaicism" in colposcopy (Figure 6.8). In HSIL cases, the punctuation and mosaicism both are coarse which is due to increased caliber of blood vessels and increased intercapillary distance. These two patterns may be superimposed to form so called umbilication.

## Histopathology

Histopathology section of HSIL exhibits atypical cells in all layers of epithelium. The immature cells extends more than lower 1/3rd of the cell layers and occupy into the upper 2/3rd of the epithelium. The atypical cells in HSIL cases show moderate nuclear enlargement, pleomorphism, irregular nuclear contour and hyperchromasia. The cytoplasm of the cell is scanty and the cells show high nucleocytoplasmic ratio. Frequent mitotic activity is seen in all the layers.

Abnormal mitotic figures are frequently seen. Polarity of the cell is remarkably lost. HSIL cases may be subdivided into CIN 2 and CIN 3 on histology section. These two lesions are distinguished on histology by the degree of immature atypical cells in the epithelial layer. In CIN 2 lesions the immature cells occupy the lower 2/3rd of the epithelium and mature epithelial cells are seen in the upper 1/3rd layer (Figure 6.9). Abnormal mitotic activities are mainly seen in the lower 2/3rd of the epithelium. In case of CIN 3, the immature atypical cells occupy almost full thickness of the epithelial layer and no mature cells are seen (Figures 6.10 to 6.12). Mitotic activity is seen in the entire epithelial cell layer. At times the endocervical glands may also show involvement by dysplastic cells (Figures 6.13 and 6.14). The HSIL may show different histological variants depending on the presence of koilocytotic cells, keratinization and the morphology of immature cells.

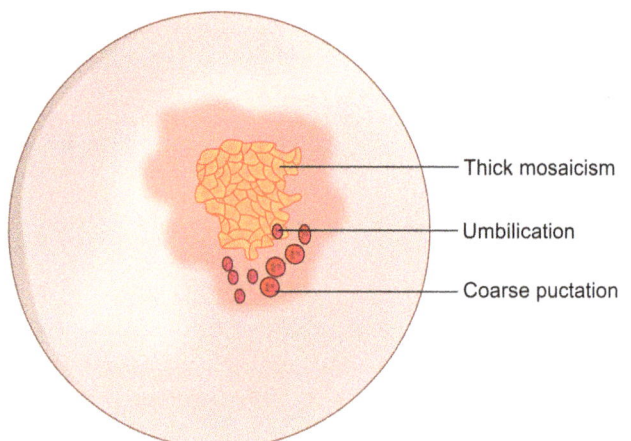

**Figure 6.8:** Colposcopic appearance of HSIL cases

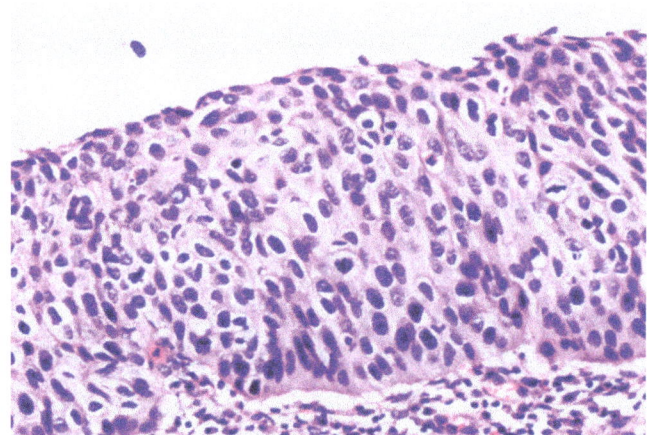

**Figure 6.10:** CIN 3: The atypical cells are present in full thickness of the epithelium

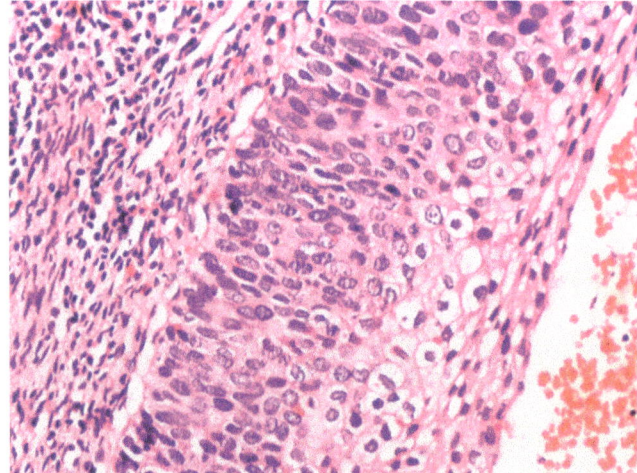

**Figure 6.9:** CIN 2: The dysplastic cells involve less than two-third of the lining epithelium

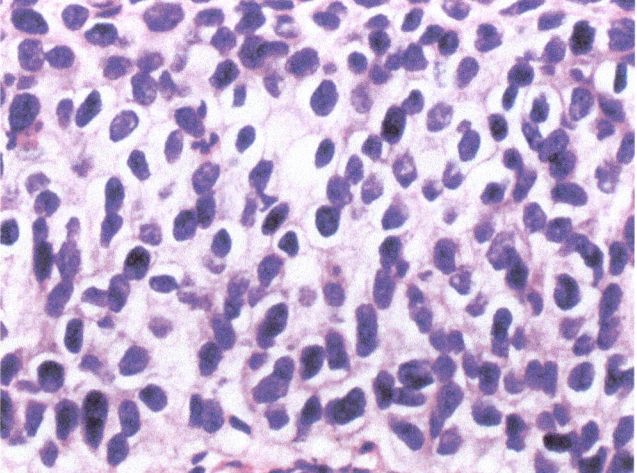

**Figure 6.11:** CIN 3: The higher magnification shows moderate nuclear atypia

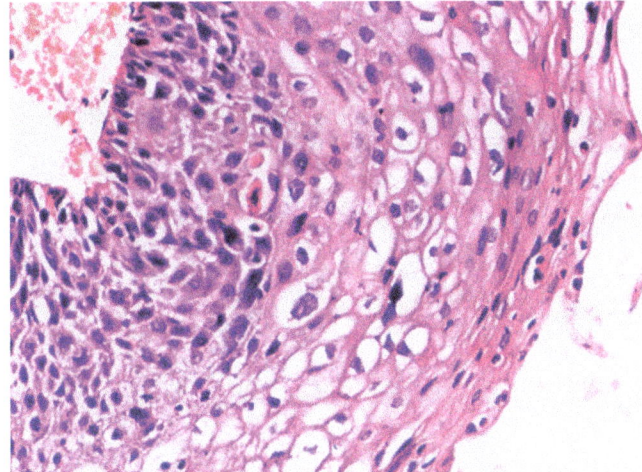

Figure 6.12: CIN 3: Koilocytotic change

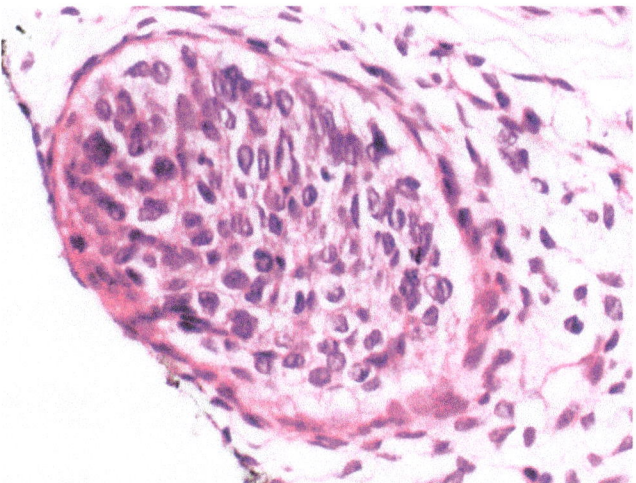

Figure 6.14: Glandular involvement of CIN: The gland is totally involved by the dysplastic cells

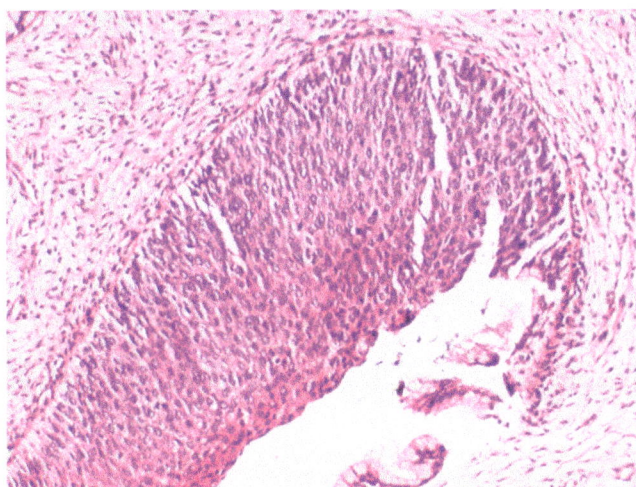

Figure 6.13: Glandular involvement of CIN: The gland is partially involved by dysplastic cells

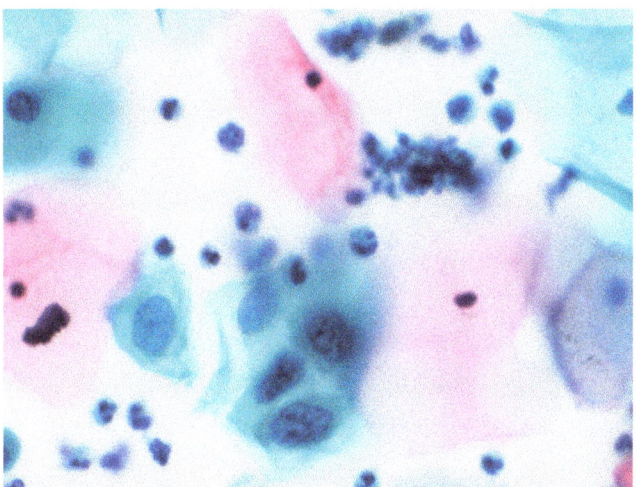

Figure 6.15: HSIL: Cells with moderately enlarged nuclei (SurePath preparation)

### Koilocytotic HSIL

In koilocytotic HSIL, the lesion contains good number of koilocytotic cells. In addition, many atypical cells are also seen in the parabasal cell layer. The koilocytotic cells show atypical nucleus. Abnormal mitosis is noted in upper part of the epithelium.

### Keratinizing HSIL

In keratinizing HSIL, prominent abnormal superficial keratinization is seen along with many atypical cells. The nuclei of the keratinized cells show enlargement, irregular nuclear contour and hyperchromasia.

### HSILs with Immature Metaplastic Differentiation

This variant of HSIL resembles reactive metaplasia in low power magnification. The lesion is composed of immature cells with scanty cytoplasm, high nucleocytoplasmic ratio and hyperchromatic nuclei in the superficial layer.

## Cytology

Cells in HSIL are usually parabasal, basal or metaplastic type. Individual cells are round to oval with scanty cytoplasm and high N/C ratio (Figures 6.15 to 6.17). Cytoplasm is dense or lacy in character. In case of keratinizing variant, there may be orangeophilia in the cytoplasm. Nuclei of the cells are enlarged, moderately pleomorphic, hyperchromatic with coarse chromatin. Nuclear contour is markedly irregular. Nucleoli are prominent.

## Differential Diagnosis

1. **Reactive atypia:** See Table 6.5.

# Preneoplastic and Neoplastic Lesions of Cervix

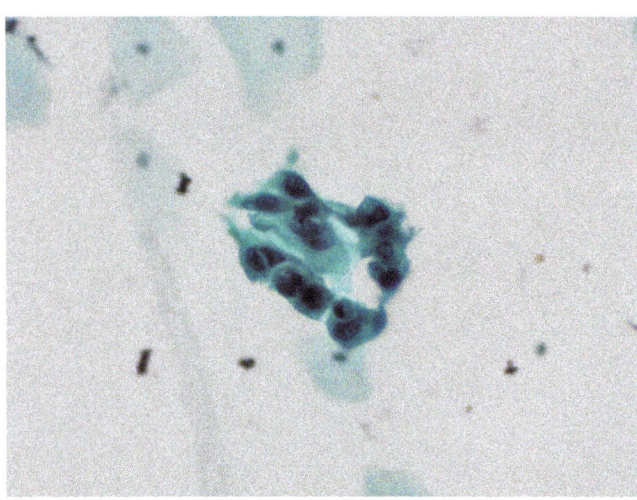

Figure 6.16: HSIL: Smear shows loosely cohesive dysplastic cells. (SurePath preparation)

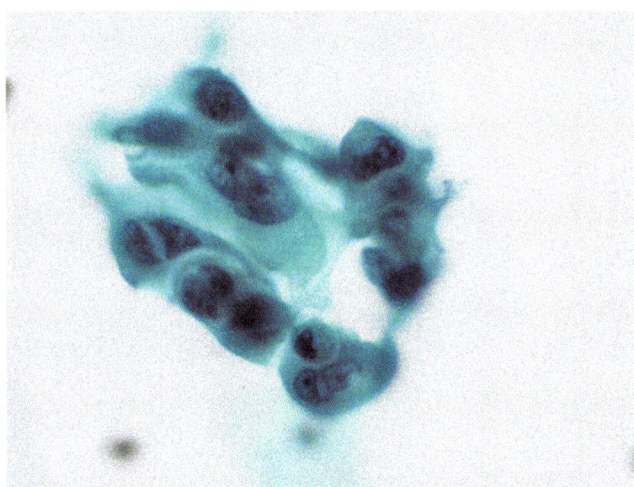

Figure 6.17: HSIL: Higher magnifications shows enlarged hyperchromatic cells. The cells occupy more than half of the cytoplasm. (SurePath preparation)

Table 6.5: Reactive atypia versus HSIL

|  | Reactive atypia | HSIL |
|---|---|---|
| Cell polarity and nuclear spacing | Maintained | Not maintained |
| Nuclear pleomorphism | Absent | Present |
| Nuclear contour | Regular | Irregular |
| Spongiosis | Present | Absent |
| Inflammatory cell infiltration | Present | Absent |

2. **Immature squamous metaplasia:** See Table 6.6.

Table 6.6: Differentiating points between immature squamous metaplasia and HSIL

|  | Immature squamous metaplasia | HSIL |
|---|---|---|
| Cell polarity | Maintained | Lost |
| Nuclear spacing | Maintained | Lost |
| Superficial mature cells | Present | Absent |
| Pleomorphism | Absent | Present |
| Chromatin | Fine | Coarse |
| Mitosis | Only in basal layer | Even in superficial layer |

3. **LSIL:** See Table 6.7.

Table 6.7: Distinguishing features of LSIL and HSIL

| Features | LSIL | HSIL |
|---|---|---|
| Age | Reproductive age: 30 to 40 | Slightly older age group: 35 to 40 |
| HPV | Mainly low risk HPV 6,11 | Mainly high risk HPV 16,18 |
| Degree of immature cells | Only basal 1/3rd | Lower 2/3rd to full thickness |
| Superficial mature cells | Present | Absent |
| Mitosis | Only in basal 1/3rd | Entire epithelial layer |
| Atypical mitosis | Absent | Present |
| Koilocytosis | Frequent | Infrequent |
| Ploidy | Diploid | Aneuploid |
| p16 | Small proportion of cases show positivity | Large proportion of cases show positivity |

4. **Atrophic changes:** Atrophic epithelium does not show any nuclear pleomorphism or mitotic activity and cell polarity is maintained.

## Prognosis of HSIL

The rate of progression of HSIL to carcinoma is higher than LSIL. Near about 5% cases of CIN 2 and 12% cases of CIN 3 progress to invasion. Forty percent cases of CIN 2 and 56% cases of CIN3 persist. Similarly, 40% CIN 2 and 33% CIN 3 may regress over the course of time.

## Management of HSIL

Overall management of cytologicaly diagnosed cases of HSIL has been highlighted in the Figure 6.18. In histopathology proved HSIL cases the entire transformation zone should be removed along with the lesion. The management of HSIL includes:

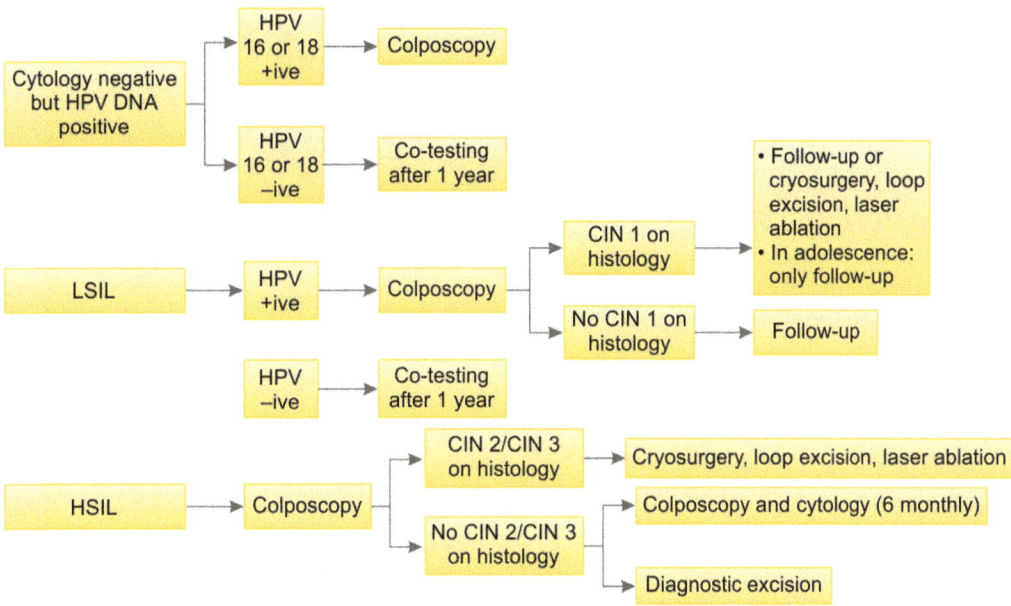

**Figure 6.18:** Management of HSIL cases

1. Cryotherapy,
2. Loop electrosurgical excision procedure (LEEP)/large loop excision of the transformation zone (LLETZ), and,
3. Cold knife conization (CKC).

### Ancillary Tests (Box 6.2)

a. p16 ink-4 immunostaining:[13] p16 ink-4 is an inhibitor of cyclin dependent kinase (CDK). Normally, CDK segregates the pRb-E2F combination and releases E2F which is necessary for cell cycle progression. HPV infection causes aberrant expression of E7 that binds with pRb protein and segregates E2F. To counteract the viral infected cells produce excessive amount of p16 ink-4, an inhibitor of CDK. Increased expression of p16 ink-4 thereby halts the cell cycle progression irreversibly and promoting apoptosis. In HPV infected cells p16 ink-4 is strongly expressed to counteract the irregular cell cycle activation. Intense diffuse positivity of p16 immunostaining is present in LSIL or HSIL and it helps to distinguish these lesions from the reactive atypical lesions. Patchy p16 staining is non-specific as it may be present in atypical epithelial cell.
b. Ki67: Ki67, the cell proliferation marker, is increased in LSIL and HSIL. More than 30% ki67 positive cell nuclei in the superficial layer of the epithelium helps in the diagnosis of SIL as the normal or atrophic epithelium shows ki67 positive cells only in basal layer.[14]
c. DNA aneuploidy: LSIL cases show diploid DNA whereas HSIL cases show DNA aneuploidy.[15]

**Box 6.2:** Ancillary tests

- p16 ink-4 immunostaining:
  - An inhibitor of cyclin dependent kinase (CDK)
  - Increased expression of p16 ink-4 halts the cell cycle progression
  - Promotes apoptosis
  - Over expressed in HSIL and also LSIL cases
  - p16 immunostaining helps to differentiate reactive atypical lesions from SIL
- Ki67:
  - Ki67 is the cell proliferation marker
  - More than 30% Ki67 positive cell nuclei in the superficial layer of the epithelium in SIL
- DNA aneuploidy:
  - LSIL: Diploid DNA
  - HSIL: DNA aneuploidy
- Cyclin:
  - A cell cycle regulatory protein
  - Cyclin D is overexpressed in low-risk HPV cases
  - No expression of cyclin D in high-risk HPV
- Telomerase:
  - It is to prevent the loss of telomere, the end sequence of chromosome
  - Increased telomerase activity was demonstrated in many HSIL cases.

d. Cyclin: In low-risk HPV cases cyclin D is overexpressed whereas in high-risk HPV there is no expression of cyclin D.[16]

e. Telomerase: Increased telomerase activity was demonstrated in many HSIL cases.[17]

## SQUAMOUS CELL CARCINOMA

### Epidemiology

Squamous cell carcinoma is the second most common cancer of the female.[18] The annual death from squamous cell carcinoma of cervix is approximately 230,000 and the majority of the death is contributed by developing countries.[18] Due to widespread cervical screening program the incidence and death rate of cervical carcinoma has declined in developed countries. The incidence of cervical cancer is widely variable in different parts of the globe. The highest incidence of this cancer is noted in East and South Africa, whereas the lowest incidence is noted in China.[19]

### Etiology

HPV and cervical cancer: The major etiological factor of cervical carcinoma is high-risk HPV infection. Other etiological factors: The other potential risk factors of carcinoma of cervix are:[20]
1. Multiple sexual partners.
2. Early age at first sexual activity.
3. Increasing parity.
4. Early age at first pregnancy.
5. Use of oral contraceptive for long duration.
   Cigarette smoking is also considered as potential risk factor of cancer cervix. Possibly, the carcinogens of tobacco act as cocarcinogenic factors with HPV. Besides the above mentioned factors the other risk factors are: poor hygiene, low socioeconomic status, associated HIV infection, and poor nutritional status.[20]

### Clinical Features

Squamous cell carcinoma of cervix may occur in any group from 20–65 year age. However, the tumor is commonly seen in 40–50 year age. The invasive carcinoma cases present mainly with postcoital bleeding. In case of advanced stage, ureter may be involved and the patient may present with anuria due to hydroureter.

### Colposcopy

Colposcopy may be helpful to detect microinvasive carcinoma. The lesions show thick and opaque acetowhite area. Punctuation and mosaicism are seen along with abnormal vessels. In case of invasive carcinoma, the acetowhite area is large, chalky white and raised from the surface. In case of invasion, the mosaic pattern is lost and irregular longitudinal vessels are seen. The pattern of atypical vessels may be like hairpin-shaped, tadpole-shaped, corkscrew like or irregular bizarre branching type (Box 6.3). The diameter of the vessels may be also variable. The lesion may be seen as red, friable growth on colposcopy.

---

**Box 6.3:** Colposcopy of carcinoma

Microinvasive: Same as HSIL

**Invasive carcinoma**
- Large, chalky white, raised irregular acetowhite area
- Irregular longitudinal blood vessel
- Atypical vessels with various pattern such as hairpin-shaped, tadpole-shaped, corkscrew like or irregular bizarre branching type
- Irregular vessel diameter
- Red and friable exophytic growth

---

### Gross Features

The exophytic cervical lesions are polypoidal and are raised from the surface. The lesion may be ulcerated. When the lesion is endophytic the growth usually invades deeper cervical stroma and endocervical canal.

### Microscopy (Figures 6.19 to 6.23)

In squamous cell carcinoma, the tumor cells are arranged in cords, trabculae and sheet. The cell are large polyhedral having moderate amount of eosinophilic cytoplasm. Nuclei show mild to moderate enlargement and pleomorphism. Nuclear chromatin is coarse. Frequent mitotic activity is seen along with atypical mitotic figures. Occasionally, adjacent lining epithelium of the tumor shows CIN changes. Keratin pearls may be noted as concentrically arranged squamous cells.

The two tier classification of squamous cell carcinoma of cervix is:
1. Keratinizing squamous cell carcinoma
2. Non-keratinizing squamous cell carcinoma

The diagnosis between keratinizing and non-keratinizing squamous cell carcinoma depends on the presence of squamous pearls and intercellular bridge in between the cells. Focal intracellular keratin may be seen in non-keratinizing squamous cell carcinoma, however the tumor lacks any squamous pearl.

The squamous cell carcinoma of cervix can be graded as:

#### Well-differentiated Carcinoma

The tumors shows large number of keratin pearls. The tumor cells look like mature squamous cells having abundant cytoplasm. The nuclei are moderately enlarged and hyperchromatic.

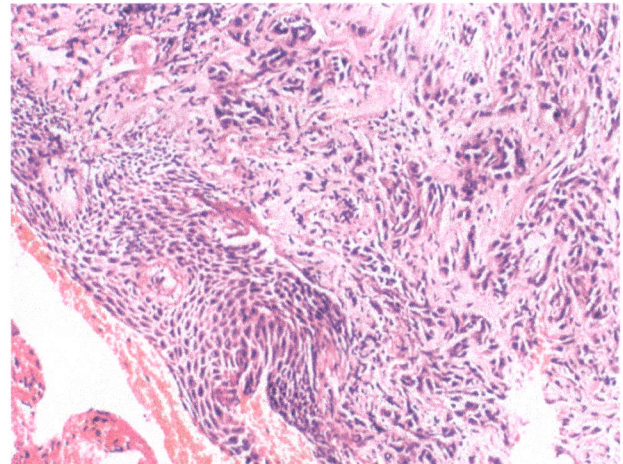

**Figure 6.19:** Keratinizing squamous cell carcinoma: Malignant squamous cells invading in the deeper tissue

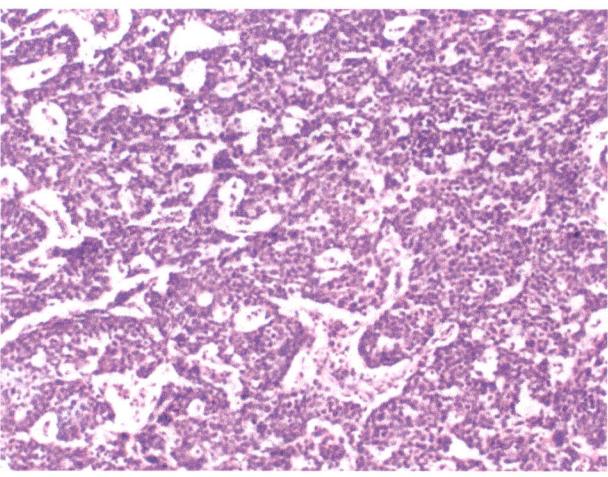

**Figure 6.22:** Non-keratinizing squamous cell carcinoma: Diffuse sheet of malignant cells

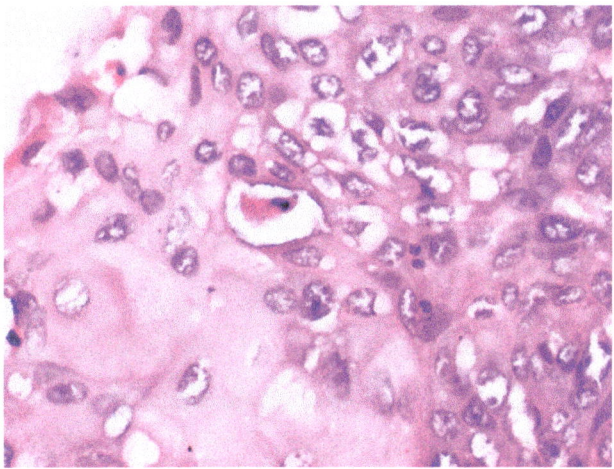

**Figure 6.20:** Keratinizing squamous cell carcinoma: Large polyhedral cells with enlarged pleomorphic nuclei along with intracytoplasmic keratinization

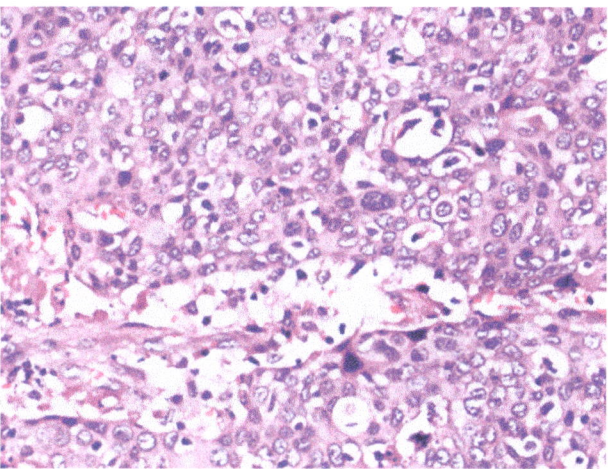

**Figure 6.23:** Non-keratinizing squamous cell carcinoma: Higher magnification shows polyhedral malignant cells with enlarged nuclei

### Moderately Differentiated Carcinoma

Here, the tumor cells contain less cytoplasm and nucleocytoplasmic ratio is relatively high. The cell to cell junction is indistinct. Nuclei are much more enlarged irregular and hyperchromatic. Mitotic activities are frequent. Rarely keratin pearls may be seen.

### Poorly Differentiated Carcinoma

The cells in this grade are much smaller in size with much higher nucleocytoplasmic ratio. The nuclei are moderate to severely pleomorphic (Figure 6.24). Frequent bi and multinucleation are seen. Mitotic activities are very high.

## FIGO Staging[21]

The staging of cervical carcinoma has been modified by International Federation of Gynecology and Obstetrics (FIGO) on 2009 (Table 6.8).

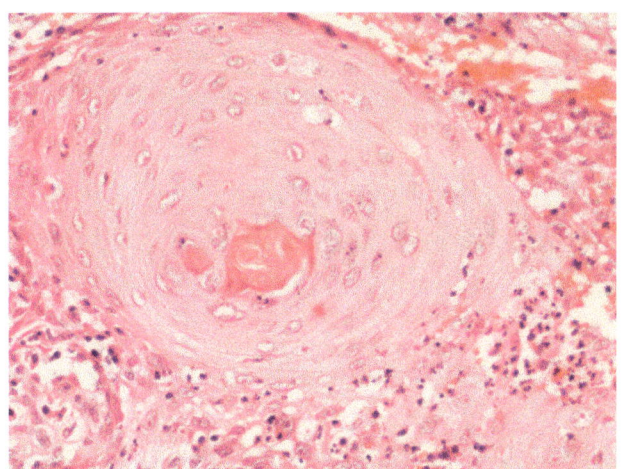

**Figure 6.21:** Keratinizing squamous cell carcinoma: Squamous pearl with keratinization

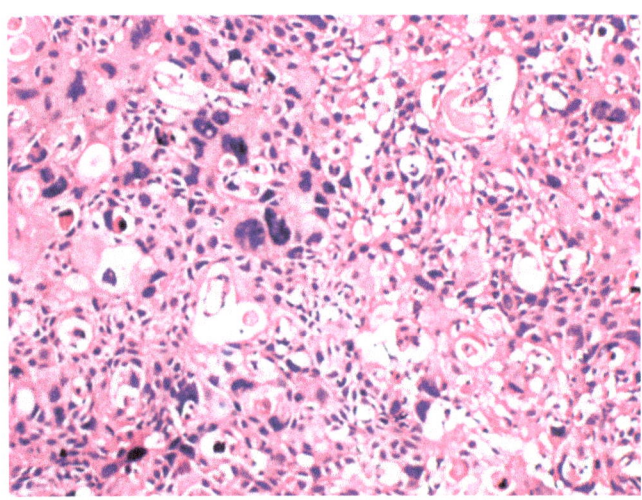

**Figure 6.24:** Squamous cell carcinoma: Poorly differentiated carcinoma shows moderate to severely pleomorphic tumor cells in sheet

### Microinvasive Carcinoma

Microinvasive carcinoma (MIC) is synonymous with early invasive carcinoma of cervix. It is defined as microscopic carcinoma with the stromal invasion limited to a maximum depth of 5 mm and greatest diameter of the tumor is lesser than 7 mm. The microinvasive carcinoma is best fitted with FIGO stage 1A carcinoma of cervix. However, according to Society of Gynecologic Oncologists (SGO) microinvasive carcinoma is defined as microscopical carcinoma with stromal invasion less than 3 mm without any lymphovascular space involvement[22] (Box 6.4).

*Feature of Invasion in Squamous Cell Carcinoma (Figures 6.25 to 6.27)*

The following features suggest the diagnosis of stromal invasion:
1. Irregular toothed margin of the tumor edge and indistinct epithelial-stromal margin.
2. Excessive eosinophilia of the overlying epithelium with keratinization in the cytoplasm.
3. Desmoplastic reaction of the underlying stroma along with inflammation.
4. Clearing of chromatin with prominent nucleoli.
5. Loss of polarity in the tumor cells in the epithelial–stromal junction.
6. Well-circumscribed nests of tumor cells within the stroma (pseudocrypt involvement).
7. Sheet like projections of tumor cells with vessels inside resembling papillary structures.

**Mimickers of invasion:**
a. **Crypt involvement by dysplastic cells**: The crypt involvement is characterized by the well-maintained polarity of the cells and sharp well-defined margin of the epithelial-stromal interphase. In addition the nests of the cells are well-separated from each other and they do not anastomose.
b. **Tangential section**: Tangential section of the epithelial cells may often mimic invasion. However, the absence of desmoplastic reaction is the helpful distinguishing feature.

**Table 6.8:** FIGO staging of cervical carcinoma

| Stage | Description |
|---|---|
| Sage I | The carcinoma is restricted to the cervix |
| IA | Invasion is seen only by microscopic examination. The stromal invasion is limited to maximum depth of 5 mm and no wider than 7 mm |
| IA1 | Stromal invasion is ≤3 mm in depth and ≤7 mm width. |
| IA2 | Stromal invasion is more than 3 mm and less than 5 mm in depth and horizontal spread or width ≤ 7 mm |
| IB | Clinical lesions confined to the cervix, or preclinical lesions greater than stage IA |
| I B1 | Clinical lesions <4 cm in size |
| IB2 | Clinical lesions >4 cm in size |
| Stage II | The carcinoma extends beyond the uterus, but has not involved the pelvic wall or to the lower third of vagina |
| IIA | Involvement of up to the upper 2/3 of the vagina. No obvious parametrial involvement |
| IIA1 | Clinically visible lesion ≤4.0 cm |
| IIA2 | Clinically visible lesion >4 cm |
| IIB | Obvious parametrial involvement but not onto the pelvic sidewall |
| Stage III | The carcinoma extends the pelvic sidewall and lower third of the vagina developing hydronephrosis or non-functioning kidney |
| IIIA | Involves lower 1/3rd of vagina but not pelvic sidewall |
| IIIB | Involves pelvic sidewall or causing hydronephrosis |
| Stage IV | The carcinoma extended beyond the true pelvis or involves the mucosa of the bladder and/or rectum |
| IVA | Spread to adjacent pelvic organs |
| IVB | Spread to distant organs |

**Box 6.4:** Microinvasive carcinoma: Criteria

**FIGO criteria**
- Stromal invasion limited to a maximum depth of 5 mm
- Greatest diameter of the tumor is lesser than 7 mm

**SGO Criteria**
- The entire lesion should be excised
- The depth of stromal invasion equal or less than 3 mm
- No lymphovascular space involvement

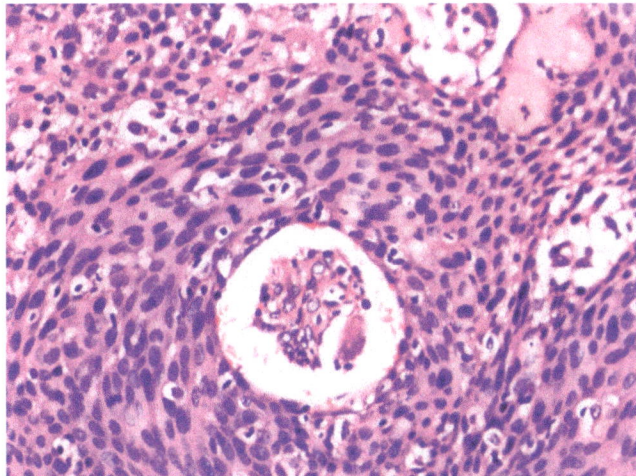

**Figure 6.25:** Features of invasion: Cluster of cells with retraction like space

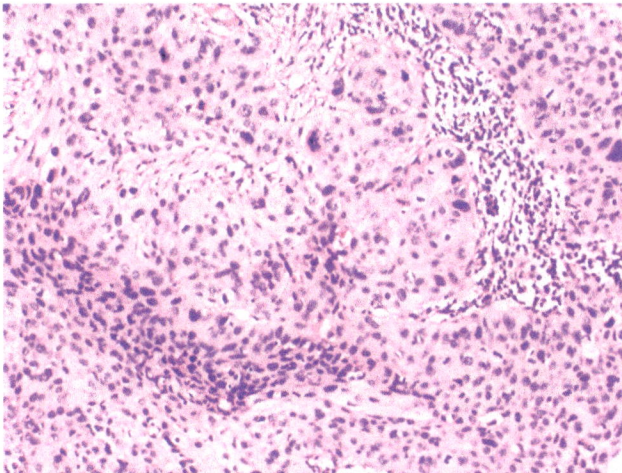

**Figure 6.26:** Features of invasion: Reduplication of the epithelium

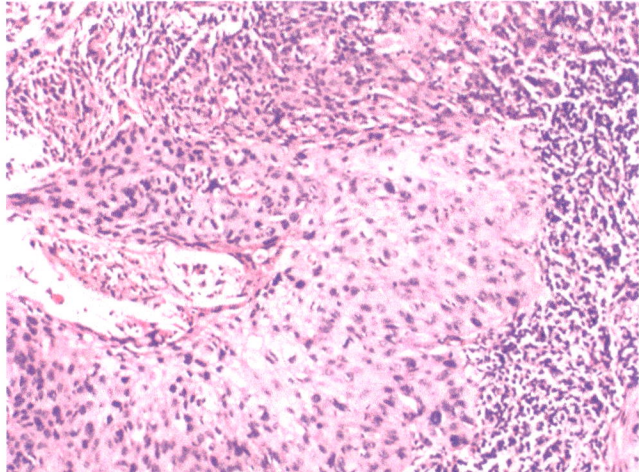

**Figure 6.27:** Features of invasion: Marked loss of polarity and abrupt maturation of the epithelial cells

c. Cautery or crushing artifact
d. Inflammatory or reactive changes.

**Features of lymphovascular involvement:** The features of lymphovascular involvement (LVI) include:
- The tumor cells surrounded by endothelial-lined space within stroma.
- The tumor cells attached with the endothelial lining cells. In case of diagnostic difficulty, the endothelial cell markers such as CD 34 or Factor VIII should be done to prove the vascular space. The mimickers of LVI are:
  - Retraction of tissue during processing mimicking vascular space, and
  - Floaters within the vascular space.

### Measurement of Depth of Invasion

The depth of invasion is estimated from the most superficial epithelial stromal interface of the adjacent epithelium up to the greatest depth of invasion.

### Reporting

In case of reporting of MIC following features should include in the histopathology report:
1. The lateral resection margins of the tissue
2. The width of the tumor
3. The exact depth of invasion
4. The presence of LVI
5. Associated CIN changes in the adjacent epithelium
6. Any glandular differentiation.

### Prognosis

Overall prognosis of MIC is excellent particularly if there is no lymphovascular space involvement. Depth of invasion is well-correlated with lymphovascular invasion. If the depth of tumor is less than 3 mm and no lymphovascular involvement is present then the chance of recurrence is just 0.6%, whereas if depth of invasion is 3–5 mm then chance of recurrence is 15%.[23]

### Treatment of MIC

Simple hysterectomy is sufficient for MIC with less than 3 mm stromal invasion. Radical hysterectomy with pelvic lymphadenectomy is the treatment of choice in case of MIC with more than 3 mm invasion or lymphovascular involvement in less than 3 mm stromal invasion.

## VARIANTS OF SQUAMOUS CELL CARCINOMA

### Basaloid Squamous Cell Carcinoma

This is a rare tumor with an aggressive behavior. The tumor cells are arranged as multiple small nests with minimal stromal reaction. The cells are small basaloid in appearance (Figure 6.28) with scanty cytoplasm and round hyperchromatic nuclei. No keratin pearls are seen.

### Warty Squamous Cell Carcinoma

Warty carcinoma is also known as condylomatous carcinoma. The tumor is very rare. The warty carcinoma shows features of HPV infection with many cells show perinuclear haloes resembling koilocytes.

### Verrucous Squamous Cell Carcinoma

This is a type of well-differentiated squamous cell carcinoma of cervix. It is a very rare tumor in cervix. The tumor presents as large sessile growth simulating condyloma. Microscopy of the tumor is similar to that of vulvo vaginal verrucous carcinoma. The tumor shows broad based bulbous pegs invading within the cervical stroma with typical pushing margin. Individual tumor cells are mature looking in appearance and do not show nuclear atypia. Mitosis and koilocytosis are absent in verrucous carcinoma.[24] This tumor is slow growing and may have local recurrence, however it does not metastasize.

*Differential Diagnosis*

a. **Condyloma accuminata**: Condyloma shows thin vascular papillae and prominent koilocytosis.
b. **Squamous cell carcinoma**: Absence of nuclear atypia in verrucous carcinoma helps to differentiate it from the well-differentiated squamous cell carcinoma.

*Treatment*

Surgical resection is the treatment of choice in this tumor.

### Papillary Squamous Cell Carcinoma

It is a rare variant of squamous cell carcinoma. The tumor is composed of papillae with fibrovascular core lined my malignant squamous cells (Figures 6.29 and 6.30). The cells may be transitional in appearance and the long axis of the tumor cells is perpendicular to the papillae. In typical squamous papillary carcinoma the cells show squamoid in appearance. The tumor shows evidence of invasion in the deeper tissue at the base of the papillae. The tumor is positive for HPV 16 and negative for HPV 6, 11 and 18.[25]

### Differential Diagnosis

Warty carcinoma: In contrast to warty carcinoma, the papillary squamous cell carcinoma shows lack of keratinization and koilocytosis.

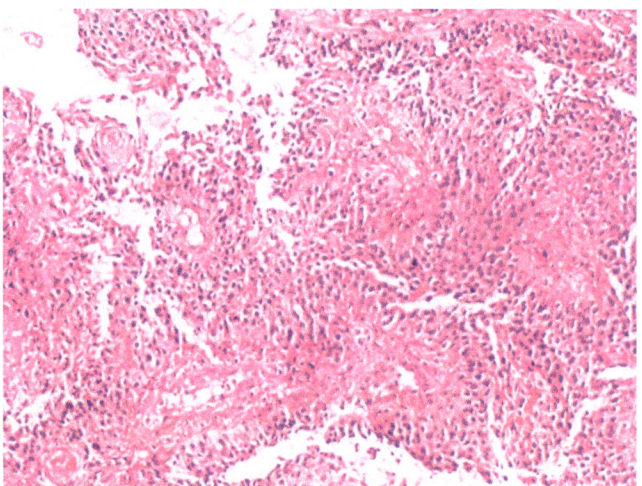

Figure 6.29: Papillary squamous cell carcinoma: Multiple papillae transversely cut

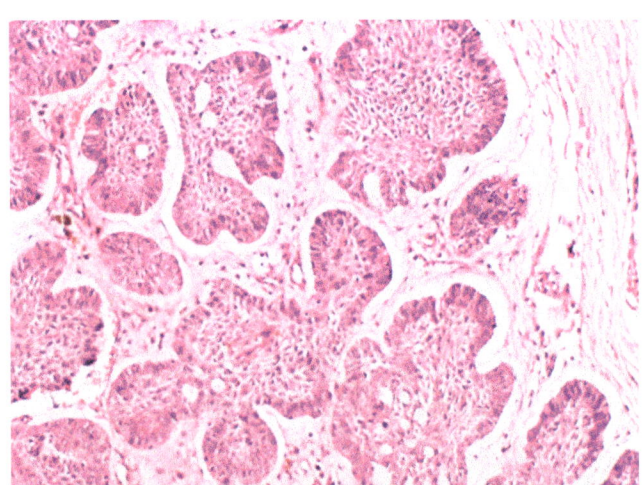

Figure 6.28: Basaloid squamous cell carcinoma: Clusters of malignant squamous cells with peripheral basaloid cells

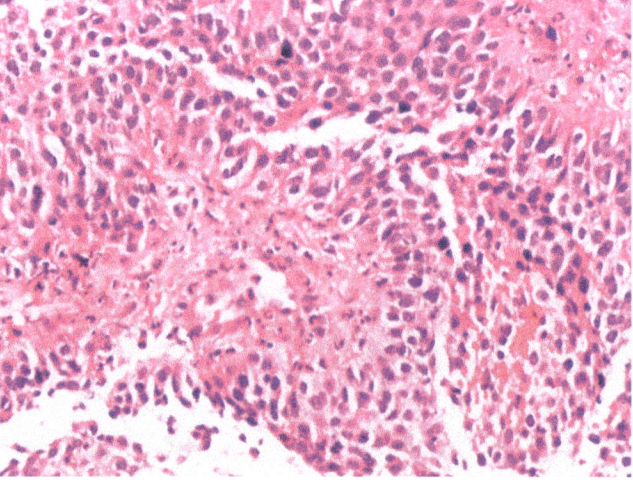

Figure 6.30: Papillary squamous cell carcinoma: Higher magnification shows central blood vessels surrounded by malignant cells

## Squamotransitional Carcinoma

This is a rare tumor and resembles urothelial cell carcinoma of urinary bladder. The tumor is composed of multiple papillary structures lined by multiple layers of atypical epithelial cells. The atypical lining cells may be of three types: clear, intermediate and basaloid cells. The clear cells contain clear vacuolated cytoplasm with centrally placed vesicular nuclei. The intermediate cells show moderate cytoplasm and basaloid cells show scanty cytoplasm with hyperchromatic nuclei. The tumor is positive for CK7 and negative for CK20 immunostaining whereas transitional cell carcinoma of bladder is positive for CK7 and CK20 both.

## Lymphoepithelioma-like Carcinomas

This tumor simulates the nasopharyngeal carcinoma of the oropharynx. The tumor shows multiple nests and sheets of malignant cells with marked lymphocytic infiltration (Figures 6.31 and 6.32). The individual cells have indistinct cytoplasmic margin and give syncytial like appearance. The cells have abundant cytoplasm along with round vesicular nuclei with single prominent nucleoli. The tumor frequently shows EBV DNA (73% cases).[26] The prognosis of this tumor appears to be better than conventional squamous cell carcinoma of cervix.

## Prognosis of Squamous Cell Carcinoma

The overall 5 year survival of squamous cell carcinoma depends mainly on the FIGO staging of carcinoma of cervix as mentioned below:[27]
Stage 1: 90–95%
Stage 2: 50–70%
Stage 3: 30%
Stage 4: 20%.

The histopathological features that are considered as independent prognostic factors include:
1. Depth of tumor invasion
2. Lymphovascular involvement
3. Size of the tumor
4. The lymph nodal and parametrial involvement.

DNA aneuploidy of the tumor along with histological grade can effectively identify the prognostically poor group of patient.[28] p53 over expression in cervical squamous cell carcinoma is associated with poor prognosis of the patient.[29]

## Treatment

Treatment of invasive squamous cell carcinoma depends largely on the FIGO staging:

**Stage IA1:** Conservative surgery such as simple hysterectomy or cone biopsy can be done.

**Stage IA2:** Modified radical hysterectomy and dissection of lymph node.

**Stage IB and IIA:** In this stage either surgery (radical hysterectomy) or radiotherapy is the treatment of choice. The 5 year survival of the patient after radical hysterectomy is almost 100%.[30]

**Stage IIB:** Radiation therapy is treatment of choice in this stage.

**Stage IIIA, B and Stage IVA:** Chemotherapy concurrent with radiotherapy is the treatment of choice.

**Stage IVB:** These patients are mostly treated by palliative therapy.

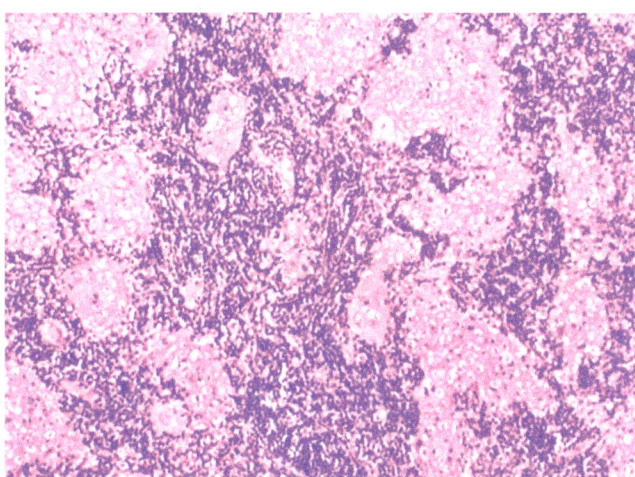

Figure 6.31: Lymphoepithelioma of cervix: Malignant squamoid cells admixed with lymphocytes

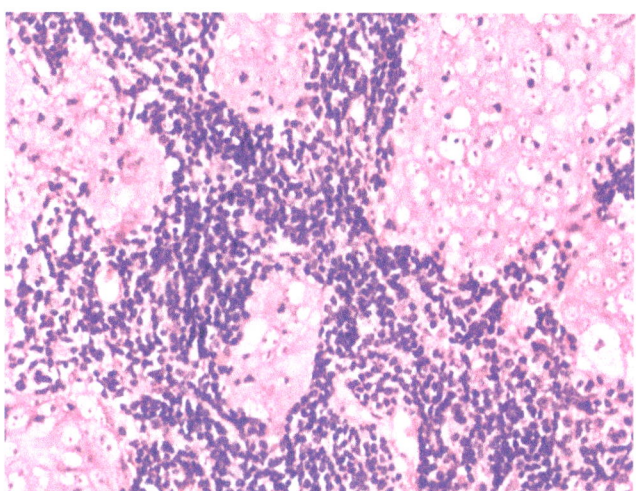

Figure 6.32: Lymphoepithelioma of cervix: Higher magnification shows better morphology of the malignant cells

## REFERENCES

1. Kurman RJ, Carcangiu ML, Herrington S, Young RH. Tumors of vulva. WHO classification of tumors of female genital reproductive organs. 4th Edition, International agency for research on Cancer, Lyon. 2014.
2. Parkin DM, Bray F. Chapter 2: the burden of HPV-related cancers. Vaccine. 2006; 24 (suppl 3):S11-25.
3. de Sanjose S, Quint WG, Alemany L, et al. Human papillomavirus genotype attribution in invasive cervical cancer: a retrospective crosssectional worldwide study. Lancet Oncol. 2010;11:1048-56.
4. Smith JS, Lindsay L, Hoots B, et al. Human papillomavirus type distribution in invasive cervical cancer and high-grade cervical lesions: a meta-analysis update. Int J Cancer. 2007 121(3):621-32.
5. Lizano M, Berumen J, Garcia-Carranca A. HPV-related carcinogenesis: Basic concepts, viral types and variants. Arch Med Res. 2009;40:428-34.
6. McLaughlin-Drubin ME, Münger K. The human papillomavirus E7 oncoprotein. Virology. 2009;384(2):335-44.
7. Ghittoni R, Accardi R, Hasan U, Gheit T, Sylla B, Tommasino M. The biological properties of E6 and E7 oncoproteins from human papillomaviruses. Viral Genes. 2010;40(1):1-13.
8. Cullen A, Reid R, Campion M, Lörincz AT. Analysis of the physical state of different human papillomavirus RNAs in intraepithelial and invasive cervical neoplasia. J Virol. 1991; 65:606-12.
9. Reagan JW, Ng ABP, Wentz WB. Concepts of genesis and development in early cervical neoplasia. Obstet Gynecol Survey. 1969;24:860-74.
10. Richart RM. Cervical intraepithelial neoplasia: a review. Pathol Ann. 1973;8:301-28.
11. Ostor AG. Natural history of cervical intraepithelial neoplasia: a critical review. Int J Gynecol Pathol. 1993;12:186-92.
12. Solomon D, Davey D, Kurman R, et al. The 2001 Bethesda System: terminology for reporting results of cervical cytology. JAMA. 2002;287(16):2114-9.
13. Zhang Q, Kuhn L, Denny LA, et al. Impact of utilizing p16INK4A immunohistochemistry on estimated performance of three cervical cancer screening tests. Int J Cancer. 2007; 120(2):351-56.
14. Alshenawy HA. Pathol Res Pract. Evaluation of p16, human papillomavirus capsid protein L1 and Ki-67 in cervical intraepithelial lesions: Potential utility in diagnosis and prognosis. 2014;210(12):916-21.
15. Melsheimer P, Vinokurova S, Wentzensen N, Bastert G, M. von Knebel Doeberitz. DNA aneuploidy and integration of human papillomavirus type 16 e6/e7 oncogenes in intraepithelial neoplasia and invasive squamous cell carcinoma of the cervix uteri, Clin Cancer Res. 2004;10(9):3059-63.
16. Southern SA, Herrington CS, Differential cell cycle regulation by low- and high-risk human papillomaviruses in low-grade squamous intraepithelial lesions of the cervix, Cancer Res. 1998;58(14):2941-5.
17. Jarboe EA, Thompson LC, Heinz D, McGregor JA, Shroyer KR, Telomerase and human papillomavirus as diagnostic adjuncts for cervical dysplasia and carcinoma. Hum Pathol. 2004;35(4):396-402.
18. Franco EL, Schlecht NF, et al. The epidemiology of cervical cancer. Cancer J. 2003;9(5):348-59.
19. Parkin DM, Bray F, et al. Global cancer statistics, 2002. CA Cancer J Clin. 2005; 55(2):74-108.
20. International Collaboration of Epidemiological Studies of Cervical Cancer. Comparison of risk factors for invasive squamous cell carcinoma and adenocarcinoma of the cervix: collaborative reanalysis of individual data on 8, 097 women with squamous cell carcinoma and 1,374 women with adenocarcinoma from 12 epidemiological studies. Int J Cancer. 2007;120(4):885-91.
21. Pecorelli S. Revised FIGO staging for carcinoma of the vulva, cervix, and endometrium. Int J Gynaecol Obstet. 2009; 105(2):103-4.
22. Ostör AG. Early invasive adenocarcinoma of the uterine cervix. Int J Gynecol Pathol. 2000;19(1):29-38.
23. Copeland LJ, Silva EG, Gershenson DM, Morris M, Young DC, Wharton JT. Superficially invasive squamous cell carcinoma of the cervix. Gynecol Oncol. 1992;45(3):307-12.
24. Zbroch T, Grzegorz Knapp P, Knapp PA. Verrucous carcinoma of the cervix--diagnostic and therapeutic difficulties with regards to HPV status. Case report. Eur J Gynaecol Oncol. 2005;26(2):227-30.
25. Brinck U, Jakob C, Bau O, Füzesi L. Papillary squamous cell carcinoma of the uterine cervix: report of three cases and a review of its classification. Int J Gynecol Pathol. 2000; 19(3):231-5.
26. Tseng CJ, Pao CC, Tseng LH, Chang CT, Lai CH, Soong YK, Hsueh S, Jyu-Jen H. Lymphoepithelioma-like carcinoma of the uterine cervix: association with Epstein-Barr virus and human papillomavirus. Cancer. 1997;80(1):91-7.
27. Benedet JL, Bender H, Jones H 3rd, Ngan HY, Pecorelli S. FIGO staging classifications and clinical practice guidelines in the management of gynecologic cancers. FIGO Committee on Gynecologic Oncology. Int J Gynaecol Obstet. 2000;70(2):209-62.
28. Bichel P, Jakobsen A, Nielsen K, Hølund B, Visfeldt J. Prediction of lymph node metastases in patients with early squamous cell carcinoma of the cervix uteri by histopathological grading and flow cytometry. Eur J Cancer. 1993; 29A(3):337-40.
29. Huang LW, Chou YY, Chao SL, Chen TJ, Lee TT. p53 and p21 expression in precancerous lesions and carcinomas of the uterine cervix: overexpression of p53 predicts poor disease outcome. Gynecol Oncol. 2001;83(2):348-54.
30. Magrina JF, Goodrich MA, Lidner TK, Weaver AL, Cornella JL, Podratz KC. Modified radical hysterectomy in the treatment of early squamous cervical cancer. Gynecol Oncol. 1999;72(2):183-6.

# Glandular and Miscellaneous Lesions of Cervix

## PRENEOPLASTIC LESION OF CERVICAL ADENOCARCINOMA

Adenocarcinoma in situ (AIS) of cervix is uncommon and it constitutes only 1% of all in situ carcinoma of cervix.

### Clinical Features

AIS is common seen in the 4th decade of life and the mean age is 26.8 years.[1] The most of the cases of AIS are asymptomatic at the time of detection. The cases are diagnosed during routine cervical smear screening. It is also seen as an incidental finding in colposcopic-guided biopsy or cone biopsy specimen. AIS is often associated with CIN (30 to 60% cases). The criteria for diagnosis of AIS are summarized as[2] (Figures 7.1 to 7.4):

1. Architectural pattern:
   a. The maintained normal glandular architecture and neoplastic glands are interspersed with normal glands,
   b. Interglandular papillary pattern.
2. Crowding of cells: Nuclei are perpendicular to the lamina with stratification and crowding.
3. Lining cells of the gland:
   a. The atypical cells involve the part or whole of the glandular lining epithelium
   b. Moderate nuclear enlargement
   c. Coarse nuclear chromatin
   d. Prominent nucleoli
   e. Cytoplasm: Acidophilic, dark granular cytoplasm with variable amount of mucin, either absent or abundant.
4. No stromal response.
5. Mitotic activity: Increased.

### AIS as Precursor Lesions of Cervix

The various evidences support that AIS is the precursor lesion of adenocarcinoma of cervix:[2]
1. The mean age of patient with AIS is 10 years less than adenocarcinoma,

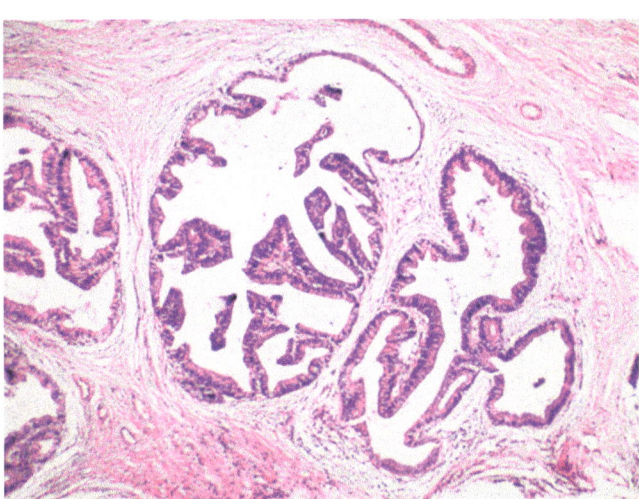

**Figure 7.1:** Adenocarcinoma in situ: The neoplastic glands are surrounded by basement membrane

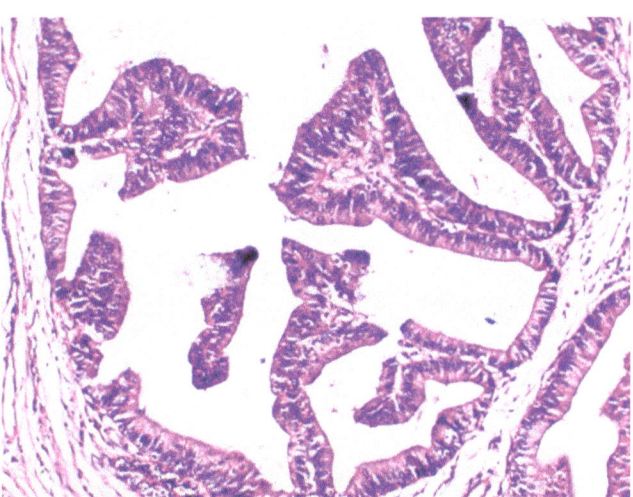

**Figure 7.2:** Adenocarcinoma in situ: Multiple papillary structures are seen

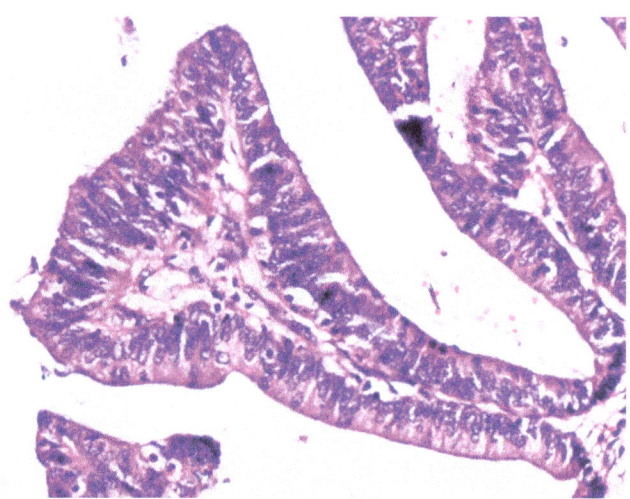

Figure 7.3: Adenocarcinoma in situ: Papillae are lined by atypical cells

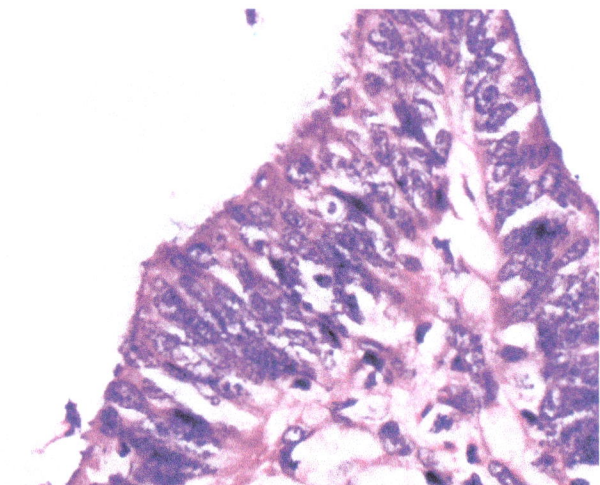

Figure 7.4: Adenocarcinoma in situ: Moderate nuclear pleomorphism and pseudostratification

2. AIS is similar to invasive adenocarcinoma on histology except the evidence of invasion,
3. AIS is often associated with invasive adenocarcinoma,
4. Same HPV types (HPV 16 and HPV 18) have been demonstrated in both AIS and invasive adenocarcinoma,
5. Untreated AIS progressed to invasive adenocarcinoma,
6. Cell cycle regulatory proteins and cell proliferation markers are altered in both AIS and invasive adenocarcinoma.[3]

## Histopathology

Various subtypes of AIS are known. These subtypes have no significant clinical relevance. These subtypes include: Endocervical, endometrial, intestinal, others such as serous type, clear cell type, and adenosquamous.

1. **Endocervical**: This is the most frequent subtype. The lesion resembles normal endocervical glands lined by mucin containing cells with vacuolated, or granular cytoplasm.
2. **Endometrioid**: The lesion simulates hyperplastic endometrial glands. The glandular cells lack any intracellular mucin. The cytoplasm of the cells are dense eosinophilic.
3. **Intestinal type**: This lesion is commonly associated with HPV 18. The lesion shows large number of intestinal goblet cells. In addition argentaffin cells and Paneth cells are also seen. Nuclear pseudostratification and pleomorphism are less recognized due to the abundant mucin in the cell. Mitotic activity is also less in this subtype of AIS. The rate of progression to invasive adenocarcinoma is higher in intestinal AIS than other subtypes.[4]
4. **Others**: Adenosquamous type of AIS shows both squamous and glandular epithelium. Otherwise the lining cells may be intermediate type with the features of both squamous and glandular cells. In lower magnification the lesion may resemble squamous intraepithelial lesion. Tubal type of AIS shows ciliated epithelial lining of fallopian tube.

## Anatomical and topographical distribution of AIS

AIS cannot be visualized by colposcopic examination. The majority of AIS develops from the transformation zone. The AIS cases develop mostly in the superficial part, neck and deep part of the glands and may be focal, multifocal or diffuse. Possibly at the initial time it starts from a single focus and then extends in lateral and horizontal direction.[2] The characteristic of multifocal AIS are: (a) Skip lesion: More than 2 mm gap of two AIS lesions with intervening normal mucosa. (b) No evidence of AIS in complete radial section in between two adjacent AIS sections.

## Immunocytochemistry

AIS shows CEA positivity in majority of the cases (67%). The tumor also shows p53 and p21 positivity.

## Differential Diagnosis

a. Reactive atypia: The following features help to differentiate it from AIS:
   1. Preserved nucleocytoplasmic ratio,
   2. Absent of mitosis, and
   3. Evenly distributed chromatin.

Table 7.1: The differential diagnosis of AIS and endometriosis

|  | AIS | Endometriosis |
|---|---|---|
| Endometrial stroma | Absent | Present |
| Hemosiderin laden histiocytes | Absent | Present |
| Small arterioles filled with blood | Absent | Present |
| P16 | Positive | Negative |
| CEA | Strongly positive | Negative |
| MIB1 | More than 30% cells are positive | Less than 10% cells are positive |
| ProExc | More than 50% cells are positive | Less than 10% cells are positive |
| CD 10 | Negative | Stromal cells are strongly positive |

b. Radiation-induced-atypia: The differentiating features between radiation atypia and AIS include:
  1. Preservation of normal endocervical glandular architecture
  2. Scanty number of glands
  3. Lack of mitosis
  4. Stratification of the lining cells of the glands
  5. Atypical cells are admixed with the normal cells of the glands.
c. Mitotically active endocervical glands: Nuclear stratification and nuclear atypia are absent in mitotically active endocervical glands.
d. Endometriosis: The cases of endometriosis may simulate AIS due to mitotically active endometrial glands with pseudostratification and presence of cytological atypia. Table 7.1 has highlighted the differentiating points in these two lesions.
e. Tubal/tubo-endometrioid metaplasia (TEM): TEM is an incidental finding that is commonly seen after conization of cervix. In this condition, the endocervical epithelium is replaced by fallopian tube like ciliated epithelium or endometrial type epithelium.

## Treatment

Conization of cervix is done in biopsy proved cases of AIS. However residual AIS has been seen in 6 to 30% cases of margin negative cone biopsy specimen who underwent subsequent hysterectomy.[5] Therefore if conization is considered as the sole therapy, then the following things should be removed: (a) Transformation zone, (b) along with 2 cm up the adjacent endocervical canal, and (c) deep part of the endocervical glands.

## EARLY INVASIVE ADENOCARCINOMA (MICROINVASIVE ADENOCARCINOMA)

Microinvasive adenocarcinoma (MIAC) has been described as the glandular tumor with stromal invasion and the invasion is so minimal that there is no risk of lymph nodal metastasis.[6] This lesion is defined as distortion of normal glandular architecture involving the deepest normal crypt and the depth of stromal invasion is less than 5 mm from the basement membrane of the surface epithelium.[7] It was also suggested that instead of one dimensional measurement, volume of the tumor should be considered to define MIAC and tumor volume of less than 500 cu mm should be kept as the definition of MIAC.[8]

### Clinical Features

MIAC is an uncommon entity. It is usually detected in the cone biopsy or hysterectomy specimen. The average age of the patient is 39 year. This lesion is not visible in colposcopy.

### Criteria of Invasion

The most reliable features of invasion include:
1. The presence of isolated cells or fragmented glands lined by malignant looking cells in the stroma.
2. Desmoplastic stromal response or inflammatory cell infiltration around the glands.

Additional criteria of invasion are:
1. Complex branching pattern of the gland
2. Cribriform pattern of glands without any intervening stroma
3. The aggregate of glands below the deep margin of normal endocervical gland. The normal endocervical glands are commonly located within the inner third of the cervical wall.

Adequate attention should be given on the cytological appearance of the glandular cells as inflammatory response may be seen in endocervicitis or microglandular hyperplasia. In a minor proportion of adenocarcinoma cases, there may not be much cytological atypia and the additional criteria mentioned above may be helpful in those cases.

### Histopathology

MIAC may show various pattern of growth such as crab like growth, cribriform pattern, papillary, villoglandular, etc. (Figures 7.5 and 7.6). These patterns may be present singly or in combination. In crab-like invasion, the irregular glands of tumor invade the surrounding stroma like claws of crab. Cribriform pattern shows complex cribriform interluminal

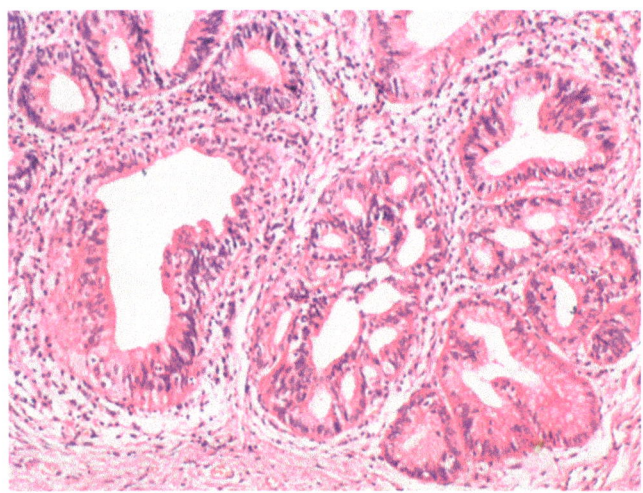

**Figure 7.5:** Microinvasive adenocarcinoma: Complex branching pattern and cribriform appearance of the glands

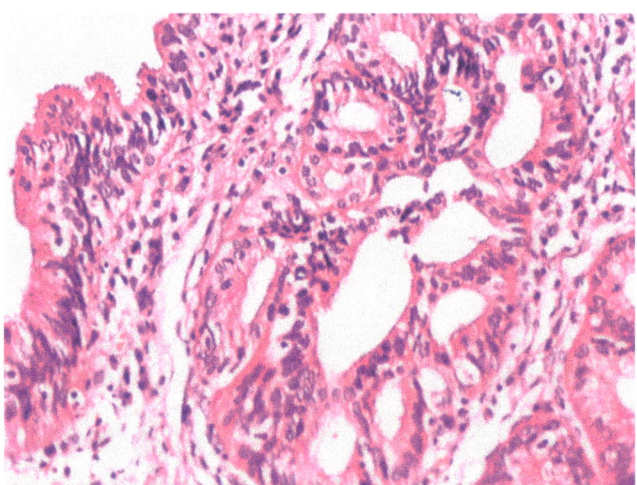

**Figure 7.6:** Microinvasive adenocarcinoma: Higher magnification of the cribriform appearance

branching of tumor cells. In villoglandular pattern, the tumor shows multiple papillary projections which are exophytic and protrude from the surface. The tumor may only show well-differentiated glands that are embedded in the deeper stroma. The adjacent fibrovascular stroma may not show any change. This pattern is difficult to recognize as adenocarcinoma however associated frank invasion may be noted in other part of the specimen.

## Differential Diagnosis

AIS: AIS should be distinguished from MIAC. The absence of complex architectural pattern of the glands and cribriform appearance along with lack of desmoplastic stromal reactivity favor AIS.

## Prognosis and Treatment

MIAC with less than 5 mm invasion usually does not show any lymph nodal metastasis. Hysterectomy completely removes the tumor. Conization of cervix is equally effective if adequate care is taken about the margins of cone and deeper endocervical glands. Conization of cervix is particularly helpful in the female who needs to preserve fertility.

## ADENOCARCINOMA

Adenocarcinoma of cervix shows various histological subtypes. Near about 60% of adenocarcinoma of cervix are mucinous carcinoma. Endometrioid carcinoma of cervix represents 30% of cervical adenocarcinoma. The other variants of adenocarcinoma constitutes the remaining bulk of the tumor.

## Endocervical Adenocarcinoma of Usual Type

### Clinical Feature

The incidence of cervical adenocarcinoma has increased over the period of time. Endocervical adenocarcinoma of cervix comprises of 70% of all cervical carcinoma and this is the most common cervical adenocarcinoma. The mean age of the patient is 55 years. The patient presents with the complaint of vaginal bleeding. The mass is detected on pervaginal examination.

### Histopathology (Figures 7.7 to 7.14)

The tumor is composed of multiple closely spaced or discerete glands. The glands show cribriform pattern or papillary projections. Occasionaly solid clusters of cells are also noted. The stroma around the gland may show desmoplastic

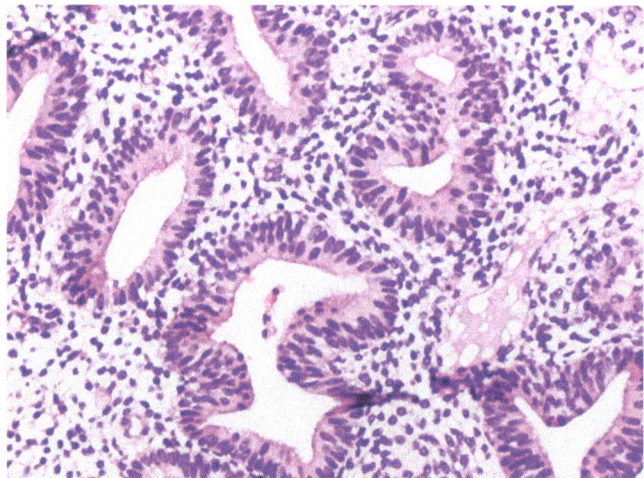

**Figure 7.7:** Endocervical adenocarcinoma: Multiple closely spaced glands

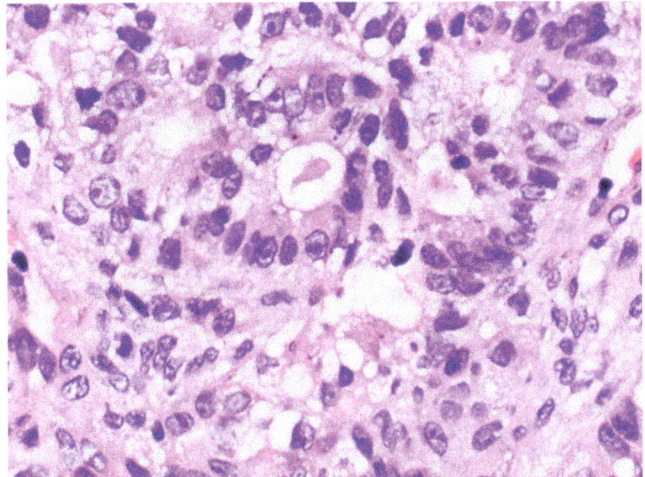

**Figure 7.8:** Endocervical adenocarcinoma: The glands are lined by moderate pleomorphic cells

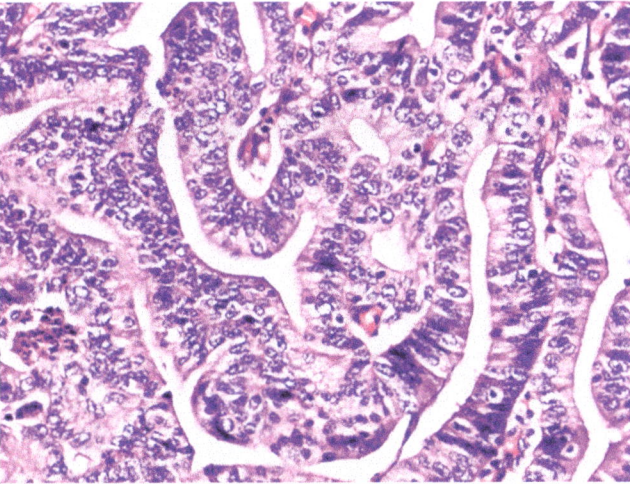

**Figure 7.11:** Higher magnification of well-differentiated endocervical adenocarcinoma

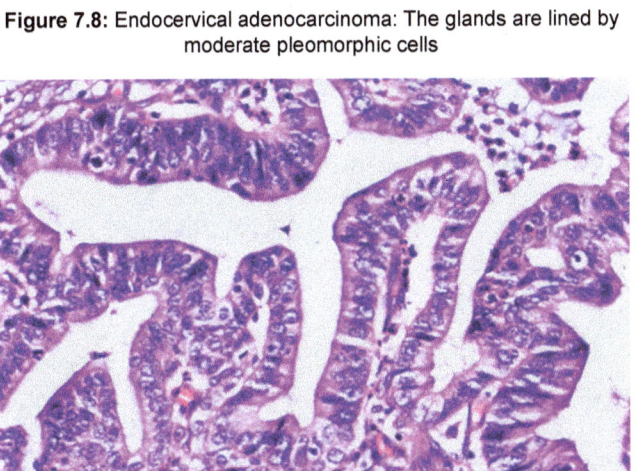

**Figure 7.9:** Endocervical adenocarcinoma: Papillary projection

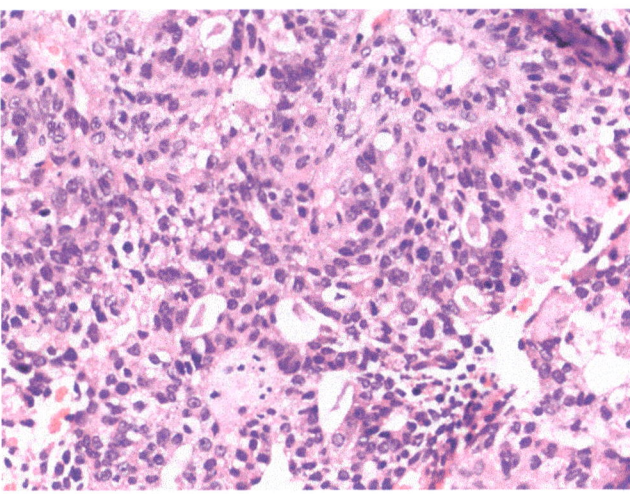

**Figure 7.12:** Moderately differentiated endocervical adenocarcinoma: Glands with solid areas

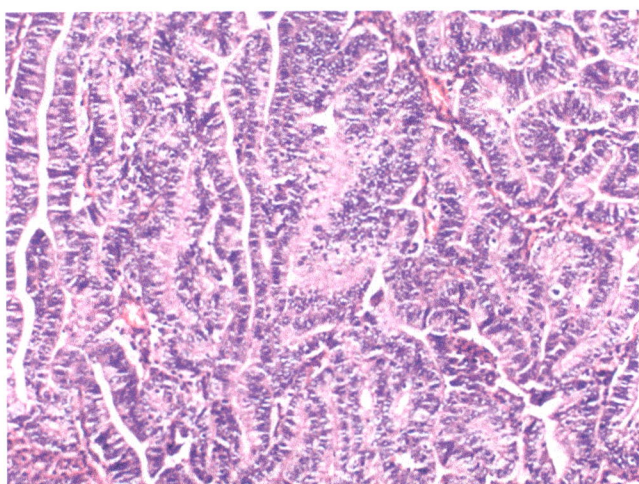

**Figure 7.10:** Well-differentiated endocervical adenocarcinoma: Closely-packed glands with no solid area

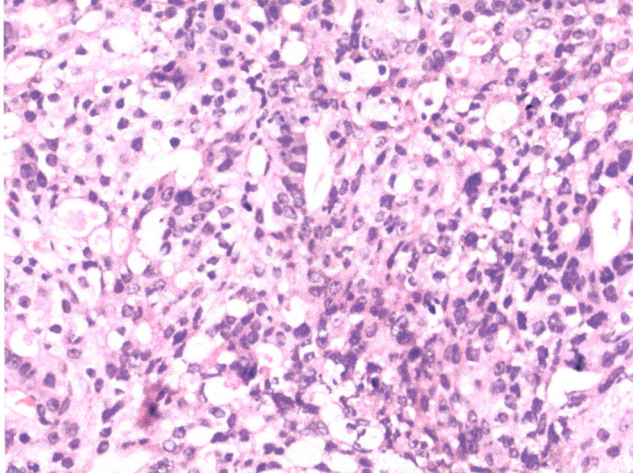

**Figure 7.13:** Poorly differentiated endocervical adenocarcinoma: Mainly solid areas along with occasional glands are seen

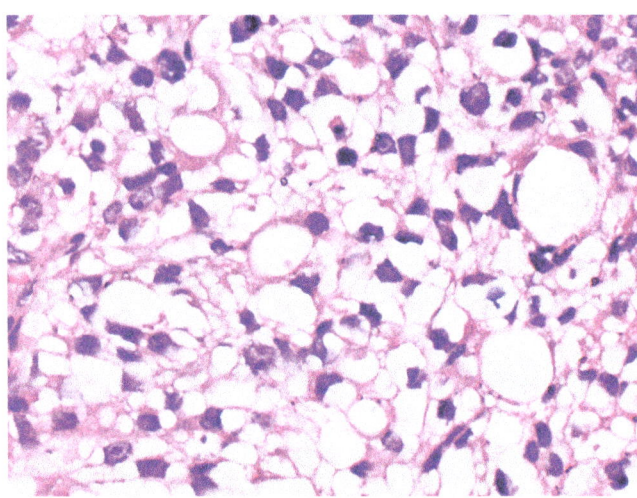

**Figure 7.14:** Higher magnification of poorly-differentiated endocervical adenocarcinoma

reaction. The glands are lined by mucin secreting endocervical cells. The individual cells are tall columnar with abundant pale cytoplasm. The nuclei are basally placed and enlarged with coarse chromatin having prominent nucleoli. The tumor shows frequent mitosis and apotosis. Pool of extracellular mucin may also be noted. The tumor is graded according to the percentage of glandular components (Table 7.2). Associated AIS changes or CIN changes may also be noted in 40% cases of endocervical adenocarcinoma.

**Table 7.2:** Grade of adenocarcinoma

| Adenocarcinoma grade | Description |
| --- | --- |
| Grade 1 | 90% of the tumor volume shows glands and only less than 10% solid component |
| Grade 2 | 11 to 49% of the tumor volume shows solid component |
| Grade 3 | More than 50% is solid component |

## Intestinal Type of Adenocarcinoma

The tumor resembles colonic adenocarcinoma. The intestinal epithelium may be present in focal areas in a mucinous tumor. The tumor frequently shows goblet cells. Uncommonly Paneth cells and neuroendocrine cells are also seen. The intestinal type of adenocarcinoma shows CDX positivity, diffuse CK 7 and variable CK 20 positivity.[9]

## Signet Ring Carcinoma

Pure signet ring carcinoma is a rare tumor. Focal signet ring type of cells are seen in poorly differentiated mucinous adenocarcinoma. Metastatic signet ring carcinoma are more common than primary signet ring carcinoma of cervix and this possibility should be excluded.

## Minimal Deviation Adenocarcinoma

Minimal deviation adenocarcinoma (MDA) is also called as adenoma malignum as the tumor resembles normal endocervical glands. The tumor represents only 1 to 3% of cervical adenocarcinoma.[10]

### Clinical Features

The average age of the patient is about 40 years. The patient presents with menorrhagia or vaginal discharge. This tumor (10 to 15% patients) is strongly related with Peutz–Jeghers syndrome.

### Histopathology

The cervix is firm and indurated and the mucosa is hemorrhagic and friable. Microscopic examination shows architecturally abnormal glands. The glands show irregular complex branching, out pouching, papillary infolding and irregular shape. The glands are typically surrounded by desmoplastic stroma. Unlike normal endocervical glands that are superficially located these glands are seen in the deeper part of cervical wall mostly in outer third. The glands are lined by bland looking tall mucous secreting columnar cells with basally placed nuclei having minimal pleomorphism. Occasional glands may show moderate nuclear atypia of the lining cells. The diagnosis of MDA is not possible on biopsy specimen and hysterectomy specimen may be needed to assess the depth of penetration of the glands.

### Immunocytochemistry

MDA is variably positive for CEA and negative for ER and PR. The tumor is also positive for HIK-1083, a marker of gastric mucosal cells.[11]

### Differential Diagnosis

a. Tunnel cluster: In tunnel cluster, the glands do not show any architectural abnormality and no atypia or mitotic activity is seen.
b. Normal endocervical glands: Normal endocervical glands are usually located within the superficial 1/3rd of the cervical wall.
c. Lobular endocervical glandular hyperplasia: The lobular endocervical glandular hyperplasia shows lobular configuration and remains within the inner half of the cervical wall.

## Villoglandular Adenocarcinoma

This is an uncommon variant of adenocarcinoma that occurs in younger woman and the average age of the patient is 33 years. Villoglandular adenocarcinoma is a type of well-differentiated adenocarcinoma characterized by multiple finger-like papillary projections from the mucosal surface. This villous like fronds resemble villi of the colon. The papillae may be short or long with central vascular structure. The lining cells of papillary structures may be endocervical, endometrioid or intestinal type. The nuclei of the cells show minimal atypia with scattered mitotic activities. The typical recognizable stromal invasion may not be detected. However, rarely deep tumor invasion is seen. The stromal invasion of villoglandular adenocarcinoma is seen as irregular branching glands in the base of the papillary surface with intervening desmoplastic stromal reaction.

*Differential Diagnosis*

a. Filiform papillary growth of AIS: The filiform papillary growth of AIS may simulate villoglandular adenocarcinoma. However typical villus like structure is absent in such lesion.
b. Papillary endocervicitis: The lesion differs from villoglandular adenocarcinoma by the complete absence of nuclear atypia.
c. Serous papillary adenocarcinoma: The multiple papillary structures of serous papillary adenocarcinoma may simulate villoglandular adenocarcinoma. However serous papillary adenocarcinoma shows much more irregular complex papillae and the tumor cells show marked nuclear enlargement and pleomorphism.
d. Papillary adenofibroma: The papillae of the papillary adenofibroma show much more stromal tissue in the central core. The lining cells are completely bland.

*Prognosis and Treatment*

The prognosis of villoglandular adenocarcinoma is overall good. In large series no metastasis have been reported when this carcinoma is treated by conization.[12] Therefore, conservative surgery such as cone biopsy can be done if there is no evidence of deep invasion or lymphovascular space involvement.

## ENDOMETRIOID ADENOCARCINOMA

Endometrioid adenocarcinoma represents near about 30% of cervical adenocarcinoma. The tumor resembles endometrial adenocarcinoma. Histopathology of the tumor shows complex glandular arrangement (Figures 7.15 to 7.17). Cribriform and papillary arrangements are also seen. The individual cells are smaller in size and contain less cytoplasm than endocervical adenocarcinoma. No mucin is seen in the cytoplasm of the cells. Foci of squamous differentiation may also be seen.

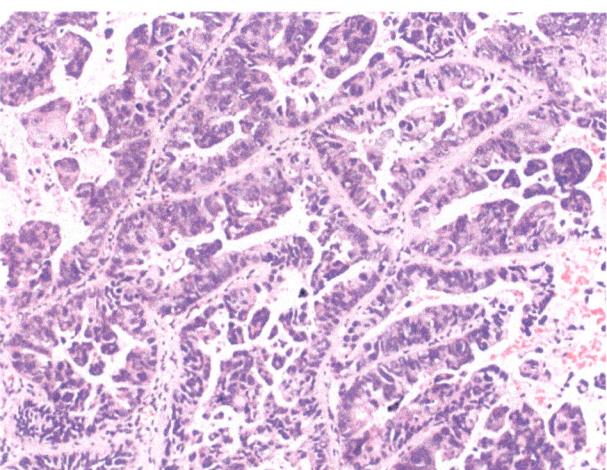

**Figure 7.15:** Endometrioid adenocarcinoma of cervix: The tumor resembles endometrial glands

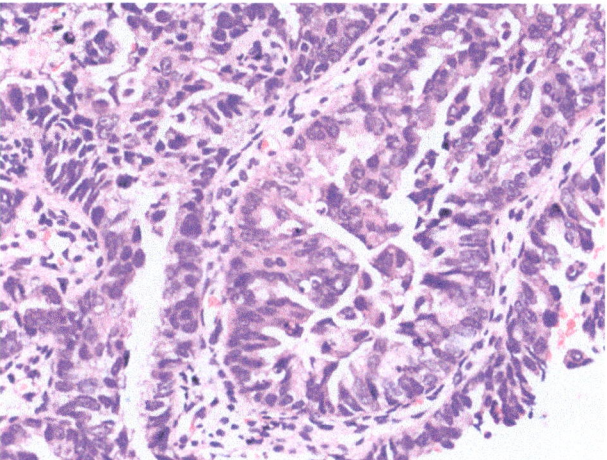

**Figure 7.16:** Endometrioid adenocarcinoma of cervix: Higher magnification shows cuboidal cells with moderate nuclear atypia

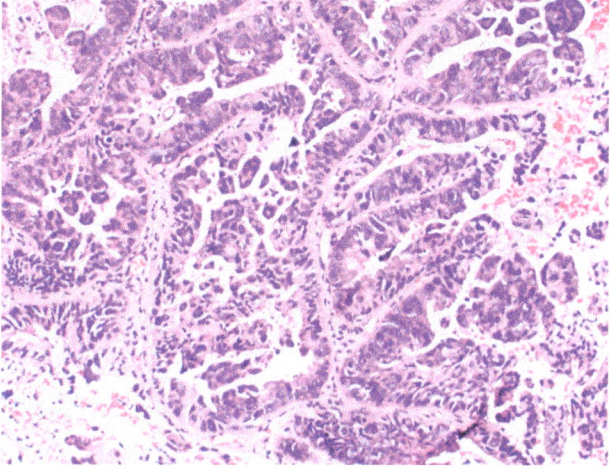

**Figure 7.17:** Endometrioid adenocarcinoma of cervix: Multiple papillary infolding of the lining epithelium

## Differential Diagnosis

Endometrioid carcinoma of uterus: In case of uterine endometrioid carcinoma, the main bulk of tumor remains in the uterus and uterus is bulky and enlarged. In primary cervical endometrioid carcinoma, the uterus is usually normal in size and the cervix shows enlargement. Fractional curettage of such tumor may show normal endometrial tissue along with endometrioid carcinoma. In addition, primary endometrioid carcinoma of uterus shows ER/PR and p16 positivity and CEA negativity.

## CLEAR CELL CARCINOMA

This is a rare tumor and represents about 4% of cervical adenocarcinoma. The tumor is related with DES exposure in uterus.[13]

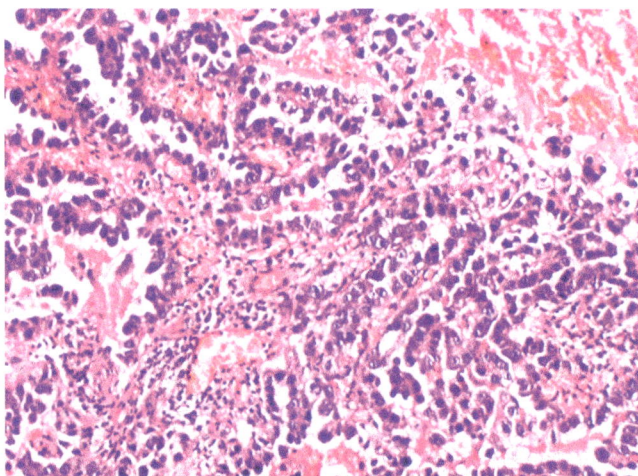

Figure 7.18: Clear cell carcinoma of cervix: Multiple papillary structures lined by tumor cells

### Histology (Figures 7.18 to 7.20)

The tumor resembles ovarian or endometrial clear cell carcinoma. The tumor shows predominantly three patterns: solid, tubulocystic and papillary. The tumor cells contain abundant clear vacuolated cytoplasm containing glycogen which can be demonstrated by PAS stain. The nuclei are enlarged, hyperchromatic with prominent nucleoli. Characteristic protrusion of nuclei from the tip of the cells, known as "hobnail appearance", is also seen.

### Differential Diagnosis

Microglandular hyperplasia: Lack of nuclear atypia in microglandular hyperplasia helps to differentiate it from clear cell carcinoma. Arias Stella reaction: Arias Stella reaction may simulate clear cell carcinoma because of the presence of clear cells. However, the lack of nuclear atypia and mitosis are helpful distinguishing features.

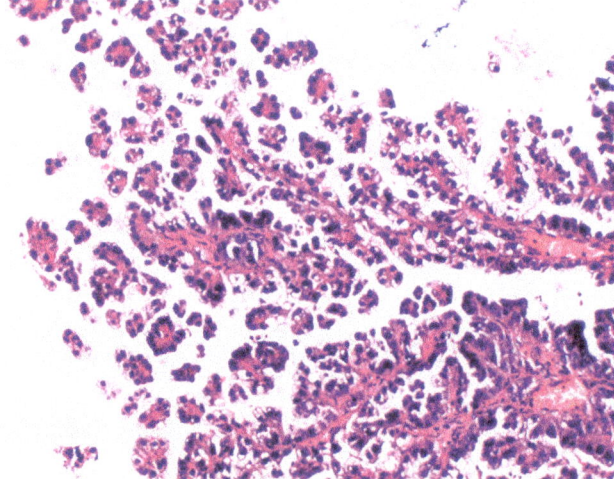

Figure 7.19: Clear cell carcinoma of cervix: Hobnail appearance

## SEROUS ADENOCARCINOMA

This is a rare tumor and represents only 1% of cervical adenocarcinoma. Before the diagnosis of primary serous adenocarcinoma of cervix the possibility of metastasis from other sites should be eliminated. Histologically the tumor simulates ovarian serous adenocarcinoma (Figures 7.21 and 7.22). The tumor consists of multiple complex papillary structures lined by cells with enlarged nuclei having prominent nucleoli. Frequent mitotic activities are also noted.[14]

## MESONEPHRIC CARCINOMA

This is a very rare carcinoma. The tumor develops from the mesonephric remnants in the lateral cervical wall. The mean age of the patient is 53 years. The patient usually complains of vaginal bleeding.

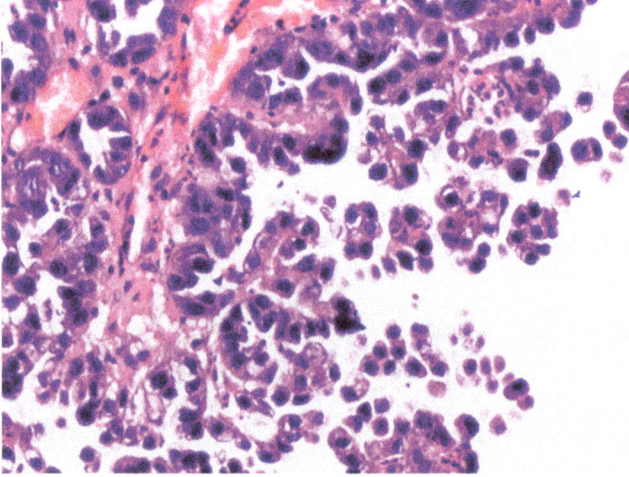

Figure 7.20: Clear cell carcinoma of cervix: Individual tumor cells show moderate amount of clear cytoplasm

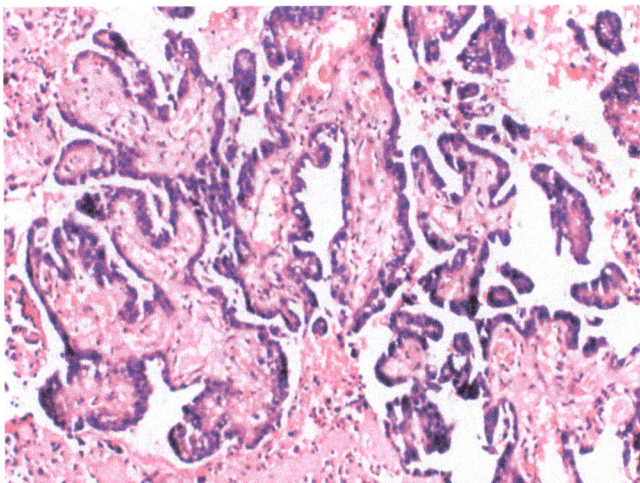

Figure 7.21: Papillary serous carcinoma of cervix: Multiple papillary structures lined by cuboidal cells

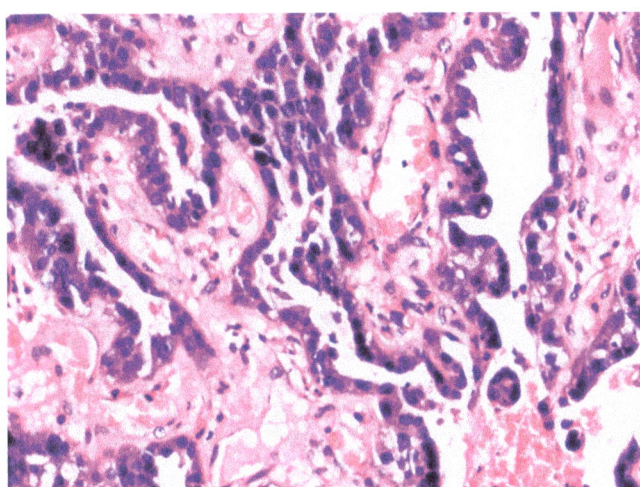

Figure 7.22: Papillary Serous carcinoma of cervix: Higher magnification shows cells with nuclear pleomorphism

## Histopathology

The tumor is typically located in the outer third or lateral wall of the cervix. Histologic pattern of mesonephric carcinoma include tubular, solid, retiform, or papillary type. Out of these patterns tubular pattern is the most commonly encountered. The tumor is composed of variable sized irregular tubules. The tubules often contain PAS positive and diastase resistant eosinophilic secretion. The tubules are lined by single to multiple layers of small columnar cells with moderate nuclear pleomorphism. Rarely, the tumor shows nonspecific malignant spindle cells component. In combination with malignant glands the spindle cells predominant tumor resembles carcinosarcoma.

## Immunohistochemistry

The cells of mesonephric carcinoma are positive for EMA, calretinin, CK7 and CD 10. The tumor is negative for ER, PR and CK 20.[15]

## Differential Diagnosis

a. Clear cell carcinoma: Mesonephric carcinoma is typically located in the outer wall of the cervix.
b. Mesonephric hyperplasia: Both the lesions are located in the lateral wall of the cervix. However, mesonephric carcinoma shows nuclear pleomorphism.
c. Carcinosarcoma: Predominant spindle cell component of mesonephric carcinoma may be confused with carcinosarcoma.

## ADENOSQUAMOUS CARCINOMA

Adenosquamous carcinoma of cervix represents about 25% of all cervical carcinoma. The mean age of the patient is 57 years.

### Histology (Figures 7.23 to 7.25)

The tumor is composed of malignant glands along with malignant squamous component. The glandular component may be of mucinous or endometrioid type. The squamous cells show intercellular bridge, intracellular keratin and squamous pearls. It has been shown that both the squamous and glandular component are originated from the common stem cell.[16]

## GLASSY CELL CARCINOMA

This is a type of adenosquamous cell carcinoma and represents less than 1% of cervical carcinoma. The glassy

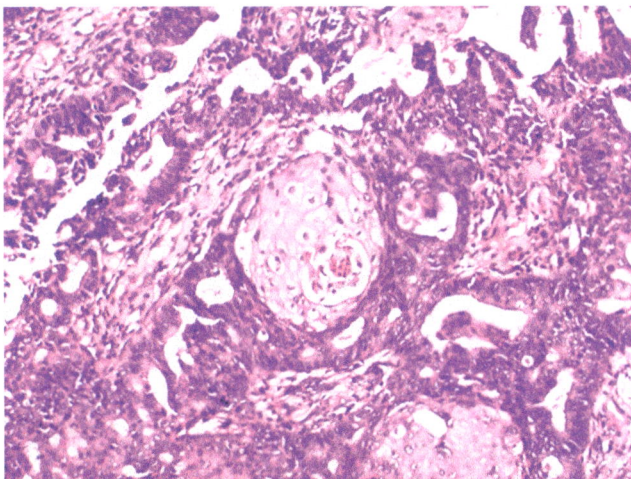

Figure 7.23: Adenosquamous carcinoma of cervix: Both glandular and squamoid cells

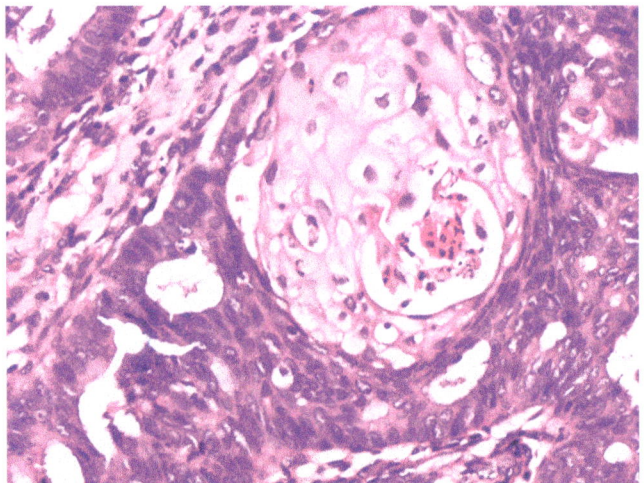

Figure 7.24: Adenosquamous carcinoma of cervix: Higher magnification shows collection of squamous cells

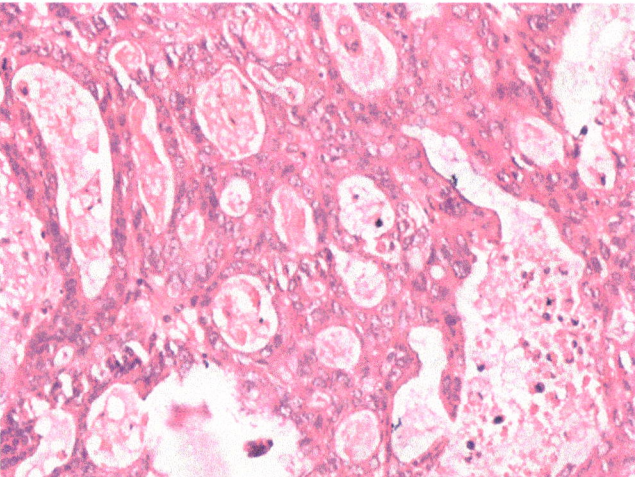

Figure 7.26: Adenoid cystic carcinoma of cervix: Multiple cribriform like glands

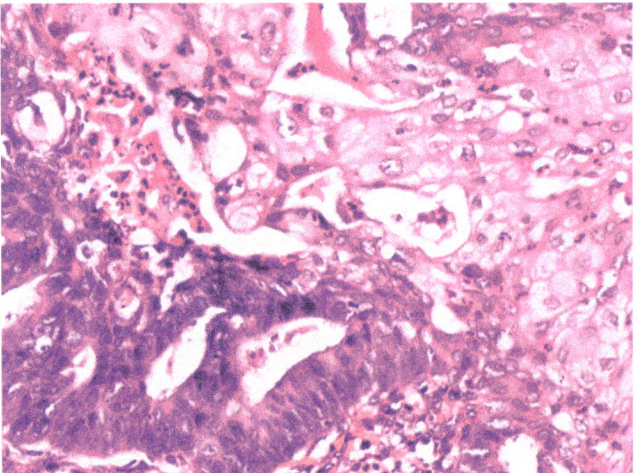

Figure 7.25: Adenosquamous carcinoma of cervix: Malignant glands and diffuse sheets of squamous cells

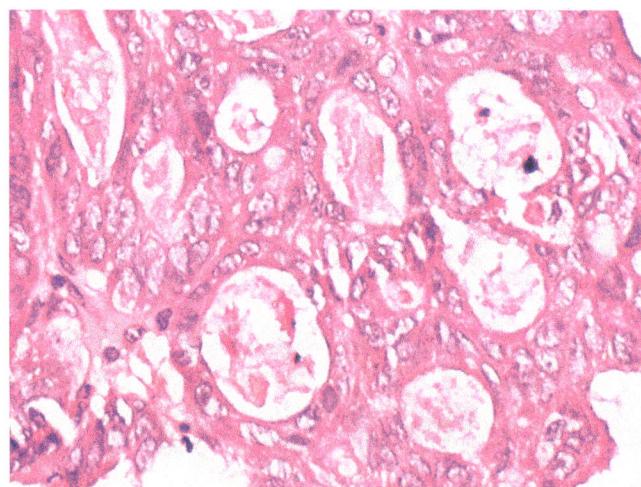

Figure 7.27: Adenoid cystic carcinoma of cervix: Higher magnification shows central pinkish material surrounded by round cells with monomorphic nuclei

cell carcinoma shows solid sheets of cells having abundant glassy cytoplasm, distinct cell border and prominent large nucleoli. The tumor is infiltrated by large number of lymphocytes and polymorphs. The tumor cells lack typical intercellular bridges and intracellular mucin.

## ADENOID CYSTIC CARCINOMA (ADC)

ADC is a rare tumor and represents less than 1% of cervical carcinoma. The tumor is commonly seen over 60 years and average of the patient is 71 years.[17]

## Histology (Figures 7.26 and 7.27)

Histology section shows cribriform, solid, or cystic pattern. The individual cells are basaloid in appearance with scanty cytoplasm and enlarged hyperchromatic nuclei. The gland like structures contain eosinophilic hyaline material that represents basal lamina and therefore positive for laminin and type IV collagen. Solid nest of cells with peripheral palisading arrangement is also seen. Focal necrosis, squamous differentiation and brisk mitosis have also been described.

## Immunohistochemistry

The tumor cells are positive for S-100, collagen IV and laminin.

## Prognosis

This is an aggressive tumor and it often shows local recurrence and distant metastasis.[18]

## ADENOID BASAL CELL CARCINOMA (ABC)

ABC is a rare tumor and represents less than 5% of cervical carcinomas. The tumor is most commonly seen elderly patients with mean age 71 years. The patient is usually asymptomatic and is detected incidentally in conization or hysterectomy specimen.[19] Both ABC and ACC originate from reserve cells however ABC is a much less aggressive carcinoma than ACC. ABC is often associated with high grade CIN. HPV 16 DNA has been demonstrated in most of the cases of ABC.

### Histopathology

The tumor shows multiple small variable-sized nests of epithelial cells composed of basaloid cells with scanty cytoplasm and bland nuclei. At the periphery of the nests, the cells are arranged in palisading manner. Mitotic activity is low in ABC. Some tumor cells show lobules like arrangement. Cords of cells and occasional cystic spaces may also be noted. The infiltrating nests of tumor cells do not show any stromal reaction. However a thin rim of stromal edema and mild lymphocytic infiltration may surround the infiltrating cells as thin rim. Squamoid differentiation is also described in the central part of the nests of cell in many cases of ABC. Extensive squamous cell differentiation in ABC may be mistaken as squamous cell carcinoma. Occasionally ABC shows cribriform appearance and simulates ADC. However unlike ADC, no eosinophilic central hyaline material is seen in the ABC.

### Differential Diagnosis

ADC: Both ADC and ABC have overlapping histological features. However extensive cribriform pattern is not seen in ABC. The typical characteristic eosinophilic material is also absent in ABC. The nodules of cells are much larger in ADC (Table 7.3).

### Prognosis

ABC has very good prognosis. Metastasis of ABC in the lymph node or other sites has not been described. In fact due to its excellent prognosis term "adenoid basal epithelioma" is suggested instead of adenoid basal carcinoma.[19] Because of its benign behavior, radical surgery or radiation therapy may not be necessary in stage I tumor and cold knife conization may be sufficient for treatment of ABC.

## NEUROENDOCRINE CARCINOMA

Neuroendocrine tumors of cervix includes: large cell neuro-endocrine carcinoma, carcinoid, atypical carcinoid and small cell carcinoma.

## SMALL CELL CARCINOMA OF CERVIX

Small cell carcinoma of cervix comprises of less than 6% of cervical carcinoma. The average age of the patient is 36 years which is much lower than cervical squamous cell carcinoma. The patients present with vaginal bleeding. Occasional patients may present with paraneoplastic syndrome. The tumor is also related with HPV 16 and 18 infections.[20]

### Histopathology (Figures 7.28 to 7.30)

The tumor may present as small ulcerated lesion to large mass. Histology section shows small nests, trabecular, solid or insular pattern of cells. The cells are small round with scanty cytoplasm. The nuclei are enlarged with fine stippled appearance and may show molding. Elongated spindle-shaped nuclei are also seen. Nuclear smudging and crushing artifact are also noted. Mitotic activity is brisk.

### Immunocytochemistry

The tumor is positive for NSE, chromogranin and synaptophysin. In addition, the cells are also positive for EMA and variable expression of low molecular weight cytokeratin.[21]

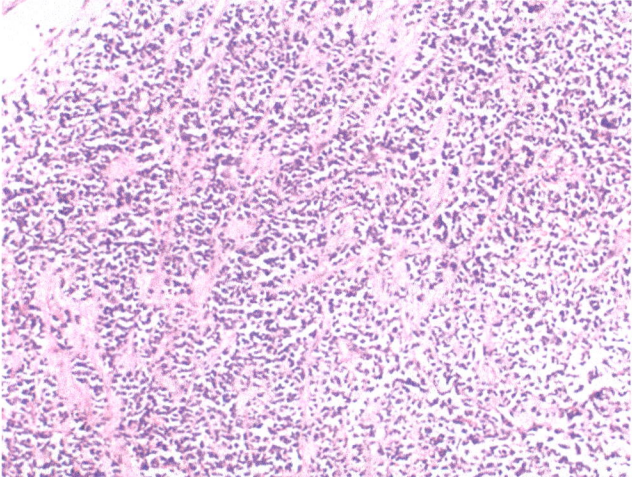

Figure 7.28: Small cell carcinoma of cervix: diffuse sheet of malignant small round cells

Table 7.3: Adenoid basal cell carcinoma versus adenoid cystic carcinoma

| Features | Adenoid basal cell carcinoma | Adenoid cystic carcinoma |
| --- | --- | --- |
| Cribriform appearance | Less frequent | More frequent |
| Eosinophilic hyaline material | Absent | Present |
| Nuclear pleomorphism | Mild | Moderate |
| Behavior | Mostly benign | Aggressive |

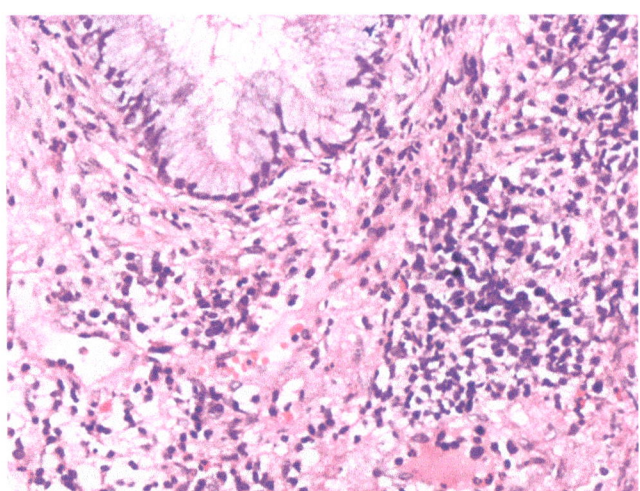

**Figure 7.29:** Small cell carcinoma of cervix: Discrete round cells in the cervical stroma

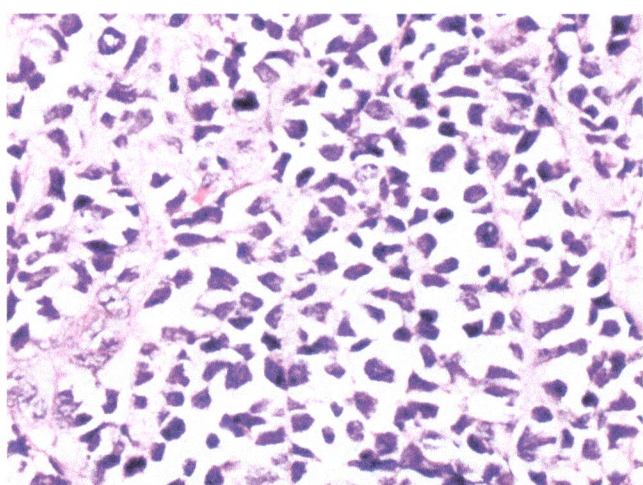

**Figure 7.30:** Small cell carcinoma of cervix: Higher magnification shows better cell morphology. The cells have hyperchromatic round nuclei with inconspicuous nucleoli

**Table 7.4:** Differences between small cell carcinoma versus non-keratinizing squamous cell carcinoma

| Features | Small cell carcinoma | Non-keratinizing squamous cell carcinoma |
|---|---|---|
| Pattern | Nests, insular, trabecular | Solid sheet |
| Crushing artifact | Present | Absent |
| Nuclear molding | Present | Absent |
| Neuroendocrine markers | Positive | May be focally positive in focal neuroendocrine differentiation |
| CK | Positive in some cases | Always positive |
| TTF-1 | Positive | Negative |
| p-63 | Negative | Positive |
| Chromogranin | Positive | Negative |

## Differential Diagnosis

Non-keratinizing squamous cell carcinoma: Differentiating points have been highlighted in Table 7.4.

## Prognosis and Treatment

It is an aggressive tumor and most patients die within one year of diagnosis. Surgery and adjuvant chemotherapy is the treatment of choice.

## CARCINOID AND ATYPICAL CARCINOID OF CERVIX

Both these tumors are very rare in cervix. The morphology of these tumors is similar as that of other regions.

## LARGE CELL NEUROENDOCRINE CARCINOMA

The tumor shows typical organoid, trabecular and cord like arrangement of cells. The individual cells are large with moderate amount of cytoplasm. The nuclei are large nuclei with prominent nucleoli. Frequent mitotic activities are seen.

### Immunocytochemistry

The tumor cells are positive for NSE, chromogranin and synaptophysin. Frequently the tumor express cytokeratin and CEA.

### Prognosis

The tumor is aggressive and behaves same as small cell carcinoma.

## METASTATIC CARCINOMA IN CERVIX

The common primary site of metastatic carcinoma of cervix is the female genital tract.[22] The metastasis may come from endometrium followed by ovary and fallopian tube. The tumor is recognized either by lymphovascular involvement or by stromal invasion. The endometrial carcinoma commonly spreads to the cervix by direct extension. Serous carcinoma from the fallopian tube or ovary may also metastasize in the cervix. The other common primary sources of metastasis are breast, lung, kidney and gastrointestinal tract. Characteristic morphology of the primary tumor and immunocytochemistry are helpful to identify the source of the tumor.

## MESENCHYMAL TUMORS

### Leiomyoma

Leiomyoma of cervix is the commonest benign mesenchymal tumor of cervix and it represents about 8% of total leiomyoma of uterus. Morphology of cervical leiomyoma is similar as that of uterine leiomyoma (Figures 7.31 and 7.32).

### Malignant Mesenchymal Tumors

The malignant mesenchymal tumors of the cervix include leiomyosarcoma, endocervical stromal sarcoma, embryonal rhabdomyosarcoma, alveolar soft part sarcoma, malignant schwannomas, and angiosarcoma. The primary sarcoma of cervix is exceedingly rare and it represents only 0.5% of all cervical malignancies.

### Leiomyosarcoma (Figures 7.33 to 7.35)

This is the commonest primary sarcoma of cervix. The patients usually presents with vaginal bleeding. Clinical examination reveals polypoidal mass in the cervix. The tumor shows interlacing bundles of oval to elongated spindle cells with moderate nuclear pleomorphism, coagulative necrosis and high mitotic activity (more than 10 per 10 high power fields). Similar to uterus, at least two criteria should be present out of these three criteria mentioned above.

### Endometrial Stromal Sarcoma

Primary endometrial stromal sarcoma of cervix is rare. The tumor is characterized by diffuse sheet of small oval to spindle cell along with network of thin blood vessels.

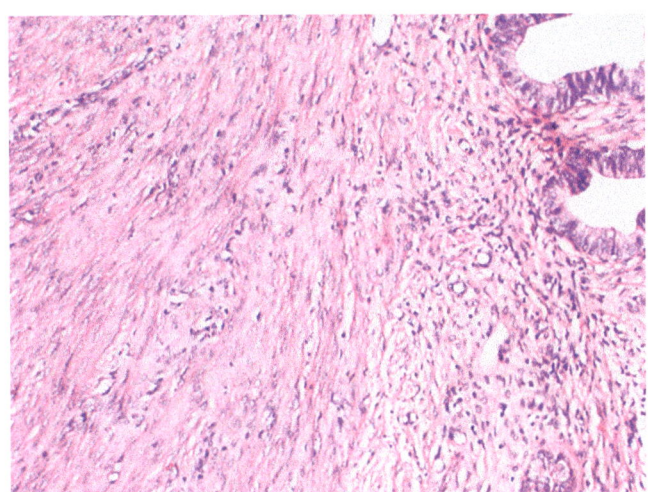

Figure 7.31: Leiomyoma cervix: Tumor presenting as endocervical polyp. Oval to spindle cells in bunch

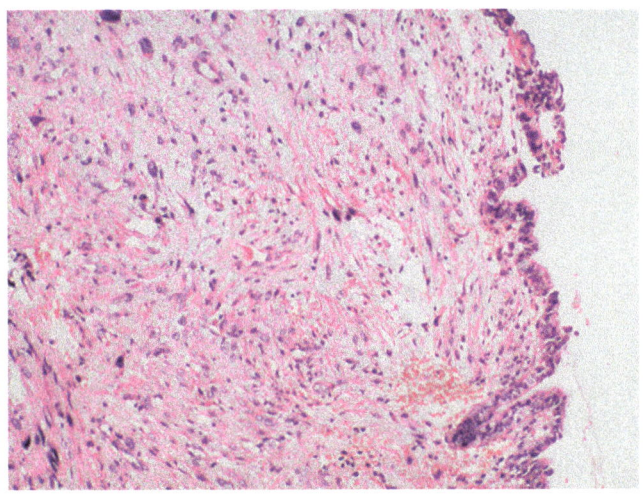

Figure 7.33: Leiomyosarcoma of cervix: The oval to spindle-shaped malignant cells in small fascicles

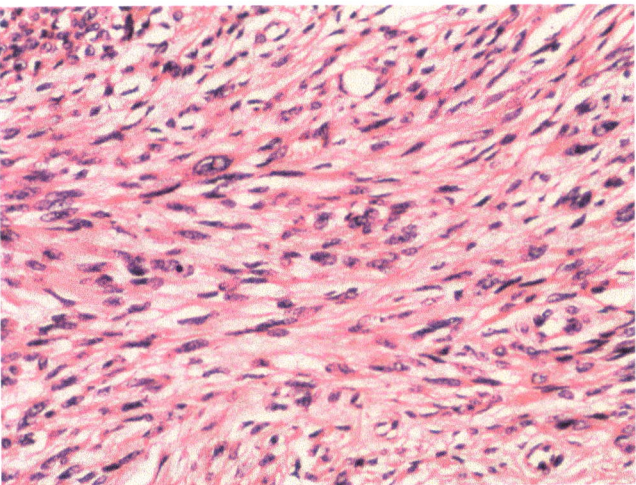

Figure 7.32: Leiomyoma cervix: Fascicles of spindle cells

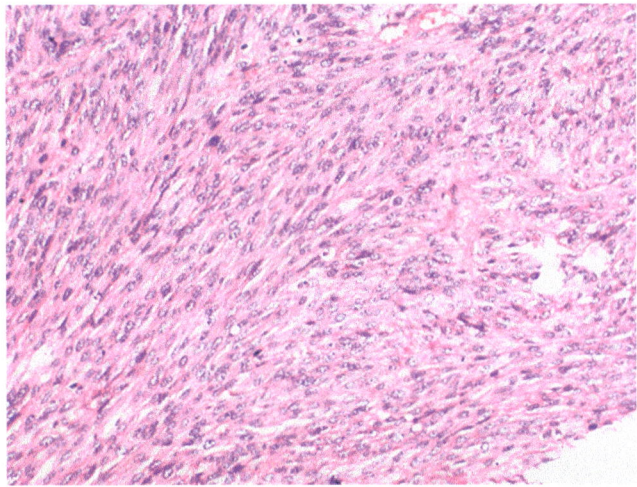

Figure 7.34: Leiomyosarcoma of cervix: Bundles of spindle cells

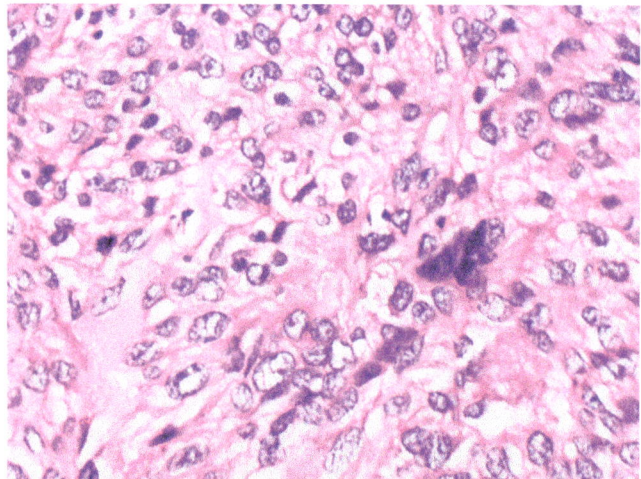

Figure 7.35: Leiomyosarcoma of cervix: Cells showing marked nuclear atypia and frequent mitosis

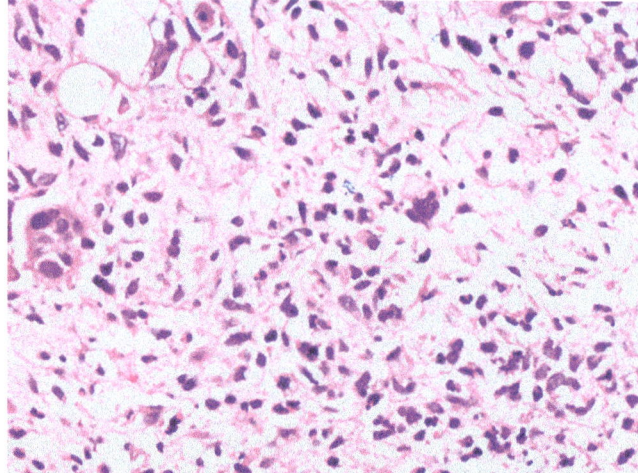

Figure 7.37: Rhabdomyosarcoma of cervix: Loosely arranged malignant round cells

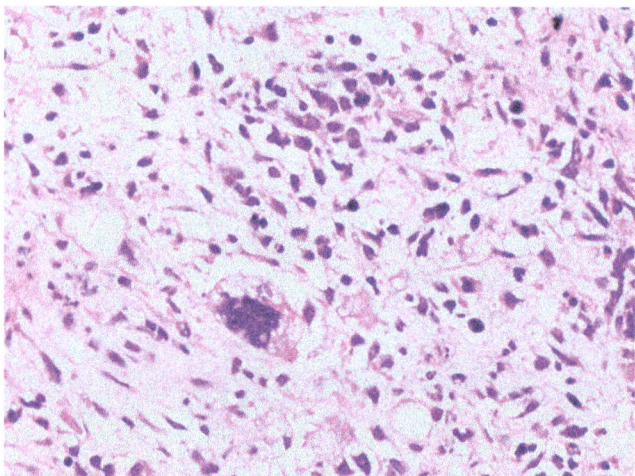

Figure 7.36: Rhabdomyosarcoma of cervix: Round cells with marked nuclear atypia

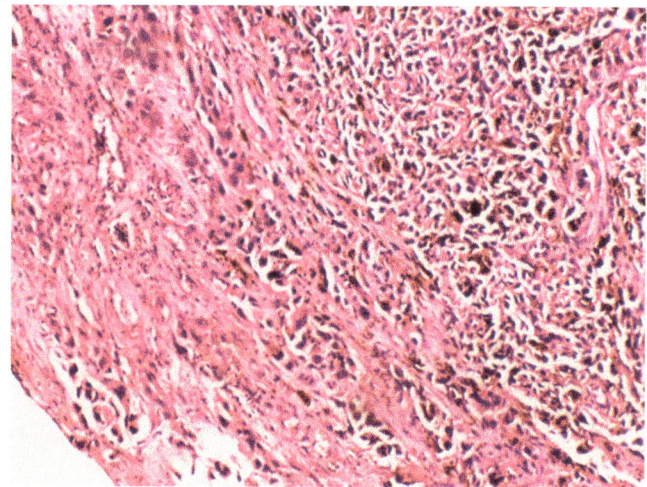

Figure 7.38: Melanoma cervix: Diffuse sheets of malignant cells containing melanin pigment

### Embryonal Sarcoma (Sarcoma Botryoides)

Embryonal sarcoma or sarcoma botryoides may rarely occur in cervix. The tumor presents as polypoidal soft mass in the cervix. The morphological features of embryonal sarcoma are similar as described in previous section (Figures 7.36 and 7.37). The tumor is characterized by oval to spindle-shaped cells with a subepithelial cambium layer.

### Alveolar Soft Part Sarcoma

This is a rare tumor in cervix. The tumor shows multiple nests of cells separated by thin fibrous septae. The central cells in the nests are loose and resembles alveoli. The individual cells show abundant granular eosinophilic cytoplasm with centrally placed large nuclei having prominent nucleoli. Occasionally PAS positive and diastase resistant crystals are seen within the cytoplasm of the cells. Prognosis of alveolar soft part sarcoma is relatively better in this region compared to other parts of the body. Overall 5 year survival is 60%.

### Nerve Sheath Tumor

Both schwannoma and its malignant counterpart malignant schwannoma are exceedingly rare in cervix. Malignant schwannoma is composed of fascicles of oval to spindle cells with elongated wavy nuclei. Mitotic activity is brisk. The tumor cells are positive for S-100 protein.

### Melanoma

Malignant melanoma of cervix is also very rare[23] (Figures 7.38 and 7.39). The presence of junctional activity is helpful to identify the primary melanoma of cervix which is

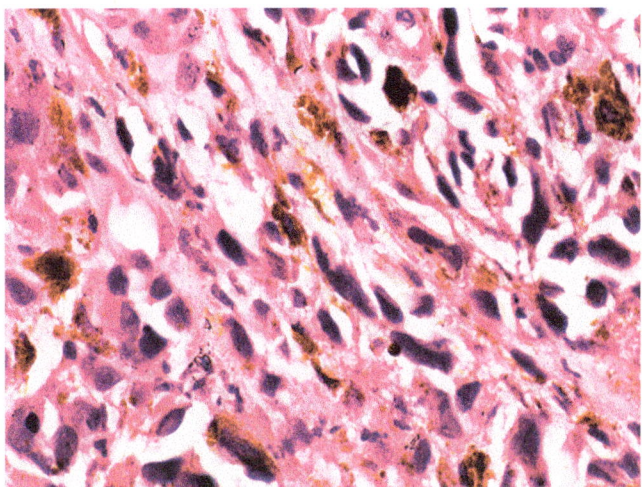

**Figure 7.39:** Melanoma cervix: Melanoma cervix: Higher magnification shows large pleomorphic tumor cells with melanin pigment

detectable in 50% of the primary cervical melanoma. HMB 45 and melan-A immunostaining are positive in melanoma and these stains help to identify the cases of amelanotic melanoma.

## LYMPHOMA OF CERVIX

Primary lymphoma of the cervix is rare and most of the lymphoma of cervix is a part of systemic disease. The patient presents with vaginal bleeding. The clinical examination shows cervical or cervicovaginal mass. Diffuse large B cell lymphoma is the most common type of lymphoma followed by follicular lymphoma and lymphocytic lymphoma. Majority of primary cervical lymphomas are B cell type.

### Differential Diagnosis

Follicular cervicitis may be misdiagnosed as follicular lymphoma. Follicular cervicitis shows a polymorphic population of cell and the follicles are widely spaced with well-defined mantle zone. Bcl-2 immunostain is strongly positive in follicular lymphoma.

## MIXED MESODERMAL TUMOR

Mixed epithelial-mesenchymal tumors include: Adenofibroma, adenomyoma, adenosarcoma and carcinosarcoma.

The glands and stromal elements both are neoplastic and the stromal elements may be benign or malignant in nature.

### Cervical Adenosarcoma

This tumor is composed of benign epithelial component along with malignant stromal component. Primary adenosarcoma of cervix is very rare.[24] The mean age of the patient is 31 years. The patient commonly complains of abnormal vaginal bleeding. Clinical examination revealed polypoid mass in the cervix.

#### Histopathology (Figures 7.40 to 7.42)

Histopathology of adenosarcoma is characterized by multiple irregular-shaped glands with condensed cellular stroma. The stroma shows nuclear pleomorphism and atypia along with frequent mitotic activities (more than 2 per 10 high power fields). In addition, heterologous elements such as striated muscle, osteoid and cartilage are also seen.

#### Differential Diagnosis

1. Atypical endocervical polyp: Atypical endocervical polyp is difficult to distinguish from adenosarcoma as the lesion often shows irregular-shaped glands and focal stromal atypia. However, the presence of increased mitotic activity and generalized nuclear atypia of the stromal cells are helpful in diagnosis of adenosarcoma.
2. Adenomyoma of cervix: The presence of smooth muscle component in adenomyoma is helpful to distinguish it from adenosarcoma.
3. Prolapsed uterine leiomyomatous polyp: Ulcerated prolapsed submucosal uterine leiomyoma may show reactive stromal cellularity and vascular proliferation. Identification of smooth muscle cells is helpful in such condition. The stromal cells are positive for CD 10 and negative for desmin.

### Carcinosarcoma

Carcinosarcoma of cervix is extremely rare tumor and it represents only 0.005% of all cervical cancer.[25] The patients are usually postmenopausal and mean age is 60 years. Vaginal bleeding is the common presenting symptoms of

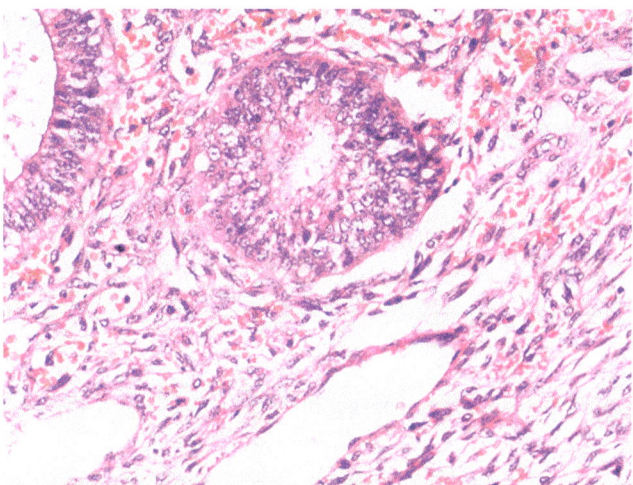

**Figure 7.40:** Adenosarcoma of cervix: Benign cervical glands surrounded by sarcomatous stroma

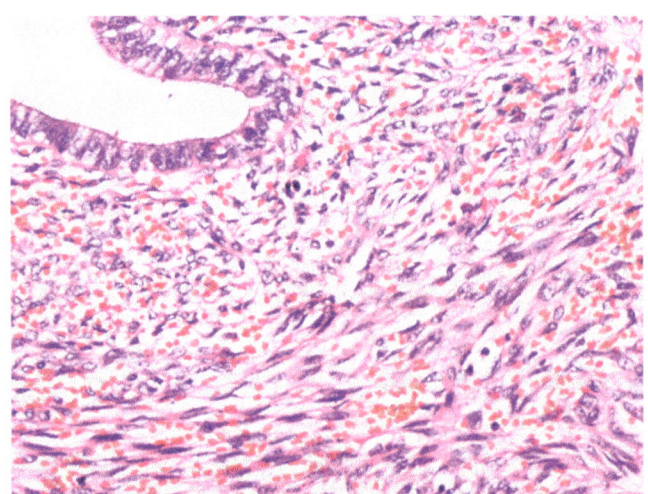

**Figure 7.41:** Adenosarcoma of cervix: The stroma shows oval to elongated cells with moderate nuclear atypia

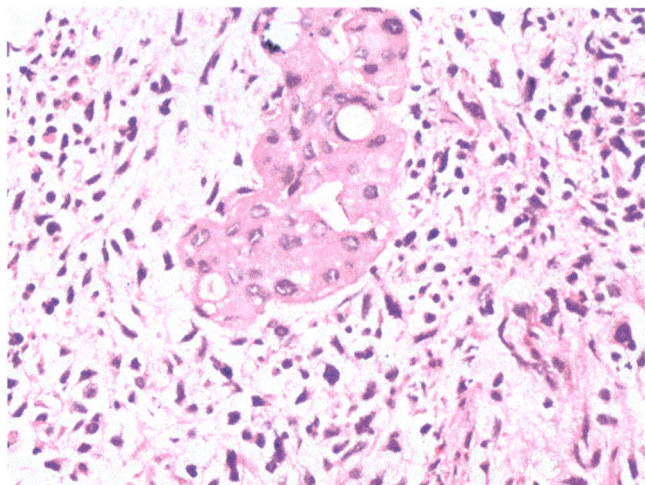

**Figure 7.43:** Carcinosarcoma of cervix: Both malignant epithelial and stromal component

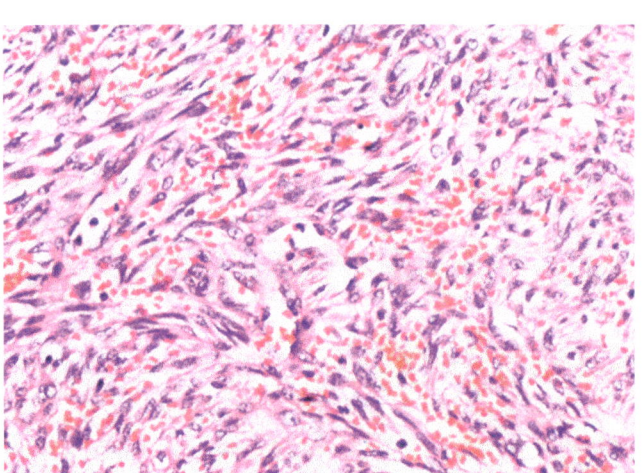

**Figure 7.42:** Adenosarcoma of cervix: Higher magnification of the stroma shows marked nuclear atypia

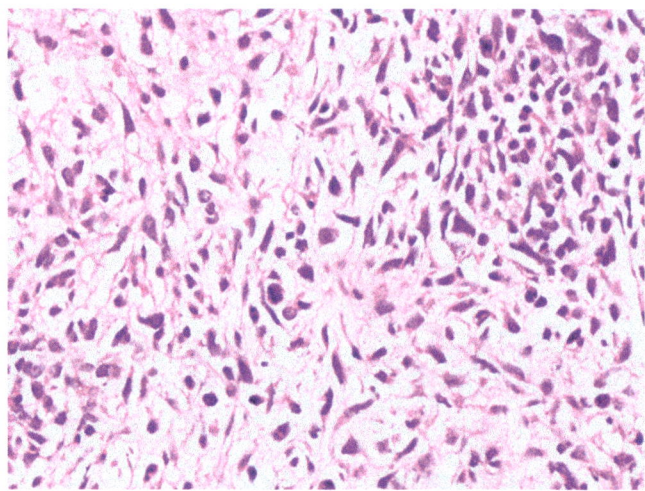

**Figure 7.44:** Carcinosarcoma of cervix: Higher magnification of the sarcomatous component

carcinosarcoma cases. Clinical examination reveals polypoidal fungating growth in the cervix.

### Histopathology (Figures 7.43 and 7.44)

Carcinosarcoma shows malignancy in both epithelial and mesenchymal elements. Unlike its uterine counterpart the epithelial component of cervical carcinosarcoma is usually squamous cell carcinoma. However, adenoid cystic, adenoid basal cell and adenocarcinoma components may also be seen. In addition adjacent superficial epithelial lining of the cervix may show dysplastic changes. The mesenchymal component of the tumor is usually homologous and shows oval to spindle cells in bundles. Heterologous elements such as rhabdomyosarcomatous and chondroid elements have also been described.[26]

### Differential Diagnosis

1. Spindle cell carcinoma: The carcinoma with predominant spindle cell component may be mistaken as carcinosarcoma.
2. Uterine carcinosarcoma with extension in cervix: In this cases, the major bulk of the tumor remains in the uterus.

### Treatment

Surgery with or without radiotherapy is the treatment of choice.

## Adenofibroma

This is a relatively uncommon tumor in the cervix than its counterpart in uterus. The tumor shows both benign epithelial and mesenchymal elements. The lesion is polypoidal lined by columnar or cuboidal epithelial cell. The glands are accompanied by spindle-shaped stroma. The stromal cells are bland and do not show mitotic activity.

## ADENOMYOMA

Adenomyoma of cervix is rare. The mean age of the patient is 40 years. The tumor presents as polypoidal lesion.

## Histopathology

In adenomyoma, the tumor is composed of benign glands and smooth muscle elements. There are three types of adenomyoma: endocervical, endometrioid, and atypical polypoid adenomyoma.

### Endocervical Adenomyoma

In this type, the glands are endocervical type. Glandular epithelial cells are tall columnar mucin secreting. Endocervical adenomyoma should be differentiated from minimal deviation adenocarcinoma. The former is better circumscribed and lack desmoplastic stromal reaction.

### Endometrioid Adenomyoma

The tumor is composed of endometrial type glands. The surrounding stroma is also endometrial type and bland in appearance. The lining cells of the glands are similar to that of proliferative endometrium.

## Atypical Polypoid Adenomyoma

In this type, the glands are variable sized with irregular, margin along with smooth muscle component.

### Treatment

Surgical excision such as polypectomy is the treatment of choice.

## REFERENCES

1. Witkiewicz A, Lee KR, Brodsky G, Cviko A, Brodsky J, Crum CP. Superficial (early) endocervical adenocarcinoma in situ: a study of 12 cases and comparison to conventional AIS. Am J Surg Pathol. 2005;29(12):1609-14.
2. Zaino RJ. Int J Gynecol Pathol. Symposium part I: Adenocarcinoma in situ, glandular dysplasia, and early invasive adenocarcinoma of the uterine cervix. 2002;21(4):314-26.
3. Riethdorf L, Riethdorf S, Lee KR, Cviko A, Löning T, Crum CP. Human papillomaviruses, expression of p16, and early endocervical glandular neoplasia. Hum Pathol. 2002;33(9):899-904.
4. McCluggage WG, Shah R, Connolly LE, McBride HA. Intestinal-type cervical adenocarcinoma in situ and adenocarcinoma exhibit a partial enteric immunophenotype with consistent expression of CDX2. Int J Gynecol Pathol. 2008;27(1):92-100.
5. Östör AG, Duncan A, Quinn M, Rome R. Adenocarcinoma in situ of the uterine cervix: an experience with 100 cases. Gynecol Oncol. 2000;79:207-10.
6. Kurman RJ, Carcangiu ML, Herrington S, Young RH: Tumours of vulva. WHO classification of tumours of female genital reproductive organs. 4th Edition, International agency for research on Cancer, Lyon 2014.
7. Christopherson W, Nealon N, Gray L. Noninvasive precursor lesions of adenocarcinoma and mixed adenosquamous carcinoma of the cervix uteri. Cancer 1979;44:975-83.
8. Buscema J, Woodruff J. Significance of neoplastic abnormalities in endocervical epithelium. Gynecol Oncol 1984;17:356-62.
9. Saad RS, Ismiil N, Dubé V, Nofech-Mozes S, Khalifa MA. CDX-2 expression is a common event in primary intestinal-type endocervical adenocarcinoma. Am J Clin Pathol. 2009;132(4):531-8.
10. Kaminski PF, Norris HJ. Minimal deviation carcinoma (adenoma malignum) of the cervix. Int J Gynecol Pathol. 1983 2(2):141-52.
11. Utsugi K, Hirai Y, Takeshima N, Akiyama F, Sakurai S, Hasumi K. Utility of the monoclonal antibody HIK1083 in the diagnosis of adenoma malignum of the uterine cervix. Gynecol Oncol. 1999;75(3):345-8.
12. Jones MW, Silverberg SG. Well-differentiated villoglandular adenocarcinoma of the uterine cervix: a clinicopathological study of 24 cases. Int J Gynecol Pathol. 1993;12(1):1-7.
13. Robboy SJ, Young RH. Atypical vaginal adenosis and cervical ectropion. Association with clear cell adenocarcinoma in diethylstilbestrol-exposed offspring. Cancer. 1984;54(5):869-75.
14. Zhou C, Gilks CB, et al. Papillary serous carcinoma of the uterine cervix: a clinicopathologic study of 17 cases. Am J Surg Pathol. 1998;22(1):113-20.
15. Silver SA, Devouassoux-Shisheboran M, Mezzetti TP, Tavassoli FA. Mesonephric adenocarcinomas of the uterine cervix: a study of 11 cases with immunohistochemical findings. Am J Surg Pathol. 2001;25(3):379-87.
16. Ueda Y, Miyatake T, Okazawa M, Kimura T, Miyake T, Fujiwara K, et al. Clonality and HPV infection analysis of concurrent glandular and squamous lesions and adenosquamous carcinomas of the uterine cervix. Am J Clin Pathol 2008;130(3):389-400.
17. Grayson W, Taylor LF, Cooper K. Adenoid cystic and adenoid basal carcinoma of the uterine cervix: comparative morphologic, mucin, and immunohistochemical profile of two rare neoplasms of putative "reserve cell" origin. Am J Surg Pathol. 1999;23(4):448-58.
18. Prempree T, Villasanta U, Tang CK. Management of adenoid cystic carcinoma of the uterine cervix (cylindroma): report of six cases and reappraisal of all cases reported in the medical literature. Cancer. 1980;46(7):1631-5.
19. Brainard JA, Hart WR. Adenoid basal epitheliomas of the uterine cervix: a re-evaluation of distinctive cervical basaloid lesions currently classified as adenoid basal carcinoma and adenoid basal hyperplasia. Am J Surg Pathol 1998;22:965-75.

20. Wang HL, Lu DW. Detection of human papillomavirus DNA and expression of p16, Rb, and p53 proteins in small cell carcinomas of the uterine cervix. Am J Surg Pathol. 2004;28(7):901-8.
21. Ambros RA, Park JS, Shah KV, Kurman RJ. Evaluation of histologic, morphometric, and immunohistochemical criteria in the differential diagnosis of small cell carcinomas of the cervix with particular reference to human papillomavirus types 16 and 18. Mod Pathol. 1991;4(5):586-93.
22. Mulvany NJ, Nirenberg A, Oster AG. Non-primary cervical adenocarcinomas. Pathology. 1996;28(4):29.
23. Mousavi AS, Fakor F, Nazari Z, Ghaemmaghami F, Hashemi FA, Jamali M. J Primary malignant melanoma of the uterine cervix: case report and review of the literature. Low Genit Tract Dis. 2006;10(4):258-63.
24. Clement PB, Scully RE. Mullerian adenosarcoma of the uterus: a clinicopathologic analysis of 100 cases with a review of the literature. Hum Pathol. 1990;21(4):363-81.
25. Wright JD, Rosenblum K, Huettner PC, Mutch DG, Rader JS, Powell MA, et al. Cervical sarcomas: an analysis of incidence and outcome. Gynecol Oncol. 2005;99(2):348-51.
26. Kadota K, Haba R, Ishikawa M, Kushida Y, Katsuki N, Hayashi T, et al. Uterine cervical carcinosarcoma with heterologous mesenchymal component: a case report and review of the literature. Arch Gynecol Obstet. 2009;280(5):839-43.

# Endometrium: Benign Lesions

## 8

## ANATOMY AND HISTOLOGY OF THE UTERUS

The uterus lies in the pelvis and is continuous with vagina below. Each fallopian tube opens into two upper corner of the uterus. The uterus is situated anterior to rectum and posterior to urinary bladder. The uterus is divided into two parts: upper two-thirds is known as body of uterus and lower 1/3rd is known as cervix. The body of the uterus is tilted or flexed towards the cervix anteriorly and is known as anteflexed. In the lower part of the uterus, the cervix is tilted anteriorly along the axis of vagina and is known as anteversion (Figure 8.1).

The peritoneum is reflected from the urinary bladder to the anterior surface of the uterus at the level of internal os. This peritoneal fold is known as uterovesical fold and it forms a pouch called as uterovesical pouch. The distended urinary bladder comes in direct contact with the uterus. Similarly reflection of peritoneum from the rectum to the posterior wall of the uterus makes rectouterine pouch which is also known as pouch of Douglas (Figure 8.1). Uterus is attached with broad ligament in the lateral surface. Each fallopian tube joins in the upper lateral corner of the uterus and the round ligament joins anteroinferior to the fallopian tube. Ovarian ligament is attached in each side of the uterus in the posteroinferior to the fallopian tube attachment.

The adult nulliparous uterus is the pear-shaped muscular tube which is near about 6 to 8 cm in length. It is wider in the fundus that measures 5 cm. The thickness of uterus is 2.5 cm. The length of the uterine cavity from the fundus to the cervix is 6 cm. Uterus is broad in the upper part and narrow in the lower part where it joins the cervical cavity. Uterine body is divided into fundus, body and isthmus (Figure 8.2). The isthmus is situated in the lower part of the uterus. The fundus lies above the level of the opening of the fallopian tubes. In between the isthmus and fundus remains the uterine body proper.

### Vascular Supply of the Uterus

The vascular supply of the uterus is from the uterine artery which is a branch of the anterior division of the internal iliac artery. The uterine artery divides into upper and lower branch in the junction of cervix and uterus. The upper branch

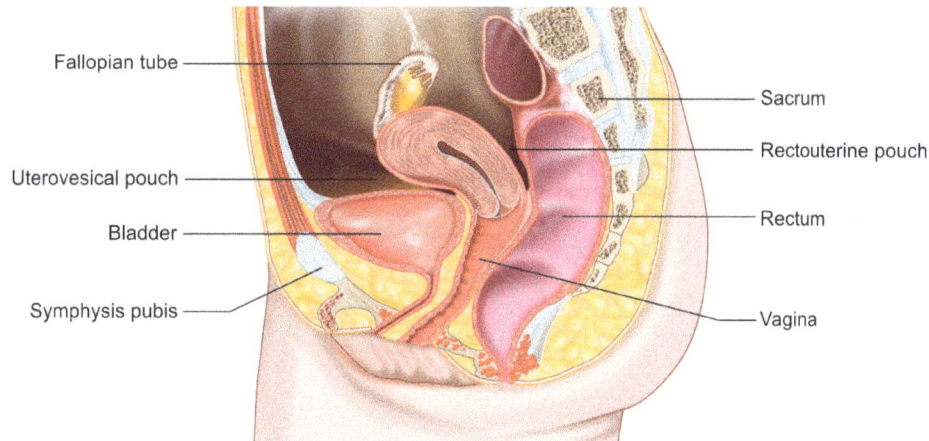

**Figure 8.1:** Schematic diagram shows anatomical position of uterus

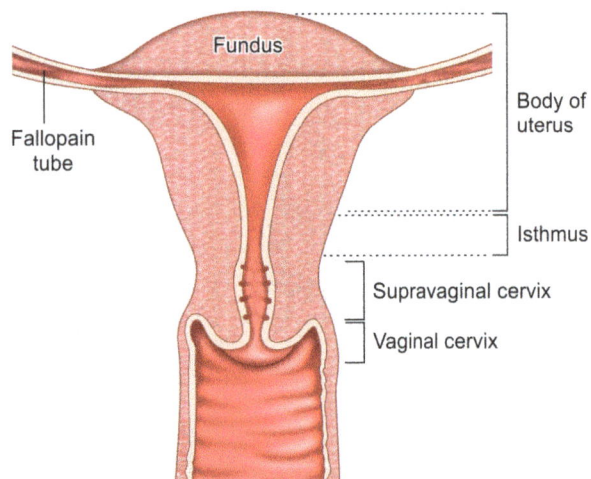

**Figure 8.2:** Detailed anatomical parts of uterus

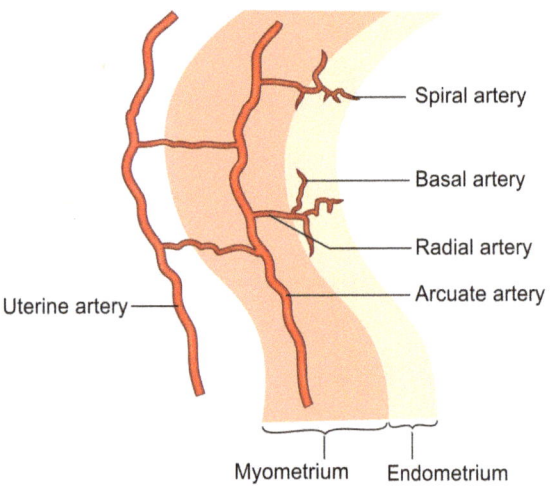

**Figure 8.3:** Uterine vascular supply

joins with the ovarian artery and lower branch joins with the vaginal artery. The myometrium of the uterus is supplied by arcuate arteries. Multiple radial arteries arise from the arcuate artery and traverse towards the endometrium (Figure 8.3). In the basal layer of the endometrium, the radial artery divides into horizontal basal artery and vertical spiral artery. The basal artery supplies the stratum basal part of endometrium and the spiral artery supplies the stratum functionalis part of the endometrium.

## Histology

Uterus is divided from outside to lumen into three parts: serosa, myometrium, and endometrium.

### Serosa

This is the thin outermost layer of the uterus which is composed of peritoneal lining epithelium and thin areolar connective tissue. The anterior part of the uterus is mostly uncovered and is devoid of any peritoneal lining epithelium.

### Myometrium

Myometrium is composed of innermost longitudinal layer, middle circular and outer longitudinal layer of smooth muscle. The myometrium contains blood vessels, nerves and lymphatic.

### Endometrium

Endometrium is divided into superficial stratum functionalis and deeper stratum basalis.

### Stratum Functionalis

This is the superficial thick functional layer that is sloughed out at the time of menstruation. The stratum functionalis part is richly vascularized by the spiral arteries.

### Stratum Basalis

This is the basal portion of the endometrium. The regeneration of the superficial endometrium after menstruation occurs from the stratum basalis.

The endometrial surface is lined by non-ciliated single layer of columnar epithelial cells. Endometrium contains multiple tubular glands surrounded by cellular endometrial stroma. The endometrial glands open into the lumen of the uterine cavity. The major part of these glands remains in the functionalis layer of the endometrium.

## CYCLIC ENDOMETRIUM

The endometrium undergoes cyclical changes consisting of proliferative phase, secretory phase and menstrual phase. Each complete endometrial cycle takes 28 days. However, it may vary from person-to-person. The duration of endometrial cycle may vary in the proliferative phase, but the time period from the ovulation to the onset of menstruation that means the secretory period is constant. The menstrual cycle is related with the growth of ovarian follicle and ovulation. The estrogen and progesterone hormone are responsible for the endometrial cycle. Four players are responsible for the game of endometrial or menstrual cycle: hypothalamus, pituitary gland, ovary and endometrium (Figure 8.4). The arcuate nuclei of hypothalamus releases gonadotropin-releasing hormone (GnRH) in a pulsatile manner. This GnRH acts on the anterior pituitary gland to release two hormones: follicular stimulating hormone (FSH) and luteinizing hormone (LH). FSH and LH both act on the primordial follicles of ovary and one of these follicles become dominant. The ovarian follicle develops and produce estrogen hormone by converting androgen to estradiol.

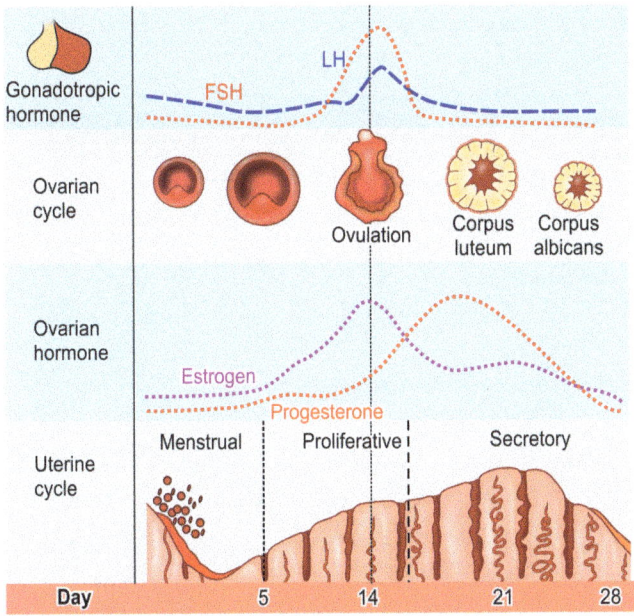

Figure 8.4: Schematic diagram of endometrial cycle

Box 8.1: Different stages of proliferative phase

➡ **Early proliferative phase**
- Small, uniform simple tubular glands
- Single layer of cuboidal epithelium
- Dense compact cellular stroma

➡ **Mid proliferative phase**
- Long and curved glands. Glands become tortuous.
- Tall columnar lining epithelial cells
- Stroma is focally edematous
- Frequent mitosis in the glands and stroma

➡ **Late proliferative phase**
- More tortuous glands
- Pseudostratified columnar epithelium
- Maximum mitosis
- Stromal edema

The estradiol helps in the development and maintenance of the proliferative phase of the endometrium. Just before ovulation, there is LH surge that causes ovulation followed by the formation of the corpus luteum. Progesterone is released from the luteinized granulose cells of the corpus luteum. The progesterone is responsible for the secretory changes in the endometrial glands and predecidual changes in the stroma. In absence of the fertilization, the corpus luteum regresses followed by the sloughing of the predecidualized stroma and secretory glands. This process of breakdown of the stroma and glands indicate the onset of menstruation. At the end of the menstruation, the glands and stroma regenerates and the proliferative phase begins.

## Proliferative phase (Box 8.1)

After the end of the menstrual phase, the proliferative phase starts and the endometrium regenerates in this phase. Endometrium thickens progressively from 0.5 to 4 mm due to the effect of estrogens produced from the granulose and theca cells of the ovarian follicles. In a 28th day cycle, the proliferative phase starts from the 5th day of the period and ends at 14th day. In this phase, the glands, stroma and blood vessels grow progressively. In the proliferative phase, the glands are regular, well-spaced and tubular in appearance (Figures 8.5 and 8.6). The glandular epithelium proliferates and becomes pseudostratified. Frequent mitotic activities are seen in the glands. The glandular epithelial cells are cuboidal with moderate amount of cytoplasm. The nuclei are round with coarse chromatin and small nucleoli. As time progresses the glands become elongated and tortuous, however the spatial

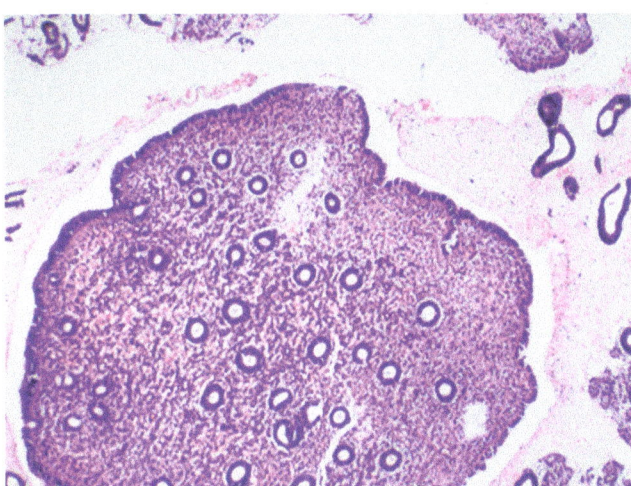

Figure 8.5: Proliferative phase: Multiple small well-circumscribed endometrial glands in a compact stroma

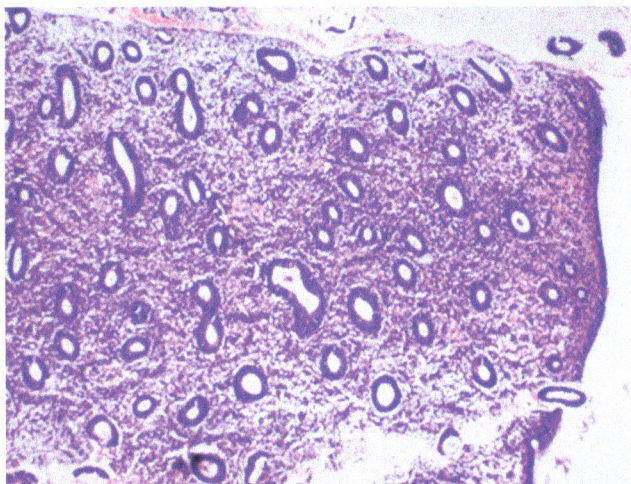

Figure 8.6: Proliferative phase: Higher magnification shows well-spaced glands lined by cuboidal cells

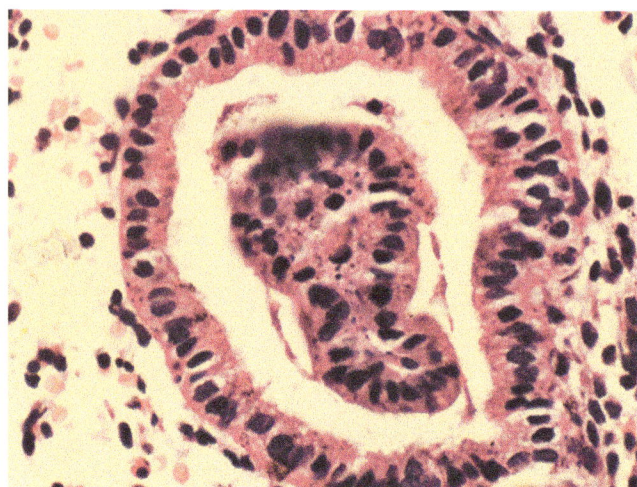

Figure 8.7: Telescoping gland: The glands within a gland

distance in between the glands are maintained. The important features of the proliferative phase are the pseudostratification of the epithelium, increased mitosis in the lining cells, regular spatial distribution and uniform shape of the glands.

Stroma in the proliferative phase is much more cellular and shows frequent mitotic activities. The stromal cells are small, round with scanty cytoplasm. The nuclei are oval to spindle shaped and condensed. Foci of edematous changes may be seen.

The exact dating of proliferative phase is not possible; however, this phase is divided into early, mid and late proliferative phase.

It is important to take care on the following matters to avoid false interpretation in proliferative phase endometrium in biopsy or endometrial curetting:
1. The tortuous proliferative showing "glands within glands" or telescoping artifact (Figure 8.7) should not be misinterpreted as hyperplastic endometrium.
2. Focal edema of the stroma should not be mistaken as predecidual stromal changes.
3. The disrupted glands may simulate focal crowding and may be misinterpreted as hyperplasia. It is important to note the orientation and distribution of the glands in relation to the surface epithelium.
4. Focal glandular secretion may not indicate secretory phase.

## Secretory Phase

The recognizable morphologic changes of endometrium begin 36 to 48 hours after ovulation. The secretory phase of the endometrial cycle starts from the 16th day of the menstrual cycle or 2nd post-ovulatory day. Exact dating is possible in each day of cycle in this phase. In secretory phase, the following changes occur:
1. Secretory activity in the glands,

> **Box 8.2:** Dating of secretory endometrium
>
> ➤ **Early secretory**
> - 16th day: Irregular subnuclear vacuolation
> - 17th day: Regular and abundant subnuclear vacuolation
> - 18th day: Both sub- and supranuclear vacuoles
> - 19th day: Uniformly arranged basal nuclei, secretions within the lumen
>
> ➤ **Mid secretory**
> - 20th day: Maximum intraluminal secretions, basally placed nuclei
> - 21st day: Stroma becomes edematous
> - 22nd day: Peak stromal edema
>
> ➤ **Late secretory**
> - 23rd day: Prominent spiral arterioles and perivascular predecidual cells
> - 24th day: The predecidual cells extend further in the stroma
> - 25th day: The predecidual cells appear beneath the surface as aggregates
> - 26th day: Confluence of the predecidual cells and they appear as large sheets
> - 27th day: Extensive predecidual cells
> - 28th day: Fibrin thrombi in the stromal blood vessels, foci of hemorrhage with extravasation of RBC, stromal granulocytes
>
> **Menstrual:** Fragments of glands, stroma, stromal granulocytes, polymorphs and necrosis

2. Stromal predecidual changes and other maturation,
3. vascular changes (Box 8.2). Secretory phase is divided into:
   a. Early secretory phase: 16th to 18th day of the cycle,
   b. Mid secretory phase: 19th to 22nd day of the cycle, and
   c. Late secretory phase: 23rd to 28th day of the cycle.

### Early Secretory Phase

The first recognizable feature of ovulation is accumulation of glycogen under the nucleus of the glandular epithelial cells indicated by subnuclear vacuolation. In 16th day of the cycle, the subnuclear vacuoles appear (Figures 8.8 to 8.10). The subnuclear vacuoles appear irregularly and may be focally in the glands of stratum functional layer. Slowly the subnuclear vacuoles become more global and all the cells in the glandular lining epithelium display the vacuoles. In the endometrial curetting it is important to have subnuclear vacuoles in more than 50% of the cells in the more than 50% of the glands to say early secretory glands. In the 17th day of the cycle, the subnuclear vacuoles are more abundant and the vacuoles are regular and continuous beneath the nucleus. In the day 18th, the vacuoles appear both sub- and supranuclear and the tip

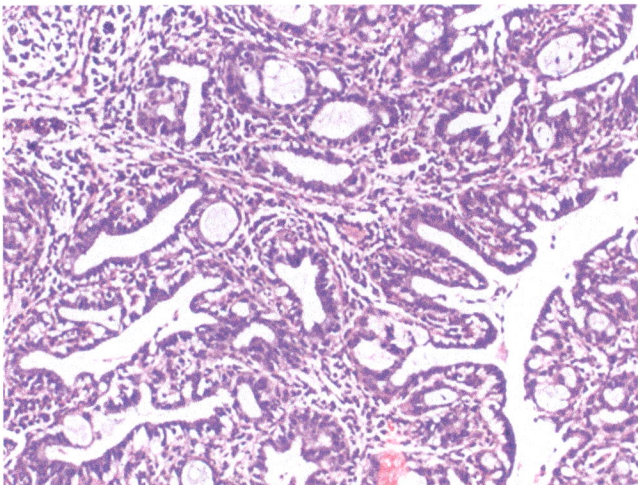

Figure 8.8: Early secretory endometrium: Subnuclear vacuolation

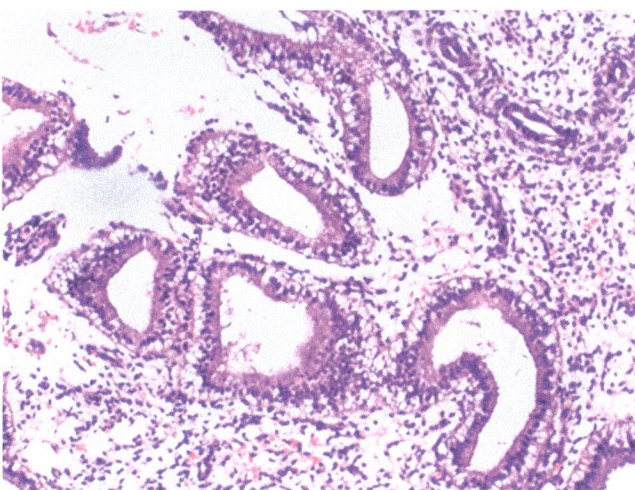

Figure 8.9: Early secretory endometrium: Regular subnuclear vacuolation

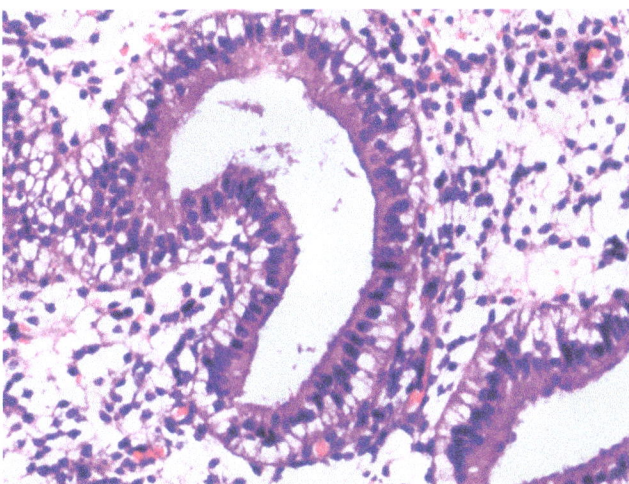

Figure 8.10: Higher magnification of the gland shows tall columnar epithelium with vacuolation under the nucleus

of the cells become ragged. The nuclear position is central within the cell. In the 19th day, the nuclei migrate again to the original basal position and the glands start secretory activities. The vacuoles are lost and mitotic activity is absent in the gland. The stroma of the early secretory phase does not differ much from the late proliferative phase.

**Following things to remember in endometrial curetting sample:**
1. Focal subnuclear vacuolation may be present in proliferative, mid or late secretory phase.
2. False crowding of the glands due to irregular gland enlargement should not be mistaken as endometrial intraepithelial neoplasm.
3. Focal edema in the stroma does not indicate any irregularity of maturation.

*Mid Secretory Activity*

In the mid secretory phase, the stromal changes are more prominent than the glandular changes. The glands are more curved and tortuous and contain luminal secretary material. Maximum intraluminal secretions are seen in the day 20th. Rarely residual subnuclear vacuolation may be noted. The stromal changes start at the day 21st and stroma becomes more edematous. The peak edema appears in the day 22nd (Figure 8.11).

*Late Secretory Endometrium (Figures 8.12 to 8.16)*

In this phase, the glands show exhausted secretory activity and become tortuous, saw tooth like appearance. The stroma shows characteristic appearance of predecidual cells. The cells are large with abundant eosinophilic cytoplasm. The cytoplasmic border is less distinct. The nuclei are central in position with fine chromatin. As these cells are not truly related with pregnancy-induced decidual cells, so they are labeled as predecidual changes. In the 23rd day, the stroma shows prominent small blood vessels and predecidual cells appear around the vessels known as perivascular cuffing. In the 24th day, the predecidual cells extends further in the stroma. In the 25th day, the predecidual cells appear beneath the surface as aggregates. In 26th day, there is confluence of the predecidual cells and they appear as large sheets. In 27th day, the predecidual cells are extensive. The stromal granular lymphocytes appear in 27th day and become more extensive in 28th day. The fibrin thrombi appear in the stromal blood vessels and foci of hemorrhage with extravasation of RBC starts.

**Menstrual Phase**

Menstrual phase starts after 28th day of the cycle and it last about 4 days. In this phase, the glands and stroma are broken

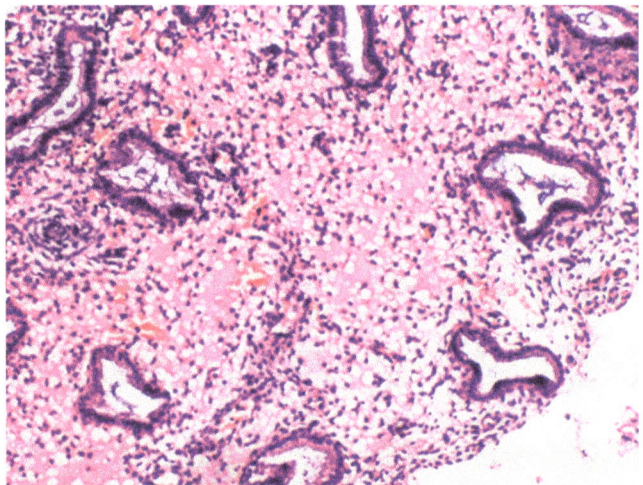

**Figure 8.11:** Mid secretory endometrium: Secretory glands with marked stromal edema

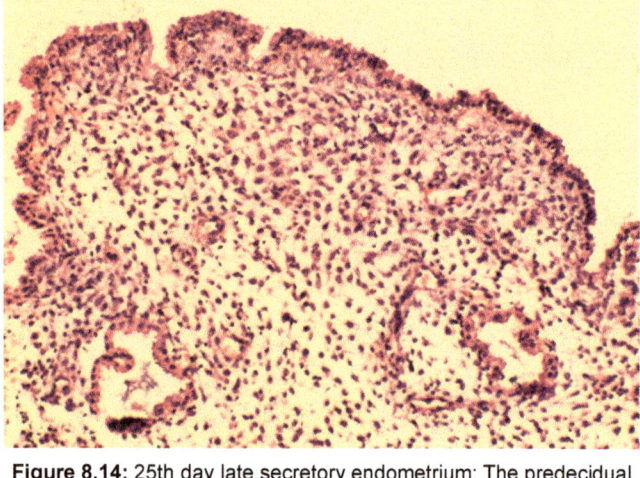

**Figure 8.14:** 25th day late secretory endometrium: The predecidual cells appear beneath the surface as aggregates

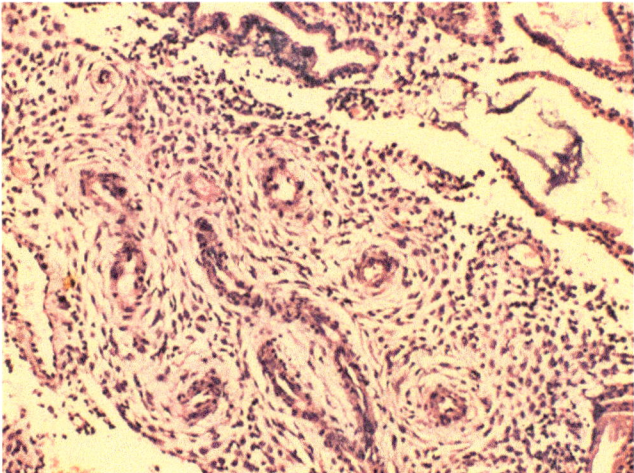

**Figure 8.12:** 23rd day endometrium: Perivascular decidualization

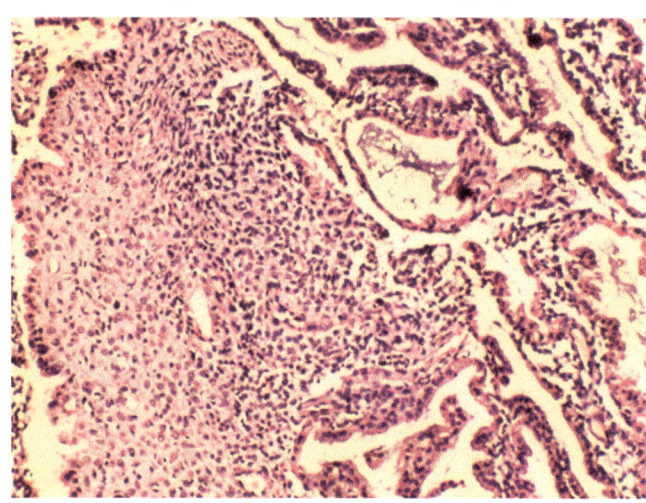

**Figure 8.15:** 26th day late secretory: Confluence of the predecidual cells and they appear as large sheets

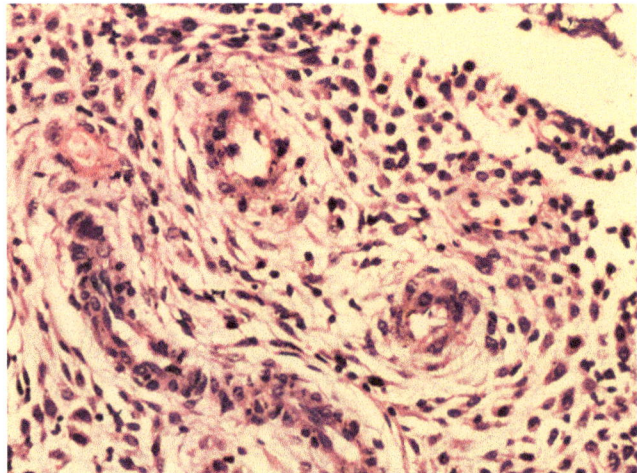

**Figure 8.13:** 23rd day endometrium: perivascular cuffing by decidual cells

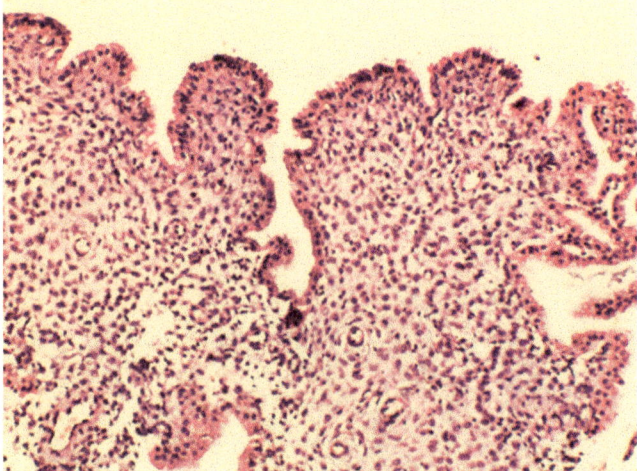

**Figure 8.16:** 27th day late secretory: Extensive predecidual cells in the surface

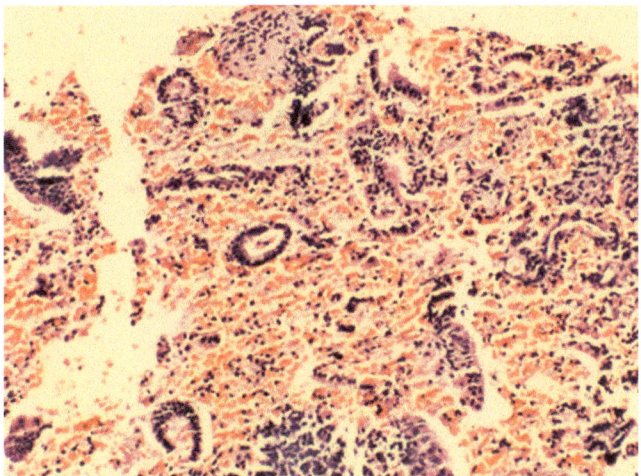

**Figure 8.17:** Menstrual endometrium: Fragmented glands and stromal break down

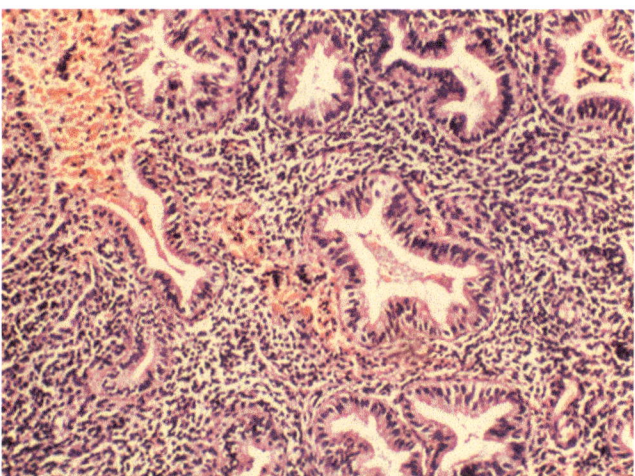

**Figure 8.19:** Lower uterine segment: Multiple endocervical glands with compact stroma

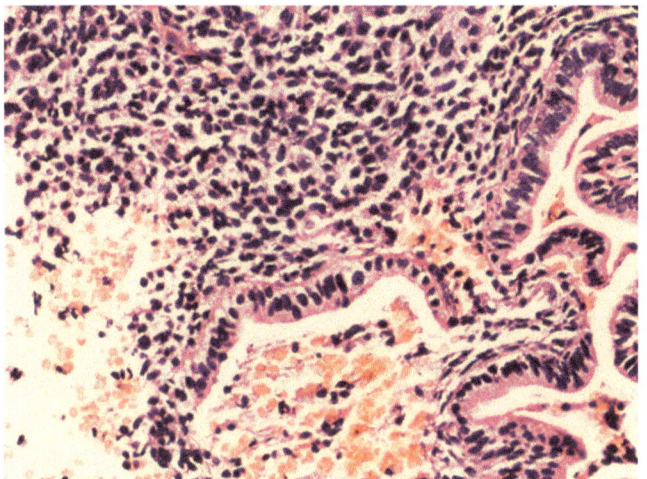

**Figure 8.18:** Menstrual endometrium: Higher magnification shows fragmented glands and stromal granulocytes

down. The glands become fragmented and the surface epithelium is also disrupted (Figures 8.17 and 8.18). The stroma breaks down and becomes condensed and collapsed. The crowding and hyperchromatic nuclei of the stromal cells may give false alarm. The blood vessels show fibrin thrombi and foci of hemorrhage are seen. The stroma shows polymorphonuclear leukocytes and necrosis.

## ENDOMETRIAL DATING AND BIOPSY

Precise endometrial dating is possible in the late secretory phase. Regarding the exact dating, the following things to remember:
1. The sampling should be procured from the upper part of the body of uterus.
2. Endometrial curetting from the lower uterine segment is insufficient or fallacious for dating (Figure 8.19).
3. The presence of surface epithelial lining in the sample is desirable.
4. Occasional cystic glands or non-reactive glands do not bear any significance.
5. The endometrial curetting should be repeated in case of scanty glands.

The span of 48 hour variation of dating from the expected date is considered as normal. During the biopsy interpretation of dating, one should consider the most advanced changes for the endometrial date. The dating may be inaccurate in case of pregnancy, exogenous hormonal therapy, chronic inflammation, uterine polyp or leiomyoma.

The estimation of the progesterone level in the luteal phase is considered as reliable test for the assessment of infertility work up.

## Indications and Contraindications of Endometrial Biopsy

The common indications and contraindications of endometrial biopsies are highlighted in Box 8.3.

## POSTMENOPAUSAL ENDOMETRIUM

In postmenopausal women, the endometrium is thinned out and the stratum functionalis layer is virtually absent. The endometrial glands are small tubular and lined by cuboidal to flattened epithelial cells. In some cases, the glands may be cystically dilated which is labeled as cystic atrophy (Figure 8.20). It differs from the hyperplastic endometrial glands by its flattened to cuboidal lining cells. The stroma in

**Box 8.3:** Endometrial biopsy and curetting

→ **Indications**
- Abnormal uterine bleeding
- Postmenopausal bleeding
- Infertility investigation
- Endometrial hyperplasia
- Follow-up cases of endometrial hyperplasia
- Evaluate the response to hormone therapy

→ **Contraindications**
- Pregnancy
- Bleeding disorder
- Severe cervical and vaginal infections
- Pelvic inflammatory disease

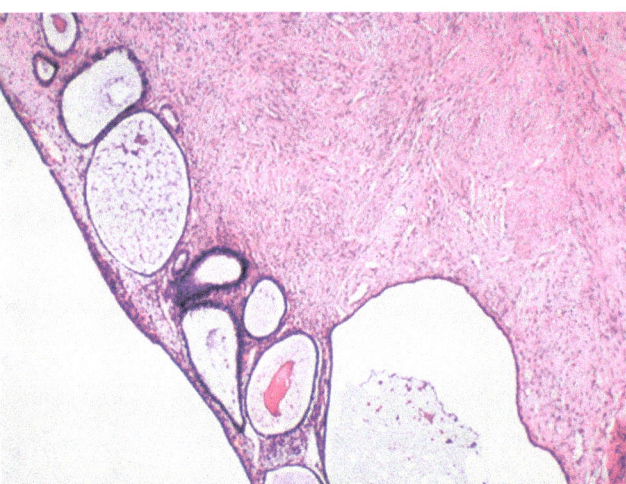

Figure 8.20: Atrophic endometrium: Cystically dilated endometrial glands lined by small cuboidal cells

postmenopausal patient is fibrous and is composed of mainly spindle cells. As the age advances, the stroma becomes increasingly hypocellular.

## PREGNANCY-INDUCED CHANGES

First three weeks of pregnancy: In early part of pregnancy, the changes in the endometrium are a bit more exaggerated phase of late secretory phase. The endometrium shows more tortuous and saw toothed like glands. The glandular luminal cells show increased secretory activity and cytoplasmic vacuolation. The stromal vessels show congestion and dilatation of the capillaries along with thick walled spiral arterioles along with decidual cells. 4th week to later part of pregnancy: As the pregnancy advances the decidua becomes more widespread. The glands become more tortuous and star shaped. The endometrium in the 4th to 12th week of pregnancy shows typical Arias-Stella reaction.[1] Arias-Stella reaction is characterized by multiple star-shaped serrated glands. These glands are lined by large cells with abundant foamy vacuolated cytoplasm (Figures 8.21 to 8.23). The nuclei of the cells are enlarged and hyperchromatic. The lining epithelial cells are often multilayered. The nuclei often show hobnailing appearance. Mitotic activity may be present.

### Ectopic Pregnancy

In ectopic pregnancy, the endometrial glands show hypersecretion. There may be focal Arias-Stella reaction. In addition, the endometrium may show decidual cells. In case of regression of the trophoblast in the ectopic site, the endometrial glands may show atrophic glands.

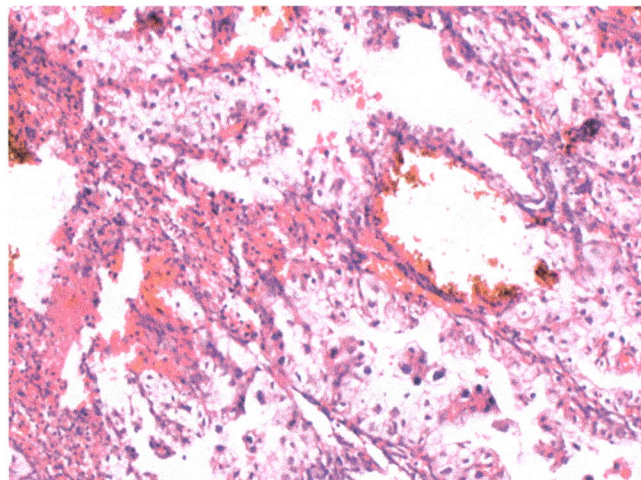

Figure 8.21: Arias-Stella reaction: Star-shaped endometrial glands

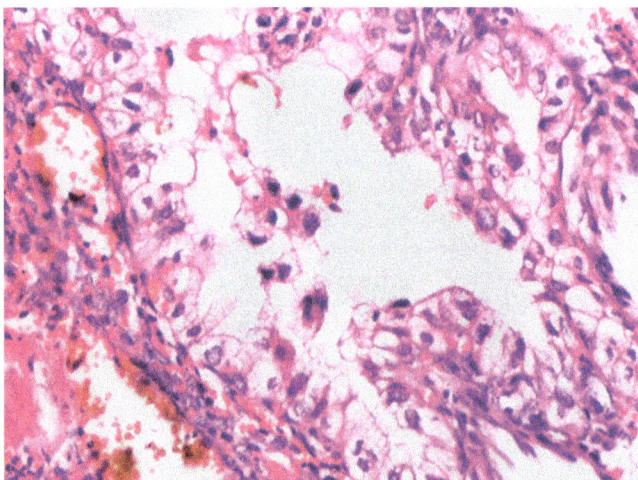

Figure 8.22: Arias-Stella reaction: Glands are lined by cells with abundant clear cytoplasm

## ARTIFACTS IN ENDOMETRIUM

Various artifacts may occur in endometrial curetting and may mislead the pathologists. These artifacts and contaminations have been described below.

### Telescoping Gland

As mentioned before glands within the glands may occur in proliferative and secretory phase due to increased tortuosity of the glands and also due to mechanical rupture and then artificial inclusion of the gland within a gland. These telescoping glands can be differentiated from hyperplasia by the lack of cytological atypia of the glandular lining cells and the normal appearing surrounding tissue.

### Collapsed Glands Simulating Crowding

The collapsed glands may come closer and simulate endometrial hyperplasia (Figure 8.24). The lack of continuous stroma and glands in the adjacent tissue is helpful to avoid mistake.

### Lower Uterine Segment

Tissue from the lower uterine segment may contaminate the endometrial curetting (Figure 8.25).

### Microglandular Hyperplasia of Cervix

Rarely the curetting may show cervical tissue with microglandular hyperplasia (Figure 8.26) and may be mistaken as

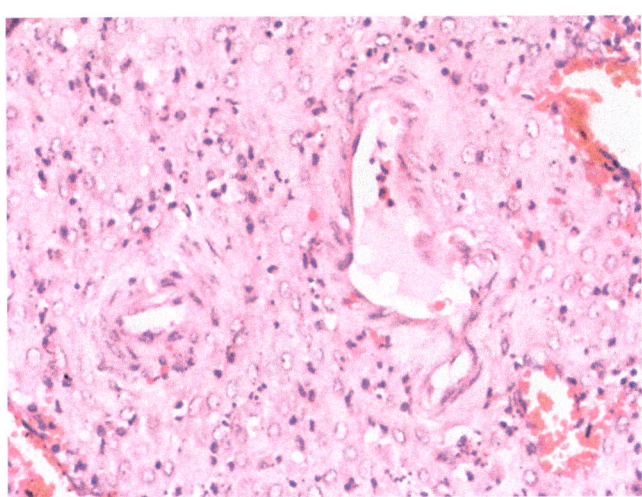

Figure 8.23: Arias-Stella reaction: abundant decidual reaction

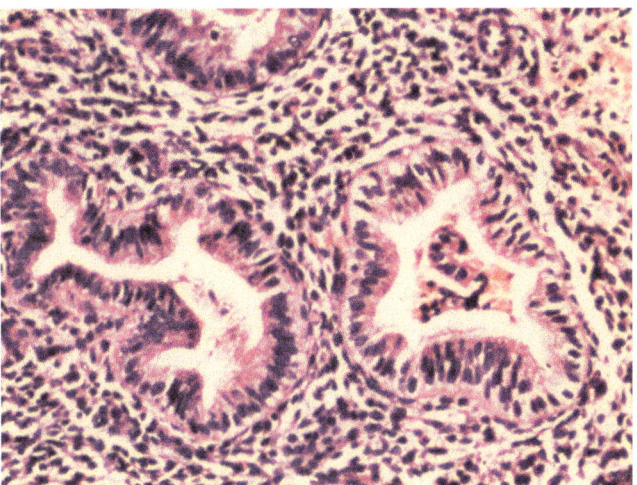

Figure 8.25: Lower uterine segment: the lining cells show endocervical glands with vacuolation that may simulate secretory changes

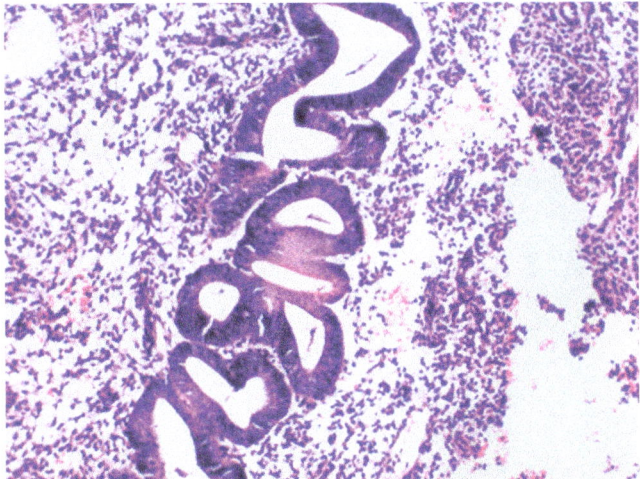

Figure 8.24: Collapsed endometrial glands simulating crowding

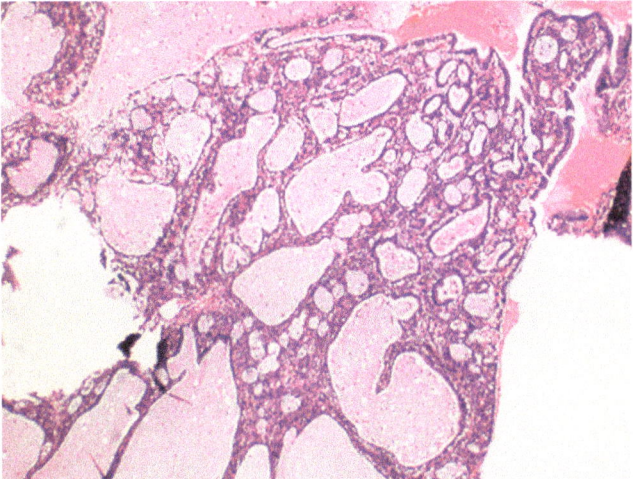

Figure 8.26: Microglandular hyperplasia of cervix: In the endometrial curetting, the microglandular hyperplasia may be mistaken as carcinoma of endometrium

endometrial carcinoma. Bland looking glandular epithelial cells and the presence of classical benign endocervical glands may be helpful to avoid such mistake.

## DYSFUNCTIONAL UTERINE BLEEDING

Normal menstrual cycle may be interfered by organic and non-organic or non-structural causes. The normal menstrual blood flow is in 28 days cycle and menstrual bleeding lasts for 4 days on average. The total blood flow in a cycle is about 30 ml and the upper limit is 80 ml.[2] Any aberration of this normal bleeding pattern is considered as abnormal uterine bleeding. The main cause of abnormal bleeding may be in the following levels:

1. Hypothalamo-pituitary axis,
2. Ovarian function, and
3. Proper response of endometrium. Dysfunctional uterine bleeding (DUB) is an abnormal bleeding in the uterus after the exclusion of the underlying pathological causes that include carcinoma, iatrogenic causes, pregnancy related diseases, medications, polyps and endometritis. There are lots of confusions regarding the terminology of DUB. Therefore the International Federation of Gynecology and Obstetrics (FIGO) recommends that this particular terminology should be discarded and the non-structural abnormal bleeding should be classified as:[3]
   a. Disturbances of endometrial origin,
   b. Disturbances of the hypothalamic-pituitary-ovarian axis and,
   c. Disturbances of hemostatic abnormality. FIGO recommends avoiding the complicated terminology such as menorrhagia, metrorrhagia, hypermenorrhea, menometrorrhagia, polymenorrhea, metropathia hemorrhagica, etc. Simple and understandable terminologies should be used (Box 8.4).

For the accurate diagnosis of DUB one has to exclude the organic causes that include:
1. Pathology in pelvis,
2. Systemic causes, and
3. Various iatrogenic causes (Box 8.5).

The two common causes of DUB are:
1. Anovulatory cycle and
2. Luteal phase abnormalities. The cause of DUB may be divided on the pathophysiological basis as Estrogen related and progesterone related DUB.

These morphological changes of glandular and stromal breakdown in DUB are non-specific as they are also found in various other conditions such as menstrual bleeding or other organic causes of bleeding.

### Glandular Changes (Box 8.6)

1. The presence of nuclear fragments in the base of the lining cells of glands.

---

**Box 8.4:** Abnormal uterine bleeding: Various definitions[3]

➡ **Disturbances of regularity**
- Irregular menstrual bleeding: It is defined as varying duration of bleeding-free intervals that is more than 17 days within a 90-day reference period
- Absent menstrual bleeding: No menstrual bleeding in 3 months

➡ **Disturbances of frequency**
- Infrequent menstrual bleeding: One or two episodes in 3 months
- Frequent menstrual bleeding: More than 4 episodes in 3 months

➡ **Disturbances of heaviness of flow**
- Heavy menstrual bleeding: Excessive menstrual blood flow that hampers the women's normal life (physical, emotional or social: it may be in combination)

➡ **Disturbances of the duration of flow**
- Prolonged menstrual bleeding: Menstrual flow of more than 8 days regularly

---

**Box 8.5:** Organic causes of uterine bleeding

➡ **Pelvic pathology**
- Leiomyoma
- Endometrial polyp
- Endometrial carcinoma
- Endometrial hyperplasia

➡ **Systemic pathology**

Coagulopathies
- Von Willebrand disease
- Hypothyroidism
- SLE

➡ **Iatrogenic causes**
- Hormonal therapy
- Contraception
- Medicine

---

**Box 8.6:** Evidences of gland and stromal breakdown

➡ **Glandular changes**
- Nuclear fragments in the base of the lining cells of glands
- Artificial crowding of the glands
- Eosinophilic epithelial cells often arranged in syncytium or pseudopapillary clusters

➡ **Stromal changes**
- Stromal collapse
- Stromal hemorrhage
- Fibrin thrombi
- Hemosiderin laden histiocytes
- Stromal fibrosis

2. Artificial crowding of the glands.
3. Eosinophilic syncytial change of the gland lining cell.[4]
4. Eosinophilic epithelial cells are often arranged in syncytium or pseudopapillary clusters in case of breakdown of glands. The pseudopapillary clusters are often infiltrated by polymorphs. The nuclei of the glandular cells are round, regular and hyperchromatic with infrequent mitotic activity. These pseudopapillary arrangements should not be over interpreted as atypia. This is a benign retrogressive change and is considered as a useful histological marker of glandular disintegration.

## Stromal Changes

1. Stromal collapse: The stromal cells collapse and form aggregate to give "stromal blue ball" appearance. The cells are often covered by surface epithelial cells. The individual stromal cell have scanty cytoplasm to strip off cytoplasm. Nuclei are round and hyperchromatic. Due to lack of cytoplasm the nuclei come close together and show nuclear molding giving false appearance of small cell carcinoma.
2. Stromal hemorrhage,
3. Fibrin thrombi: The stromal vessels show fibrin thrombi in the spiral arterioles or in small capillaries causing vascular stasis and bleeding,
4. Hemosiderin laden histiocytes
5. Stromal fibrosis in chronic bleeding.

## DUB due to Anovulatory Cycle

Anovulatory cycle is the most common cause of DUB. This is frequently occurs in perimenarcheal period. There is defect in hypothalamo-pituitary-ovarian axis and the ovarian follicle persists for long time.

This follicle continuously produce estrogen hormone causing the persistent proliferative changes in endometrium. Ultimately the follicle becomes atrophic and there is fall of estrogen level causing destabilization of the lysosomal membrane and vasoconstriction followed by endometrial breakdown and bleeding. This is also labeled as estrogen withdrawal bleeding. In case of breakthrough bleeding, the persistent estrogen may cause endometrial proliferation in such a degree that the endometrial tissue becomes deficient in vascular supply and finally sheds out.

### Changes in the Endometrium

The endometrium shows exuberant proliferative changes in the gland and stroma along with evidence of breakdown of the glands (Box 8.7). Endometrial glands are focally dilated and may show metaplastic changes. In case of long standing estrogen stimulation, the endometrial glands become more tortuous and dilated. Focal crowding of the glands may

---

**Box 8.7:** Changes of endometrium in anovulatory cycle

- Abundant proliferative endometrium
- Evidences of glandular and stromal breakdown
- Focal dilatation of the gland

In long standing cases
- More dilated glands
- More tortuous glands
- Focal crowding
- Tubal and eosinophilic metaplasia

Differential diagnosis: Simple hyperplasia

---

**Box 8.8:** Progesterone effect

➡ **Luteal phase defect: Defective corpus luteum**
- Lag period for more than 48 hours
- Discordance of glands and stroma
- Variable pattern of secretory changes

➡ **Persistent corpus luteum**
- Irregular shedding of endometrial tissue
- Mixed pattern of both secretory and proliferative endometrium in the 5th day of the menstrual cycle

---

also be noted. Focal and irregular subnuclear vacuolization may appear due to the effect of estrogen and the exact interpretation may be problematic.

### Differential Diagnosis

Simple hyperplasia: The glands are less crowded and show evidences of breakdown in case of disordered proliferative phase.

## Progesterone-related Disorder

The progesterone-related disorders may be due to: (1) Luteal phase defect, and (2) Persistent luteal phase.

### Luteal Phase Defect (Box 8.8)

In case of luteal phase defect the ovulation occurs, but there is deficient corpus luteum and inadequate production of progesterone hormone. The exact etiology of the deficient corpus luteum is not known. Possibly this is due to the defect of hypothalamo-pituitary axis and less production of FSH and LH.

**Endometrial changes:** As ovulation occurs in the luteal phase defect, so the glands and stroma both show secretory activity. However, there is lag period of the dating of the secretory endometrium for more than 48 hours. The glands and stroma may show discordance such as the glands may have saw toothed appearance and secretory changes, but the stroma may not show any predecidual changes.

In addition, the endometrium may show varying pattern of secretory changes such as early secretory changes along with predecidual reaction.

*Persistent Corpus Luteum (Box 8.8)*

The presence of persistent corpus luteum may cause irregular shedding of endometrial tissue. This will be represented by the mixed pattern of both secretory and proliferative endometrium. The diagnosis of irregular shedding is made when this mixed pattern is demonstrated in the 5th day of the menstrual cycle.

## HORMONE-INDUCED CHANGES

The variable type of hormones in varying combinations is used for different purposes and may have different effects on endometrium (Box 8.9).

### Estrogenic Hormone

The continuous use of estrogen shows endometrial proliferation and the effects simulate disordered proliferation as described in anovulatory cycle. There is high risk of endometrial hyperplasia and carcinoma in case of estrogen therapy alone.[5]

### Oral Contraceptives (OCP)

Both estrogen and progesterone is used in combination in oral contraceptives. The risk of ovarian and endometrial cancer is negligible in case of OCP. The endometrial curetting shows small tubular glands in a spindly stroma. The glands are lined by cuboidal cells.

### Progesterone Effect

Progesterone hormone therapy is used in case of DUB due to anovulatory disorders or in endometrial hyperplasia. In fact, the progesterone effect may show three types of patterns that includes—(1) decidual pattern, (2) secretory changes, and (3) atrophic changes.

*Decidual Changes*

The endometrium shows abundant predecidual changes. The marked predecidual changes may give rise to polypoid appearance. The glands show marked secretory activity.

*Secretory Changes (Figures 8.27 and 8.28)*

The stroma shows relatively abundant predecidual changes along with scattered secretory glands.

*Atrophic Changes*

This pattern is mainly seen in prolonged use of progesterone. The glands become small tubular and atrophic with weak

**Box 8.9:** Endometrial changes in hormonal therapy

→ **Estrogenic hormone**
- Tortuous proliferative glands
- Dilatation of the gland
- Simulates disordered proliferation

→ **Oral contraceptives**
- Small tubular glands
- Cuboidal lining with occasional vacuoles
- Spindly stroma

→ **Progesterone effect**
- Decidual changes
  - Extensive predecidual cells
  - Glands show marked secretory activity
- Secretory changes
  - Abundant predecidual changes
  - Scattered secretory glands
- Atrophic changes
  - Small tubular and atrophic gland
  - Weak secretory activity
  - Spindle-shaped stromal cells

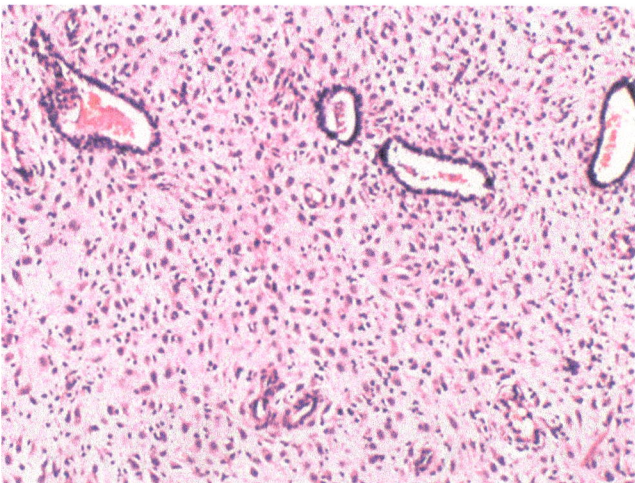

**Figure 8.27:** Progesterone effect: Secretory glands with abundant predecidual change

secretory activity. The glands are lined by low cuboidal epithelial cells. The stromal cells are spindle-shaped containing moderate amount of cytoplasm.

### Gonadotropin Releasing Hormone

Gonadotropin releasing hormone (GnRH) initially stimulates pituitary gland to release FSH and LH. Later on the pituitary becomes desensitized and the release of FSH and LH are decreased. Therefore, the ovarian hormone is also decreased. The endometrium shows marked atrophic changes. The glands become small tubular lined by low cuboidal cells.

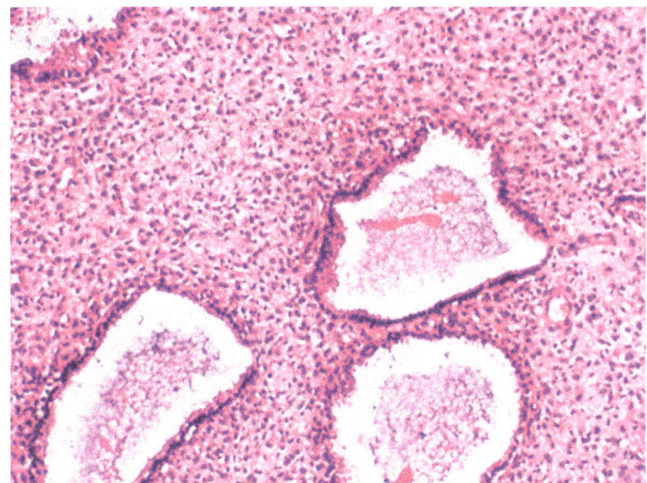

Figure 8.28: Progesterone effect: higher magnification shows slit like glands lined by cuboidal cells

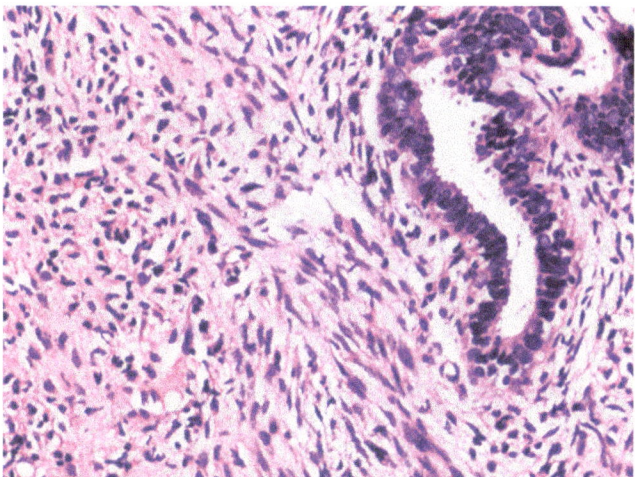

Figure 8.29: Chronic endometritis: Endometrial glands with lymphoplasmacytic infiltration in the stroma

## Tamoxifen

Tamoxifen is a non-steroidal antiestrogenic hormone which has also partial estrogenic agonistic action. In postmenopausal patients, tamoxifen mainly causes atrophic endometrium and occasionally proliferative changes. Endometrial hyperplasia and carcinoma may occur due to tamoxifen therapy.

## ENDOMETRITIS

Endometritis is often associated with recent pregnancy, use of intrauterine contraceptive device, instrumentation, and the presence of endometrial polyp or leiomyoma. The patient commonly complains of vaginal bleeding or heavy menstrual bleeding. The endometritis may be divided into acute and chronic phase. Practically speaking the endometritis is a continuous spectrum and therefore, there may be overlapping features and so it is not always possible to label the lesion acute or chronic.

## Nonspecific Endometritis

In case of acute endometritis, there is acute inflammatory cell infiltration in the glandular lumen and within the epithelial cells of the glands. The stroma is more spindle-shaped and may show collection of neutrophils with microabscess formation. The neutrophils are also seen beneath the surface of the endometrium. The endometrial surface and the glands show breakdown. The diagnosis of acute endometritis is complicated as it shares the same morphologic features of menstrual endometrium. In chronic endometritis, there is infiltration of lymphocytes, plasma cells and histiocytes. Rarely lymphoid follicles may be present. The presence of plasma cells is the indicator of chronic endometritis (Figures 8.29 and 8.30).

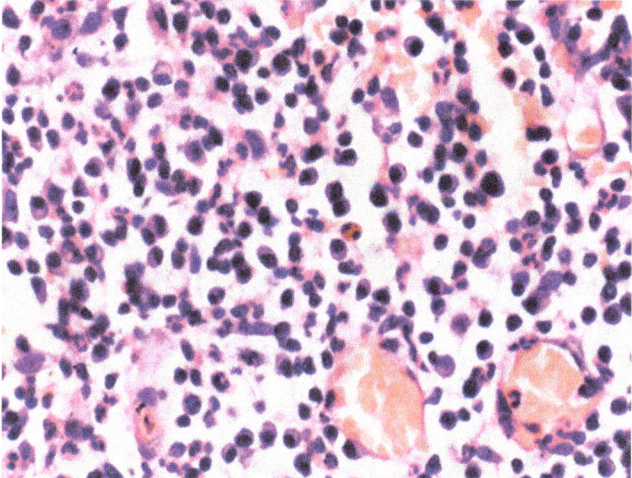

Figure 8.30: Chronic endometritis: Plasma cells and lymphocytic infiltration in the stroma

Stroma of the endometritis show bipolar spindle-shaped cells. The cells often show interlacing arrangement. The glands are underdeveloped and usually atrophic small tubular with weak proliferative activity. In case of secretory endometrium, the glands show lagging and weak secretory activity. In addition, the glands may show squamous, tubular or eosinophilic metaplasia.

## Specific Endometritis

It may be due to actinomycosis, herpes simplex, mycoplasma and tuberculosis.

### Tuberculosis

*Mycobacterium tubercle* infection of uterus may be either blood-borne or by direct extension from the fallopian tube or cervix. Tuberculosis of uterus is common in Indian subcontinent.[6] The patient usually presents with infertility. The postmenopausal patient may have menorrhagia. Histopathology of the endometrium show epithelioid cell granulomas and multinucleated giant cells (Figures 8.31 and 8.32). Caseous necrosis is usually not present. The endometrial glands are usually poorly developed and show lagging. It is necessary to have acid fast stain to demonstrate the bacilli or culture of mycobacteria.

## ENDOMETRIAL POLYP

Endometrial polyp represents 25% of all abnormal uterine bleeding.[7] The polyp occurs more commonly in 4th and 5th decade and rarely seen after 60 years. Patients with endometrial polyps are asymptomatic or may present with metrorrhagia, menorrhagia, postmenopausal bleeding and rarely with infertility.[7] Near about 2.5% of uterine polyps are malignant and malignancy occurs mainly in postmenopausal patient.[8] The risk factors of development of endometrial polyps are hormone replacement therapy and tamoxifen administration.[9] Polyps are detected and assessed by transvaginal ultrasound examination. Hysteroscopy also helps to detect and localize the endometrial polyp.

### Gross

Polyp is fleshy soft gray-white mass covered with surface epithelial lining in three surfaces. Polyps are variably sized and may be single or multiple, sessile or pedunculated.

### Histopathology

The essential characteristics of polyp in the microscopical examinations are:
1. Thick-walled stromal blood vessels.
2. Architectural abnormalities of the glands: The glands are dilated, branched and show focal crowding. The long axis of the glands is often parallel to the surface epithelium.
3. Dense and fibrotic stroma: The stroma is hypercellular and consists of spindle-shaped cells.
4. Simultaneous presence of normal uterine glands along with fragments of polypoid tissue with different glandular pattern. In addition, the glands may show squamous, tubular, ciliated or eosinophilic metaplasia.

The various histological patterns of endometrial polyps have been described that include hyperplastic (proliferative), atrophic, mixed endometrial and endocervical, and functional polyp.

a. Hyperplastic polyp: Mainly composed of many variable sized, irregular, dilated proliferative endometrial glands with focal crowding in a fibrous stroma. The histopathological features simulate like hyperplastic endometrium. The presence of normal appearing endometrium is helpful to diagnose such polyp (Figure 8.33).
b. Atrophic: The polyp shows many cystically dilated endometrial glands lined by small cuboidal cells. This pattern is commonly seen in postmenopausal patients (Figure 8.34).
c. Functional: The glands in the polyp are hormone sensitive and show cyclical changes (Figure 8.35). The glands may be proliferative or secretory, however, they are out of phase and shows poor secretory activity. The orientation of the glands are abnormal and this is the main clue of diagnosis such polyp. In addition, the presence of thick-walled vessels is also helpful diagnostic feature.
d. Mixed endometrial and endocervical polyp: This pattern shows combined feature of endometrial and endocervical polyp.

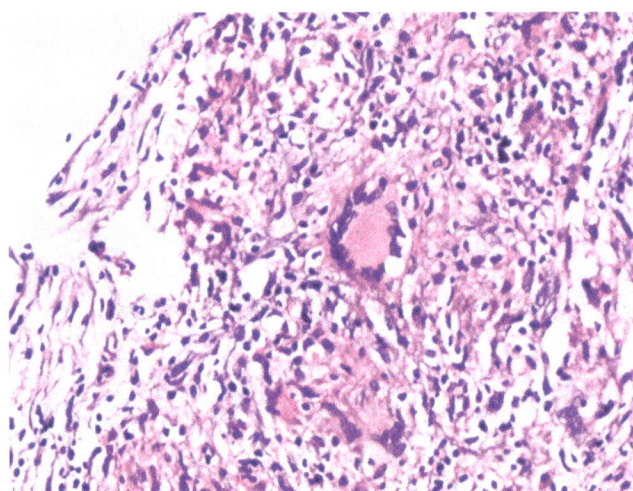

**Figure 8.31:** Tuberculosis of endometrium: Epithelioid cell granuloma in the endometrium

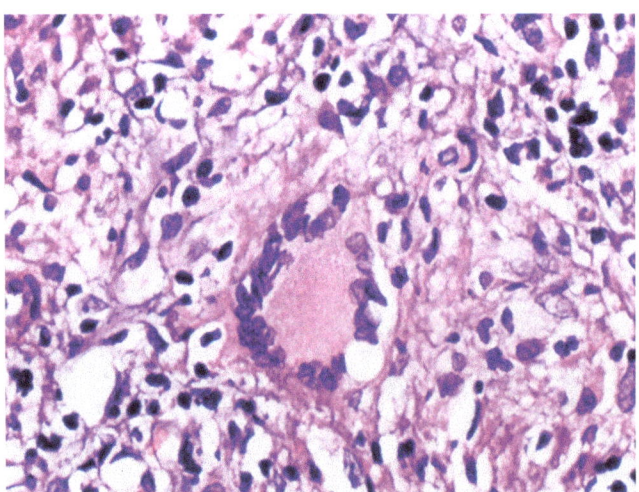

**Figure 8.32:** Tuberculosis of endometrium: Higher magnification shows Langhans giant cell

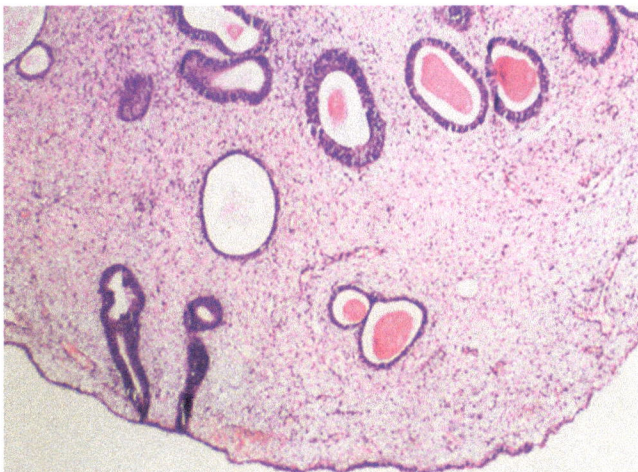

Figure 8.33: Endometrial hyperplastic polyp: Polyp lined by small cuboidal cells

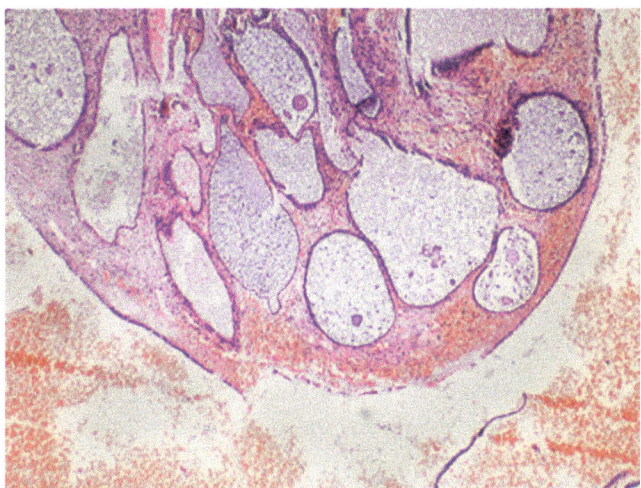

Figure 8.34: Endometrial atrophic polyp: Polyp lined by flat cells

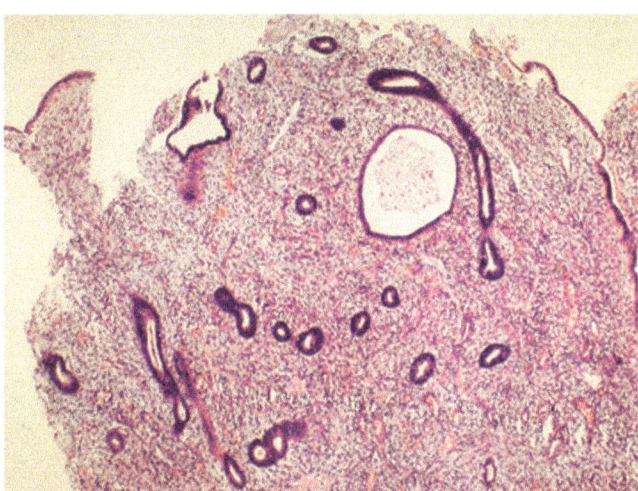

Figure 8.35: Endometrial functional polyp: Multiple endometrial glands in proliferative phase

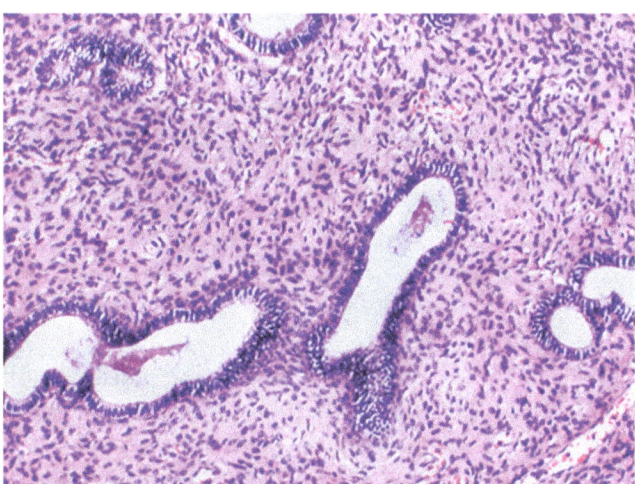

Figure 8.36: Adenomyomatous polyp: Endometrial glands surrounded by smooth muscle cells

## ADENOMYOMATOUS POLYP

In this polyp, the glands are encircled by spindle-shaped smooth muscle cells (Figure 8.36). The glands may be hyperplastic or functional and often show metaplastic changes.

## ATYPICAL POLYPOID ADENOMYOMA (APAM)

APAM is an uncommon tumor of uterus and the average age of the patient is 40 years. The tumor is rarely reported in postmenopausal patient.[10] The patient of APAM usually complains of vaginal discharge, abnormal uterine bleeding and post-coital bleeding.[10]

### Gross

APAM is commonly seen in the lower uterine segment. The lesion is of variably sized and is well circumscribed polypoidal mass with or without stalk.

### Microscopy

The tumor shows biphasic pattern consisting of atypical looking endometrial glands and smooth muscle cells surrounding the glands. The glands are of variable sized and irregular in shape with complex branching pattern. The glands are lined by cuboidal to columnar epithelial cells with moderate amount of cytoplasm. The nuclei are round and show mild to moderate atypia. The stroma shows smooth muscle cells in small interlacing fascicles. Unlike normal myometrium the smooth muscle component in APAM is more cellular, present in short fascicles along with small amount of fibrous tissue. More than 90% cases of APAM show the characteristic squamous metaplasia.

## Differential Diagnosis

1. Well-differentiated adenocarcinoma; The atypia of the glandular lining cells in APAM is less severe than adenocarcinoma and the stroma shows lack of desmoplastic reaction in APAM.
2. Malignant mixed Mullerian tumor (MMMT): The patients of APAM are younger than MMMT. The stromal component of APAM does not show significant pleomorphism and mitosis.

## Treatment

APAM is a benign tumor with indolent behavior. Simple removal of the polyp and follow-up of the patient is usually the treatment of choice. There is small risk of malignancy in APAM cases.[11] Therefore, hysterectomy is advised in patients of APAM who have completed their family or APAM diagnosed on fragmented curetting material.

## ENDOMETRIAL METAPLASTIC AND REACTIVE CHANGES

The terminology metaplasia indicates replacement of one group of mature cells to another group of mature cells that are not normally found in that organ. Endometrial Metaplastic changes (EMC) and reactive changes may be epithelial and stromal metaplasia in the endometrium.

The epithelial metaplasia includes: squamous, tubal, mucinous, eosinophilic, clear cell and hobnail variant. The stromal metaplasia may be osseous, smooth muscle and cartilaginous metaplasia (Box 8.10).

### Origin of the Metaplastic Cells

The metaplastic cell probably is originated from the endometrial stem cells. These cells probably remain in the stratum basal and stratum functional layer.

**Box 8.10:** Types of endometrial metaplasia

- **Epithelial**
  - Squamous
  - Tubal
  - Mucinous
  - Eosinophilic
  - Clear cell
  - Hobnail variant
  - Morula
- **Stromal**
  - Osseous
  - Smooth muscle
  - Cartilaginous metaplasia

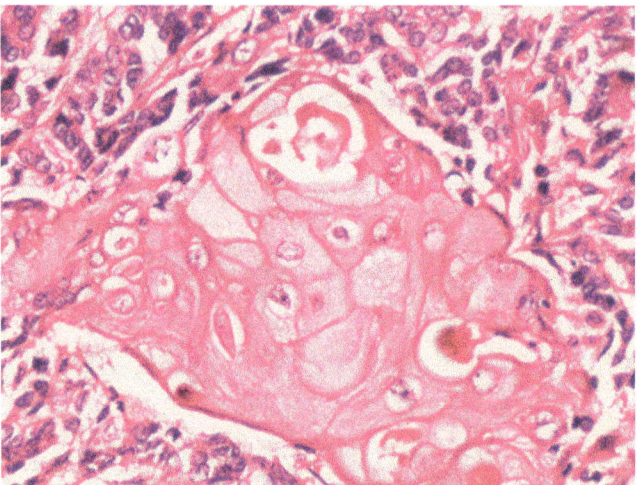

**Figure 8.37:** Squamous metaplasia: Cells with polyhedral appearance and centrally placed nuclei

### Significance

It is important to identify the various EMC as the presence of some of the EMCs has potential risk of carcinoma. Such as morules like EMC is always associated with malignancy. Ciliary and mucinous metaplasia have frequent association of carcinoma. Clear cell metaplasia is never related with any malignancy.

### Squamous Metaplasia

Endometrial squamous metaplasia (ESM) is one of the commonest EMC and is commonly seen in menopausal patient or patient undergoing investigation of infertility. The cases are usually asymptomatic. ESM is often associated with endometrioid carcinoma, endometrial hyperplasia, endometrial polyps, chronic irritation, pyometritis, etc. In case of ESM, there are sheets of non-keratinized mature polyhedral squamous cells with obvious intercellular bridge (Figure 8.37). The keratin may evoke giant cell reaction. ESM is usually focal. However, the whole of the uterine surface may be involved by diffuse ESM which is known as ichthyosis uteri.[12] Ichthyosis uteri commonly occurs in long standing obstruction in the uterine passage.

*Differential Diagnosis*

Whenever ESM is detected in curetting sample, the possibilities of atypical endometrial hyperplasia, well-differentiated endometrioid carcinoma and atypical polypoid adenomyoma should be excluded.

### Morules

This is a type of ESM and morphologically characterized by round to oval well circumscribed mass of cells within the glandular lumen. The individual cells show abundant eosinophilic cytoplasm, ill-defined cell border with monomorphic oval nuclei.

The central cells of morules may undergo necrosis and may form comedo pattern. Morules are often considered as the morphological variant of ESM.

*Differential Diagnosis*

The morular cells may be confused with: (a) Epithelioid cell granuloma, (b) Smooth muscle lesions.

## Ciliated and Tubular Metaplasia

Ciliated and tubular metaplasia (CTM) is one of the commonest metaplasia among EMCs. Normally the proliferative endometrium may show focal ciliated lining of endometrial surface. Therefore, CTM is considered when the majority of the glands and surface epithelium is replaced by the ciliated epithelial cells (Figure 8.38). The tubular metaplasia is characterized by the presence of three types of cells that include ciliated, clear and intercalary. CTM is seen in association with endometrial hyperplasia, adenocarcinoma, in atrophic endometrium, endometriosis and endometrial polyp.

*Immunocytochemistry*

CTM shows positivity for LhS28, the antibody of ciliary cells and p16INK4A. The cells show weak positivity for p53 stain.[13]

## Mucinous Metaplasia

Endometrial mucinous metaplasia (EMM) is relatively uncommon and is usually noted in perimenopausal and postmenopausal patients. EMM is commonly associated with tamoxifen-induced polyps, adenofibroma, adenosarcoma, endometriosis.[14] EMM is characterized by focal or diffuse replacement of the endometrial cells by abundant intracytoplasmic mucin. The tip of normal endometrial cells may contain mucin. The mucin containing cells are tall columnar with endocervical look. Rarely intestinal metaplasia may be seen characterized by the presence of goblet cell, neuroendocrine cells and columnar cells with the presence of brush borders. The cells of intestinal metaplasia show positivity for villin, chromogranin, CK 20 and CDX.[15]

*Differential Diagnosis*

1. Mucinous differentiation of endometrial carcinoma: The presence of foam cells and other fragment with complex hyperplasia usually favor adenocarcinoma.
2. Microglandular hyperplasia: The microglandular hyperplasia does not show complex branching pattern and cytological atypia.

## Clear Cell Metaplasia

The clear cell metaplasia (CCM) is uncommon and is usually seen in pregnancy, hyperplastic endometrium and progesterone therapy. It is characterized by replacement of the endometrial cells by clear cell with abundant vacuolated cytoplasm (Figure 8.39). The CCM should be distinguished from clear cell carcinoma. The bland nuclear morphology and lack of structural abnormality of the endometrial glands help to confirm the diagnosis of CCM.

## Hobnail Metaplasia

Hobnail metaplasia is rare and is usually seen in endometrial polyp and in pregnancy-induced change. The hobnail metaplasia is characterized by the cells with eosinophilic cytoplasm with nuclei protrude out into the glandular lumen.

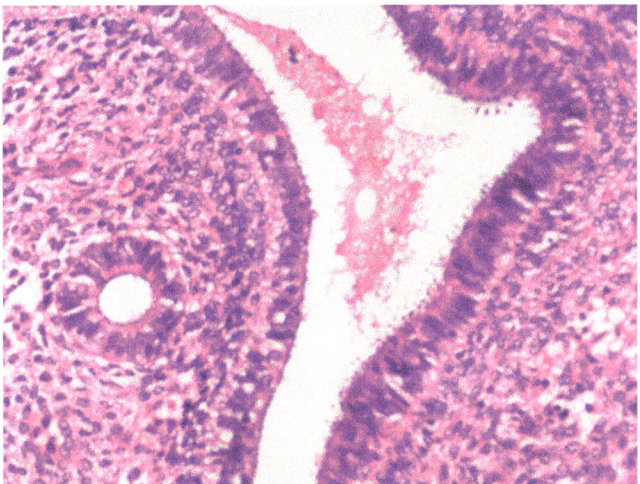

Figure 8.38: Tubal metaplasia: The endometrial glandular epithelium shows ciliate lining of the columnar cells

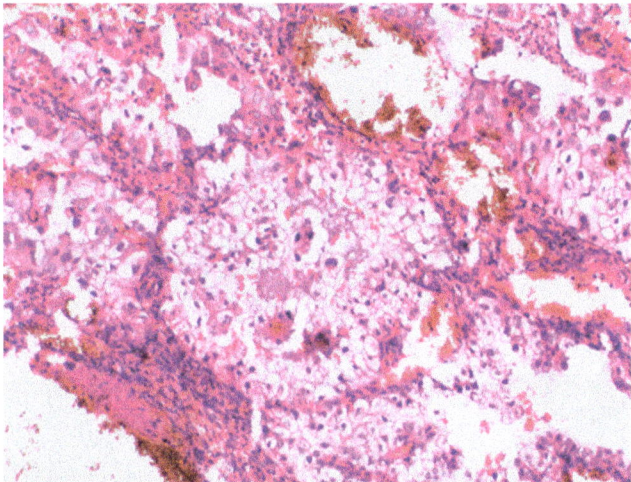

Figure 8.39: Clear cell metaplasia: The glandular epithelial cells show abundant clear cytoplasm with central nuclei

## Eosinophilic Metaplasia (Oncocytic Metaplasia)

Eosinophilic metaplasia is usually seen in endometrial polyp and endometritis. It is characterized by endometrial glandular cells with abundant eosinophilic cytoplasm (Figures 8.40 and 8.41). The cells contain abundant mitochondria in the electron microscopy. The differential diagnosis of eosinophilic metaplasia is oncocytic variant of endometrioid adenocarcinoma. The absence of nuclear atypia, no glandular architectural abnormality and no gross tumor eliminate the possibility of tumor.

## Papillary Syncytial Metaplasia

Papillary syncytial metaplasia (PCM) is a reactive changes and not a true metaplasia. This is seen in endometrial cyclic breakdown, endometrial polyp and hyperplasia. PCM is characterized by the proliferation of eosinophilic cells as small tufts. The clusters of cells often show micropapillary like arrangement with central fibrovascular core. Glandular lumen may be present in the aggregates of cells. The cells may show nuclear atypia and mitosis.

*Differential Diagnosis*

Papillary serous carcinoma: PCM may be confused with papillary serous carcinoma. The glands do not show any structural abnormality in PCM.

## Stromal Metaplasia

Stromal metaplasia is a rare incidental finding without much clinical significance. Osseous metaplasia and cartilaginous metaplasia both are very uncommon[16] and MMMT should be excluded before such diagnosis. The presence of adipose tissue is a reactive process and is usually seen along with endometrial carcinoma.

## ASHERMAN'S SYNDROME

Asherman's syndrome is characterized by intrauterine adhesion and is usually noted after trauma of endometrium during curettings, endometritis or abortion. The patient usually presents with infertility, menstrual abnormality (amenorrhea and hypomenorrhea) and recurrent abortion. The patients may also have various complications in pregnancy such as placenta previa or placenta accreta.

### Risk Factors

Miscarriage curetting, abortion, chronic endometritis, uterine myomectomy, and hysteroscopic surgery.

### Histology

Endometrial cavity is lined by single layer of cuboidal epithelial cells. The endometrial stroma is fibrosed and often calcified. There is marked reduction of endometrial layer and both stratum functionalis and stratum basalis shrinks.

### Diagnosis

Hysterosalpingography or transvaginal USG.

### Treatment

Hysteroscopic surgery: The method of choice. Here the adhesion of the uterine wall is broken down by the tip of the hysteroscope by direct view.

## ENDOMETRIOSIS

Endometriosis is characterized by the presence of endometrial tissue consisting of both glands and stroma outside the uterine cavity.

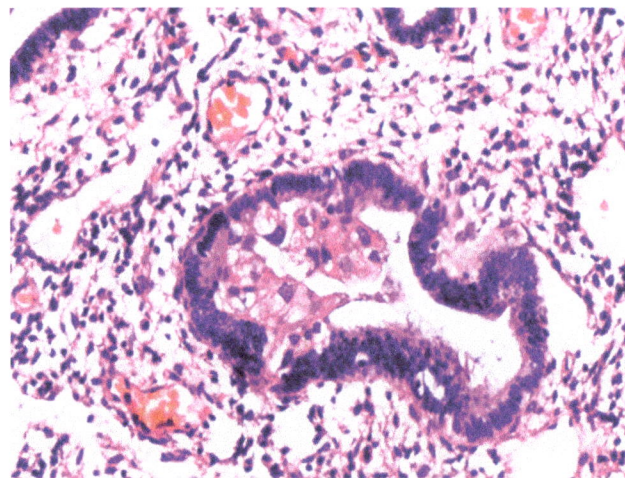

**Figure 8.40:** Eosinophilic metaplasia: Cell with moderate to abundant eosinophilic cytoplasm

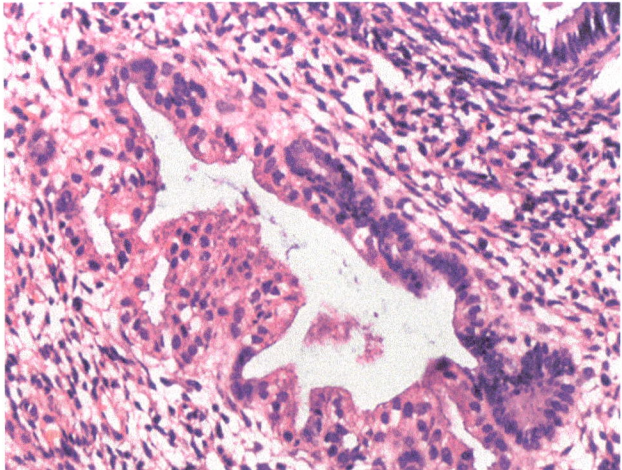

**Figure 8.41:** Eosinophilic metaplasia: Higher magnification of the eosinophilic metaplastic cells of glandular lining epithelium

## Etiology and Pathogenesis

There are two main theories of endometriosis:
1. Metastatic theory: This theory suggests that due to retrograde menstrual flow through the fallopian tube the endometrial tissue is implanted on the peritoneal surface followed by growth.[17]
2. Metaplastic theory: The metaplastic theory suggests that metaplasia of the peritoneal epithelium is the source of endometriosis.[18]
3. Other factors: Various other etiological factors such as genetic cause, hormonal factor and immunological factors are also blamed for endometriosis.[19]

## Clinical Features

The exact incidence of endometriosis is difficult to ascertain as many patients are asymptomatic. However, the overall prevalence of endometriosis is 10 to 15%. The disease predominantly occurs in the reproductive age group. Endometriosis commonly affects ovary, uterine ligaments, and rectovaginal septum. In addition, it may involve skin, cervix, vagina, vulva, gastrointestinal tract, and umbilicus. The patients commonly complain of pelvic pain, cyclical dyspareunia, dysmenorrhea and infertility. Rarely endometriosis of lung may present with catamenial pneumothorax.

## Gross

Grossly, the lesion presents as small reddish nodule or cyst over the surface of the organ. It may also appear as dense white scar due to long standing lesion. In ovary, endometriosis may cause repeated hemorrhage and thereby may form large cyst filled with reddish brown chocolate colored material known as "chocolate cyst".

## Histopathology (Figures 8.42 to 8.44)

The characteristic histological triad of endometriosis includes:
1. The presence of endometrial like glands.
2. Typical endometrial stroma: Typical spindle-shaped endometrial stroma is easily identifiable.
3. Hemosiderin laden macrophages indicating old hemorrhage.

The typical three features may not be found in all cases of endometriosis. The endometrial glands and stroma may be obscured by repeated hemorrhage.

In ovary, the endometriotic foci may be small and superficial or it may produce cystic lesion. The endometriotic cyst in the ovary may be large and lined by only single layer of cuboidal epithelial cell. Careful examination may reveal endometrial stroma. Occasionally both the lining of endometrial gland and stroma may be totally obscured

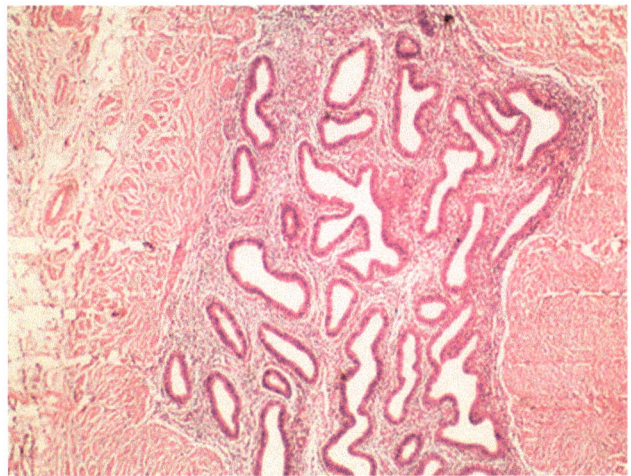

**Figure 8.42:** Tubal endometriosis: Endometrial glands and stroma in fallopian tube

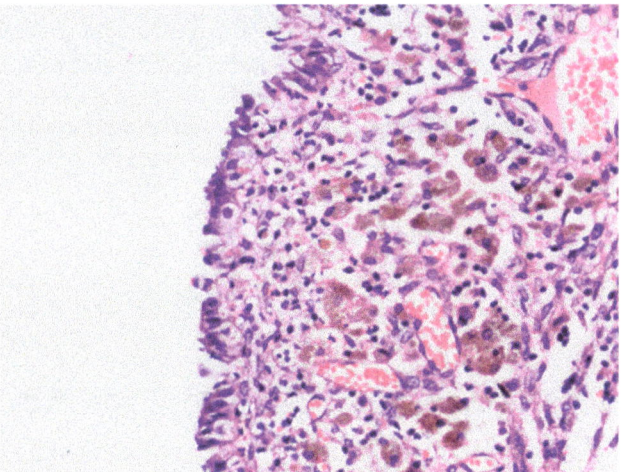

**Figure 8.43:** Ovarian endometriosis: Endometriotic cyst in ovary is lined by cuboidal epithelium with pigment laden macrophages underneath the lining

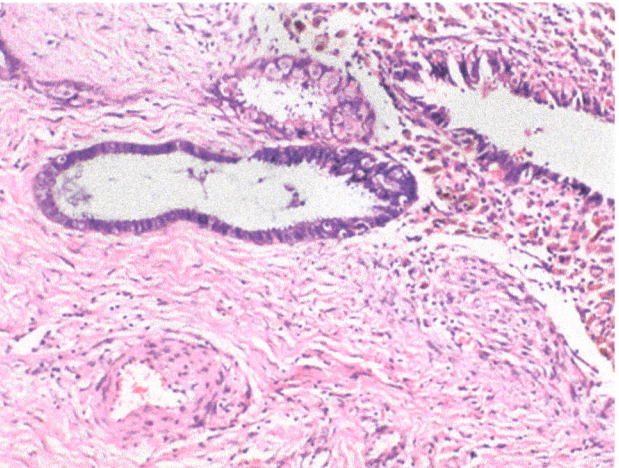

**Figure 8.44:** Ovarian endometriosis: Endometrial gland within the ovarian stroma

and only hemosiderin laden macrophages along with dense fibrosis are seen.

## Differential Diagnosis

a. Endosalpingiosis: In endosalpingiosis, the epithelial cells of the glands are bland looking and ciliated. No endometrial stroma is seen.
b. Metastatic adenocarcinoma: Metastatic adenocarcinoma shows significant atypia of the glandular epithelial cells and absence of any endometrial stroma.
c. Endometrioid stromal sarcoma (ESS): Endometrial stromal sarcoma lacks typical endometrial glands.

## Prognosis and Management

Endometriosis is a chronic disease and complete remission is difficult to obtain. The patient is treated both by medically and also by surgically. The medical treatment includes use of estrogen antagonists, androgenic agents, progestins, and gonadotropin releasing hormone (GnRH) analogs.[20] The disease may recur after cessation of medical therapy. Surgical ablation of the endometriotic foci and removal of endometriotic cyst followed by medical therapy are also recommended.

## REFERENCES

1. Beswick IP, Gregory MM. The Arias-Stella phenomenon and the diagnosis of pregnancy. J Obstet Gynaecol. 1971;78:143-8.
2. Treloar AE, Boynton RE, Behn BG, Brown BW. Variation of the human menstrual cycle through reproductive life. Int J Fertil. 1967;12(1 Pt 2):77-126.
3. Fraser IS, Critchley HO, Broder M, Munro MG. The FIGO recommendations on terminologies and definitions for normal and abnormal uterine bleeding. Semin Reprod Med. 2011;29(5):383-90.
4. Shah SS, Mazur MT. Endometrial eosinophilic syncytial change related to breakdown: immunohistochemical evidence suggests a regressive process. Int J Gynecol Pathol. 2008;27:534-8.
5. Grady D, Rubin SM, Petitti DB, Fox CS, Black D, Ettinger B, et al. Hormone therapy to prevent disease and prolong life in postmenopausal women. Ann Intern Med. 1992;117:1016-37.
6. Mondal SK. Histopathologic analysis of female genital tuberculosis: a fifteen-year retrospective study of 110 cases in eastern India.Turk Patoloji Derg. 2013;29(1):41-5.
7. Van Bogaert LJ. Clinicopathologic findings in endometrial polyps. Obstet Gynecol. 1988;71(5):771-3.
8. Armenia CS. Sequential relationship between endometrial polyps and carcinoma of the endometrium. Obstet Gynecol. 1967;30:524-9.
9. Bakour SH, Gupta JK, Khan KS. Risk factors associated with endometrial polyps in abnormal uterine bleeding. Int J Gynaecol Obstet. 2002;76:165-8.
10. Young RH, Treger T, Scully RE. Atypical polypoid adenomyoma of the uterus: a report of 27 cases. Am J Clin Pathol. 1986;86:139-45.
11. Heatley MK. Atypical polypoid adenomyoma: a systematic review of the English literature. Histopathology. 2006;48:609-10.
12. Brown D Jr, Spjut HJ. Extensive squamous metaplasia of the endometrium (ichthyosis uteri). South Med J. 1982;75:593-5.
13. Horree N, Heintz AP, Sie-Go DM, et al. p16 is consistently expressed in endometrial tubal metaplasia. Cell Oncol. 2007;29:37-45.
14. Deligdisch L, Kalir T, Cohen CJ, et al. Endometrial histopathology in 700 patients treated with tamoxifen for breast cancer. Gynecol Oncol. 2000;78:181-6.
15. Wells M, Tiltman A. Intestinal metaplasia of the endometrium. Histopathology. 1989;15:431-3.
16. Courpas AS, Morris JD, Woodruff JD. Osteoid tissue in utero. Report of 3 cases. Obstet Gynecol. 1964;24:636-40.
17. Sampson JA. Peritoneal endometriosis due to menstrual dissemination of endometrial tissue into the peritoneal cavity. Am J Obstet Gynecol. 1927;14:422-69.
18. Lauchlan SC. The secondary müllerian system. Obstet Gynecol Surv. 1972;27:133-46.
19. Steele RW, Dmowski WP, Marmer DJ. Immunologic aspects of human endometriosis. Am J Reprod Immunol. 1984;6:33-6.
20. Olive DL. Medical therapy of endometriosis. Semin Reprod Med. 2003;21(2):209-22.

# Uterus: Preneoplastic Lesions and Carcinoma

**9**

## WHO CLASSIFICATION OF THE TUMORS OF THE UTERINE CORPUS[1]

### Epithelial tumors and precursors

Precursors
- Hyperplasia without atypia
- Atypical hyperplasia/Endometrioid intraepithelial neoplasia

Endometrial carcinoma
Endometrioid carcinoma
- Squamous differentiation
- Villoglandular
- Secretory

Mucinous carcinoma
Serous carcinoma
Clear cell carcinoma
Neuroendocrine tumors
- Low-grade neuroendocrine tumor
  - Carcinoid tumor
- High-grade neuroendocrine carcinoma
  - Small cell neuroendocrine carcinoma
  - Large cell neuroendocrine carcinoma

Mixed adenocarcinoma
Undifferentiated carcinoma
Dedifferentiated carcinoma
Tumor-like lesions
- Polyp
- Metaplasia
- Arias-Stella reaction
- Lymphoma like lesion

Mesenchymal tumors
Leiomyoma
- Cellular leiomyoma
- Leiomyoma with bizarre nuclei
- Mitotically active leiomyoma
- Hydropic leiomyoma
- Apoplectic leiomyoma
- Lipomatous leiomyoma
- Epithelioid leiomyoma
- Myxoid leiomyoma
- Dissecting leiomyoma
- Diffuse leiomyomatosis
- Intravenous leiomyomatosis
- Metastasizing leiomyoma

Smooth muscle tumor of uncertain malignant potential
Leiomyosarcoma
- Epithelioid leiomyosarcoma
- Myxoid leiomyosarcoma

Endometrial stromal and related tumors
- Endometrial stromal nodule
- Low-grade endometrial stromal sarcoma
- High-grade endometrial stromal sarcoma
- Undifferentiated uterine sarcoma
- Uterine tumor resembling ovarian sex cord tumor

Miscellaneous mesenchymal tumors
- Rhabdomyosarcoma
- Perivascular epithelioid cell tumor
  - Benign
  - Malignant

Others

### Mixed epithelial and mesenchymal tumors
- Adenomyoma
- Atypical polypoid adenomyoma
- Adenofibroma
- Adenosarcoma
- Carcinosarcoma

### Miscellaneous tumors
- Adenomatoid tumor
- Neuroectodermal tumor
- Germ cell tumor

### Lymphoma and myeloid tumors
### Secondary tumor

## ENDOMETRIAL HYPERPLASIA

Endometrial hyperplasia is a group of diseases of uterus that consist of benign disease to premalignant conditions.[1] The term endometrial hyperplasia indicates non-physiologic non-invasive proliferation of the endometrium that encompasses benign changes due to hormonal influence to a premalignant condition.[1] In 1994, WHO classified endometrial hyperplasia mainly on the basis of "atypia" (Table 9.1).

**Table 9.1:** World Health Organization classification of endometrial hyperplasia (1994)

| Typical endometrial hyperplasia |
| --- |
| • Simple |
| • Complex |
| Atypical endometrial hyperplasia |
| • Simple |
| • Complex |

However, the practical application of this classification has been criticized[2] because of: (1) poor reproducibility, (2) the category simple hyperplasia with atypia is almost non-existent and it is very difficult to differentiate simple atypical hyperplasia from complex atypical hyperplasia. Therefore in 2014 classification, WHO divided hyperplasia into two groups:[1]

a. Hyperplasia without atypia
b. Atypical hyperplasia/Endometrioid intraepithelial neoplasia.

### Clinical Features

Endometrial hyperplasia (EH) is usually detected during the work up of infertility patients. A significant fraction of the patients are asymptomatic and remain undetected. The patient may also complain of abnormal uterine bleeding. EH occurs due to unopposed estrogenic stimulation of endometrium in case of: (1) anovulatory cycle, (2) Stein Leventhal syndrome, (3) excess estrogen secretion in estrogen producing ovarian tumors, and (4) exogenous estrogen administration.

### Histopathology

*Non-Atypical Hyperplasia*

**Simple hyperplasia:** In simple hyperplasia (SH), the glands are variable sized and well separated by cellular stroma (Figures 9.1 and 9.2). The glands may be cystically dilated and tortuous and give Swiss-cheese pattern. Occasional out pouching of the glands are also seen. The glandular lining cells may show focal tufting and pseudostratification. The nuclei of the cells are round monotonous with inconspicuous nucleoli and fine chromatin. Frequent tubal metaplasia and ciliated metaplasia are also noted. The stroma is dense and cellular. The gland versus stromal ratio is not much altered. Stroma and glands both show mitotic activity.

*Differential diagnosis:* (a) Cystic atrophy: The lining epithelium of cystic atrophy are low cuboidal to flattened and the stroma is dense fibrotic in cystic atrophy, (b) endometrial polyp: The polyps are covered in by surface epithelium in all the three surfaces and may show a separate fragments of normal endometrium, (c) disordered proliferation: This is a less defined subjective diagnosis. The lack of increased number of glands, significant size variation and absence of crowding helps to diagnose disordered proliferation, (d) chronic endometritis: the presence of plasma cells in the stroma is a diagnostic clue of chronic endometritis.

**Complex hyperplasia:** In complex hyperplasia (CH), the gland versus stromal ratio is increased (more than 2:1). The glands are variable sized and show frequent out pouching

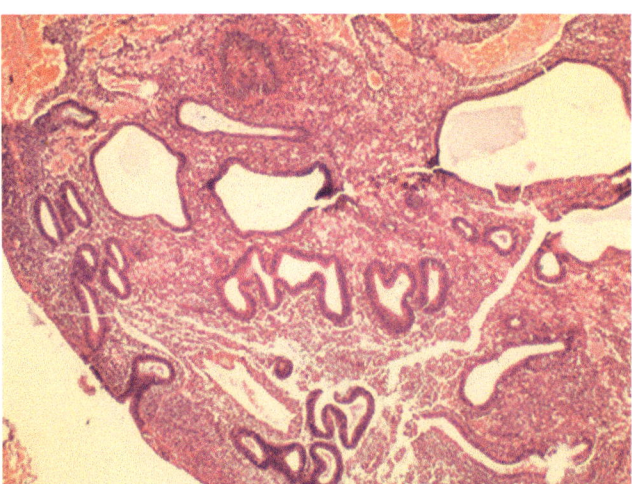

**Figure 9.1:** Simple hyperplasia: Multiple cystically dilated glands with dilatation and crowding

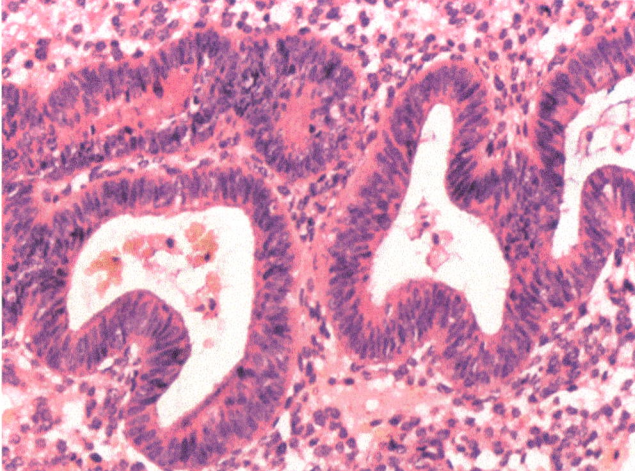

**Figure 9.2:** Simple hyperplasia: Higher magnification shows dilated glands lined by cuboidal epithelium with pseudostratification

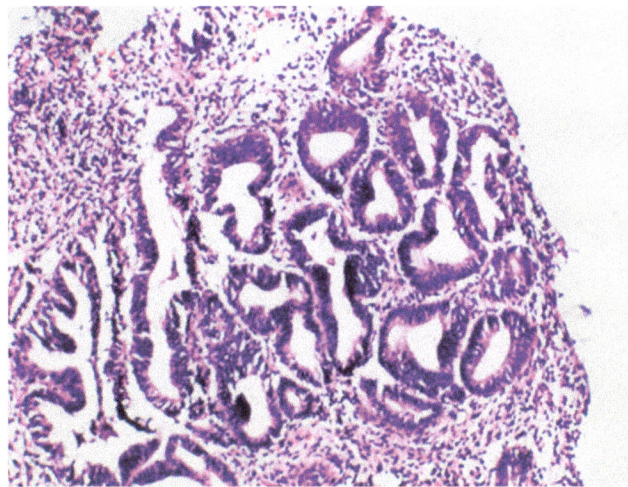

Figure 9.3: Complex hyperplasia without atypia: Complex branching of the glands

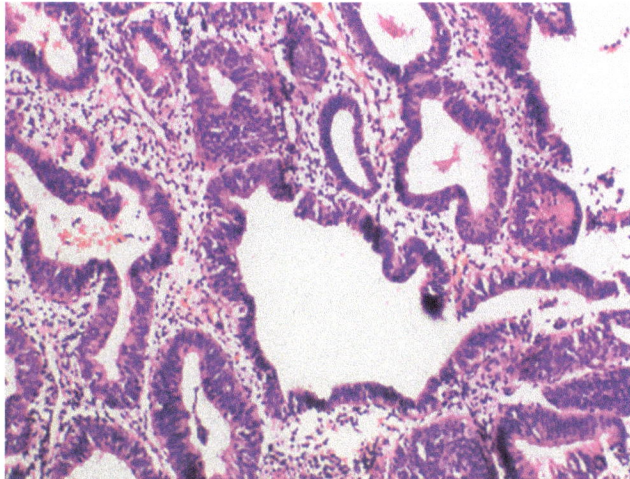

Figure 9.4: Complex hyperplasia without atypia: The cells of lining epithelium do not show any atypia

and complex branching pattern. Glands show significant crowding and back-to-back appearance (Figures 9.3 and 9.4). The glandular crowding is an important feature to diagnose complex hyperplasia. In addition, the glands may show tubular, squamous and clear cell metaplastic changes.

*Differential diagnosis of CH:* (a) all the differential diagnostic entities of SH, (b) SH: the distinguishing features between SH and CH are mainly glandular crowding (Table 9.2), (c) atypical polypoid adenomyoma (APAM): APAM is a single polypoid lesion and shows small interlacing bundle of smooth muscles around the gland.

Table 9.2: Differential features of simple hyperplasia versus complex hyperplasia

| Features | Simple hyperplasia | Complex hyperplasia |
| --- | --- | --- |
| Gland versus stromal ratio | Less | More |
| Glandular crowding | Usually less and focal | Significant |
| Glandular branching | Simple branching | Complex branching |

**Atypical Hyperplasia**

*Simple atypical hyperplasia:* Here the glands do not have any architectural complexity; however, the glandular lining cells show nuclear atypia.

*Complex atypical hyperplasia:* Complex atypical hyperplasia (CAH) shows marked increase of gland versus stromal area. The glands are overcrowded and have back-to-back appearance with little intervening stroma (Figures 9.5 and 9.6). Each gland retains the basement membrane. The glands are of variable shape and size with complex branching pattern. The lining epithelium of the glands shows true stratification. The orientation of nuclei is altered and there is loss of polarity. The cells show enlarged round nuclei with

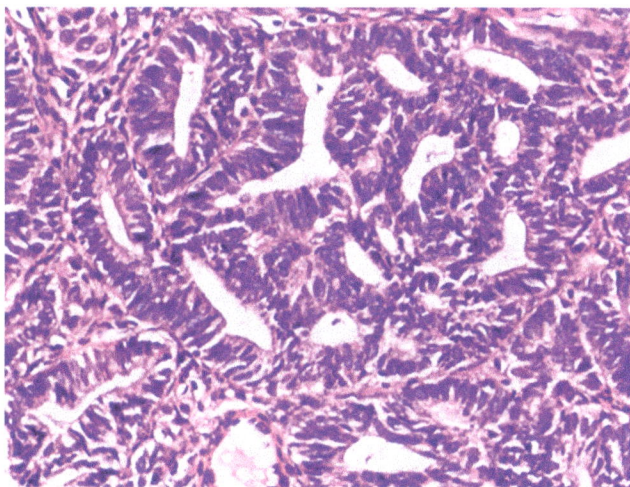

Figure 9.5: Atypical complex hyperplasia: The glands show crowding and branching

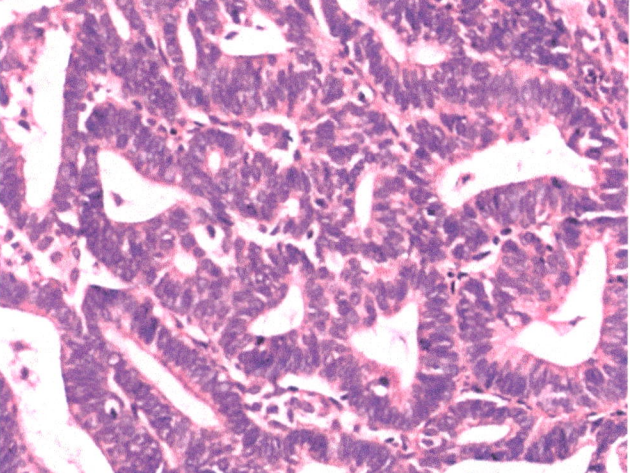

Figure 9.6: Atypical complex hyperplasia: The glandular lining epithelial cells show nuclear atypia

moderate pleomorphism having irregular membrane and coarse granular chromatin. Nucleoli are prominent. Frequent mitotic activities are also noted. In addition the glands show frequent squamous metaplastic changes.

*Differential diagnosis of CAH:* (a) atypical polypoid adenomyoma, (b) chronic endometritis, (c) metaplastic changes: squamous, eosinophilic, ciliated and mucinous metaplasia may be seen in normal endometrium and also in hyperplastic endometrium. (d) well-differentiated adenocarcinoma (WDAC): It is extremely difficult to differentiate CAH from WDAC on endometrial curetting based on morphology. The following features may be helpful in diagnosis of WDAC:[3] (1) back-to-back gland with almost no intervening stroma, (2) stromal desmoplasia, and (3) papillary projections of epithelial lining of the glands.

*Prognosis:* The different studies emphasized the greater risk of progression in atypical hyperplasia than typical hyperplasia. Architectural crowding without atypia may also progress to carcinoma but in much lower rate. The progression of carcinoma was seen in 1% cases of SH, 3% cases of CH and 29% cases of atypical hyperplasia (Table 9.3).[4] It was noted that most of the cases of SH and CH are regressed and the regression rate of SH, CH and CAH is 74–80%, 75–80% and 31–57% respectively.[4]

Table 9.3: Progression rate of different hyperplasia to carcinoma

|  | SH (%) | CH (%) | SAH (%) | AH (%) |
|---|---|---|---|---|
| Kurman[4] | 1 | 3 | 8 | 28.6 |
| Baak[5] | 0 | 16.7 | 7 | 45.4 |
| Lacey JV Jr[6] | 2 | 2.8 | - | 51.8 |

*Abbreviations*: SH, Simple hyperplasia, CH, Complex hyperplasia, AH, Atypical hyperplasia

*Treatment:* The management and treatment of EH depends on the type of hyperplasia, and age of the patient (Figure 9.7).

**Premenopausal:** The cases of EH are estrogen dependent therefore progesterone therapy is used to regress the tumor. The glandular volume regresses by apoptosis. SH and CH in premenopausal patient can be treated with progestogen and the patients should be followed up further by repeat curetting.[7]

**Postmenopausal**: CH in postmenopausal patients can also be managed by conservative therapy by administering progestogens and to do follow-up curetting and sonography at regular interval. In case of persistence of the lesion hysterectomy can be done.

**Atypical hyperplasia**: The CAH should be managed by simple hysterectomy in postmenopausal patients. In surgically high-risk patients the combined treatment with progestogens and gonadotropin-releasing hormone analogues has been successfully used and regression was noted in 84% patients of CAH.[8]

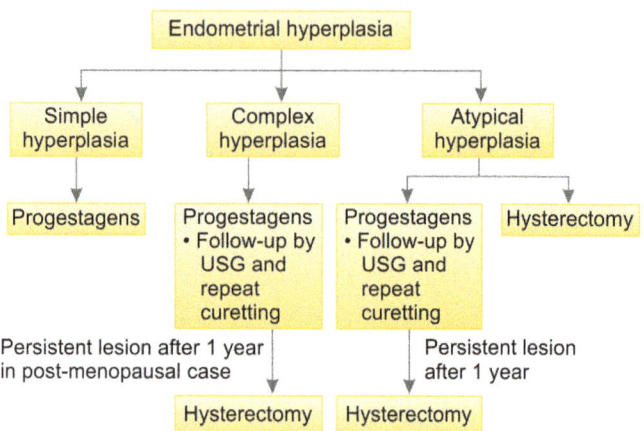

Figure 9.7: Management of endometrial hyperplasia

## ENDOMETRIAL INTRAEPITHELIAL NEOPLASIA

Endometrial intraepithelial neoplasia (EIN) is a monoclonal proliferation of architecturally and cytologically altered glands that carry high risk to undergo transformation to adenocarcinoma.[9] If untreated, then 30 to 50% EIN may develop into invasive adenocarcinoma. EINs are always noninvasive and they include most of the cases of CAH.

### Genetic Changes in EIN

*PTEN*

Phosphatase and tensin homolog (PTEN), a tumor suppressor gene, is most active in the proliferative glands. The expression of PTEN is diminished in the mid and late secretory glandular epithelial cells. PTEN is inactivated in proliferative (43%), persistent proliferative (56%), and EIN diagnostic categories (63%).[10] PTEN loss should always correlate with the morphology of the endometrium before any diagnosis of EIN.

*PAX2*

PAX-2 gene is responsible for Müllerian tract differentiation and morphogenesis. There is progressive loss of PAX-2 from normal endometrium (36%) to EIN (71%). Coexistent loss of PAX-2 and PTEN is more common in EIN (31%) compared to normal endometrial tissue (21%).[11]

*p-53*

Mutation of p53 gene is usually demonstrated by diffuse strong nuclear stain of p53 in immunocytochemistry. Both immunostain and p53 mutation is well correlated. The

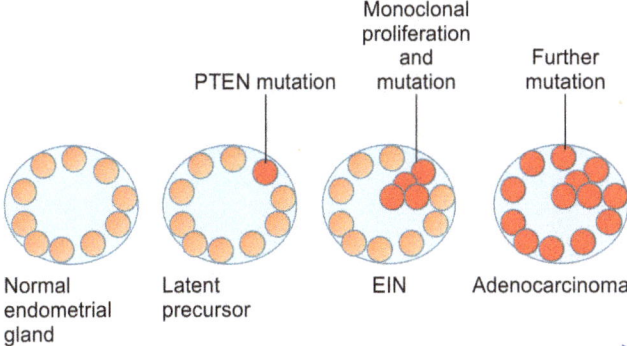

**Figure 9.8:** Schematic diagram shows the development of endometrial carcinoma from normal to preneoplastic gland

identical p53 gene mutation has been demonstrated in the synchronous EIN and endometrial carcinoma.[12]

*Others*

Microsatellite instability and K-ras mutation have been also demonstrated in 15 to 20% cases of EIN.[13]

## Pathophysiology

The occasional endometrial gland of endometrial hyperplasia at first shows loss of PTEN expression of the normal looking glands. These glands are often labeled as "latent precursors" as other additional genetic damage is needed to develop morphological recognizable lesion (Figure 9.8). Possibly continuous long-term exposure of the glands by estrogen acts as stimulation for further genetic changes. The epithelial cells develop PAX-2 mutation and other genetic changes such as microsatellite instability. These genetically altered glands show morphologically recognizable abnormality and is labeled as EIN. Possibly further mutational changes are responsible for the development of adenocarcinoma.

## Histopathology

The histopathological diagnostic criteria of EIN include:
1. Architecture: The glands are crowded, irregular in shape and size and may show branching. Importantly the gland area exceeds that of stroma and the volume percentage of the gland should exceed more than 50%. It is important to assess the gland volume in the area with intact stroma as stromal collapse may give false impression of excess gland area.
2. Cytology: The cells show nuclear enlargement, pleomorphism, high nucleo-cytoplasmic ratio and prominent nucleoli. The nuclear polarity along the basement membrane of the glandular lumen is altered.
3. Size: An EIN lesion must be greater than 1 mm diameter.
4. Exclusion of mimickers: The various mimickers of EIN must be excluded before diagnosis of EIN. These mimickers include: (a) Benign endometrial hyperplasia, (b) Reactive changes: Epithelial piling and loss of polarity may occur in reactive changes of the gland resulting from recent instrumentation, or infection. (c) Endometrial polyp in fragment, (d) Stromal breakdown: Stromal breakdown may mimic EIN due to artificial crowding, piling up of glandular lining cells and loss of polarity.
5. Exclusion of cancers: Solid areas, cribriform appearance and myoinvasion indicate invasive carcinoma.

## Treatment

Due to high risk of malignant transformation and possibility to miss an occult carcinoma in endometrial curetting, it is advisable to do hysterectomy in case of EIN. However, the young patient who wants to preserve the fertility, progestin hormone can be given.

## ENDOMETRIAL CARCINOMA

Endometrial carcinoma is the most common carcinoma of the female genital tract in the developed countries. There are about 34,000 new cases of endometrial cancer in every year in the USA.[14] The incidence rate of this cancer varies widely in the globe. Based on demographic, histopathology and molecular genetic features the endometrial carcinoma is divided into two broad groups: Type I and type II carcinoma (Table 9.4):

**Table 9.4:** Endometrial carcinoma: Two pathogenetic subsets

| Features | Type I | Type II |
| --- | --- | --- |
| Age | 50 to 60 years | 60 to 70 years |
| Estrogenic stimulation | Present | Absent |
| Obesity | Common | Uncommon |
| Precursor | Atypical hyperplasia | Endometrial intra-epithelial neoplasm |
| Transition | Slow | Rapid |
| Grade | Low | High |
| Histological type | Endometrioid carcinoma | Serous and clear cell carcinoma |
| Myoinvasion | Minimal | Deep |
| Spread | Lymph node | Peritoneum |
| Molecular genetics | Microsatellite Instability PTEN and k-RAS mutations Loss of PAX 2 | P53 mutation, Loss of heterozygosity |
| Prognosis | Good | Bad |

These two groups are not air tight compartments and there may be overlapping features in type I and type II carcinomas. High grade type I carcinoma may show p-53 genetic mutation and may be immunophenotypically similar to type II carcinoma.

### Etiology and Risk Factors

The common risk factors of endometrial carcinoma are:
a. Obesity: The obese patients get more endogenous estrogen by the converting androstenedione to estrone with the help of the enzyme aromatase present in adipose tissue. There is 10-fold risk of EC if the patient is more than 23 kg overweight.[15]
b. Early menarche and late menopause,
c. Nulliparity and diabetes: Both nulliparity and diabetes have two-fold increased risk of malignancy.
d. Estrogen: Continuous estrogen hormone is one of the important risk factors for EC. High estrogen level may be endogenous or exogenous. Endogenous causes of high estrogen level include Stein Leventhal syndrome, estrogen producing ovarian tumors and cirrhosis of liver. Exogenous causes of high estrogen are mainly due to the use of estrogen therapy in postmenopausal patient and tamoxifen therapy in breast carcinoma.
e. Ethnicity: Whites have two times more incidence of EC than African-American woman.[15] However, the disease progression is worse in black and they have four times higher risk of dying than white population.

### Molecular Genetics of Endometrial Cancer

Different genes are responsible for endometrial cancer (Table 9.5).

Table 9.5: Genes responsible for endometrial carcinoma

| Gene | Mode of action | Frequency |
|---|---|---|
| PTEN | Tumor suppressor gene, Inactivated by somatic or germ line mutation or methylation. It converts PIP3 to PIP2 and causes inhibition of cell proliferation | 83% cases of endometrial carcinoma |
| K-RAS | Oncogene. Inactivated by somatic or mutation. K-RAS has intrinsic GTPase activity and it breaks down GTP to its inactive form GDP | 22% cases of endometrial carcinoma |
| P53 | Tumor suppressor. Inactivated by mutation. Causes cell survival and proliferation | 10 to 20% cases of endometrial carcinoma |
| hMSH2, hMSH6, hMSH3, hMLH1, hPMS1 and hPMS2 | DNA repair. Inactivated either by mutation or methylation. Mutation of these genes causes microsatellite instability | 10 to 45% cases of endometrial carcinoma |

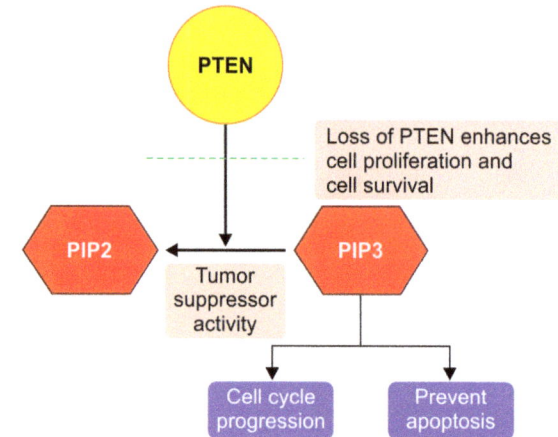

Figure 9.9: Mechanism of action of PTEN gene in the development of endometrial carcinoma

### PTEN (Phosphatase and Tensin Homolog)

The PTEN protein enzyme removes the phosphate from phosphatidylinositol-3,4,5-triphosphate (PIP3) and converts it into phosphatidylinositol bi-phosphate (PIP2). Normally the PIP3 is related with cell cycle progression and increased cell survival (Figure 9.9). Therefore, the conversion of PIP3 to PIP2 by PTEN acts as inhibitor of cell proliferation and survival. PTEN mutation has been noted in 18 to 55% cases of endometrial hyperplasia and 83% cases of EC.[16] The loss of PTEN in endometrial hyperplasia with atypia indicates that this tumor suppressor gene plays in early part of endometrial carcinogenesis.

### KRAS Proto-oncogene

K-RAS is a G protein and is located in the inner aspect of the cell membrane. K-RAS encodes a protein that has intrinsic GTPase activity and it breaks down GTP to its inactive form GDP (Figures 9.10A and B). In case of mutation of K-RAS, there is no catalytic activity and the active form of 'GTP bound RAS protein' function is continuously on. In 10 to 30% of EC cases, KRAS proto-oncogene is demonstrated.[17]

### P53

P53 mutation is commonly seen in type II EC such as serous and clear cell type and overall 10 to 20% of EC is affected by p53 mutation.[18] Mutation of p53 was demonstrated in all grades of adenocarcinoma and it was more frequent in stage III and IV EC (41%).[19] p53 mutation is a late event in endometrial carcinogenesis.

### Epidermal Growth Factor (EGF)

EGF and its receptor (EGFR) are associated with the cell proliferation. EGFR is normally seen in the epithelial cells

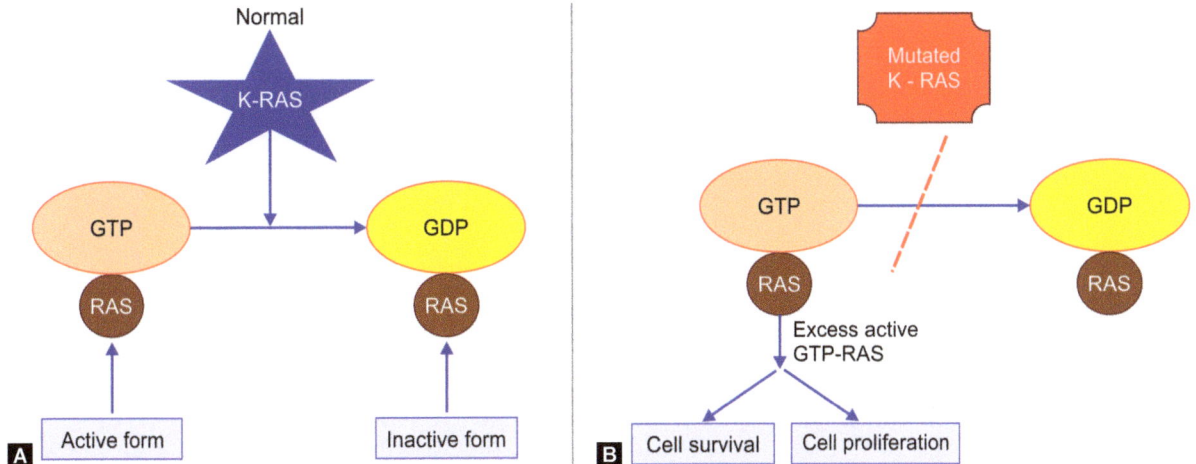

**Figures 9.10A and B:** (A) Normal action of K-RAS gene in the endometrial cell; (B) Mutated K-RAS is unable to block GTP and thereby cells survive and proliferate

of normal endometrial gland. Loss of EGFR has been demonstrated in 34% of grade II and 90% of grade III EC.[20]

*DNA Mismatch Repair Gene*

Microsatellite instability (MSI) means alteration of the pattern of polymorphic short tandem repeat segments of DNA. This MSI is also associated with the mutation of several DNA mismatch repair genes such as hMSH2, hMSH6, hMSH3, hMLH1, hPMS1 and hPMS2. Microsatellite instability has been demonstrated in 10 to 45% cases of EC.[21] MSI has also been demonstrated in complex hyperplasia with atypia.

## Clinical Features

Endometrial carcinoma predominantly occurs in the age group of 55–65 years of age. Near about 75% of endometrial carcinoma occurs in postmenopausal patients. The median age of endometrial carcinoma is 63 years age. The common presentation of endometrioid carcinoma is post-menopausal bleeding per vagina. The premenopausal patients present with menorrhagia or menometrorrhagia.

## Gross Features

The uterus is enlarged in majority of the cases. The tumor is usually exophytic and the growth may be of variable sized. The tumor is sold and gray white with friable surface (Figure 9.11). Areas of necrosis and hemorrhage may be seen. The cut section of the uterus shows the area of infiltration in the myometrium. The invasion usually appears as sharply demarcated area from the adjacent myometrium. The tumor may have pushing or infiltrating margin. Rarely no visible growth is seen and the malignancy is detected on histopathology section.

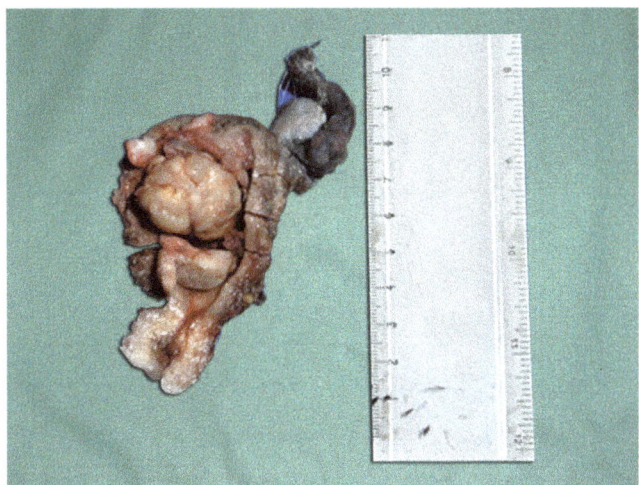

**Figure 9.11:** Gross photograph of endometrioid carcinoma. The tumor is polypoidal and projecting into the endometrial lumen

## Classification

WHO classified this tumor as mentioned in the beginning of the present chapter.

## Histopathology

*Endometrioid Carcinoma (Figures 9.12 to 9.15)*

Endometrioid carcinoma (EC) constitutes the main bulk of the endometrial adenocarcinoma of uterus (80%). This tumor in its well-differentiated form resembles normal endometrium and therefore it is called as endometrioid carcinoma. The tumor is composed of multiple glands arranged in back-to-back appearance and simulates complex hyperplasia. The glands may show complex branching pattern. Significant

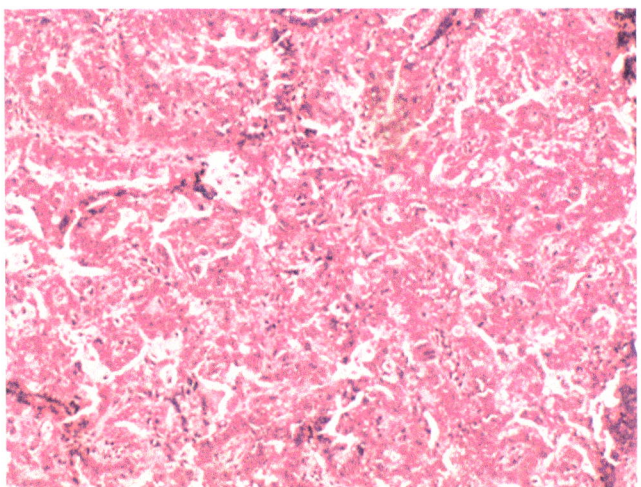

Figure 9.12: Endometrioid carcinoma: The tumor is composed of multiple glands arranged in back-to-back appearance complex branching pattern is seen

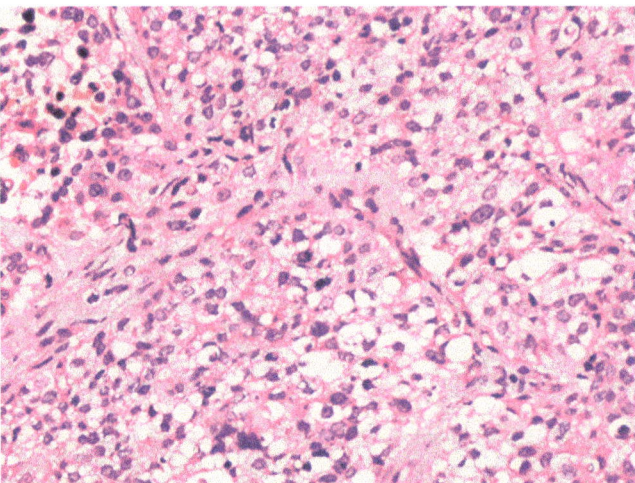

Figure 9.14: Endometrioid carcinoma: Solid area

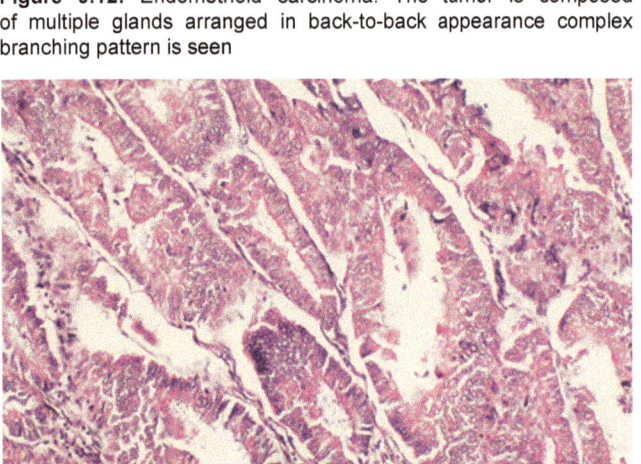

Figure 9.13: Endometrioid carcinoma: Large atypical lining epithelial cells

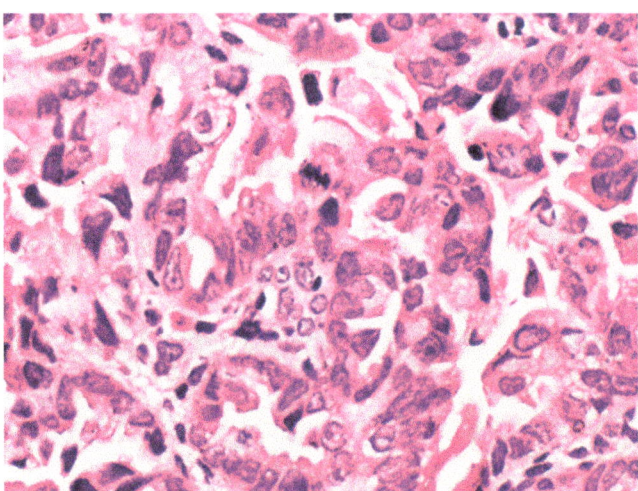

Figure 9.15: Endometrioid carcinoma: Frequent mitotic figures

solid areas are seen in poorly differentiated carcinoma. The lining cells of the glands are larger than normal cells of proliferative endometrial glands. The cells are cuboidal in shape with round moderately pleomorphic nuclei having prominent nucleoli. Frequent mitotic activities and apoptosis are also seen.

Grading of endometrioid carcinoma is done based on architectural grade and nuclear grade (Figures 9.16 to 9.20). Table 9.6 highlights the criteria of grading of endometrial carcinoma.

The tumor grade will increase one grade more in the presence of significant nuclear atypia.[22]

Nuclear grade of EC is determined by nuclear pleomorphism, shape, nucleoli and chromatin. Grade 1 nuclei: Mildly enlarged, pleomorphic nuclei with prominent small nucleoli having fine chromatin. Grade 2 nuclei: in between Grade 3 nuclei and Grade 1 nuclei. Grade 3 nuclei: markedly enlarged pleomorphic with large prominent nucleoli and coarse chromatin.

Regarding the grading of the tumor, it should be always remembered that solid nests of cells with squamous differentiation or morular component should be ignored for grading purpose. There may be considerable variation of architectural grade from area-to-area in hysterectomy specimen and in that case the grade should be allotted by seeing the overall appearance of the tumor. Obermair et al.[23] demonstrated that the grading of EC on curetting is well correlated in 79% cases on subsequent hysterectomy specimen. There was upgrading from grade I to grade II tumor in 21% cases.

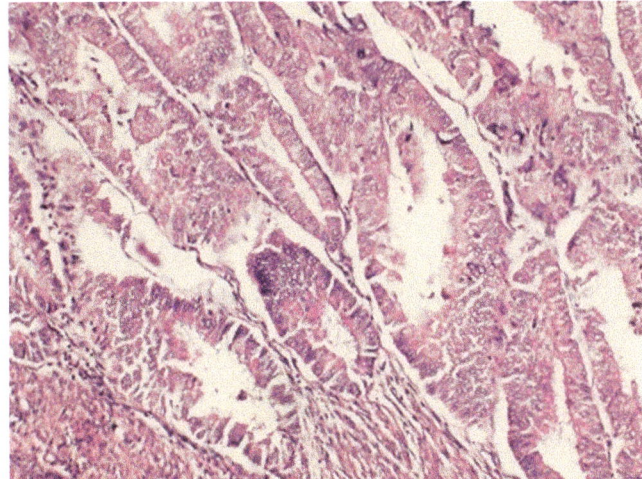

Figure 9.16: Grade 1 endometrioid carcinoma: Multiple glands with solid area less than 5%

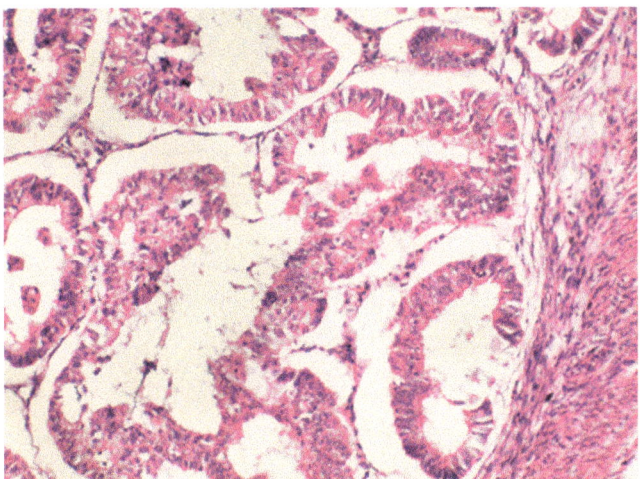

Figure 9.17: Well-differentiated endometrioid carcinoma (grade 1): The nuclei show minimal pleomorphism

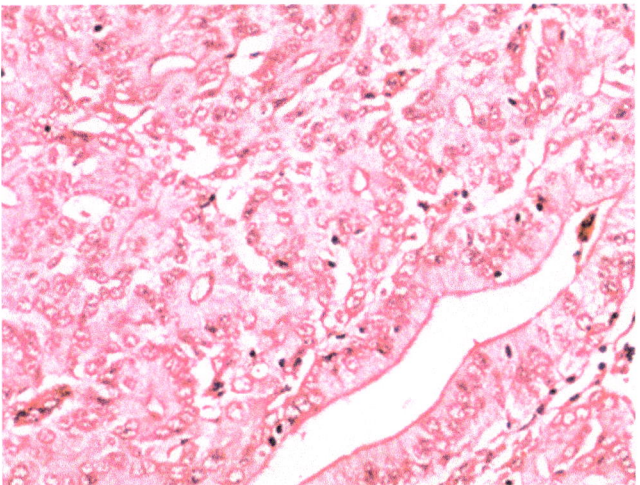

Figure 9.18: Moderately differentiated endometrioid carcinoma: Solid component is from 6–49% along with glandular area in the remaining part

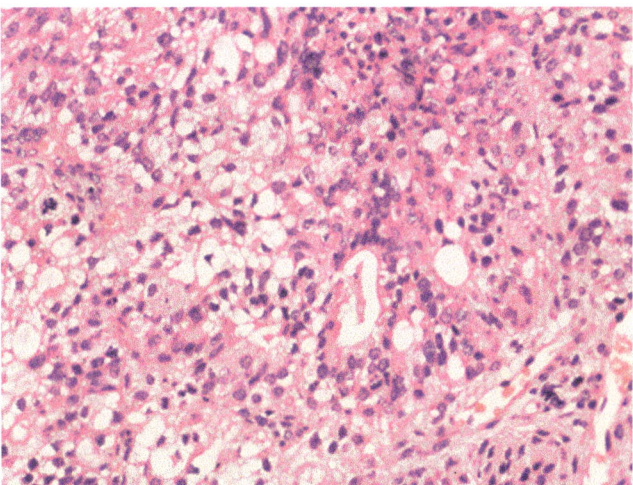

Figure 9.19: Poorly-differentiated endometrioid carcinoma: Architecturally grade 3 carcinoma with predominant solid component

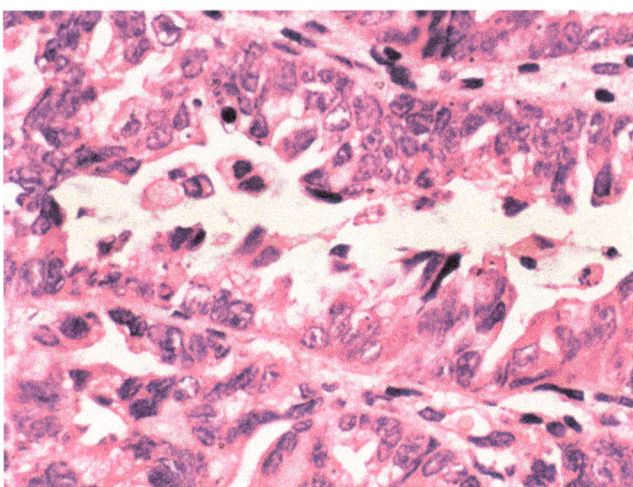

Figure 9.20: Endometrioid carcinoma: High-grade nucleus

Table 9.6: Grade of endometrial carcinoma

| Grade | Amount of solid growth excluding squamous differentiated area |
| --- | --- |
| Grade 1 | Less than 5% |
| Grade 2 | 6 to 50% |
| Grade 3 | Over 50% |

## Differential Diagnosis of EC

a. Atypical polypoid adenomyoma (APAM): The following features support the diagnosis of APAM: (1) less severe atypia, (2) lobular architectural pattern, (3) lack of desmoplastic and inflammatory response, (4) lack of myometrial invasion and (5) lack of CD 10 expression in the myofibromatous stromal component.
b. Epithelial metaplasia: Various metaplastic changes such as squamous metaplasia, mucinous metaplasia, clear cell changes, etc. may mimic malignancy.

c. **Arias–Stella reaction:** The following features are helpful to diagnose Arias–Stella reaction: (1) History of pregnancy, (2) Young patient, (3) Multifocal, (4) Admixed with decidual and secretory glands, and (5) Lack of cribriform appearance.
d. **Artifacts:** At times, the epithelial cells may be clumped together and may mimic carcinoma in endometrial curetting specimen. The distinguishing features from malignancy include: (1) Young age of the patient, (2) Bland nuclei of the epithelial cells, and (3) Admixture of benign secretory glands.
e. **Endocervical adenocarcinoma (Table 9.7):** At times, it is difficult to distinguish EEC from endocervical adenocarcinoma in small biopsies and even in hysterectomy specimen. The following histological type may overlap: (1) Endometrioid carcinoma of uterus and mucinous carcinoma of cervix. (2) Mucinous type of endocervical adenocarcinoma and EEC with focal mucinous differentiation. (3) Endometrioid type of uterine and cervical adenocarcinoma, (4) Very rarely pure primary squamous cell carcinoma of uterus with squamous cell carcinoma of cervix. Table 9.7 highlighted the salient points to distinguish these two entities. Rarely minimal deviation endometrioid adenocarcinoma of cervix shows benign looking endometrial glands within the cervix and do not evoke any stromal response. The glands are large and show lack of cytological atypia.

A panel of three markers consisting of vimentin, hormone receptor (ER/ PR) and a HPV marker (p16, HPV in situ hybridization or ProExC) may resolve the problem of origin of adenocarcinoma (Box 9.1).[24] It is difficult to do HPV in situ hybridization in many laboratories so p16 or ProExC immunostaining is suggested. These panels may not be suitable in cases of USC or CCC of uterus.

f. **Endometrioid carcinoma versus pseudoglandular serous carcinoma:** The important diagnostic features of USC include: (1) Architectural and cytological discrepancy: USC shows well-differentiated glands but the individual cells show moderate to marked nuclear atypia, (2) Atrophic endometrium in adjacent endometrium, (3) Presence of focal papillary structure, (4) Strong and diffuse p53 positivity and, (5) Strong and diffuse p16 positivity.
g. **Malignant mixed Müllerian tumors (MMMT):** The following features are helpful to distinguish EEC and MMMT: (1) heterologous elements in EEC are always benign, (2) spindle cell component in EEC does not show much pleomorphism, (3) abrupt keratinization within the spindle cell component and, (4) epithelial cell component merges with the spindle cell component.

**Box 9.1:** Panel recommended distinguishing ECC versus endocervical adenocarcinoma

1. Vimentin
2. Hormone receptor marker (ER or PR)
3. One HPV marker (p16, HPV in situ hybridization or ProExC)

**Table 9.7:** Differentiating points between ECC versus endocervical adenocarcinoma

| Feature | Endometrial adenocarcinoma | Endocervical adenocarcinoma |
|---|---|---|
| Mass present in the center of uterine body | Favors | Not favors |
| Foamy histiocytes in the stroma | Yes | No |
| Associated atypical hyperplasia | Yes | No |
| Squamous morules | Yes | No |
| The marked stromal desmoplastic reaction | No | Yes |
| Glands showing adenocarcinoma in situ | No | Yes |
| Associated dysplastic squamous epithelial fragments | No | Yes |
| Immunostain | | |
| Vimentin | + | − |
| P16 | − | + |
| ProExC | − | + |
| ER/PR | + | − |
| CEA | − | + |
| HPV DNA | − | + |

## VARIANTS OF ENDOMETRIOID CARCINOMA

### Endometrioid Adenocarcinoma with Squamous Differentiation (Figures 9.21 to 9.23)

Squamous differentiation in the endometrioid carcinoma may be noted in 20 to 50% cases. At least 10% area of the carcinoma should have squamous differentiation to categorize the lesion as endometrioid carcinoma with squamous differentiation. The squamous area may be benign or malignant in appearance. The degree of the differentiation of the glandular component should be considered in grading such tumor and the squamous component should be just mentioned as metaplastic change.

Squamous component is present as solid sheet of cells along with adenocarcinoma component. The cells are polyhedral having intercellular bridge. The cytoplasm of the cell is eosinophilic. The nuclei are monomorphic with inconspicuous to absent nucleoli. Keratin pearls or

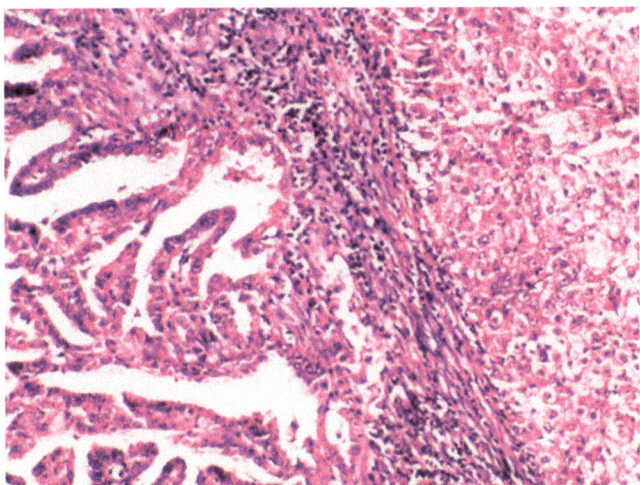

**Figure 9.21:** Endometrioid carcinoma with squamous differentiation: Both adenocarcinoma and squamous component

keratin-induced granulomas may also be seen. According to WHO group,[25] the criteria for identification of squamous differentiation are: (1) Keratinization noted by standard staining preparation, (2) The presence of intercellular bridges, and (3) Three or more of the criteria mentioned below: (a) Solid sheet of cells with no demonstrable gland, (b) Well-defined sharp cell margin, (c) Eosinophilic cytoplasm and, (d) Low nucleocytoplasmic ratio of the cells.

## Villoglandular Variant (Figures 9.24 to 9.27)

This tumor represents about 15 to 30% of adenocarcinoma. The tumor shows multiple slender villi like structures with thin fibrovascular core inside. The papillae are lined by columnar cells with moderate atypia. The nuclei of the cells are perpendicular to the basement membrane and show pseudostratification. The prognosis of this tumor is similar to that of conventional endometrioid carcinoma. However, this

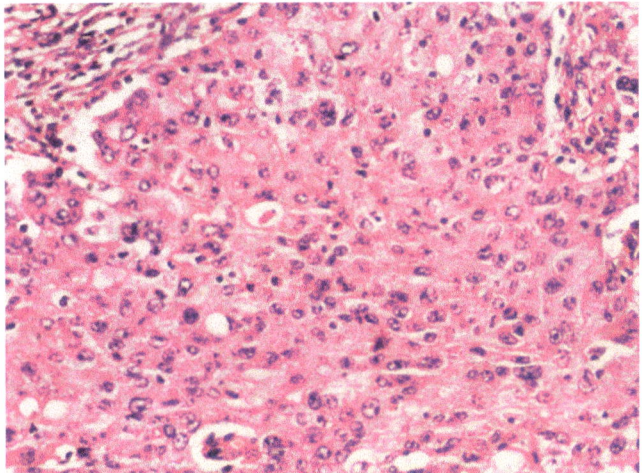

**Figure 9.22:** Endometrioid carcinoma with squamous differentiation: Malignant squamous element

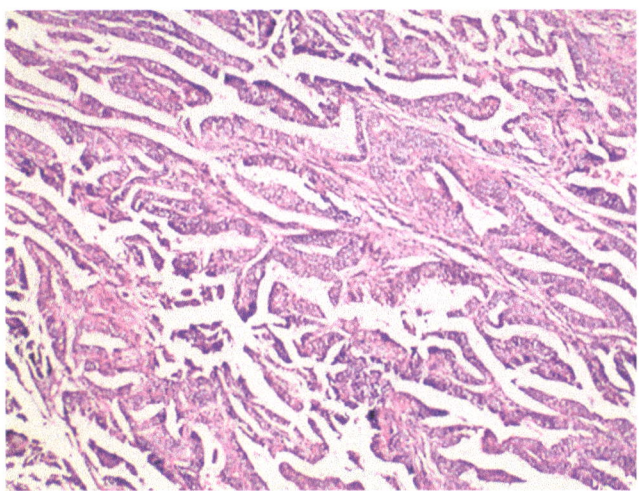

**Figure 9.24:** Villoglandular endometrioid carcinoma: Both glands and villi

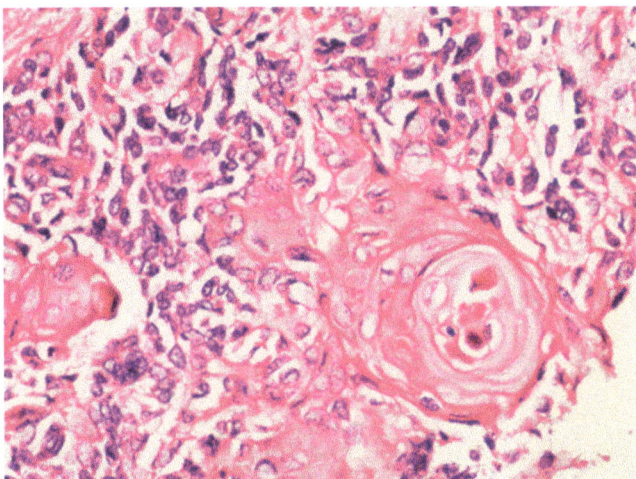

**Figure 9.23:** Endometrioid carcinoma with squamous differentiation: Squamous pearls

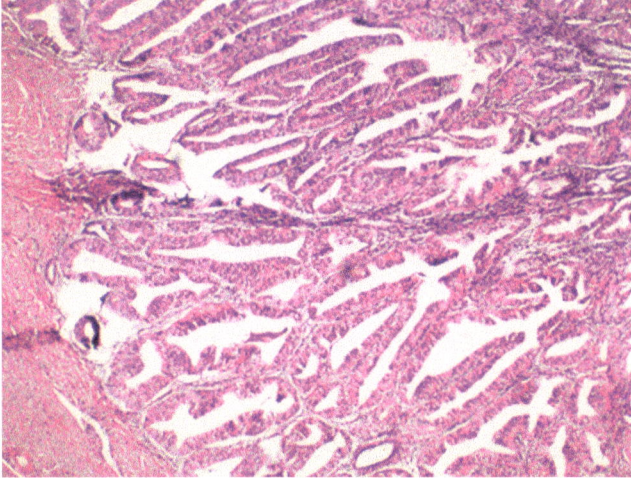

**Figure 9.25:** Villoglandular endometrioid carcinoma: Tumor is composed of multiple slender villi like structures with thin fibrovascular core inside

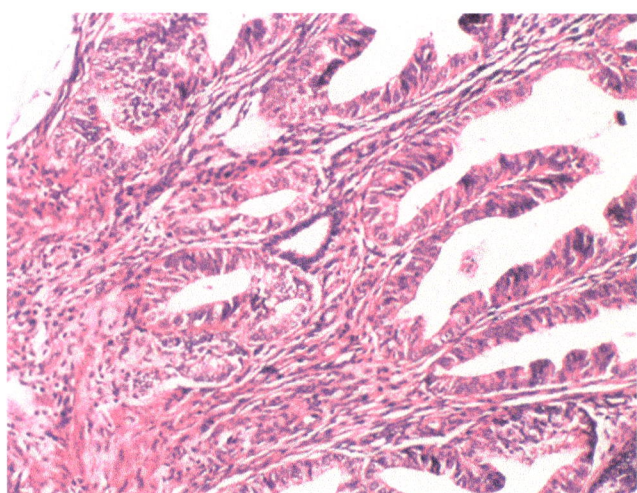

**Figure 9.26:** Villoglandular endometrioid carcinoma: The papillae are lined by columnar cells with pseudostratification

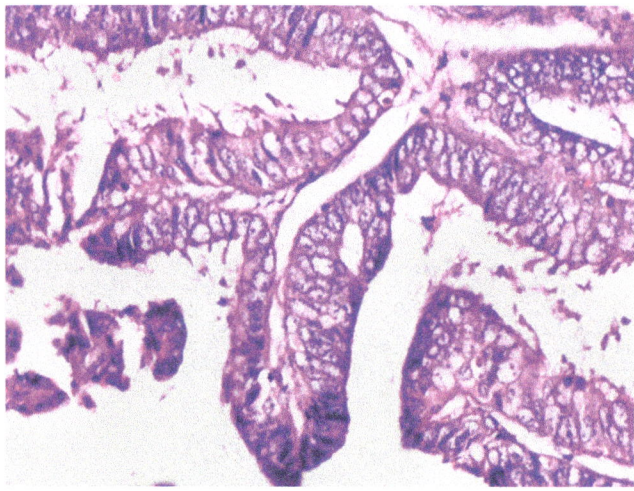

**Figure 9.27:** Villoglandular endometrioid carcinoma: Higher magnification shows bland looking cells

tumor usually shows superficial invasion in myometrium. Lymphovascular invasion is common in villoglandular pattern.

### Differential Diagnosis

Uterine serous carcinoma (USC): The differentiating features of villoglandular variant of endometrioid carcinoma from USC are highlighted in Table 9.8.

## Secretory Carcinoma (Figures 9.28 to 9.30)

This is an uncommon carcinoma and represents less than 1% of endometrial carcinoma. The morphology of secretory carcinoma resembles early secretory endometrium.[26] The tumor is composed of multiple glands lined by tall columnar epithelial cells with prominent subnuclear vacuoles containing glycogen. The nuclei show mild pleomorphism. The secretory carcinoma has no relation with any progesterone effect. The tumor may be coexisting with conventional endometrioid carcinoma. The secretory carcinomas are usually well-differentiated and bears similar prognosis as that of well-differentiated endometrioid carcinoma.

### Differential Diagnosis

Clear cell carcinoma: The following features are helpful to diagnose secretory carcinoma over clear cell carcinoma:

**Table 9.8:** Distinguishing features of villoglandular variant of endometrioid carcinoma versus serous carcinoma

| Features | Villoglandular variant of endometrioid carcinoma | Serous carcinoma |
|---|---|---|
| Papillae | Tall, slender, finger like | Short, broad, stout |
| Nuclear atypia | Mild | Moderate to severe |
| Nuclear polarity | Maintained | Not maintained |
| Nucleoli | Small | Large, cherry red macronucleoli |
| Apical luminal border | Smooth | Ragged |
| Micropapillary structure | Absent | Present |
| **Immunostaining** | | |
| P53 | Negative | Strong and diffuse |
| ER/PR | Usually positive | Usually negative |
| P16 | Weak and focal positivity | Strong and diffuse positivity |
| Ki 67 | Low index | High Ki 67 index |

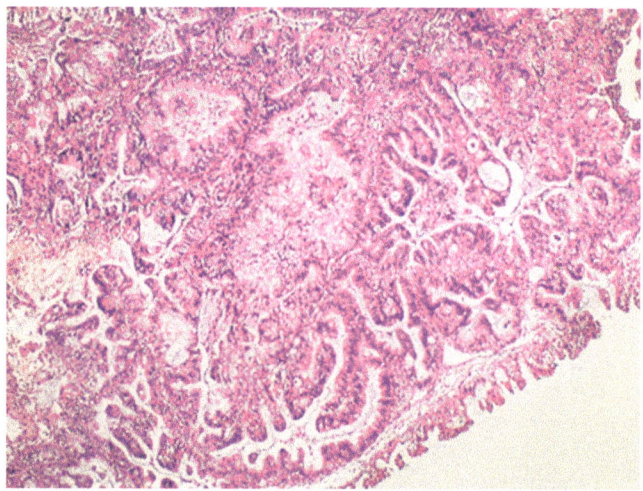

**Figure 9.28:** Secretory carcinoma: The tumor is composed of multiple glands that resembles secretory endometrium

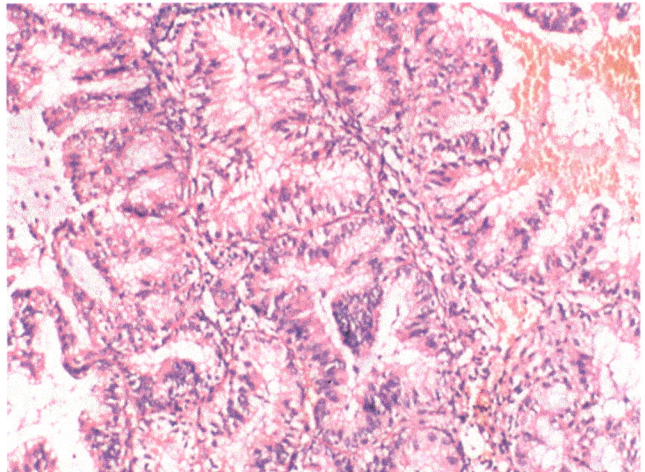

Figure 9.29: Secretory carcinoma: Higher magnification shows prominent subnuclear vacuoles

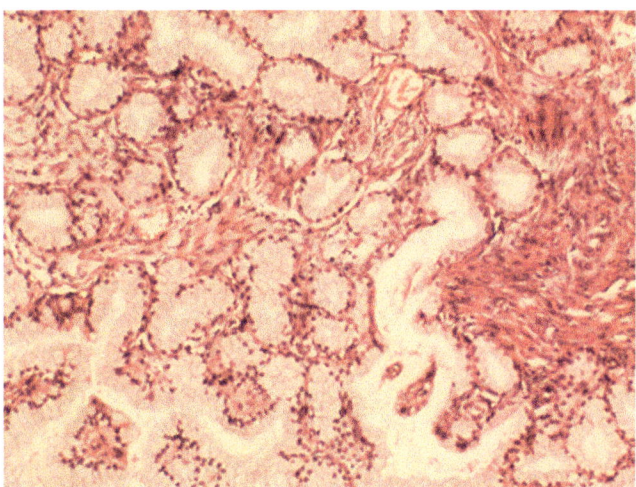

Figure 9.31: Mucinous carcinoma: The tumor is composed of multiple mucus secreting glands

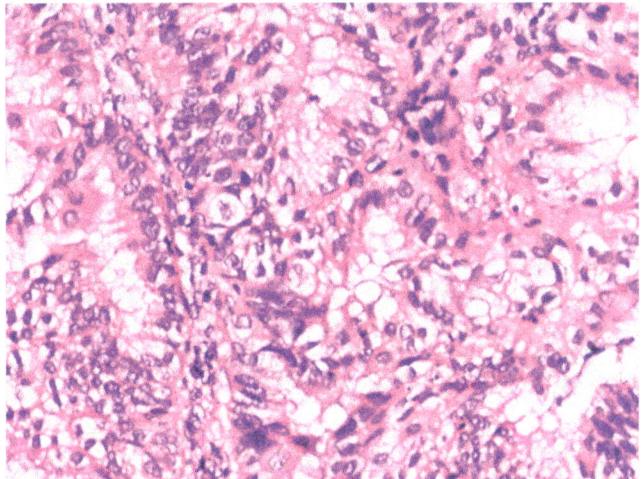

Figure 9.30: Secretory carcinoma: The cells show nuclear enlargement and pleomorphism

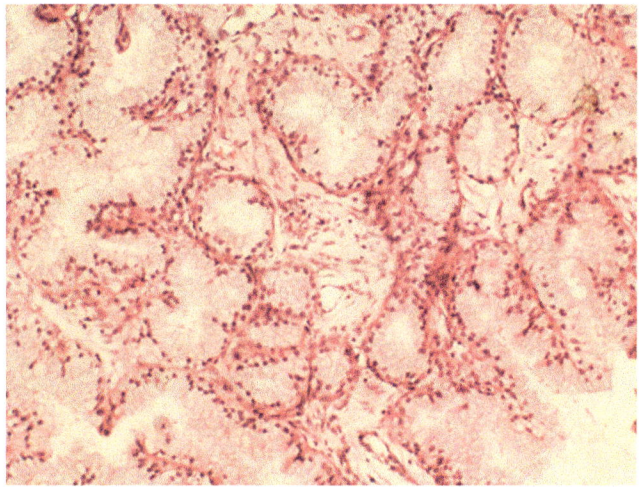

Figure 9.32: Mucinous carcinoma: Crowded glands

(1) low nuclear grade, (2) subnuclear vacuoles, and (3) the columnar cell morphology.

### Ciliated Carcinoma

This is rare variant of endometrioid carcinoma. The ciliated variant is composed of multiple glands arranged in cribriform pattern. The glands are lined by cells with eosinophilic cytoplasm having cilia on the luminal surface.[27] The nuclei show moderate pleomorphism and coarse chromatin. This tumor behaves similar as conventional endometrioid carcinoma.

### Mucinous Carcinoma (Figure 9.31 to 9.34)

Mucinous carcinoma is rare and represents less than 10% of EEC. To diagnose a case as mucinous adenocarcinoma, at least 50% of the tumor cells should have intracytoplasmic mucin.

The mucin is PAS positive and diastase resistant. Mucinous adenocarcinoma resembles mucinous adenocarcinoma of cervix. The tumor consists of multiple glands with papillary fronds and foci of cribriform appearance. The glands show tall columnar mucin secreting cells with stratification. The nuclear pleomorphism is minimal. The glandular lumen is filled with mucinous material. The tumor is often associated with typical neutrophilic infiltrate.

*Differential Ddiagnosis*

1. Endocervical mucinous carcinoma: The morphological distinction between endometrial mucinous carcinoma and endocervical mucinous carcinoma is very difficult. Immunocytochemistry may be helpful in this aspect and has been discussed in the differential diagnosis of EEC.

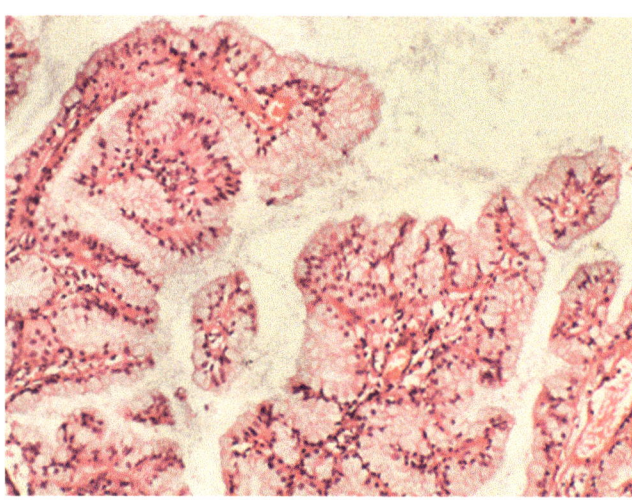

**Figure 9.33:** Mucinous carcinoma: Multiple papillary fronds

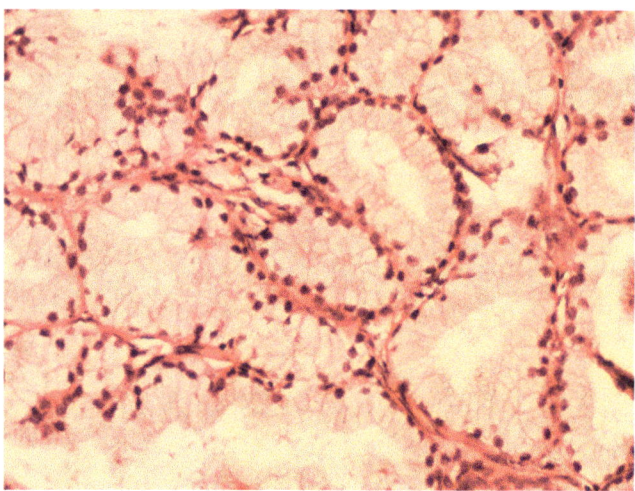

**Figure 9.34:** Mucinous carcinoma: Higher magnification shows tall columnar mucin secreting epithelium. The nuclei show minimal pleomorphism

2. Clear cell carcinoma (CCC): The distinguishing features of mucinous carcinoma and CCC is highlighted in Table 9.9.

## SEROUS CARCINOMA

Uterine serous carcinoma (USC) is the typical prototype of type II EC and represents 10% of all EC. This tumor is unrelated with estrogenic stimulation and there is no relation with prior hyperplasia of the endometrium. USC is often accompanied with synchronous serous carcinoma in ovary, fallopian tube or peritoneum.

### Clinical Features

The tumor occurs typically in postmenopausal patients in 7th decade. High incidence of this tumor is reported in African-American women. The patient commonly complains of serosanguinous vaginal bleeding. Occasionally, the patients show raised serum CA 125 and carcinoembryonic antigen.[28]

**Table 9.9:** Differentiating mucinous carcinoma versus clear cell carcinoma

| Feature | Mucinous carcinoma | Clear cell carcinoma |
|---|---|---|
| Architecture | Glandular and papillary | Always papillary or solid pattern |
| Hobnailing | Absent | Present |
| Cell morphology | Columnar | Polygonal |
| PAS followed by diastase | PAS positive diastase resistant | PAS positive diastase sensitive |

### Gross Finding

The uterus is usually enlarged. However as the patients are postmenopausal and uterus is atrophic, so the uterus may be small in size. The tumor is usually exophytic. Uncommonly, the tumor may be present only within the endometrial polyp.

### Histopathology (Figures 9.35 to 9.39)

The architectural pattern of USC is variable and the various patterns may coexist in the same tumor. The characteristic patterns are:

(a) Papillary structures: The tumor predominantly shows complex irregular papillary pattern with primary and secondary branching papillae. The papillae are broad, stout and irregular with central fibrovascular core. There is characteristic sloughing of the papillary cells forming isolated free floating islands of cells known as micropapillary structures. In addition, intraglandular micropapillary structures are also seen.

(b) Slit-like glands: In low power magnification the tumor often shows slit-like spaces. The compact growths of the papillae make them less well-defined and the cords of epithelium are divided by narrow slit-like spaces in between them.

(c) Solid growth: The tumor may show confluent solid nests of cells with abundant eosinophilic cytoplasm having marked nuclear atypia.

(d) Organized fibrous stroma: The tumor consists of narrow angular glands with intervening fibrosis.

(e) Microcystic pattern: The tumor shows many small cystic spaces lined by malignant cells.

### Tumor Cells

The lining cells of the papillae are columnar to polygonal cells. The individual cells have abundant eosinophilic cytoplasm and round nuclei. The nuclei show moderate to marked pleomorphism with large prominent nucleoli.

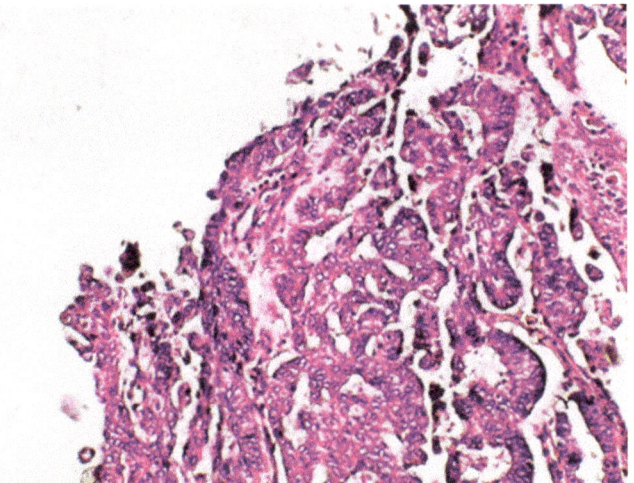

**Figure 9.35:** Serous carcinoma: complex irregular papillary pattern

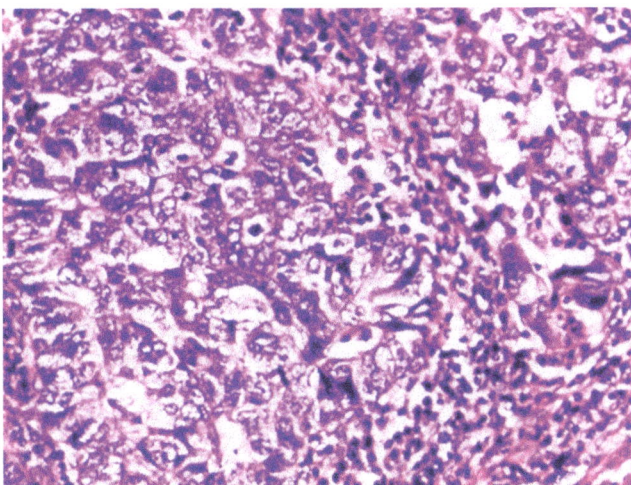

**Figure 9.38:** Solid area of serous carcinoma: confluent solid nests of cells

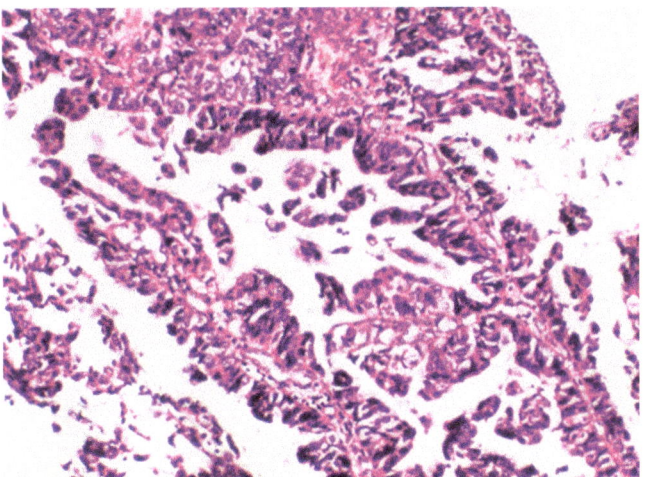

**Figure 9.36:** Serous carcinoma: isolated free floating islands of cells forming micropapillary structures

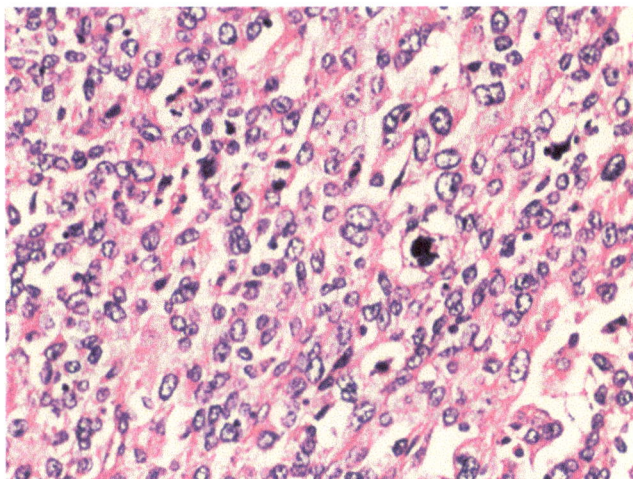

**Figure 9.39:** Solid area of serous carcinoma: moderate to marked nuclear atypia

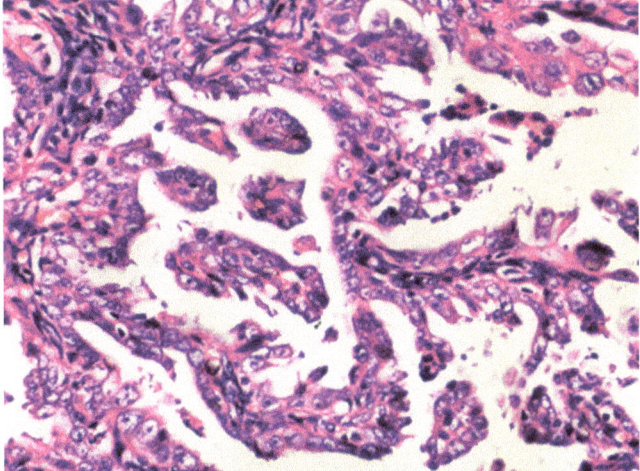

**Figure 9.37:** Serous carcinoma: sloughed out papillae in the lumen of the gland

Occasional nuclei may be angulated with deep convolution. Multinucleated tumor giant cells and bizarre nuclei are also seen. Increased mitotic activity and atypical mitosis are also noted.

*Other Features*

Marked hobnail appearance is also noted. One-third of the USC may show psammoma bodies. The endometrium adjacent to USC almost always shows atrophic changes unlike the EEC that shows hyperplastic endometrium.

It is important to note that USC consists of prominent papillary structures resembling well-differentiated carcinoma however, the cells always show high nuclear grade. The tumor is often deeply infiltrating within the myometrium and even in absence of deep myometrial invasion, there may be extensive lymphovascular invasion and extrauterine tumor deposit. The USC may be associated with endometrioid or clear cell carcinoma in one-third cases. The presence of more than 25% tumor volume of serous component is necessary to diagnose a USC.[29]

## Serous Endometrial Intraepithelial Carcinoma

Serous endometrial intraepithelial carcinoma (SIC) is considered as precursor lesions of the USC. In this condition, the uterine surface and glands are lined by highly malignant cells. In majority of the cases SIC is also accompanied by invasive serous or clear cell adenocarcinoma. The tumor cells may be limited to the surface lining of the uterus without any evidence of invasion but there may be extensive dissemination of the tumor in the peritoneum. The most important prognostic factor of SIC is the presence of extrauterine dissemination at the time of presentation.[30]

## Immunohistochemistry of USC

More than 90% of USC shows strong diffuse positivity of p53 protein indicating p53 gene mutation. Even the tumors with p53 negative immunostaining also exhibit p53 mutation. This is due to truncated p53 protein that cannot be demonstrated by commercially available antibodies. USC also shows diffuse positivity of p16. The tumor shows weak or absent ER and PR positivity. In addition, USC also express CK, EMA, BER EP4, vimentin and IMP3, an insulin-like growth factor II messenger RNA-binding protein 3. The strong positivity of IMP3 is helpful to differentiate USC from high grade endometrioid carcinoma.[31]

## Differential Diagnosis

a. Endometrioid carcinoma villoglandular carcinoma versus serous carcinoma: Discussed before in villoglandular variant part.
b. Endometrioid carcinoma versus serous pseudoglandular serous carcinoma: Discussed before in EEC part.
c. Grade III Endometrioid carcinoma: FIGO grade III carcinomas and USC both are considered as high-grade carcinomas. However, the outcome of these two groups is different and these tumors should be distinguished from each other. The differentiating features of these two entities are highlighted in Table 9.10.

Clear cell carcinoma (CCC) (Table 9.11): CCC and USC have certain overlapping histological features that include the presence of papillary structures, prominent hobnailing, psammoma bodies and clear cell morphology. Both the tumors show atrophic endometrium in the adjacent normal area. In addition, Ki 67 proliferative index is high in both USC and CCC. The differentiating features between CCC and USC are highlighted in Table 9.11.

Table 9.10: Grade III endometrioid carcinoma versus serous carcinoma

| Features | Grade III endometrioid carcinoma | Serous carcinoma |
|---|---|---|
| Architectural | More than 50% solid area | Papillary areas in addition to solid area |
| Cell morphology | Grade III nuclear changes | Marked atypia and morphology similar in the cells of solid and papillary area |
| Glands | Cells maintain nuclear polarity | Loss of nuclear polarity |
| Psammoma bodies | Absent | Present in 1/3rd cases |
| P53 | Positive | Positive |
| P16 | Significantly less positive | Strong and diffuse positive |
| ER/PR | Less positive | Negative |
| Ki-67 index | High | High |

Table 9.11: Clear cell carcinoma versus uterine serous carcinoma

| Features | Clear cell carcinoma | Serous carcinoma |
|---|---|---|
| Papillae | Small round | Large, complex branching |
| Micropapillae | Absent | Present |
| Core of papillae | Edematous and hyalinized core | Fibrovascular |
| Lining cells | No pseudo-stratification | Prominent pseudostratification |
| Cells | Well-defined border with good amount of cytoplasm | Round to polygonal with high nucleocytoplasmic ratio |
| Hyaline globules | Present | Absent |
| HNF-1β | Positive | Negative |
| P53 | Focal weak positivity | Strong and diffuse positivity |
| Ki-67 proliferative index | Relatively low | Very high |

## CLEAR CELL ADENOCARCINOMA

Clear cell carcinoma is considered as a prototype of type II endometrial carcinoma. Pure clear cell carcinoma (CCC) is rare and represents 5% of all EEC. This tumor occurs in postmenopausal patient and the mean age is 65 years. The uterine CCC has no relation with diethylstilbestrol exposure. The patients of CCC usually complain of postmenopausal bleeding.

## Gross

The gross feature of CCC is nonspecific. Grossly, the uterus is enlarged and tumor shows a soft fleshy grey white mass. The tumor may show as polypoid mass.

## Histopathology (Figures 9.40 to 9.45)

The CCC show papillary, solid and tubular and cystic pattern.[32] In papillary pattern, the tumor shows multiple small round papillae with fibrovascular core. The core of the papillae frequently shows edema and hyalinization (69%). Unlike USC, the exfoliation or sloughing of the papillae are not seen in CCC. Cellular tufting and budding are usually absent. The papillae are lined by single to double layer of cuboidal cells with clear cytoplasm containing glycogen which is PAS positive and diastase sensitive. The nuclei show moderate to marked atypia. Typical hobnail appearance of the nuclei is also noted in papillary pattern.

In glandular pattern, the tumor exhibits multiple irregular-shaped glands with intervening fibrous stroma. The glandular lumen may contain eosinophilic materials. The lining cells of the glands are cuboidal. Hobnailing nuclei are also seen.

In solid pattern, the cells show solid nests of cells separated by thin fibrous septa. The individual tumor cells are large, polygonal with clear vacuolated cytoplasm. The cystic pattern is uncommon in uterus and the cysts are lined by flattened cells.

Nearly 75% of CCC shows round eosinophilic hyaline material. These eosinophilic globules simulate endodermal sinus tumor and are PAS positive but diastase resistant. Psammoma bodies are seen in 32% cases of CCC.

## Immunohistochemistry

CCCs are negative for ER and PR; and positive for CK7, BER EP4, Leu-M1, vimentin, and CA-125. The tumor also shows high Ki 67 proliferation index, p16 positivity and p53 overexpression. In addition, the cases of CCC show positive HNF-1β staining.[33]

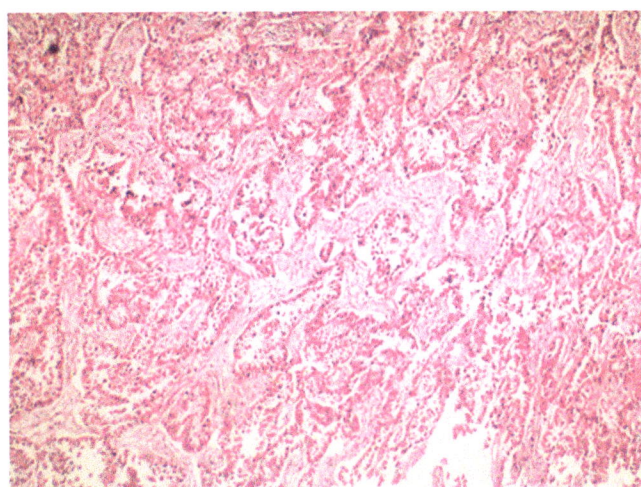

Figure 9.40: Clear cell carcinoma: Multiple glands and papillary structures

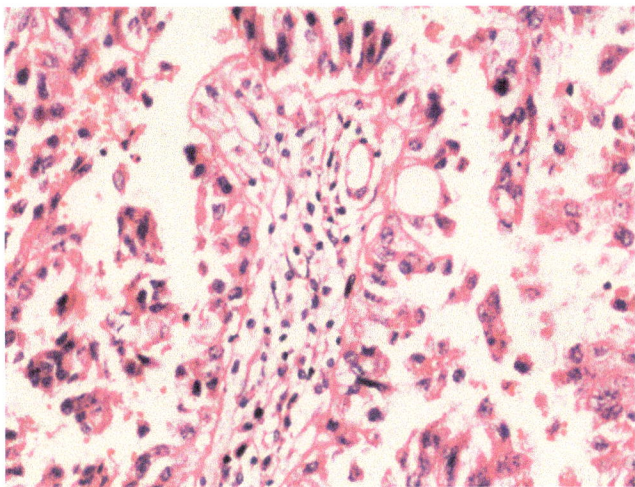

Figure 9.42: Clear cell carcinoma: The papillae are line by the cells with abundant clear cytoplasm having moderately pleomorphic nuclei

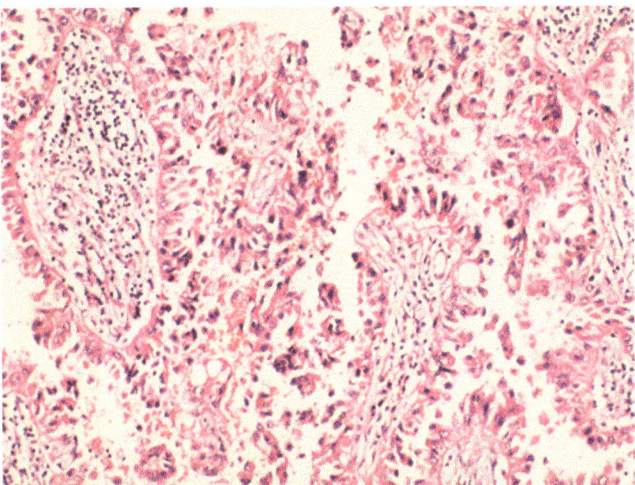

Figure 9.41: Clear cell carcinoma: The papillae with central fibrovascular core

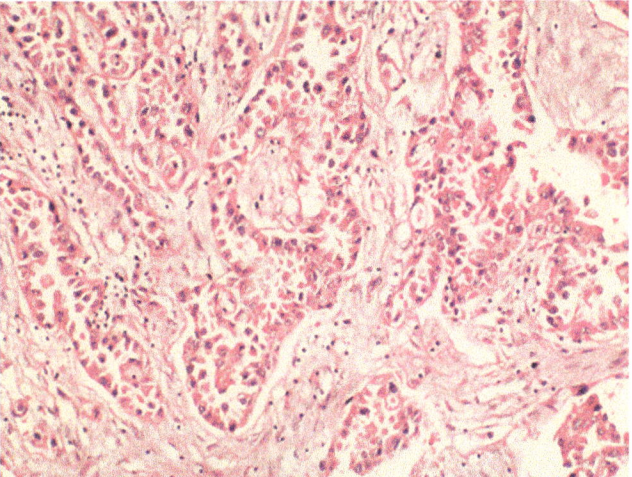

Figure 9.43: Clear cell carcinoma: Multiple glandular structures

Uterus: Preneoplastic Lesions and Carcinoma

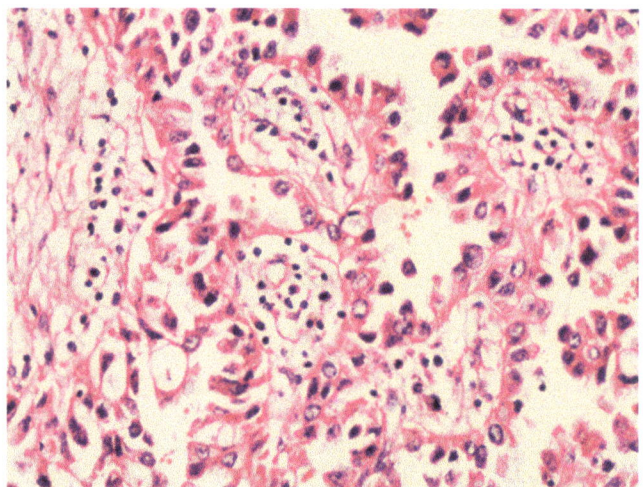

Figure 9.44: Clear cell carcinoma: Hobnail appearance

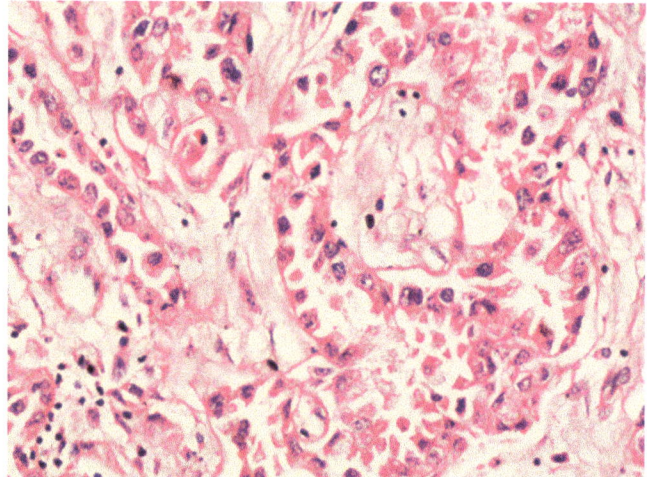

Figure 9.45: Clear cell carcinoma: Eosinophilic pinkish material in the glandular lumen

## Differential Diagnosis

a. Serous carcinoma: Discussed before in serous carcinoma part.
b. Secretory carcinoma: Discussed before in secretory carcinoma part.
c. Mucinous carcinoma: Discussed before mucinous carcinoma part.
d. Yolk sac tumor: Yolk sac tumor is extremely rare in endometrium. The following features favor the diagnosis of Yolk sac tumor: (1) Young age, (2) High alpha feto-protein level, and (3) Presence of Schiller-Duval bodies.

## MIXED TYPES OF CARCINOMA

Mixed types of carcinoma comprises of both type I and type II endometrial carcinoma and according to World Health Organization classification, the minor type must constitutes at least 10% of the total tumor volume.[34] In case of more than 25% serous component in a mixed carcinoma, the overall prognosis is bad.

## SQUAMOUS CELL CARCINOMA

The primary squamous cell carcinoma of uterus is rare and comprises less than 0.5% of all EC. This occurs mainly in postmenopausal patient. The tumor is often associated with cervical stenosis, pyometra and history of pelvic radiation. It is important to exclude the squamous cell carcinoma of cervix before the diagnosis of primary carcinoma in uterus.
Differential diagnosis: (A) Squamous cell carcinoma of cervix: The following features are helpful in conformation a primary squamous cell carcinoma of uterus: (1) No preexisting squamous cell carcinoma of cervix, (2) No associated adenocarcinoma, (3) No anatomical continuity between the carcinoma in the body of uterus and cervical squamous epithelium.

## TRANSITIONAL CELL CARCINOMA

Transitional cell carcinoma (TCC) of the uterus is very rare. According to WHO for the diagnosis of TCC of uterus, the tumor should have at least 90% area of transitional cell carcinoma, otherwise the tumor should be labeled as mixed carcinoma.[35]

## Histopathology

The tumor shows multiple broad exophytic papillary structures lined by multiple layers of transitional cells. The tumor resembles urothelial carcinoma of bladder.

## Immunohistochemistry

TCC of uterus is positive for CK 7 and negative for CK 20 and thrombomodulin.

## SMALL CELL CARCINOMA

Small cell carcinoma (SCC) of uterus is very uncommon and comprises less than 1% of all EC. The tumor resembles small cell carcinoma of lung. The tumor is composed of sheets of small to intermediate cells with scanty cytoplasm and round nuclei having stippled chromatin. The tumor cells are positive for neuroendocrine markers: NSE, CD 56, synaptophysin and chromogranin.

## OVARIAN CARCINOMA ALONG WITH UTERINE CARCINOMA

About 10% ovarian carcinoma patients may have synchronous or independent endometrial carcinoma. Similarly endometrial

carcinoma may also be associated with ovarian carcinoma (5%). If the endometrial carcinoma is small and associated with atypical hyperplasia then probably the two tumors are independent. It is difficult to distinguish USC from an ovarian serous carcinoma in small biopsies. However, the following features are helpful to suggest primary endometrial carcinoma:
1. Papillary serous tumor with high nuclear grade,
2. Mucosal and deep myometrial invasion,
3. Small (less than 5 cm diameter ovary) tumor size,
4. Involvement of both ovaries,
5. Negative for WT1 nuclear expression.

## Prognostic Markers of Endometrial Carcinoma

Various prognostic factors of EC (Box 9.2) include:

**Box 9.2:** Prognostic markers

- FIGO staging: Most important
- Histological grading
- Myometrial invasion
- Peritoneal cytology
- Lymphovascular invasion: Associated with higher risk of para-aortic lymph node metastasis
- Lymph node involvement: Pelvic and para-aortic lymph node involvement
- Histological type: Type I versus type II
- Cervical involvement
- DNA ploidy
- Hormone receptors: ER and PR
- Tumor cell proliferation
- Tumor suppressor genes: PTEN and p53
- Microsatellite instability

### Stage

FIGO staging (Table 9.12) is the most important prognostic factors of uterine endometrial carcinoma.[36] The five year disease free survival in stage I, II and III endometrial carcinoma is 90%, 83% and 43% respectively.

### Histological Grading

Prognostic importance of the grading of EC is well recognized. Details of this grading system have been mentioned before. This is a three tier grading and is applied for mainly type I endometrial carcinoma as all type II EC are considered as high grade tumor.

### Myometrial Invasion

In low-stage (stage I and stage II) EC, depth of myometrial invasion is the important prognostic marker and there is

**Table 9.12:** FIGO staging of endometrial carcinoma[36]

| Stage | Features |
|---|---|
| I | Tumor restricted to the corpus uteri |
| IA | Tumor limited to less than half of myometrium |
| IB | Tumor extended more than half of myometrium |
| II | Tumor extends in the cervical stroma but is limited within the uterus |
| IIIA | Tumor invades the serosa of the corpus uteri and/or adnexae |
| IIIB | Vaginal and/or parametrial involvement |
| IIIC<br>IIIC1<br>IIIC2 | Metastases to pelvic and/or para-aortic (PA) lymph nodes<br>Positive pelvic lymph node<br>Positive para-aortic lymph nodes |
| IVA | Tumor involves bladder and/or bowel mucosa |
| IVB | Distant metastases to intra-abdominal and/or inguinal lymph nodes |

positive correlation between the depth of myometrial invasion and aortic lymph node metastasis.[37] Microscopically, the myometrial invasion can be determined by:
1. Assessing the proportion of the involvement of the myometrium such as more than half or less than half of the myometrial wall.
2. Measuring the distance from the deeper part of invasion to serosa of the uterine wall.

Following difficulties may arise in the assessment of myometrial invasion:
a. Adenomyosis involved by EC: The features favoring the involvement of adenomyotic foci are
   1. Well-circumscribed smooth outline of glands,
   2. Benign glands within the same focus,
   3. Absence of surrounding desmoplastic reaction, and
   4. Presence of adenomyosis in other sections.
b. Unusual infiltrative pattern: Occasionally, EC may show infiltration without any stromal response or inflammation and no atypia is seen in glandular lining cell. This peculiar pattern of infiltration is labeled as "diffusely infiltrating," "adenoma malignum," or "minimum deviation" type.

### Peritoneal Cytology

Positive peritoneal cytology is removed from the revised FIGO staging of EC. The peritoneal fluid cytology positivity is well correlated with histological grade, and pelvic lymph node metastasis.

### Lymphovascular invasion

Lymphovascular space invasion is associated with higher risk of para-aortic (PA) lymph node metastasis.[38] The histological characteristics of lymphovascular invasion are:
1. The island of tumor cells surrounded by the lymphatic space.

2. Smooth margin of the clusters, and
3. Perivascular lymphocytic infiltration. Occasionally, there may be artefactual lymphatic space involvement due to defect in sectioning. In this condition a large chunk of tumor tissue or whole gland is surrounded by vascular space.

### Lymph Node Involvement

Para-aortic lymph nodal involvement is related with deep myometrial invasion, higher grade of tumor and positive peritoneal cytology. The pelvic lymph nodal metastasis increases the chance of para-aortic (PA) lymph nodal metastasis.[39] Lymphovascular space involvement also increases the chance of PA lymph nodal metastasis.

### Histological Type

Histological type is one of the important prognostic factors of EEC. Type II non-endometrioid carcinomas are far more aggressive than type I EC. The estimated 5-year survival of USC and clear cell carcinoma patient is 42% and 27% respectively compared to 74–93% in endometrioid carcinoma.[40]

### Cervical Involvement

Cervical involvement is related with higher risk of recurrence, lymph nodal involvement and poor survival.

### DNA Ploidy

Diploid DNA tumors are less aggressive and have higher survival than the aneuploid tumor.[41]

### Tumor Cell Proliferation

Studies have shown significant correlation between Ki 67 proliferation index with FIGO staging, histological type and prognosis.[42]

### Tumor Suppressor Genes

a. PTEN: PTEN expression by immunostaining is not considered as a prognostic marker.
b. p53. Abnormal expression of p53 indicates mutation of p53. P53 overexpression is correlated with advanced stage and poor survival of EC.

Microsatellite instability (MSI): There is no association of MSI and prognosis of EC.[43]

## Management

### Type I carcinoma

Total hysterectomy with bilateral salpingo-oophorectomy is the treatment of choice in case of EC. At the time of operation peritoneal fluid examination and careful palpation or observation of abdomen should be done. In case of endometrioid carcinoma with poor prognostic factors postoperative radiotherapy is given.

### Type II Carcinoma

Uterine serous and clear cell carcinomas are initially managed by total hysterectomy with bilateral salpingo-oophorectomy and omentectomy along with surgical staging. After optimal cytoreduction platinum-taxane based adjuvant chemotherapy improves survival. Local radiation therapy may be used for local control of the cancer.[44] Pelvic lymphadenectomy has doubtful effect on survival of the patient.

## TUMORS OF THE EPITHELIAL AND MESENCHYMAL COMPONENT (MIXED MÜLLERIAN TUMOR)

These tumors are composed of both the epithelial and mesenchymal tissues. WHO has classified these tumors into six broad categories: (1) Carcinosarcoma (malignant mixed Müllerian tumor), (2) Adenosarcoma, (3) Carcinofibroma, (4) Adenofibroma, (5) Adenomyoma, (6) Atypical polyploid variant.

### Malignant Müllerian Mixed Tumor (Carcinosarcoma)

By definition, the tumor is composed of both carcinoma and malignant mesenchymal component. According to WHO classification, this tumor is labeled as carcinosarcoma rather than the older terminology Malignant Mixed Mesodermal Tumor. Uterine carcinosarcoma (UCS) is a relatively uncommon tumor and consists of less than 5% uterine malignancies. The clinical, immunocytochemistry and molecular genetic studies indicate that these tumors are nothing but high grade uterine carcinoma with mesenchymal metaplasia.[45] The carcinoma and sarcomatous component of the tumor are monoclonal in origin and the same genetic changes have been demonstrated in both the epithelial and mesenchymal components of the carcinosarcoma by gene mutation analyses, and loss of heterozygosity studies.[46]

### Etiology

Both the endometrial carcinoma and UCS bear almost same risk factors such as marked obesity, exogenous estrogen use, and tamoxifen therapy.

### Clinical Features

UCS usually occurs in postmenopausal patient and the mean age is 65 year. The common complaint of the patient is bleeding per vagina. Occasional the patient may present with protruding mass from the vaginal orifice.

## Gross Features

Grossly UCS is large and polypoid mass. The mass often fills the uterine cavity and protrudes from the cervical os. The presence of cartilage or bone may give hard consistency. The surface of the tumor often shows ulceration and necrosis.

## Histopathology (Figures 9.46 to 9.50)

UCSs show biphasic tumor and composed of both carcinoma and sarcoma components. Usually both these components are homogenously admixed with each other. However, the either elements may be present focally. Therefore, extensive sampling should be done in a high grade carcinoma or even pure sarcoma. Occasionally, the tumor shows distinct separation of the two elements and may simulate as collision tumor. The carcinoma element of the tumor is commonly high-grade endometrioid carcinoma. However, it may show non-endometrioid carcinoma such as serous or clear cell carcinoma. Occasionally, the carcinoma element may show mucinous or undifferentiated adenocarcinoma components. The sarcomatous component of UCS is composed of either homologous or heterologous elements. The homologous component may show leiomyosarcoma, endometrial stromal sarcoma, undifferentiated sarcoma, and malignant fibrous histiocytoma. The heterologous component is present in 50% of UCS and it commonly consists of rhabdomyosarcoma and occasionally chondrosarcoma. Rarely the heterologous element shows osteosarcoma or liposarcoma. Immunohistochemistry: Immunohistochemistry is only helpful in doubtful cases. The carcinoma component is positive for cytokeratin, and epithelial membrane antigen. Mesenchymal component is positive for vimentin. Homologous sarcomatous components are positive for CD 10 and CD 34. Leiomyosarcoma is positive for smooth muscle actin and may also show epithelial membrane antigen expression. Rhabdomyosarcoma shows desmin and myogenin positivity. Chondrosarcoma element is positive for S-100. Higher percentage of UCS also show p16 positivity.

## Differential Diagnosis

a. Sarcomatoid endometrioid carcinoma: The sarcomatoid type of endometrioid carcinoma lacks any heterologous component.
b. Endometrioid carcinoma with heterologous elements: Endometrioid carcinoma may show benign heterologous elements such as cartilage or osteoid material and may pose diagnostic confusion with UCS.
c. Dedifferentiated endometrial carcinoma: This tumor shows typical glandular elements of grade 1 or grade 2 adenocarcinoma along with diffuse sheets of undifferentiated cells that gives rise to the impression of sarcoma. It is usually seen in lower age group and lack the spindle cell component of sarcoma.

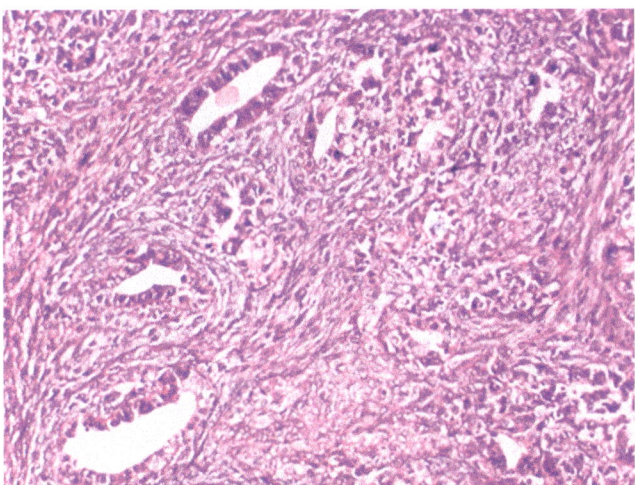

**Figure 9.46:** Carcinosarcoma: The tumor shows both malignant glands and homogenously admixed sarcomatous element

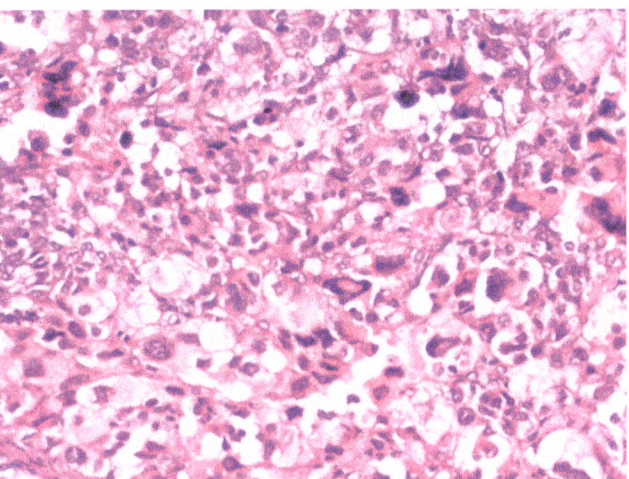

**Figure 9.47:** Carcinosarcoma: Diffuse sheets of large pleomorphic cells

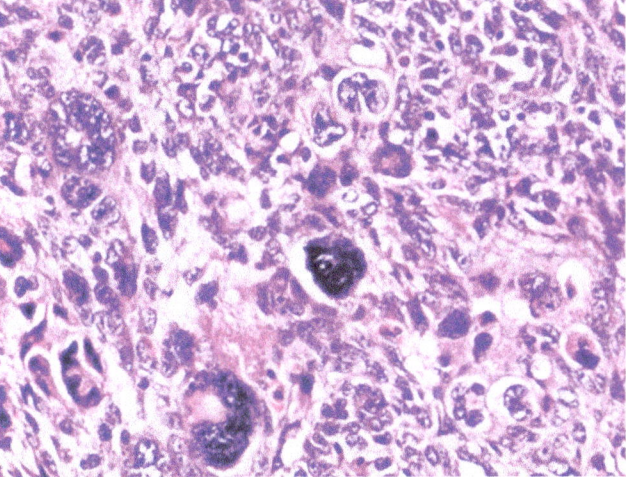

**Figure 9.48:** Carcinosarcoma: Higher magnification shows large multinuclear and mononuclear bizarre malignant cells

Uterus: Preneoplastic Lesions and Carcinoma

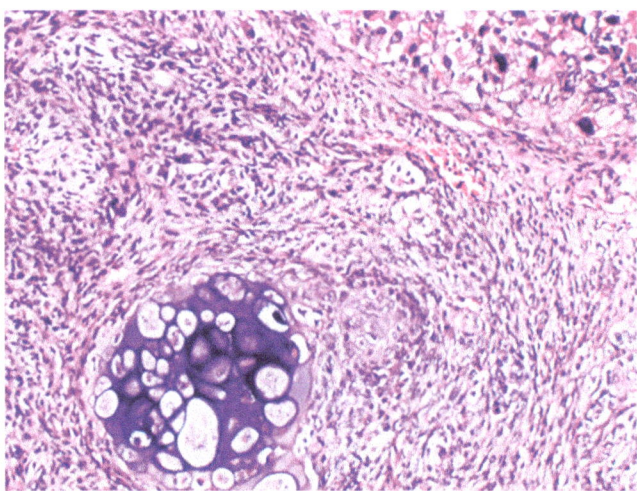

Figure 9.49: Carcinosarcoma: Foci of cartilaginous component present

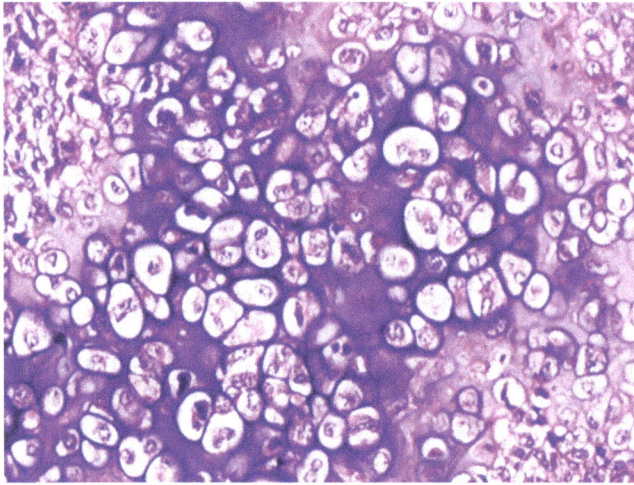

Figure 9.50: Carcinosarcoma: Higher magnification shows malignant cartilaginous component

d. Pleomorphic rhabdomyosarcoma
e. Low-grade Müllerian adenosarcoma: In case of UCS both the sarcomatous and epithelial components are of high grade.

## Prognosis and Survival

Overall prognosis of UCS is poor with 5 year survival rate is less than 35%. In stage I and II UCS cases, the 5 year survival rate is 50%.[85] The behavior of UCS in FIGO stage I is poor compared to serous or clear cell carcinoma in the FIGO stage I.[47] The prognosis of UCS greatly depends on deep myometrial invasion, lymphovascular space involvement, high-grade tumors and the presence of non endometrioid carcinomatous components (serous or clear cell).

## Treatment

The treatment of UCS is total hysterectomy and bilateral salpingo-oophorectomy with pelvic and para-aortic lymph node dissection and peritoneal cytology examination. The role of adjuvant chemotherapy or radiotherapy is unclear.

## Low-grade Müllerian Adenosarcoma

This is a rare variant of mixed Müllerian tumor and consists of only 8% of uterine sarcoma. This tumor is composed of benign glands along with sarcomatous element. Adenosarcoma usually occurs in the postmenopausal patients with mean age 58 years. The one third of the patients may be premenopausal age group. The patient commonly presents with vaginal bleeding, along with pain abdomen, enlarged uterus or mass protruding out from vagina.

### Gross Features

The adenosarcoma commonly presents with a solitary polypoid growth in the uterine lumen. The mass may be sessile or pedunculated. The tumor is grey white and soft on cut surface. Small cystic foci or hemorrhagic areas may also be seen.

### Histopathology

The tumor shows biphasic pattern with benign glandular elements and low-grade sarcomatous elements. The glands are slit and leaf like in low power microscopical examination. The stromal cells are condensed around the glands. This arrangement of the stromal cells is typically known as "periglandular collaring". In this area, the stromal cells show mitotic activity and atypia. The glandular epithelial cells are benign looking. However, mild atypia may be seen in the lining epithelium. The glandular lining epithelial cells show focal mucinous, squamous or hobnail type of metaplastic changes. The mesenchymal component of adenosarcoma is usually low grade type heterologous component that consists of endometrial stromal sarcoma or fibrosarcoma. The stroma is hypocellular and often shows myxoid changes in the other areas. The mitotic count should be assessed in the hypercellular area. The mean mitotic rate of adenosarcoma is 9/10 high power field. The criteria for the diagnosis of adenosarcoma are: (1) Two or more mitotic figures per 10 HPFs, (2) Increased stromal cellularity, and (3) Significant stromal cell atypia. Sex cord like tubules are seen within the stroma in 10% cases of adenosarcoma. The cells are arranged in cords, tubules and trabeculae.

### Immunocytochemistry

The mesenchymal component of adenosarcoma is positive for vimentin, CD10, WT1, ER and PR. The tumor cells also variably express smooth muscle actin, desmin and caldesmon. Epithelial element of adenosarcoma is positive for cytokeratin.

*Differential Diagnosis*

a. Cellular endometrial polyps: The endometrial polyps is homogenously cellular and does not show any mitotic activity or atypia.
b. Müllerian adenofibroma: This is an extremely rare tumor. Here both the epithelial and stromal components are benign.

*Prognosis*

Adenosarcoma is a low-grade malignant tumor. The local recurrence of the tumor in vagina or pelvic region is seen in 25% of the tumor. About 5% of the tumor shows distant metastasis and in 70% of the cases, the metastatic element is sarcoma. The poor prognostic indicators are: (1) More than half of myometrial invasion of the tumor, (2) Extrauterine spread, (3) Sarcomatous overgrowth.

*Treatment*

The patient is treated by total abdominal hysterectomy and bilateral salpingo-oophorectomy. The exact role of post-surgical adjuvant therapy in adenosarcoma is not known.

## Carcinofibroma

This is an extremely uncommon type of tumor that is composed of carcinoma with benign stromal component. The mesenchymal component is usually fibrous. Occasionally heterologous elements have been described. Only a few case reports have been reported on this rare tumors.

## Adenofibroma

Adenofibroma of the uterus is a rare tumor. It is composed of both benign glandular and mesenchymal elements. The tumor is grossly polypoid in appearance. Histopathology section shows multiple cleft like glands surrounded by connective tissue stroma. The glandular lining epithelium is benign and the cells are cuboidal or columnar. The stroma is composed of endometrial stromal cells. Smooth muscle cells may also be seen.

*Prognosis and Treatment*

Adenofibroma is a benign tumor and simple polypectomy is the treatment of choice.

## REFERENCES

1. Kurman RJ, Carcangiu ML, Herrington S, Young RH. WHO classification of tumors of female genital reproductive organs. 4th Edition, International agency for research on Cancer, Lyon 2014.
2. Skov BG, Broholm H, Engel U, Franzmann MB, Nielsen AL, Lauritzen AF, et al. Comparison of the reproducibility of the WHO classifications of 1975 and 1994 of endometrial hyperplasia. Int J Gynecol Pathol. 1997;16:33-37.
3. Kurman RJ, Norris HJ. Evaluation of criteria for distinguishing atypical endometrial hyperplasia from well–differentiated carcinoma. Cancer. 1982;49:2547-57.
4. Kurman RJ, Kaminski PF, Norris HJ. The behaviour of endometrial hyperplasia. Along-term study of "untreated" hyperplasia in 170 patients. Cancer. 1985;56:403-12.
5. Baak JP, Wisse-Brekelmans EC, Fleege JC, et al. Assessment of the risk on endometrial cancer in hyperplasia, by means of morphological and morphometrical features. Pathol Res Pract. 1992;188:856-9.
6. Lacey JV Jr, Ioffe OB, Ronnett BM, Rush BB, Richesson DA, Chatterjee N, et al. Endometrial carcinoma risk among women diagnosed with endometrial hyperplasia: the 34-year experience in a large health plan. Br J Cancer. 2008;98(1):45-53.
7. Figueroa-Casas PR, Ettinger B, Delgado E, et al. Reversal by medical treatment of endometrial hyperplasia caused by estrogen replacement therapy. Menopause. 2001;8:420-3.
8. Pérez-Medina T, Bajo J, Folgueira G, et al. Atypical endometrial hyperplasia treatment with progestogens and gonadotropin-releasing hormone analogues: long-term follow-up. Gynecol Oncol. 1999;73:299-304.
9. Spiegel GW. Endometrial carcinoma in situ in postmenopausal women. Am J Surg Pathol. 1995;19:417-32.
10. Mutter GL, Ince TA, Baak JP, Kust GA, Zhou XP, Eng C. Molecular identification of latent precancers in histologically normal endometrium. Cancer Res. 2001;61(11):4311-4.
11. Monte NM, Webster KA, Neuberg D, Dressler GR, Mutter GL. Joint loss of PAX2 and PTEN expression in endometrial pre-cancers and cancer. Cancer Res. 2010;70(15):6225-32.
12. Tashiro H, Isacson C, Levine R, et al. p53 gene mutations are common in uterine serous carcinoma and occur early in their pathogenesis. Am J Pathol. 1997;150:177-85.
13. Mutter GL, Wada H, Faquin WC, et al. K-ras mutations appear in the premalignant phase of both microsatellite stable and unstable endometrial carcinogenesis. Mol Pathol. 1999;52:257-62.
14. Jemal A, Siegel R, Ward E, Hao Y, Xu J, Murray T, Thun MJ. Cancer statistics, 2008. CA Cancer J Clin. 2008;58(2):71-96.
15. Rose PG. Endometrial carcinoma. N Engl J Med. 1996;335(9):640-9. Review. Erratum in: N Engl J Med. 1997;336(18):1335.
16. Boruban MC, Altundag K, Kilic GS, Blankstein J. From endometrial hyperplasia to endometrial cancer: Insight into the biology and possible medical preventive measures. Eur J Cancer Prev. 2008;17:133-8.
17. Boyd J, Risinger JI. Analysis of oncogene alterations in human endometrial carcinoma: prevalence of ras mutations. Mol Carcinog. 1991;4:189-95.
18. Lax SF, Kendall B, Tashiro H, Slebos RJ, Hedrick L. The frequency of p53, K-ras mutations, and microsatellite instability differs in uterine endometrioid and serous

carcinoma: evidence of distinct molecular genetic pathways. Cancer. 2000;88:814-24.
19. Kohler MF, Nishii H, Humphrey PA, Sasaki H, Boyd JA, Marks JR, et al. Mutation of the p53 tumor-suppressor gene is not a feature of endometrial hyperplasias. Am Obstet Gynecol. 1993;169:690-4.
20. Reynolds R, Talavera FR, Hopkins M, Menon K. Characterization of epidermal growth factor receptor in normal and neoplastic human endometrium. Cancer. 1990;66:1967-73.
21. Helland A, Børresen-Dale AL, Peltomäki P, Hektoen M, Kristensen GB, Nesland JM, et al. Microsatellite instability in cervical and endometrial carcinomas. Int J Cancer. 1997;70:499-501.
22. Creasman WT. Announcement. FIGO stages: 1988 revision. Gynecol Oncol. 1988;35:125-7.
23. Obermair A, Geramou M, Gücer F, Denison U, Graf AH, Kapshammer E, et al. Endometrial cancer: accuracy of the finding of a well differentiated tumor at dilatation and curettage compared to the findings at subsequent hysterectomy. Int J Gynecol Cancer. 1999;9:383-6.
24. Kong CS, Beck AH, Longacre TA. A panel of 3 markers including p16, ProExC, or HPV ISH is optimal for distinguishing between primary endometrial and endocervical adenocarcinomas. Am J Surg Pathol. 2010;34:915-26.
25. Siverberg SG, Kurman RJ. Atlas of tumor pathology. Tumors of the uterine corpus and gestational trophoblastic disease. AFIP: Washington DC, 1992.
26. Tobon H, Watkins GJ. Secretory adenocarcinoma of the endometrium. Int J Gynecol Pathol. 1985;4:328-35.
27. Hendrickson MR, Kempson RL. Ciliated carcinoma –a variant of endometrial adenocarcinoma: a report of 10 cases. Int J Gynecol Pathol. 1983; 2:1–12.
28. Fukuma K, Miyamura S, Thoya T, et al. Uterine papillary serous carcinoma with high levels of serum carcinoembryonic antigen. Response to combination chemotherapy. Cancer. 1987;59:403-5.
29. Sherman ME, Bitterman P, Rosenshein NB, et al. Uterine serous carcinoma. A morphologically diverse neoplasm with unifying clinicopathologic features. Am J Surg Pathol. 1992;16:600-10.
30. Rabban JT, Zaloudek CJ. Minimal uterine serous carcinoma: current concepts in diagnosis and prognosis. Pathology. 2007;39(1):125-33.
31. Mhawech-Fauceglia P, Herrmann FR, Rai H, et al. IMP3 distinguishes uterine serous carcinoma from endometrial endometrioid adenocarcinoma. Am J Clin Pathol. 2010;133:899-908.
32. Fadare O, Zheng W, Crispens MA, Jones HW, Khabele D, Gwin K, et al. Morphologic and other clinicopathologic features of endometrial clear cell carcinoma: a comprehensive analysis of 50 rigorously classified cases. Am J Cancer Res. 2013;3(1):70-95.
33. Yamamoto S, Tsuda H, Aida S, et al. Immunohistochemical detection of hepatocyte nuclear factor 1beta in ovarian and endometrial clear-cell adenocarcinomas and nonneoplastic endometrium. Hum Pathol. 2007;38:1074-80.
34. Silverberg SG, Kurman RJ, Nogales FF, et al. Tav: Epithelial tumors and related lesions, in Tavassoli F and Devilee P (eds): WHO Classification of Tumors: Pathology and Genetics: Tumors of the Breast and Female Genital Organs. Lyon, IARC Publishing Group, 2003, pp 221-32.
35. Lininger RA, Ashfaq R, Albores-Saavedra J, et al. Transitional cell carcinoma of the endometrium and endometrial carcinoma with transitional cell differentiation. Cancer. 1997;79:1933-43.
36. Pecorelli S. Revised FIGO staging for carcinoma of the vulva, cervix, and endometrium. Int J Gynecol Obstet. 2009;105:103-4.
37. Morrow CP, Bundy BN, Kurman RJ, Creasman WT, Heller P, Homesley HD, et al. Relationship between surgical-pathological risk factors and outcome in clinical stage I and II carcinoma of the endometrium: a Gynecologic Oncology Group study. Gynecol Oncol. 1991;40:55-65.
38. Watanabe M, Aoki Y, Kase H, Fujita K, Tanaka K. Low risk endometrial cancer: a study of pelvic lymph node metastasis. Int J Gynecol Cancer. 2003;13(1):38-4.
39. Mariani A, Keeney GL, Aletti G, Webb MJ, Haddock MG, Podratz KC. Endometrial carcinoma: paraaortic dissemination. Gynecol Oncol. 2004;92(3):833-8.
40. Abeler VM, Kjørstad KE. Serous papillary carcinoma of the endometrium: a histopathological study of 22 cases. Gynecol Oncol. 1990;39:266-71.
41. Britton LC, Wilson TO, Gaffey TA, Lieber MM, Wieand HS, Podratz KC—Flow cytometric DNA analysis of stage I endometrial carcinoma. Gynecol Oncol. 1989;34:317-22.
42. Geisler JP, Wiemann MC, Zhou Z, Miller GA, Geisler HE. Proliferation index determined by MIB-1 and recurrence in endometrial cancer. Gynecol Oncol. 1996;61:373-7.
43. MacDonald ND, Salvesen HB, Ryan A, Iversen OE, Akslen LA, Jacobs IJ. Frequency and prognostic impact of microsatellite instability in a large population-based study of endometrial carcinomas. Cancer Res. 2000;60:1750-2.
44. Boruta DM 2nd, Gehrig PA, Fader AN, Olawaiye AB. Management of women with uterine papillary serous cancer: a Society of Gynecologic Oncology (SGO) review. Gynecol Oncol. 2009;115(1):142-53.
45. McCluggage WG. Malignant biphasic uterine tumors: carcinosarcomas or metaplastic carcinomas? J Clin Pathol. 2002;55:321-25.
46. Gorai I, Yanagibashi T, Taki A, et al. Uterine carcinosarcoma is derived from a single stem cell: an in vitro study. Int J Cancer. 1997;72:821-7.
47. Ferguson SE, Tornos C, Hummer A, et al. Prognostic features of surgical stage I uterine carcinosarcoma. Am J Surg Pathol. 2007;31:1653-61.

# Mesenchymal Tumor of Uterus

## 10

Uterine mesenchymal tumors are developed from the endometrial stromal cells and uterine smooth muscles.

## ENDOMETRIAL STROMAL TUMORS

Endometrial stromal tumors (EST) are constituted of cells that simulate the endometrial stroma of the non-neoplastic proliferative phase of uterus. They are comprised of less than 10% of uterine tumors.

## Classification

In the year 2014, WHO reclassified endometrial stromal tumor as[1] (Table 10.1): (1) Endometrial stromal nodule (ESN), (2) Low-grade endometrial stromal sarcoma (ESS), (3) High-grade endometrial stromal sarcoma, (4) Undifferentiated endometrial sarcoma (UES).

## Endometrial Stromal Nodule

Endometrial stromal nodule (ESN) is a relatively uncommon benign endometrial stromal tumor and comprises of 0.2% of all uterine malignancies. The tumor commonly occurs in 5th and 6th decade of life and the median age is 47 years. The patients present with abnormal uterine bleeding. Less commonly the patient may have pain in abdomen.

### Gross

The tumor may be in the submucosal or intramural location. ESN is solitary and well-circumscribed round to oval nodule and yellowish to tan appearance. The size of the tumor varies from few mm to several cm and the mean size is 7 cm in diameter. The cut surface of the tumor shows whitish grey to orange appearance.

### Histopathology

Endometrial stromal nodule (ESN) is characterized by well-circumscribed growth with sharp discrimination between the tumor cells and the myometrium (Figure 10.1). Rarely small finger-like projections may be noted from the main nodule towards the myometrium. However, these projections should be within the 3 mm area of the main nodule. The tumor shows sheets of round cells with scanty cytoplasm having round monomorphic nuclei (Figure 10.2). The cells simulate endometrial stromal cells. ESN is usually vascular and shows multiple thin walled vascular channels. The tumor cells often show whorling appearance around such capillaries. Occasionally, the vessels show thick muscular wall particularly towards myometrial side of the tumor. Thin reticulin network encircles single or group of tumor cells. It was suggested that well-defined nodule, thin reticulin

Table 10.1: Classification of endometrial stromal tumor: WHO 2014[2]

| Type | Margin and myoinvasion | Nuclear pleomorphism | Lymphovascular invasion | Mitosis | Comments |
|---|---|---|---|---|---|
| ESN | Well-circumscribed | No | Absent | Less than 5/10 HPF | |
| ESS-low grade | Infiltrating finger like | Minimal | Present | Less than 5/10 HPF | |
| ESS-high grade | Infiltrating finger like | Moderate | Present | More than 10/10 HPF | Specific YWHAE-FAM22 gene rearrangement |
| Undifferentiated ESS | Destructive | Severe | Present | More than 10/10 HPF | |

ESN, Endometrial nodule, ESS, Endometrial stromal sarcoma

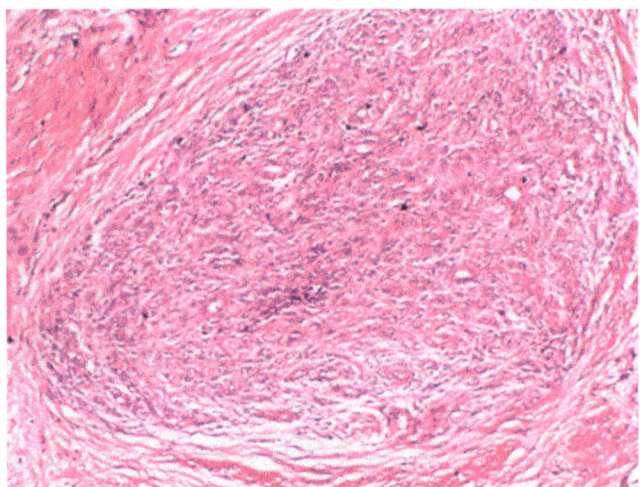

Figure 10.1: Endometrial stromal nodule: Well-circumscribed nodular growth

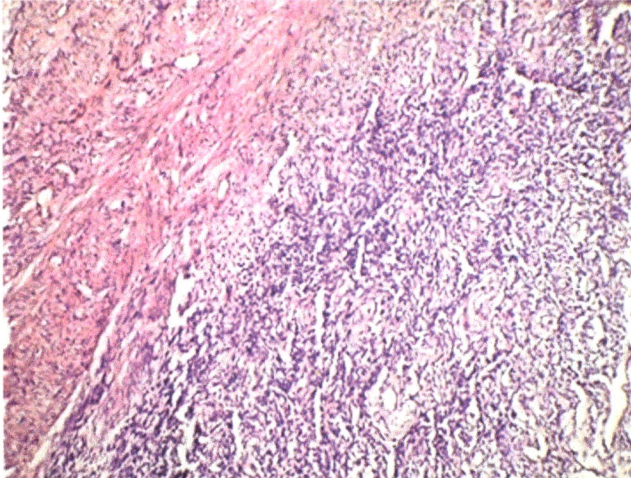

Figure 10.2: Endometrial stromal nodule: Round to oval cells

network, vascular channels and lack of vascular invasion are the characteristic features of ESN.[2] The tumor usually shows less than 3 mitotic figures per 10 high power fields. However, mitosis may be upto 5 per 10 high power fields in 10% of ESN. The sex cord-like tubular differentiation in the form of tubules or cords may also be seen in two third of ESN. Extensive smooth muscle differentiation may give wrong impression of myoinvasion of ESN. Foci of myxoid changes and cholesterol clefts may also be noted.

*Immunocytochemistry*

ESN is positive for smooth muscle actin (SMA), desmin and caldesmon. The tumor is also positive for CD10 and this is a good marker to differentiate ESN from smooth muscle tumor. In addition the tumor cells show nuclear positivity for WT1, estrogen receptor (ER) and progesterone receptor (PR).

*Differential Diagnosis*

1. *Cellular leiomyoma*: The areas of spindle cells with fascicular arrangement and lack of multiple small vessels help to differentiate this tumor from ESN. The cells of leiomyoma are always positive for SMA and desmin; and are negative for CD10.
2. *Low-grade ESS*: This tumor is diffuse unlike well circumscribed nodular growth of ESN. Low-grade ESS shows finger-like infiltrating growth pattern. Lymphatic invasion may also be noted in low-grade ESS.

*Prognosis and Treatment*

ESN is a benign tumor. No recurrence is seen after the complete removal of the tumor.[2] However, hysterectomy may be needed in case of incomplete removal of the tumor.

## Low-Grade ESS

This is an uncommon tumor and represents 0.2% of all malignant tumors of the genital tract and 10% of all uterine malignancies.

*Clinical Features*

The patients are mainly of lower age group than that of other uterine sarcomas. The average age of the patient is 40–55 years. The patients mostly present with vaginal bleeding or pain abdomen. About 25% patients may be completely asymptomatic.

*Gross Examination*

Majority of low-grade ESS are intramural growth. The tumor may present as nodule in the myometrium or less well-circumscribed lesion permeating within the adjacent myometrium. Occasionally, the myometrium may be diffusely thickened with no definite macroscopical growth. The tumor may also present as soft polypoidal mass in the endometrial cavity. The cut surface of the tumor is soft, fleshy, bulging, yellowish rather than firm whorled appearance of leiomyoma.

*Histopathology (Figures 10.3 to 10.6)*

The section shows a densely cellular tumor. In lower magnification diffuse sheets, irregular tongue-shaped areas and islands of cells are seen. The cells look monotonous in appearance in lower magnification and resemble endometrial stroma of proliferative phase. Individual cells are round to oval with scanty cytoplasm. Nuclear pleomorphism is minimal. However, rarely the cells show moderate nuclear pleomorphism and bizarre nuclei. The tumor shows prominent vascular structures that are homogenously distributed within the tumor. The tumor cells are often concentrated around these vascular channels forming concentric whorl

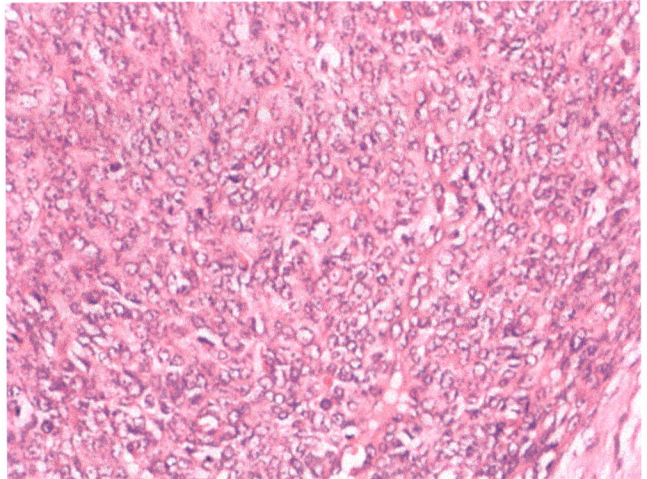

**Figure 10.3:** Low-grade endometrial stromal sarcoma: Diffuse sheets of cells that resemble endometrial stromal cells

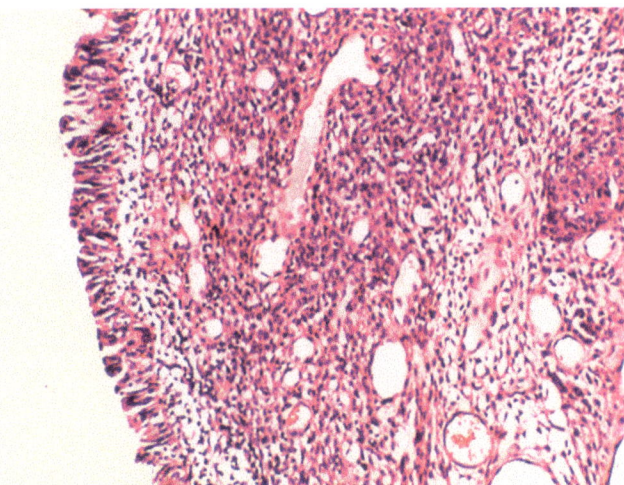

**Figure 10.5:** Low-grade endometrial stromal sarcoma: Low-grade tumor underneath the epithelium presenting as polyp

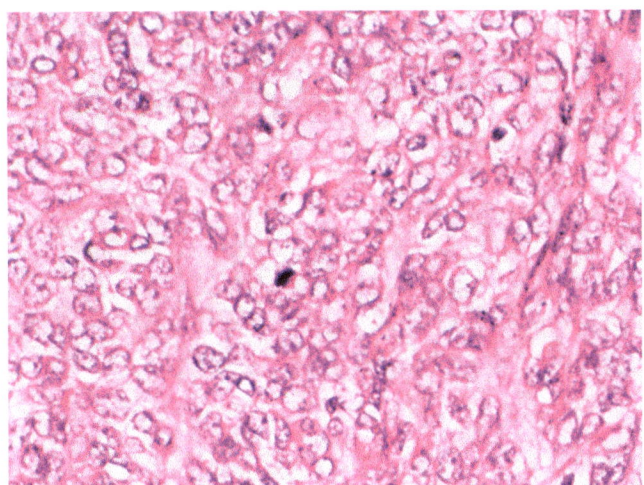

**Figure 10.4:** Low-grade endometrial stromal sarcoma: Higher magnification of the cells. Individual cells are round to oval. Occasional mitotic figures are seen

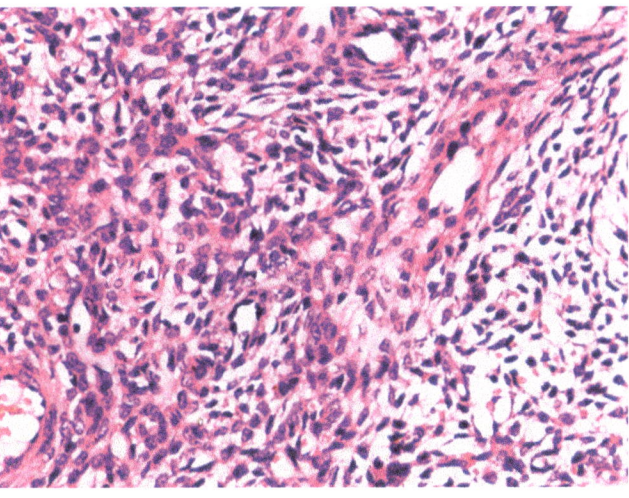

**Figure 10.6:** Low-grade endometrial stromal sarcoma presenting as polyp: Higher magnification shows individual cell morphology

like arrangement. Reticulin stain shows dense network around group of cells or individual cells. Occasional ESS shows predominant spindle cells. ESS may show large cells with abundant clear cytoplasm having small eosinophilic intracytoplasmic inclusion. Rhabdoid, fatty metaplasia and smooth muscle metaplasia is also noted. If more than 30% area of the tumor shows smooth muscle component then the tumor should be categorized as combined smooth muscle - ESS tumor.[3] Myxoid variant of ESS shows prominent myxoid degeneration. Near about 70% cases of low-grade ESS may have sex cord like differentiation and shows tubules, cord and trabeculae like cells. The mitotic activity of the tumor is usually less than 3 per 10 HPF.

*Immunocytochemistry*

The tumor cells are strongly positive for CD10. In addition, the cells of ESS are occasionally positive for desmin, actin and occasionally CK 19.

*Differential Diagnosis*

1. ESN: Discussed before,
2. High grade ESS (undifferentiated endometrial sarcoma): discussed later,
3. Highly cellular leiomyoma (HCL): The following features are helpful to distinguish this tumor from ESS: (1) The soft and fleshy appearance of ESS, (2) Typical spindle

cells with interlacing fascicular areas in the periphery of the tumor in leiomyoma. (3) Cleft-like spaces in HCL. (4) Thin vascular channels in ESS compared to thick muscular wall of the vessels of leiomyoma. (5) Strong CD10 positivity in ESS.
4. Intravenous leiomyomatosis (IVL): The following features may be helpful: (1) Thick-walled blood vessels, (2) Slit-like spaces within the tumor, (3) Spindle-shaped nuclei with blunt ends, (4) Interlacing fascicles, (5) Low mitotic figures.
5. Tumors of perivascular epithelioid cells (PEComas): The cells of PEComas are epithelioid or spindle-shaped containing moderate eosinophilic cytoplasm. These cells are positive for HMB45 and smooth muscle markers, and characteristically negative for CD10.

*Behavior and Prognosis*

Low-grade ESS is a slow growing indolent tumor and 5 year survival rate is 80%. The median survival of ESS is near about 11 years. The patient may have recurrence and the median interval of recurrence is 3–5 years. The prognosis of the tumor mainly depends on the stage of the tumor. Even after metastasis or relapse the tumor may remain stable for long time by appropriate therapy.

*Treatment*

The patient of ESS is treated with total abdominal hysterectomy with bilateral salpingo-oophorectomy. Removal of the ovary is needed as the tumor is estrogen sensitive and the presence of ovary may have adverse effect of the behavior of the tumor. The masses of tumor outside the uterus should be removed by surgery followed by either radiation therapy or hormone therapy (progestational agent).

## High-Grade Endometrial Stromal Sarcoma (HG-ESS) (Figures 10.7 and 10.8)

This tumor shows atypical cells that simulate endometrial stromal cells, however the pleomorphism of the cells are not marked as UES.[4] HG-ESS shows round to oval cells with more nuclear atypia than LG-ESS. HG-ESS usually shows high mitotic figures (more than 10/10HPF), necrosis and vascular invasion. Unique YWHAE-FAM22 gene rearrangement is seen in HG-ESS.

## Undifferentiated Endometrial Sarcoma (UES)

This tumor was previously labeled as high-grade ESS or poorly differentiated ESS. UES represents only 6% of all uterine sarcomas. This tumor represents a high-grade sarcoma with no specific differentiation. This is a diagnosis of exclusion of other sarcomas such as leiomyosarcoma, carcinosarcoma and adenosarcoma of uterus.

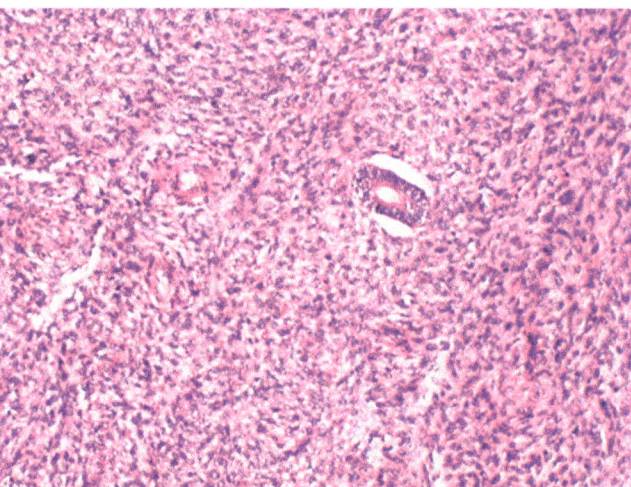

**Figure 10.7:** High-grade endometrial stromal sarcoma: Diffuse sheets of cells encircling the endometrial glands

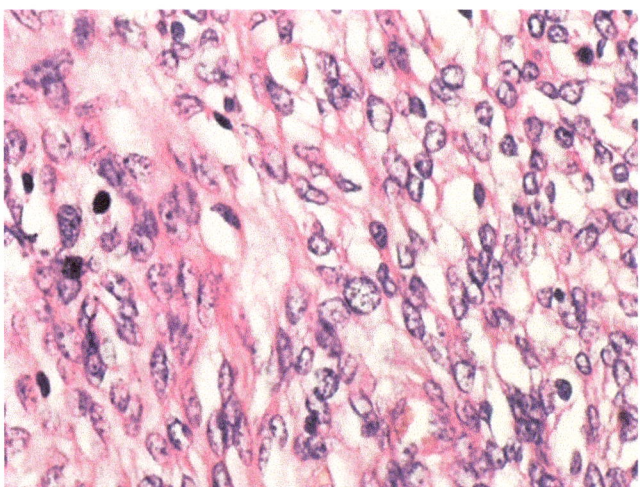

**Figure 10.8:** High-grade endometrial stromal sarcoma: Mild nuclear pleomorphism and excess mitosis are seen

*Clinical Feature*

The patients of UES are postmenopausal. The mean age of the patient is 55 years and median age is 58.2 years. Abnormal vaginal bleeding along with pelvic mass due to uterine enlargement is the common presentation of the patients.

*Gross*

The tumor appears as soft, fleshy and polypoid mass filling the whole uterine cavity. The cut surface of the mass is fleshy and often shows areas of hemorrhage and necrosis.

*Histopathology*

The tumor shows diffuse sheets of cells with destructive infiltration into the myometrium unlike infiltrative pattern of growth in low-grade ESS. The tumor shows haphazard collection of variably sized blood vessel in contrast to uniform small blood vessels in ESS. UES may show relatively monomorphic or polymorphic histologic variants. However, these variants have no special clinical significance. The cells show moderate amount of cytoplasm having moderate nuclear enlargement and pleomorphism. Many bizarre cells are also seen. Multinucleated giant cells are also present. The nuclei show prominent nucleoli with fine to coarse chromatin. Abundant mitotic figures are seen and the count is usually more than 10 per 10 high powered fields up to 20 per 10 high power fields. Many atypical mitotic figures may also be seen. Foci of low-grade ESS may also be associated with UES that suggests the evolution of UES from the ESS component.

*Immunohistochemistry*

CD10 is focal and weakly positive in UES. The tumor does not express any SMA and h-caldesmon. Some cases are completely negative for CD10. ER and PR are also focal and weakly positive in this tumor. EMA is focal and patchy positive in UES. Ki67 index is usually high and more than 10% in UES.

*Differential Diagnosis*

1. Low-grade ESS: The following features are helpful in distinguishing these two tumors:
   - Growth pattern: Low-grade ESS shows infiltrating growth within the myometrium whereas UES shows destructive pushing margin.
   - Vascular channels: The vascular channels are small and homogenously distributed in low-grade ESS in comparison to variable sized haphazard vascular channels in UES.
   - Pleomorphism: The cells of UES show moderate to marked nuclear pleomorphism compared to mild nuclear pleomorphism in low-grade ESS.
   - Resemblance to endometrial stromal cells: The cells of UES are poorly differentiated and may not simulate endometrial stromal cells.
2. Leiomyosarcoma: Following features help in the diagnosis of leiomyosarcoma: (1) Myometrial location, (2) Focal areas of fascicles of oval to spindle cells. (3) Actin, desmin, and caldesmon positivity and CD10 negativity.
3. Rhabdomyosarcoma: The presence of rhabdomyoblasts and myogenin positivity helps in the diagnosis of rhabdomyosarcoma.
4. Carcinosarcoma: The presence of malignant epithelial component may help in the diagnosis of carcinosarcoma.

*Prognosis*

This is an aggressive tumor. Five year survival rate of the patient depends on the initial stage of the tumor at the time of presentation. The majority of stage 1 UES dies within 2 years.[4] The patients with initial extrauterine extension or metastasis show multiple recurrence and dies shortly.[4]

## Molecular Genetics of Endometrial Stromal Tumor

Endometrial stromal tumor shows different genetic alterations (Box 10.1). The most frequent genetic change in ESN and LG-ESS is t(7;17)(p15;q21) translocation. This chromosomal translocation produces a fusion gene known as JAZF1-SUZ12. The JAZF1-SUZ12 gene fusion is mainly noted in the classical pattern of LG-ESS and not in the variant of ESS.[9] Less frequently PHF1-JAZF1 t(6;7)(p21;p15), and EPC1-PHF1 t(6;10;10)(p21;q22;p11.2) are noted in ESN and LG-ESS.

In case of HG-ESS, an unique translocation of t(10;17)(q22;p13) occurs. This results in the formation of YWHAE-FAM22 gene fusion. YWHAE-FAM22 translocation is particularly seen only in HG-ESS and no other uterine sarcomas such as LG-ESS, UES, carcinosarcoma or leiomyosarcoma show this gene fusion.

**Box 10.1: Genetic alteration in EST**

**ESN and LG-ESS**
- JAZF1-SUZ12 t(7;17)(p15;q21)
- PHF1-JAZF1 t(6;7)(p21;p15)
- EPC1-PHF1 t(6;10;10)(p21;q22;p11.2)

**HG-ESS**
- YWHAE-FAM22 t(10;17)(q22;p13)

**UES**
- JAZF1-SUZ12 t(7;17)(p15;q21) Rare

## SMOOTH MUSCLE TUMORS

WHO classified smooth muscle tumors as three broad heading that include: leiomyoma, leiomyosarcoma and smooth muscle tumor of uncertain potential[1] (Table 10.2).

**Table 10.2:** Classification of smooth muscle tumor

| Benign | Uncertain | Malignant |
|---|---|---|
| • Leiomyoma<br>• Variants<br>  - Epithelioid<br>  - Cellular<br>  - Myxoid<br>  - Atypical<br>  - Lipoleiomyoma<br>• Growth pattern<br>  - Intravenous leiomyomatosis<br>  - Diffuse leiomyomatosis | Smooth muscle tumor of uncertain malignant potential | • Leiomyosarcoma usual<br>• Variant<br>  - Epithelioid<br>  - Myxoid |

## Leiomyoma

Leiomyoma is the most common uterine tumor. It is seen in near about 20% of the female below the age of 30 years. Leiomyoma is present in 77% of the hysterectomy specimen and 84% leiomyoma in uterus are multiple in number.[5]

### Clinical Features

The patients with symptomatic leiomyoma are usually middle aged women around 35 years. This tumor is less frequent in young patients. Near about 25% patients with leiomyoma are asymptomatic. The symptoms of leiomyoma depend on the location and size of the tumor. The common symptoms include abnormal uterine bleeding, pain, pressure symptoms and various dysfunctions related to pregnancy. Abnormal vaginal bleeding is mainly associated with submucosal leiomyoma. The menorrhagia in leiomyoma may be severe and may produce anemia. In addition, the submucosal leiomyoma may also cause various reproductive dysfunction such as infertility, spontaneous abortion and fetal malformation. Large intramural leiomyoma may produce pressure symptoms and pain. The large uterus may give pressure in nearby structure and may cause constipation, urinary incontinence and even ureteric obstruction resulting in hydronephrosis. Subserosal pedunculated leiomyoma may often be detached from the uterus due to torsion and may be secondarily infected causing fever. Leiomyoma may rapidly enlarge and may give rise to suspicion of malignant transformation. However, malignant transformation is rare in leiomyoma and should not be the first diagnosis. Intravenous leiomyoma may metastasize in the heart resulting in different cardiac manifestation.

### Gross Features

Leiomyoma is well-circumscribed mass and is easily recognizable from the surrounding myometrium. The tumor is firm and rubbery in consistency. The cut surface is grey white in appearance and shows typical whorled appearance (Figure 10.9). Leiomyoma may often show degenerative changes such as cystic degeneration, necrosis, calcification and ossification. Submucosal leiomyoma may bulge in the endometrial cavity and may show surface ulceration and hemorrhage. Subserosal leiomyoma may be pedunculated and due to torsion may often be separated from the uterus. Very rarely this leiomyoma may often be attached with the other structure and acts as a parasitic leiomyoma.

### Histopathology (Figures 10.10 to 10.13)

Leiomyoma is mostly well-circumscribed and consists of interlacing fascicles of bland looking spindle cells. The cells show elongated spindle-shaped nuclei with moderate amount of eosinophilic cytoplasm. The nuclei are cigar-shaped with blunt ends having fine chromatin and small nucleoli. The tumor cells may be cut transversely and may show round shaped nuclei. The tumor often shows hyalinization in postmenopausal patients. In addition there may be edema, cystic degeneration, myxoid change and hemorrhage. Hyaline deposit is noted in variable extent in most of the leiomyoma. Except severe hyalinization this feature may not draw adequate attention to the pathologist. Occasionally, leiomyoma may show many large vascular channels and this tumor may be labeled as vascular leiomyoma or angiomyoma. Foci of hematopoietic cells containing lymphocytes, histiocytes, eosinophils and mast cells may be seen. This is specially seen in case of patients receiving GnRH therapy. Occasionally, large amount of lymphoid cells may be infiltrated in the tumor and may simulate lymphoma. Leiomyoma located near submucosa may often show ulceration and necrosis. Unlike coagulative necrosis in leiomyosarcoma, here the necrosis is accompanied with acute inflammatory cells. The outline of the cells is not seen at all

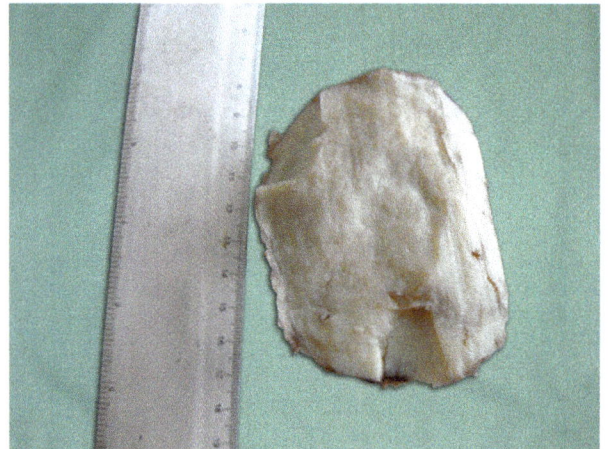

**Figure 10.9:** Leiomyoma gross photo: Greyish white surface shows whorled appearance

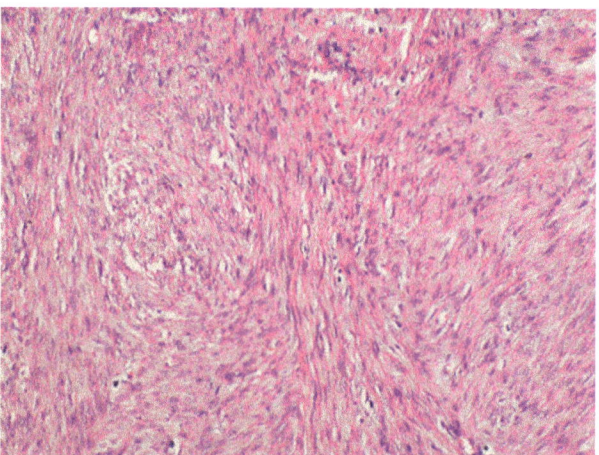

**Figure 10.10:** Leiomyoma: Oval to spindle-shaped cells with interlacing fascicles

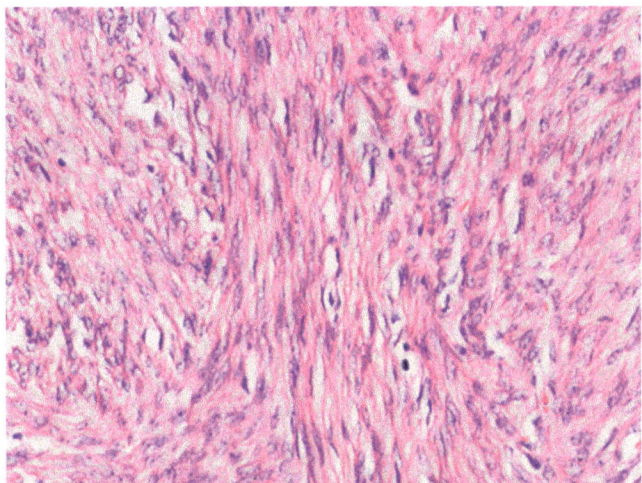

Figure 10.11: Leiomyoma: The individual cells have spindle-shaped nuclei

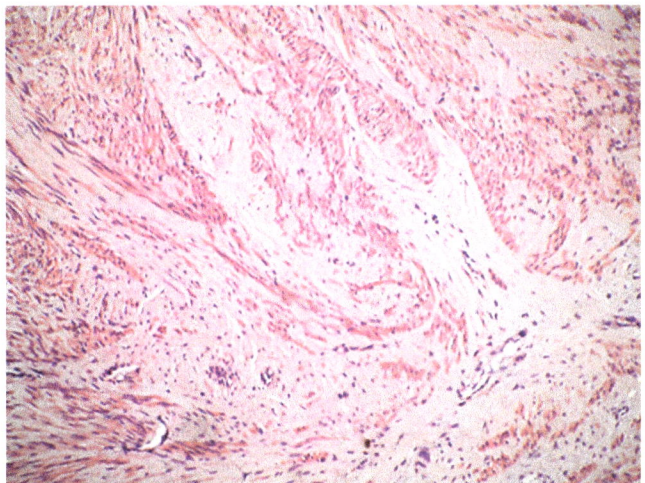

Figure 10.12: Hyaline change in leiomyoma: Acellular pinkish hyaline material

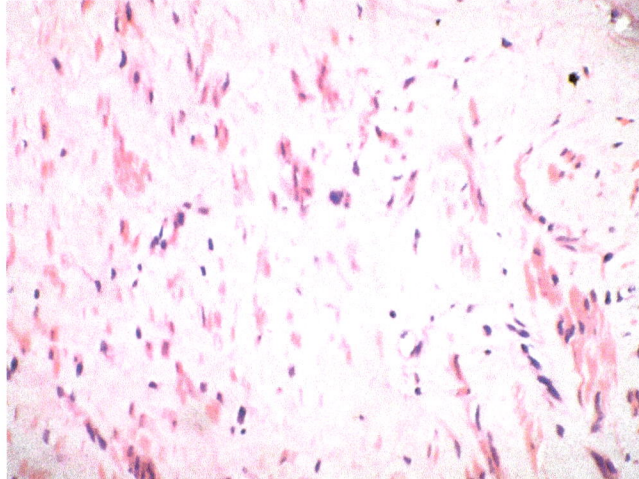

Figure 10.13: Hyaline change in leiomyoma: Higher magnification shows acellular pinkish material with scattered cells

in necrosis of leiomyoma. Occasionally, leiomyoma may be present as dissecting or infiltrating pattern with infiltration of the tumor cells in the adjacent myometrium.

### Ancillary Studies

**Immunocytochemistry:** Leiomyomas are positive for desmin, smooth muscle actin, HDCA8 and h-caldesmon, ER and PR. The cells are variably positive for CD10. Leiomyoma often shows cytokeratin positivity and is usually negative for EMA.

**Cytogenetics:** Studies on random inactivation of X chromosome showed that uterine leiomyoma is monoclonal in origin.[6] Near about 40% of leiomyoma of uterus shows cytogenetic abnormalities and translocation of chromosome 12 and 14 resulting t(12;14)(q15;q23–24) is the most common chromosomal aberration.

## Specific Variants of Leiomyoma

### Cellular Leiomyoma

The cellular leiomyoma (CL) is defined as significantly more cellular tumor than the surrounding normal myometrial tissue in an otherwise typical leiomyoma.[7] There may be nuclear crowding and overlapping. However, CL lacks tumor cell necrosis, mitosis or atypia. Highly cellular leiomyoma (HCL) shows highly cellular dense collection of cells and the cellularity is comparable to endometrial stromal tumors.

**Gross Features:** CL and HCL usually resemble leiomyoma however they are less well-circumscribed and are often fleshy, soft and more tan to yellowish on cut surface.

**Histopathology (Figures 10.14 and 10.15):** On histology section, the tumor shows small interlacing fascicles of spindle cells. The individual cells contain scanty cytoplasm and spindle-shaped nuclei. The tumor contains thick walled blood vessels and split like spaces. The periphery the tumor has irregular margin and blends with the surrounding myometrium. As mentioned before both CL and HCL lack nuclear atypia and mitotic activity.

**Differential diagnosis:** (a) Endometrial stromal tumor (EST): Discussed before. (b) Leiomyosarcoma: The following features help to distinguish leiomyosarcoma from HCL and CL: (a) Mitosis: the mitotic count is more than 10 per 10 HPFs in leiomyosarcoma; (b) Coagulative necrosis: Coagulative necrosis is always absent in HCL and CL; (c) Atypia: Atypia is rarely present in HCL and CL. In contrast atypia is often seen in leiomyosarcoma.

### Mitotically Active Leiomyoma

Mitotically active leiomyoma (MAL) is defined as smooth muscle tumor with typical morphological appearance of

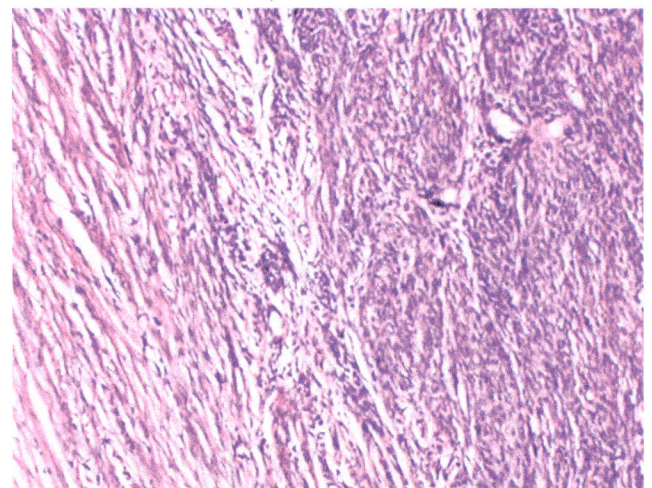

Figure 10.14: Cellular leiomyoma: Tumors shows abundant cellularity

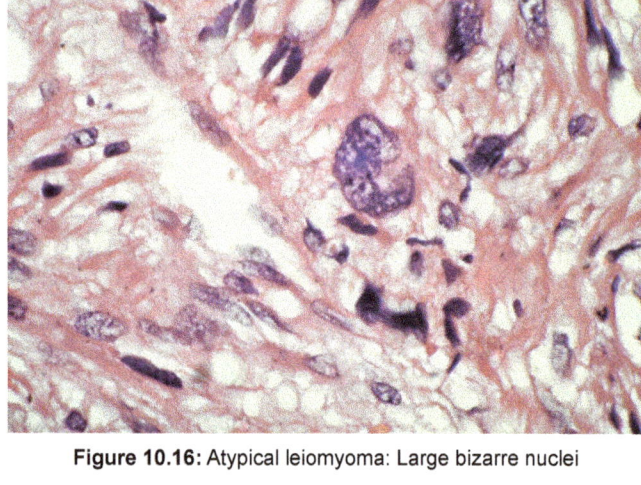

Figure 10.16: Atypical leiomyoma: Large bizarre nuclei

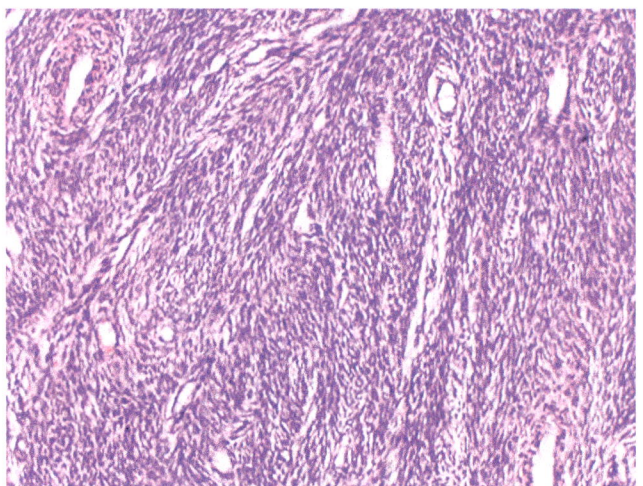

Figure 10.15: Cellular leiomyoma: Higher magnifications of densely crowded cells

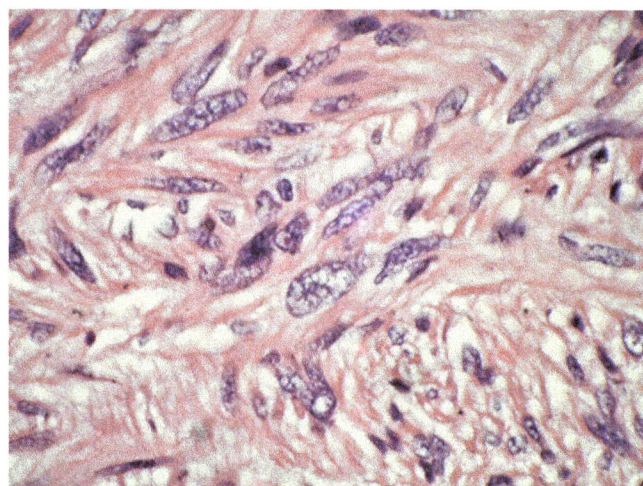

Figure 10.17: Atypical leiomyoma: Many large atypical cells are seen

leiomyoma except high mitotic figures ranging from 5–15 per 10 HPFs.[8]

**Clinical features:** MAL patients have same clinical features of classical leiomyoma. Patients with secretory phase of endometrial cycle may show high mitotic count. Similarly use of exogenous progesterone may cause increased proliferation of cells of leiomyoma.

**Histopathology:** The mitotic count of MAL varies from 5–15 per 10 HPFs. However, Bell et al, reported more than 20 mitotic figures per 10 HPFs in bland looking MAL.[8] MAL does not show any significant atypia or coagulative necrosis. Morphologically, MAL looks similar to ordinary leiomyoma.

### Atypical Leiomyoma (Bizarre Leiomyoma/Pleomorphic Leiomyoma, Symplastic Leiomyoma)

The atypical leiomyoma (AL) shows large atypical cells containing bizarre-shaped nuclei and many multinucleated or mononuclear giant cells in an otherwise ordinary leiomyoma. The clinical features and gross appearance of the AL does not differ from ordinary leiomyoma.

**Histopathology (Figures 10.16 and 10.17):** The tumor shows diffuse or focal distribution of bizarre cells. The number of such atypical cells varies from 5–60%. The individual cells are large with variable amount of eosinophilic cytoplasm. The nuclei are pleomorphic with irregular nuclear margin having prominently clumped chromatin. In addition large intranuclear cytoplasmic inclusions are also seen. The tumor also shows many large multinucleated and mononuclear giant cells. Mitotic activity of AL may be variable and ranges from 0–7 per 10 HPFs.

### Hemorrhagic Cellular Leiomyoma

This distinct type of leiomyoma is usually noted in the postpartum patients or the women who are using oral contraceptives.[9]

Hemorrhagic cellular leiomyoma is usually rapidly enlarging and the patients often present as acute abdomen with rapid uterine enlargement and abdominopelvic pain.

**Histology:** The tumor is heavily cellular and consists of oval to spindle cells with central area of hemorrhage and edema. The tumor is more cellular around the area of hemorrhage. Necrosis is usually absent. Mitotic activity is infrequent.

### Epithelioid Leiomyoma

Epithelioid Leiomyoma (EL) is less known in uterus. EL is defined as a leiomyoma that contains more than 50% round or polygonal cells appearing as "epithelial cells".[10] Plexiform leiomyomas are type of epithelioid leiomyoma that show predominantly plexiform pattern with cord or nest of cells separated by a hyalinized stroma. If this tumor is less than 10 mm in diameter then it is designated as plexiform tumorlets.

**Clinical features:** EL shows similar presentation as leiomyomas. Majority of the tumor show whorled appearance in cut section.

**Histology (Figures 10.18 and 10.19):** The tumor cells are arranged in large sheets, cords or nests rather than fascicles. However in 50% of cases the tumor also shows spindle cells arranged in fascicles along with sheets of epithelioid cells. The individual cells are round to polygonal with centrally placed enlarged round nuclei. Nuclei show small nucleoli and fine chromatin. Occasionally, the tumor cells show clear cytoplasm and the vacuoles may push the nucleus to the periphery giving a signet ring-like appearance. In certain cases the cytoplasmic vacuolization is extensive and produces completely clear appearance. When major portion of the tumor shows such clear cell, the tumor is designated as clear cell leiomyoma. The clear cells of the tumor show glycogen and some mucin.

**Behavior:** Small EL with no atypia or mitosis behaves as a benign tumor.

### Myxoid Smooth Muscle Tumor

These are very rare tumor of uterus and only a handful of such cases have been reported.[11] Microscopically, the tumor shows abundant myxoid material in between the spindle or epithelioid cells. The margin of the tumor is well-circumscribed. The tumor does not show any cytological atypia. Mitotic rate of this tumor is low and usually less than 2 per 10 HPFs.

The myxoid stromal material appears as pale or basophilic in hematoxylin and eosin stain. This material consists of hyaluronic acid rich glycosaminoglycans and this material is positive for Alcian blue. Myxoid degeneration may also be seen focally in ordinary leiomyoma. This is particularly noted around the area of infract.

Pathological assessment of malignancy in myxoid smooth muscle tumor is very difficult. The standard criteria of malignancy are not applicable in myxoid leiomyoma and mitotic count of malignant tumor may be low. Large tumor with infiltrating margin with the presence of cytological atypia is suggestive of malignancy. However, the infiltration of the tumor may be deceptive because myxoid area with the surrounding cellular area may give false impression of infiltration. It is therefore, advisable to take multiple sections from the periphery of the tumor.

### Vascular Leiomyoma

Vascular leiomyomas are usually well-circumscribed and along with spindle cells in fascicle they also show many large

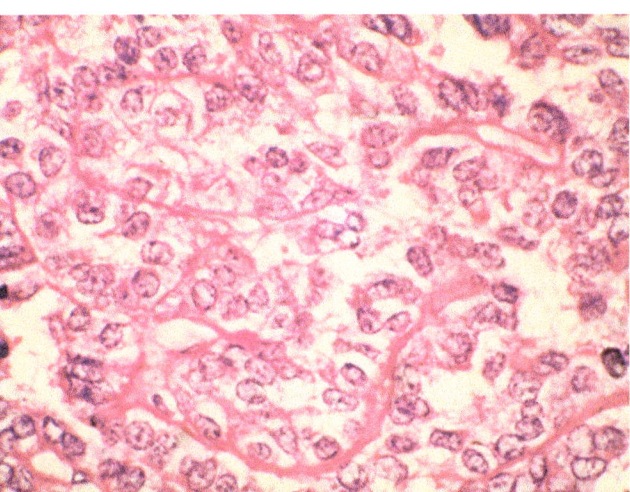

**Figure 10.18:** Epithelioid leiomyoma: Polyhedral cells with round monomorphic nuclei

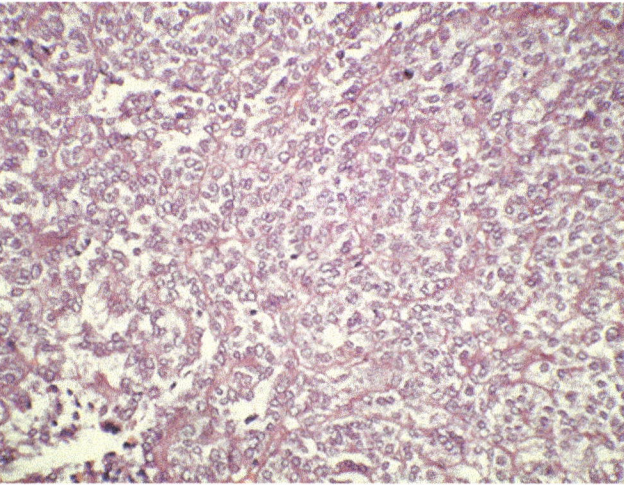

**Figure 10.19:** Epithelioid leiomyoma: Diffuse sheet of polyhedral cells

blood vessels with muscular wall. This tumor may simulate hemangioma which is extremely uncommon in uterus.

### Leiomyoma with Lymphoid Infiltrate

Leiomyoma with lymphoid infiltrate is rare and may be seen in case of GnRH agonist therapy cases.[12] The tumor shows focal or diffuse infiltration by small lymphoid cells in varying intensity. The infiltrate may also show plasma cells and eosinophils along with occasional germinal centers.

### Growth Pattern

*Intravenous Leiomyomatosis of Uterus*

Intravenous leiomyomatosis of uterus (IVL) is a rare condition and shows proliferation of benign smooth muscle cells within the lumina of the myometrial vessels.[13] The most of the patients are young and the mean age is 44 years. No predisposing factors have been described in this tumor. The tumor is usually associated with multiple leiomyomata in uterus. It may involve inferior vena cava and heart. Cardiac involvement is known in IVL and IVL affecting right heart may produce congestive cardiac failure.

**Histopathology (Figures 10.20 and 10.21):** Microscopically the tumor shows smooth muscle cells arranged in fascicles within the venous channel. The tumor cells are surrounded by thin layer of endothelial cells.

*Diffuse Uterine Leiomyomatosis*

This is characterized by multiple variable sized benign leiomyomatous nodules that merge with each other and causing symmetrically enlarged uterus.[14] The patient commonly presents with pain in lower abdomen and abnormal vaginal bleeding. The tumor is commonly seen in reproductive age period. The tumor shows benign smooth muscle cells that blend with the surrounding smooth muscle of myometrium. The cells are bland looking and show lack of any mitotic activity.

*Dissecting Leiomyoma*

This is a rare growth pattern of leiomyoma characterized by proliferation of smooth muscle cells of leiomyoma in dissecting pattern within the adjacent myometrium.. At times the tumor may simulate placental tissue due to marked edema and congestion and is designated as "cotylednoid" dissecting leiomyoma.[15]

*Benign Metastasizing Leiomyoma (BML)*

BML is characterized by the presence of benign smooth muscle tumors in the extra uterine sites and commonly in lung. The diagnosis of such entity should only be done after a careful exclusion of leiomyosarcoma in uterus or any other sites. This tumor mostly behaves in benign fashion. However the tumor may grow progressively in lung and may cause death due to respiratory failure.[16] The patients of BML are usually elderly women. The patents have always history of prior hysterectomy for leiomyoma. The median interval of the hysterectomy and the presence of BML is 15 years. Histologically, BML is composed of oval to spindle cell with interlacing fascicles. The tumor does not show any cytological atypia or mitotic activity.

## LEIOMYOSARCOMA

Leiomyosarcoma consists of 1–2% of uterine malignancies. It is considered as the malignant counterpart of leiomyoma. However malignant transformation of leiomyoma to leiomyosarcoma is very uncommon and the incidence is less than 1%.

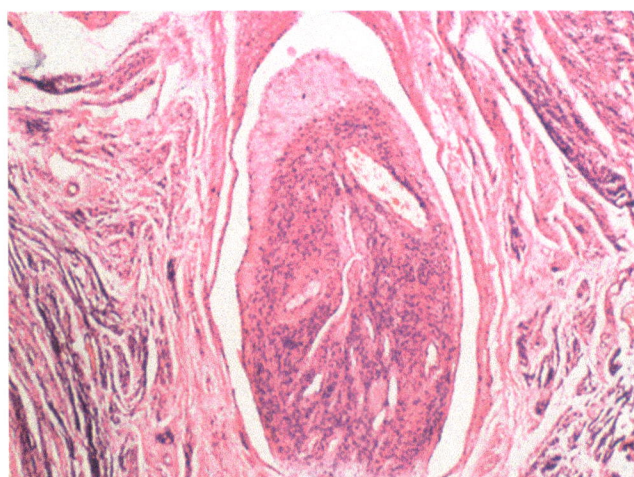

Figure 10.20: Intravenous leiomyoma: Leiomyomatous nodule within the blood vessel

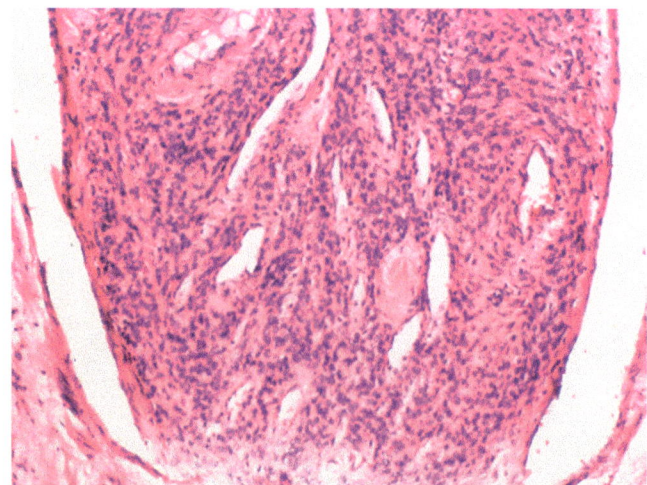

Figure 10.21: Intravenous leiomyoma: Higher magnification shows smooth muscle cells in small fascicles within the vascular channel

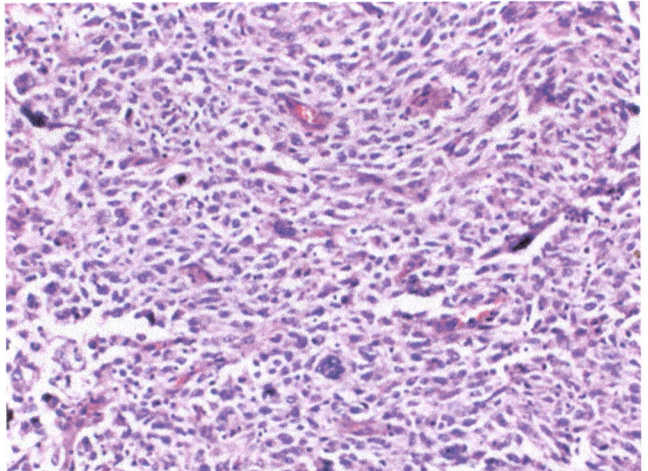

Figure 10.22: Leiomyosarcoma: Sheets of malignant cells

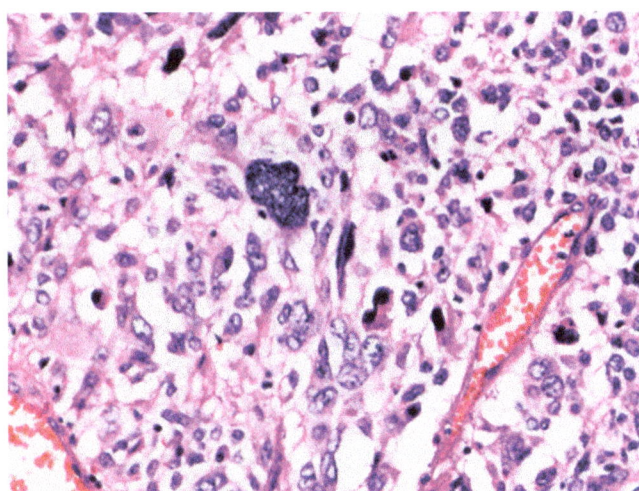

Figure 10.24: Leiomyosarcoma: Large bizarre tumor giant cells

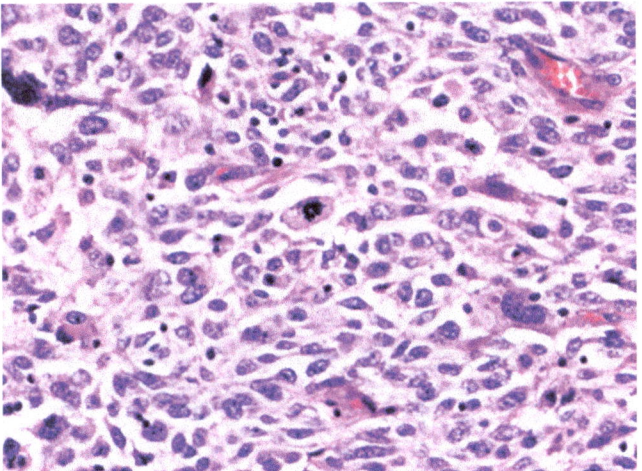

Figure 10.23: Leiomyosarcoma: Moderate nuclear atypia and frequent mitotis

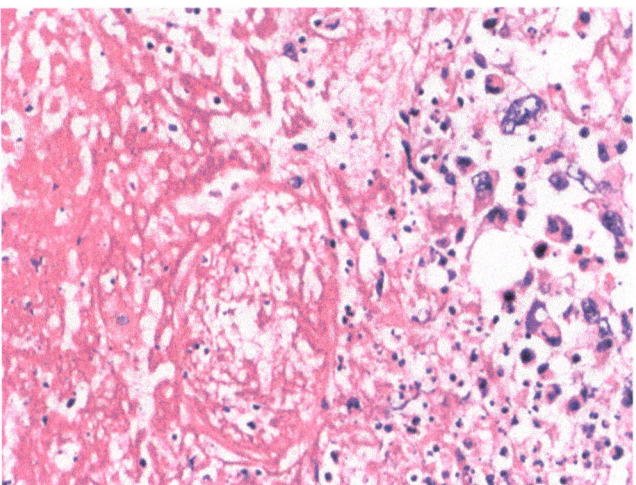

Figure 10.25: Leiomyosarcoma: Coagulative necrosis

## Clinical Features

Leiomyosarcoma commonly occurs in the elderly patient with a mean age of 55 years and the median age is 50–55 years.[17] The patients are usually 10 years older than the patients of leiomyoma. The patient commonly complaints of vaginal bleeding, lower abdominal mass and pain. It is difficult to distinguish leiomyosarcoma and leiomyoma preoperatively. However, rapid tumor growth in the postmenopausal women who are not receiving any hormonal therapy may indicate the presence of leiomyosarcoma.

## Gross Features

The majority of the leiomyosarcomas are intramyometrial in location. The leiomyosarcomas are mostly large tumor and average size is 10 cm in diameter. The tumor is usually poorly circumscribed and the tumor margins intermingle with the adjacent myometrium. The cut surface of the tumor is fleshy and grayish in color. Frequently hemorrhage and necrotic areas are also seen.

## Histopathology (Figures 10.22 to 10.25)

Leiomyosarcoma shows bundle of long intersecting fascicles composed of oval to spindle cells. The tumor cells often infiltrate the surrounding normal smooth muscle of uterus. The individual cells have eosinophilic cytoplasm and elongated spindle-shaped nuclei with blunt ends giving a cigar-shaped appearance. The nuclei are hyperchromatic with coarse chromatin having prominent nucleoli. The tumor cells shows moderate to marked nuclear atypia. The mitotic activity is high in most of the cases and usually exceeds 10 per 10HPFs. Most of the leiomyosarcomas show characteristic coagulative necrosis. There is sudden

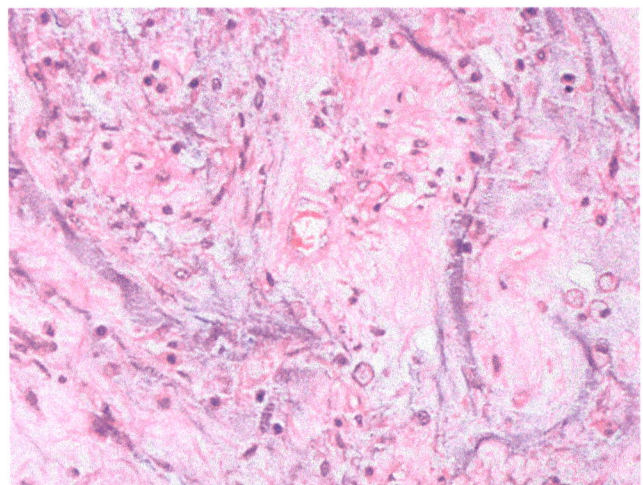

Figure 10.26. **Myxoid leiomyosarcoma:** Higher magnification shows oval to elongated cells with abundant cytoplasm

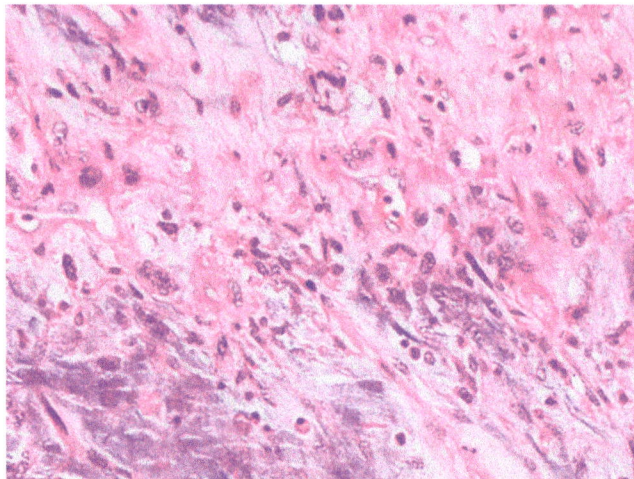

Figure 10.28: Myxoid leiomyosarcoma: The tumor shows focally increased cellularity

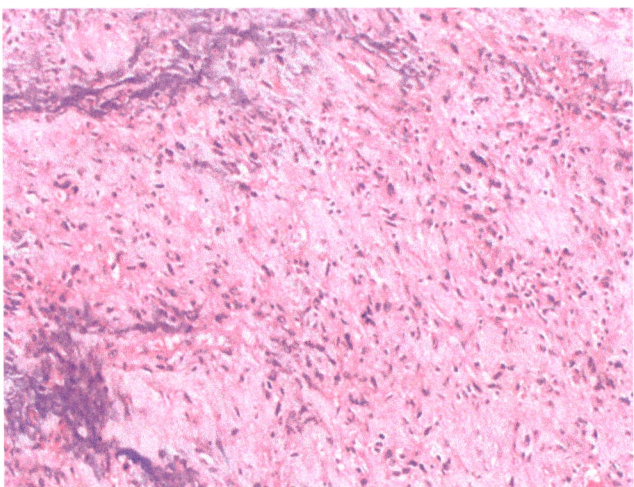

Figure 10.27: Myxoid leiomyosarcoma: Discrete tumor cells in the myxoid background

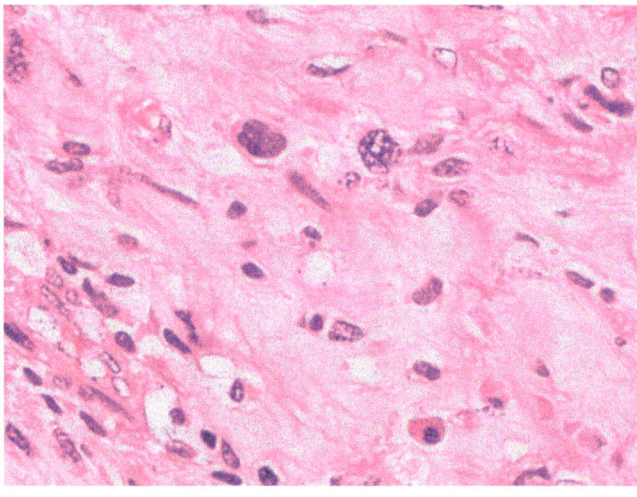

Figure 10.29: Myxoid leiomyosarcoma: The tumor cells are oval to spindle-shaped with moderately pleomorphic nuclei

transition from viable cellular area to necrotic foci without any intervening granulation tissue or fibrosis. The necrotic foci may contain occasional viable tumor cells. In one-fourth of leiomyosarcoma cases vascular invasion by tumor cells are noted. In addition, many multinucleated giant cells resembling osteoclast like giant cells are also seen.

To diagnose leiomyosarcomas any two of the following features are needed: (1) Mitosis more than 10 per 10 HPFs, (2) Significant nuclear atypia, and (3) Foci of coagulative necrosis.

## MYXOID VARIANT (FIGURES 10.26 TO 10.29)

In myxoid variant of leiomyosarcomas the tumor shows abundant myxoid material in between the tumor cells. The tumors are often paucicellular.[18] The cells are spindle-shaped and arranged in interlacing fascicles. The cytoplasm of the cells is scanty. The nuclei are spindle-shaped with small inconspicuous nucleoli. The nuclei show mild to moderate atypia. Mitosis of myxoid leiomyosarcomas may be variable and usually more than 5 per 10 HPFs. However, the tumor may show low mitotic activity. Any myxoid tumor with atypia should be suspected for malignancy regardless of the count of mitotic figures.

## EPITHELIOID LEIOMYOSARCOMAS (FIGURES 10.30 TO 10.32)

The tumor shows diffuse sheets, cords and nests of cell comprising more than 50% of the tumor. The individual cells are oval to polyhedral in shape having ample eosinophilic cytoplasm and centrally placed round nuclei. The nuclei

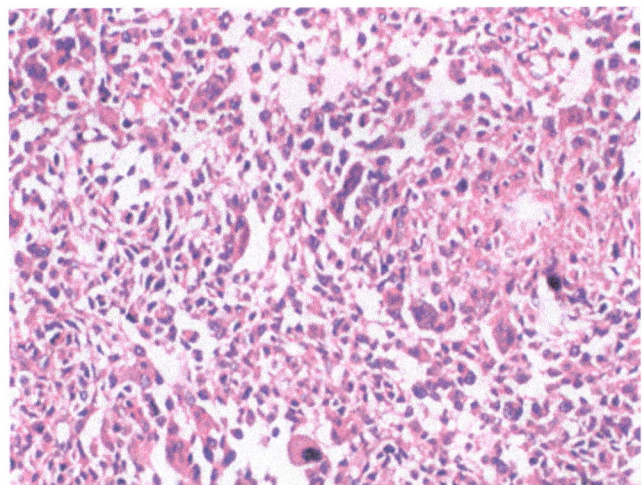

**Figure 10.30:** Epithelioid leiomyosarcoma: Discrete tumor cells

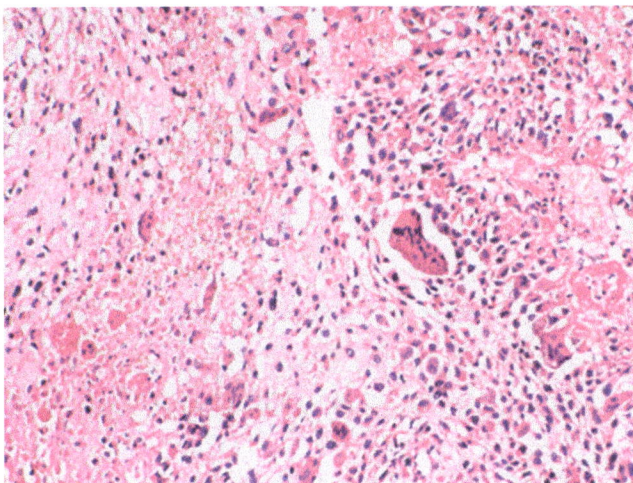

**Figure 10.31:** Epithelioid leiomyosarcoma: Tumor with areas of coagulative necrosis

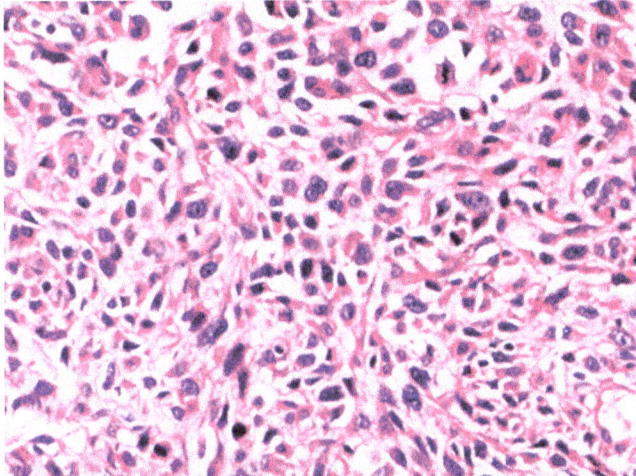

**Figure 10.32:** Epithelioid leiomyosarcoma: Oval cells with central pleomorphic nuclei

show moderate atypia. Mitotic activity is usually more than 5 per 10 HPFs. The criteria of epithelioid leiomyosarcomas include (1) nuclear atypia, (2) mitosis more than 5 per 10 HPF and (3) coagulative necrosis.[19]

## Immunohistochemistry

Leiomyosarcomas are positive for desmin, SMA and HDCA8. The tumor cells are often positive for CD 10. Near about 40% of the cases are positive for ER and PR. In addition, the tumor cells may also show p16 positivity, high MIB 1 and p53. CD 117 positivity has also been seen in leiomyosarcoma cases.

## FIGO Staging

FIGO staging of leiomyosarcoma has been highlighted in Table 10.3.

**Table 10.3:** FIGO staging of leiomyosarcoma[20]

| Stage I | Tumor limited to uterus |
|---|---|
| IA | Tumor 5 cm or less in greatest diameter |
| IB | More than 5 cm in greatest diameter |
| Stage II | Tumor spreads to the pelvis |
| IIA | Adnexal involvement by tumor |
| IIB | Tumor extends to extrauterine pelvic tissue |
| Stage III | Tumor extends abdominal tissues |
| IIIA | One site |
| IIIB | More than one site |
| IIIC | Metastasis to pelvic and/or para-aortic lymph nodes |
| IVA | Tumor invades bladder and/or rectum |
| IVB | Distant metastasis |

## UTERINE SMOOTH MUSCLE TUMORS OF UNCERTAIN MALIGNANT POTENTIAL

Uterine smooth muscle tumors of uncertain malignant potential (STUMP cannot be unequivocally diagnosed as benign or malignant on the basis of known histological criteria. In a large study of uterine smooth muscle tumor Bell et al[21] tried to identify this group of tumor based on the presence or absence of (1) coagulative necrosis, (2) significant nuclear atypia, and (3) mitotic activity. The following combination of histopathological features may be seen in STUMP:

1. Tumor cell necrosis present, no significant nuclear atypia, and mitosis less than 10 per 10 HPFs.
2. Tumor cell necrosis absent, significant nuclear atypia and mitosis less than 10 per 10 HPFs.
3. Tumor cell necrosis absent, no atypia, and mitosis more than 20 per 10 HPFs.

Table 10.4: Criteria of uterine smooth muscle tumors of uncertain malignant potential

| Tumor cell necrosis | Nuclear atypia | Mitosis (per 10 high power fields) |
|---|---|---|
| Present | No | Less than 10 |
| Absent | Yes | Less than 10 |
| Absent | No | More than 20 |
| Present | Yes | Less than 10 |

4. Tumor cell necrosis present, significant nuclear atypia, and mitosis less than 10 per 10 HPFs.

## Clinical Features

The clinical features of STUMP are similar to leiomyosarcomas and leiomyoma. The patient commonly presents as pelvic mass, bleeding per vagina and pain abdomen. The mean age of the patient is 44 years.

## Diagnosis

The histopathologic diagnosis of leiomyosarcomas depends on the any two criteria that include tumor cell necrosis, nuclear atypia and ≥ 10 per 10 HPFs. If the tumor partially fulfils these criteria then the diagnosis of STUMP should be considered (Table 10.4). The role of p53, p16 and Ki 67 has doubtful role in the area of STUMP.

## PERIVASCULAR EPITHELIOID CELL TUMORS

Perivascular epithelioid cell tumors (PECOMA) are developed from the perivascular epithelioid cells.[22] PECOMAs are rare tumors. In the female genital tract the tumor commonly occurs in the fundus of the uterus. The tumors are commonly associated with lymphangioleiomyomatosis and tuberous sclerosis. The patient is adult female in fourth decade and commonly presents with uterine bleeding.

## Gross

Grossly, the tumor may vary from few mm to several cm in diameter. The tumor is mostly single and well-tcircumscribed. However, occasionally the margin of PECOMA may be infiltrative.

## Histopathology

The tumor is composed of nests and sheets of cells. PECOMA is divided morphologically in two groups. In first group the tumor resembles low-grade endometrial stromal sarcoma. The cells show tongue like infiltrative growth. The individual cells are oval to polyhedral with abundant clear, eosinophilic or granular cytoplasm. The cell border is well-defined. Nuclei are round with minimal nuclear pleomorphism and placed centrally. Spindle cells may be intermingled with the epithelioid like cells. The tumor shows diffuse positivity of melanin marker HMB 45 and focal positivity of various smooth muscle markers.

The second group of tumor does not look similar to endometrial stromal tumor. The tumor and myometrial border is usually smooth. The epithelioid cells have less cytoplasm compared to other group. The cytoplasm of the cell is dense and eosinophilic and clear cell is less prominent. The tumor often shows hyalinized stroma. The tumor cells show focal HMB 45 positivity and strongly positive for SMA and desmin (Table 10.5).

Table 10.5: Immunocytochemistry of PECOMA

| Groups | HMB45 | Melan A | SMA | Desmin |
|---|---|---|---|---|
| First group | Strong positive | Weak positive | Weak positive | Weak positive |
| Second group | Weak, focal positive | Negative | Strong positive | Strong positive |

PECOMAs may be benign or malignant in nature. The following features are related with aggressive behavior of PECOMAs: (1) Large size (more than 5 cm in diameter), (2) Highly cellularity, (3) infiltration in the myometrium, (4) Coagulative tumor necrosis, (5) High nuclear grade, (6) More than 1 mitosis per 50 HPFs, and (7) Lymphovascular invasion of the tumor.

## Differential Diagnosis

1. ESS: PECOMA often resembles ESS. However, ESS is always negative for HMB 45.
2. Melanoma: Due to positivity of HMB 45 the tumor may be reported as metastatic melanoma. However, melanomas are negative for SMA and desmin.
3. Epithelioid smooth muscle tumor: PECOMAS are positive for CD 1a immunostaining.[23]

## ADENOMATOID TUMOR

Adenomatoid tumor of the uterus is noted incidentally in the hysterectomy specimen. The tumor may also occur in the fallopian tube and ovary.[24] This tumor is of mesothelial in origin and is distinct from leiomyoma.

## Clinical Features

The median age of patients is 45 years. The patients are asymptomatic and the tumor is detected after hysterectomy.

## Gross

The tumor is usually subserosal in location and the size varies from few mm to 1 cm. The cut surface of the tumor is tan white to yellow and is less well-circumscribed than leiomyoma.

## Histopathology (Figures 10.33 and 10.34)

The tumor is composed of multiple tubules and pseudovascular structures lined by flattened to cuboidal epithelial cells. The cytoplasm of the cells is abundant and pale with centrally placed nucleus having monomorphic bland look. These tubular spaces are surrounded by collagen and smooth muscle fibers. The epithelial cells of the tubular lining may be flattened and may give false appearance of vascular tumor.

## Immunohistochemistry

The epithelial cells of the tumor are positive for calretinin, D2-40 and WT1. The tumor cells are negative for factor VIII related antigen, CD 31, CEA and BER-EP4.

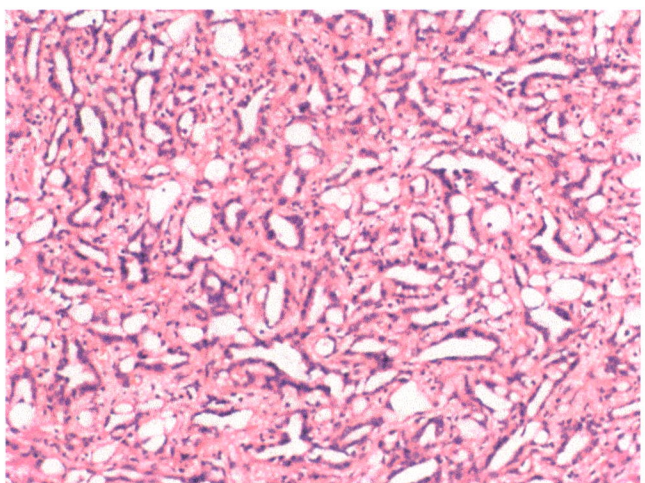

Figure 10.33: Adenomatoid tumor: Multiple tubules and pseudovascular spaces

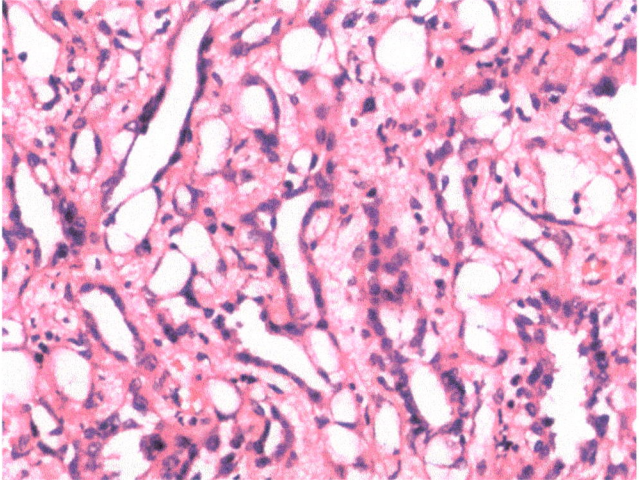

Figure 10.34: Adenomatoid tumor: The pseudovascular spaces are lined by cuboidal to flattened cells

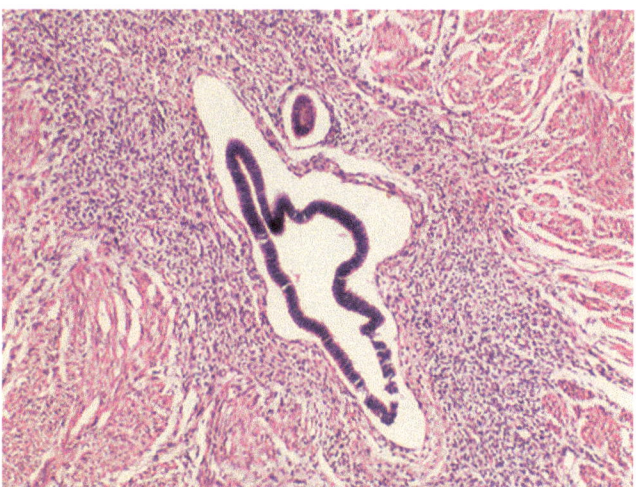

Figure 10.35: Adenomyosis: Both endometrial glands and stroma are present deep in the myometrium

## ADENOMYOSIS AND ADENOMYOMA

Adenomyosis is characterized by ectopic presence of endometrial glands and stroma deep within the myometrium.[25]

## Clinical Features

Adenomyosis is common in uterus and near about 30% of the uterine specimen shows feature of adenomyosis. The mean age of the patient is 46 year. The patient commonly complains of menorrhagia and dysmenorrhea. Near about one-third of the patient remains asymptomatic.

## Gross Features

The uterus in adenomyosis is diffusely enlarged. The cut surface of the uterus shows trabeculated appearance. No well-circumscribed nodule is seen in adenomyosis.

## Microscopy

The exact depth of endometrial glands and stroma in the myometrium is debatable. However, 2.5 mm is considered as the minimum distance between the lower border of the endometrium and the adenomyosis. In practice the glands should be present in the depth of more than the width of 10 X objective of the microscope. There may be single gland to multiple endometrial glands within the myometrium (Figure 10.35). The glands and stroma simulate proliferative endometrium. However, the endometrial glands of the adenomyosis may undergo hormonal changes and may show secretory changes. Adenomyosis may coexist with uterine leiomyoma.

Adenomyoma is a tumor like well-circumscribed mass of adenomyosis. The mass may be recognized on cut surface of the uterus. Adenomyoma is usually present within the myometrium and occasionally may be seen in the submucosal location.

## UTERINE TUMORS RESEMBLING OVARIAN SEX CORD-LIKE ELEMENTS

Uterine tumors resembling ovarian sex cord-like elements (UTROSCT) are uncommon tumors of uterus with distinct histological features. This tumor is characterized by the presence of ovarian sex cord-like elements in more than 10% areas. Previously, this tumor was believed as endometrial stromal tumor but WHO in 2003 classified them as sex cord like tumors.[7] This tumor is divided in two types:

### Type 1 Tumor

Endometrial stromal tumors with the focal presence of epithelial like differentiation that simulates ovarian sex cord stromal tumor-like elements (ESTCLE). Type I tumor shows characteristic JAZF1–JJAZ1 gene fusion.[26]

### Type 2 Tumor

This group of tumor shows mainly sex cord-like elements in the histopathology. This group of tumor is abbreviated commonly as UTROSCT that means uterine tumor resembling ovarian sex cord tumor. This tumor does not show the JAZF1–JJAZ1 gene fusion.[27]

### Clinical Features

The patients are usually in reproductive age period or postmenopausal with mean age of 50 years. The patients commonly complain of abnormal uterine bleeding or uterine enlargement. The patients may be completely asymptomatic.

### Gross

The tumor may be located intramural, subserosal or submucosal. The mass is usually present in the fundus and is well-circumscribed. Occasionally, the tumor shows pushing or infiltrating margin. The tumor may be polypoidal and may project as polyp within the endometrial cavity. The size of the tumor varies from 1–15 cm in diameter and average tumor diameter is 6 cm. On cut section the tumor shows grey white and fleshy in appearance.

### Histogenesis

The tumor cells are positive for both epithelial and myoid markers and the expression of these markers suggest that the tumor is originated from the pleuripotential mesenchymal uterine cells. These stem cells have the capability of differentiate into epithelial, stromal and muscle cells.

### Histopathology

Type 1 tumor: ESTCLE shows endometrial sex cord-like areas along with foci of sex cord stromal elements. The epithelial elements are arranged in trabeculae, anastomosing cords, small tubules and nest-like pattern. The individual epithelial cells of the sex cord elements are small cuboidal in appearance. The cells have scanty eosinophilic cytoplasm and round monomorphic nuclei.

Type 2 tumor: UTROSCT shows 10–40% areas of ovarian sex cord elements. The sex cord elements are present diffusely in all the areas of the tumor. The tumor cells are arranged in small cords of two cells thick, trabeculae, plexiform or as hollow tubules. The tubules are lined by small cuboidal cells with bland nuclei. Mitotic activity is sparse to nil. Occasional glomeruloid-like structures, prominent retiform pattern and cystic changes have also been described. Occasionally, anastomosing cords of cells along with Call-Exner like bodies resembling granulose cell tumor may be noted. Variable amount of hyaline-like or fibrous stroma occupying almost 50% area of the tumor may be seen. The foci of stromal cells with lipid material may be seen.

### Immunohistochemistry

ESTCLE shows variable positivity for CK, actin and desmin. These tumors also show sex cord markers particularly calretinin and also variable expression of inhibin and CD 99. Sex cord elements of UTROSCT tumor show positivity of calretinin, inhibin, CD 99, Melan A, EMA, WT1, CD 56, vimentin and occasionally desmin.[28] The expression of calretinin and inhibin is consistent with sex cord elements of the ovarian tumor.

### Differential Diagnosis

The differential diagnosis of UTROSCT includes endometrioid carcinoma, perivascular epithelioid cell tumor, epithelioid leiomyomas, endometrial stromal tumors and epithelioid leiomyomas.

### Prognosis

Well-circumscribed ESTSCLE tumor behaves as benign tumor. However, tumor with infiltrating margin behaves as endometrial stromal sarcoma of low-grade type. Most of the cases of UTROSCT behave in benign manner and rarely the tumor may show recurrence.[29]

## REFERENCES

1. Kurman RJ, Carcangiu ML, Herrington S, Young RH. WHO classification of tumours of female genital reproductive organs. 4th Edition, International agency for research on Cancer, Lyon; 2014.

2. Tavassoli FA, Norris HJ. Mesenchymal tumors of the uterus. VII. A clinicopathological study of 60 endometrial stromal nodules. Histopathology. 1981;5:1-10.
3. McCluggage WG, Date A, Bharucha H, Toner PG. Endometrial stromal sarcoma with sex cord-like areas and focal rhabdoid differentiation. Histopathology. 1996 Oct;29(4):369-74.
4. Evans HL. Endometrial stromal sarcoma and poorly differentiated endometrial sarcoma. Cancer. 1982;50:2170-82.
5. Cramer SF, Patel A. The frequency of uterine leiomyomas Am J Clin Pathol. 1990;94(4):435-8.
6. Linder D, Gartler SM. Glucose-6-phosphate dehydrogenase mosaicism: utilization as a cell marker in the study of leiomyomas. Science. 1965;150(3692):67-9.
7. Hendrickson MR, Tavassoli FA, Kempson RL, et al. Mesenchymal tumours and related lesions. In: Tavassoli FA, Devilee P (eds). World Health Organization Classification of Tumours: Pathology and Genetics of Tumours of the Breast and Female Genital Organs. Lyon: IARC Press; 2003:236-43.
8. Bell SW, Kempson RL, Hendrickson MR. Problematic uterine smooth muscle neoplasms. A clinicopathologic study of 213 cases. Am J Surg Pathol. 1994;18:535-58.
9. Myles JL, Hart WR. Apoplectic leiomyomas of the uterus. A clinicopathologic study of five distinctive hemorrhagic leiomyomas associated with oral contraceptive usage. AmJ Surg Pathol. 1985; 9:798-805.
10. Kurman RJ, Norris HJ. Mesenchymal tumors of the uterus. VI. Epithelioid smooth muscle tumors including leiomyoblastoma and clear-cell leiomyoma: a clinical and pathologic analysis of 26 cases. Cancer. 1976;37:1853-65.
11. Peocock G, Archer S. Myxoid leiomyosarcoma of the uterus. Am J Obstet Gynecol 1989;160;1515-19.
12. Bardsley V, Cooper P, Peat DS. Massive lymphoid infiltration of uterine leiomyomas associated with GnRH agonist treatment. Histopathology, 1998;33;80-82.
13. Norris HJ, Parmley TH. Mesenchymal tumours of the uterus (V). Intravenous leiomyomatosis: a clinical and pathologic study of 14 cases. Cancer 1975;36;2164-78.
14. Clement PB, Young RH. Diffuse leiomyomatosis of the uterus: a report of four cases. Int. J. Gynecol. Pathol. 1987;6;322-330.
15. Roth LM, Reed RJ, Sternberg WH. Cotyledonoid dissecting leiomyoma of the uterus: the Sternberg tumour. Am. J. Surg. Pathol. 1996;20;1455-61.
16. Kayser K, Zink S, Schneider T, et al. Benign metastasizing leiomyoma of the uterus: documentation of clinical, immunohistochemical and lectin-histochemical data of ten cases. Virchows Arch. 2000;437:284-92.
17. Giuntoli RL, Metzinger DS, et al. Retrospective review of 208 patients with leiomyosarcoma of the uterus: prognostic indicators, surgical management, and adjuvant therapy. Gynecol Oncol. 2003;89(3):460-9.
18. King ME, Dickersin GR, Scully RE. Myxoid leiomyosarcoma of the uterus: a report of six cases. Am J Surg Pathol. 1982;6:589-98.
19. Kurman RJ, Norris HJ. Mesenchymal tumors of the uterus. VI. Epithelioid smooth muscle tumors including leiomyoblastoma and clear cell leiomyoma: a clinical and pathological analysis of 26 cases. Cancer. 1976;37:1853-65.
20. Prat J. FIGO staging for uterine sarcomas. Int J Gynaecol Obstet. 2009;104:177-8.
21. Bell S, Kempson RL, Hendrickson MR. Problematic uterine smooth muscle neoplasms: a clinicopathologic study of 213 cases. Am J Surg Pathol. 1994;18;535-58.
22. Vang R, Kempson R L. Perivascular epithelioid cell tumor ('PEComa') of the uterus: a subset of HMB-45-positive epithelioid mesenchymal neoplasms with an uncertain relationship to pure smooth muscle tumors. Am J Surg Pathol. 2002;26:1-13.
23. FadareO, Liang SX. Epithelioid smooth muscle tumors of the uterus do not express CD1a: a potential immunohistochemical adjunct in their distinction from uterine perivascular epithelioid cell tumors. Ann Diagn Pathol. 2008;12(6):401-05.
24. Nogales F F, Isaac M A, Hardisson D et al. Adenomatoid tumors of the uterus: an analysis of 60 cases. Int J Gynecol Pathol. 2002;21:34-40.
25. Bergeron C, Amant F et al. Pathology and physiopathology of adenomyosis. Best Pract Res Clin Obstet Gynaecol. 2006;20(4):511-21.
26. Hrzenjak A, Moinfar F, Tavassoli FA, Strohmeier B, Kremser ML, Zatloukal K, Denk H. JAZF1/JJAZ1 gene fusion in endometrial stromal sarcomas: molecular analysis by reverse transcriptase-polymerase chain reaction optimized for paraffinembedded tissue. J Mol Diagn 2005;7(3):388-95.
27. Staats PN, Garcia JJ, Dias-Santagata DC, Kuhlmann G, Stubbs H, McCluggage WG, et al. Oliva E.Uterine tumors resembling ovarian sex cord tumors (UTROSCT) lack the JAZF1-JJAZ1 translocation frequently seen in endometrial stromal tumors. Am J Surg Pathol. 2009;33(8):1206-12.
28. Baker RJ, Hildebrandt RH, Rouse EV, et al. Inhibin and CD99 (MIC2) expression in uterine stromal neoplasms with sex-cord-like elements. Hum Pathol. 1999;30:671-9.
29. Clement PB, Scully RE. Uterine tumors with mixed epithelial and mesenchymal elements. Seminars Diagn Pathol. 1988; 5:199-222.

# Anatomy, Histology and Non-neoplastic Lesions of Ovary

## 11

It is necessary to have detailed knowledge of ovarian histology to provide report on non-neoplastic ovarian lesions. In this chapter, the anatomy, histology and salient non neoplastic lesions of ovary have been discussed.

## ANATOMY OF THE OVARY

Ovary is located outside the pelvic cavity in new born. It descends progressively and lies on each side of the uterus in prepubertal period. Adult ovary is suspended in the broad ligament of the uterus by the mesovarium. The adult ovary is dull white in color with a dimension of $4 \times 3 \times 2$ cm. The weight of normal ovary is near about 14 g. The lateral surface of the ovary faces the parietal peritoneum and the medial surface faces the uterus. The upper extremity of the ovary is near the fimbrial end of the fallopian tube and the inferior extremity is directed towards the floor of the pelvis. The anterior margin of the ovary is attached with the mesovarium to the posterior part of the broad ligament. The superior and lateral pole of the ovary is attached with the lateral pelvic wall by the infundibulopelvic ligament. Utero-ovarian ligament attaches medial pole of each ovary to the uterine cornu.

### Blood Supply

*Arterial Supply*

The ovary gets it blood supply from the ovarian artery, a branch of the abdominal aorta. The branches of the ovarian artery enter through the ovarian hilum and proceeds towards the medulla and cortex.

*Venous Supply*

The veins of the ovary form a pampiniform plexus and emerge as single vein that passes through mesovarium and suspensory ligaments. The ovarian vein accompanies ovarian artery. The right and left ovarian vein enters into inferior vena cava and left renal vein respectively.

*Lymphatic Drainage*

Lymphatics of the ovary accompany the ovarian vein and drains into the para-aortic lymph node. Lymphatic drainage may also pass through the pelvic lymph node to para-aortic lymph node.

## HISTOLOGY

The external surface of the ovary is covered by single layer of cuboidal cells. The cells may be completely flattened. A thick connective tissue stroma known as tunica albuginea remains underneath the epithelium.

Ovary is divided into two parts: Cortex and medulla.

### Cortex

The ovarian cortex is composed mainly of specialized stromal cells arranged in small bundles in whorls and storiform pattern. The individual cells are spindle shaped with scanty cytoplasm. With the use of special stain lipid droplets can be demonstrated within the stromal cells. In the reproductive age small cortical nodules may be seen in the cortex. The size of such nodules are always less than 1 cm and thereby readily distinguishable from small fibroma. The cortex also contains primordial follicles, primary follicles, secondary follicles, Graffian follicles, corpus luteum and atretic follicle.

### Medulla

Medulla of the ovary is highly vascular area and is composed of loose fibroblasts, large blood vessels, lymphatics and nerves.

## FOLLICLE AND DERIVATIVES

### Primordial Follicles

Primordial follicles show central primary oocyte surrounded by single layer of flat granulosa cells (Figures 11.1 and 11.2). They are present since birth.

## 158  Essentials of Gynecologic Pathology

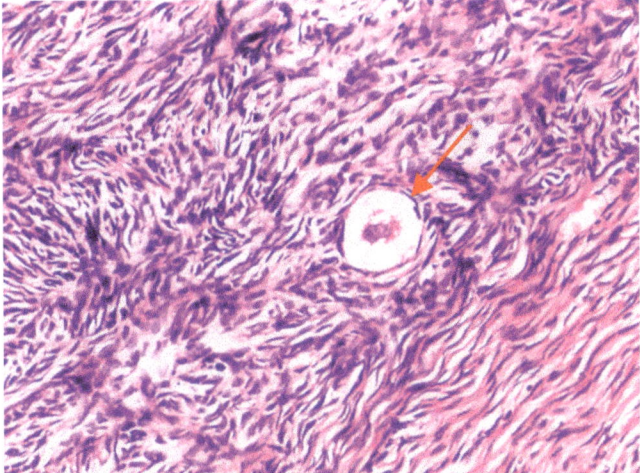

Figure 11.1: Primordial follicle: Central primary oocyte surrounded by single layer of flat granulosa cells

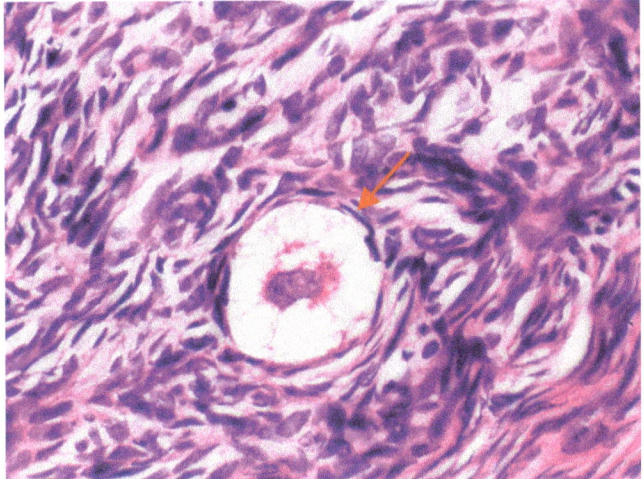

Figure 11.2: Primordial follicle: Higher magnification

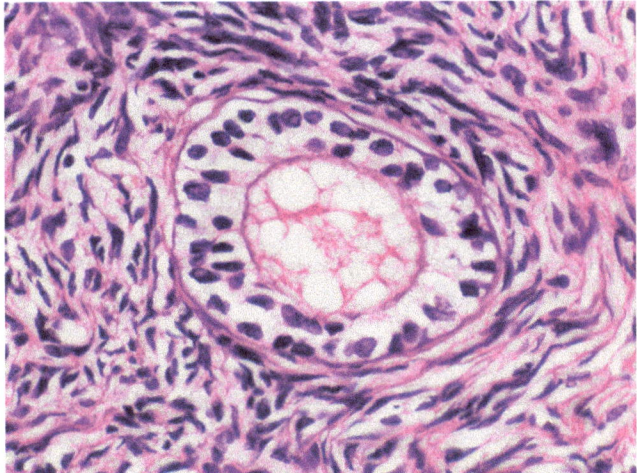

Figure 11.3: Early primary follicle: Two to three layered granulosa cells

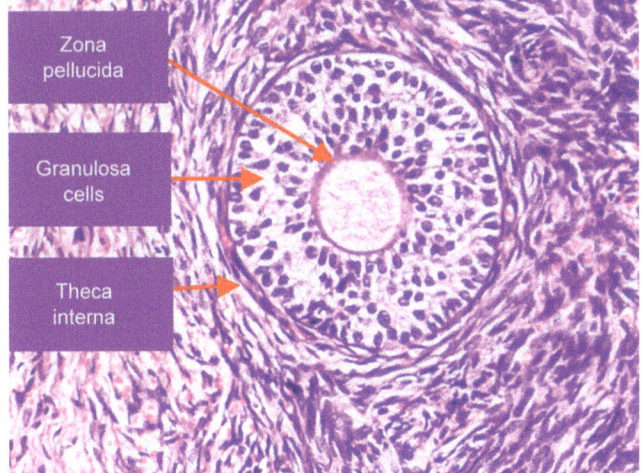

Figure 11.4: Secondary follicle: The granulosa cells proliferate into several layers

## Primary Follicles

Primordial follicle develops to the primary follicle in course of time (Figure 11.3). The following changes occur in the primary follicle:
1. The oocyte enlarges,
2. The surrounding granulosa cells are changed from flat to cuboidal in appearance,
3. Granulosa cells become multilayered, and
4. The oocyte now is surrounded by PAS positive proteoglycan-rich eosinophilic layer of zona pellucida.

## Secondary Follicle

Secondary follicle or preantral follicle is formed from the primary follicle. The following changes are seen in the secondary follicles (Figure 11.4):
1. The proliferation of the granulosa cells continues,
2. External to the granulosa cell layer the adjacent stromal cells differentiate into spindle-shaped theca interna cells.
3. Theca interna layer is surrounded by the thick fibrous stroma known as theca externa.
4. A fluid filled cavity is formed within the granulosa cell and is known as antrum.
5. Antrum is surrounded by multiple layers of granulosa cells. In one corner, the number of granulosa cells is more and these cells surround the oocyte forming cumulus oophorus.

## Tertiary (Graafian) Follicle

In the first week of menstrual cycle, out of many secondary follicles only one tertiary or Graafian follicle develops (Figures 11.5 and 11.6). Following changes occur in tertiary follicle:
1. More amount of fluid is accumulated within the antrum and the follicle becomes bigger in size (near about 2 cm).

Anatomy, Histology and Non-neoplastic Lesions of Ovary

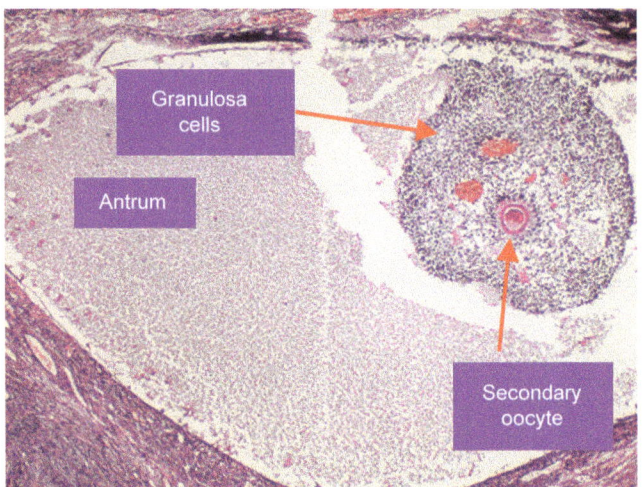

Figure 11.5: Tertiary follicle (Graafian follicle): Antral cavity, granulosa cells and secondary oocyte

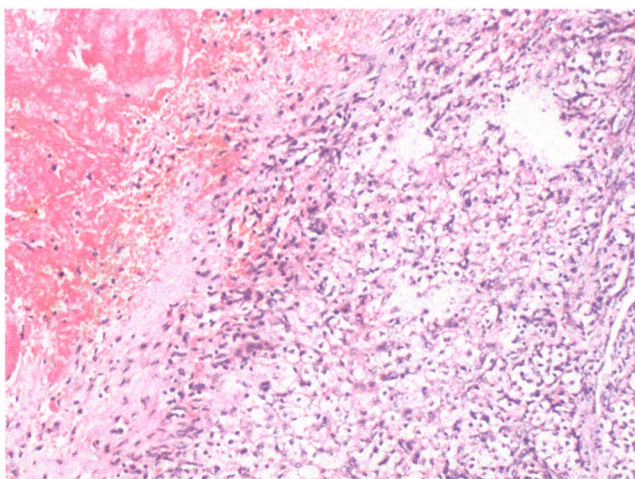

Figure 11.7: Corpus luteum: Corpus luteal cells

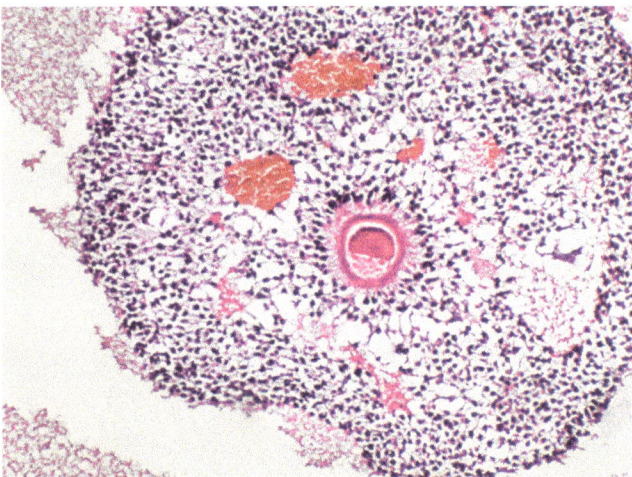

Figure 11.6: Tertiary follicle (Graafian follicle): Higher magnification shows secondary oocyte and corona radiate

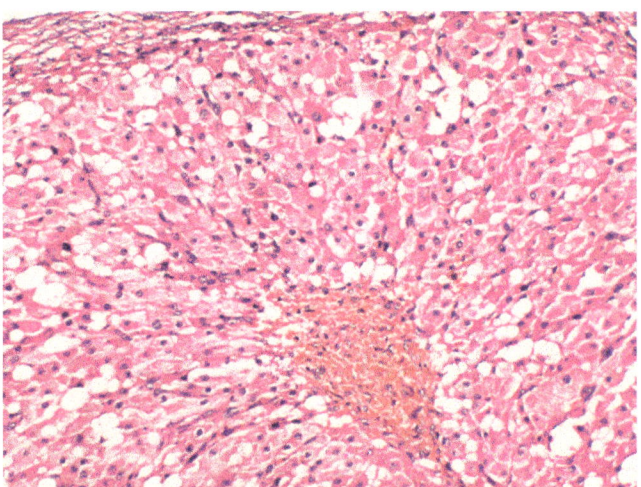

Figure 11.8: Corpus luteum: Cells with abundant granular eosinophilic cytoplasm and centrally placed nuclei

2. The oocyte is detached and freely floats with ring of adjacent granulosa cells known as corona radiate.
3. The primary oocyte completes the first meiotic division, and secondary oocyte (haploid chromosome) and a small first polar body are formed.
4. The secondary oocyte undergoes second meiotic division and is halted in the metaphase till fertilization.
5. The follicle moves to the superficial cortex.
6. The tertiary follicle degenerates when no fertilization occurs.

## Atretic Follicle

The atretic follicle develops when no ovulation occurs. The basement membrane in between the granulosa cells and the theca interna becomes hyalinized. The granulosa cells are slowly replaced by fibrous tissue. The follicular space disappears and the whole follicle becomes slit like atretic channel. The increased number of atretic follicle is mainly seen in polycystic ovarian disease.

## Corpus Luteum

After ovulation, the Graaffian follicle is converted into corpus luteum. Grossly the corpus luteum is yellowish in color with a small cyst in the center.

Microscopically the corpus luteum shows large polygonal granulosa cells containing abundant cytoplasm (Figure 11.7 and 11.8). The cells contain lipid droplets. The nuclei of the cells are round with prominent nucleoli. Small number of theca cells are admixed with the granulosa cells. Granulosa cells secrete progesterone and theca cells secrete estrogen hormone. Both granulosa and theca cells undergo apoptotic changes at the onset of menstruation. After one or two

### Corpus Albicans

This is a scar like structure that develops in the corpus luteum (Figure 11.9). In course of time, the corpus albicans also disappears.

### Corpus Luteum of Pregnancy

In case of pregnancy, the corpus luteum persists and enlarges. The characteristic eosinophilic droplets appear within the cytoplasm of the cells. The corpus luteum regresses after pregnancy.

### Surface Inclusion Cyst

Surface inclusion cyst develops due to invagination of the surface lining of the ovary within the cortex. The lining epithelial cells of the cysts is ciliated columnar and rarely mucinous or endometrioid type (Figures 11.10 and 11.11). The inclusion cysts are microscopical in size. If the diameter of the cyst exceeds more than 1 cm then it is labeled as cystadenoma.

## INFECTIONS OF OVARY

### Non-granulomatous Infection

The majority of the bacterial infections of the ovary are related to pelvic inflammatory diseases and secondary to salpingitis. The common organisms causing salpingo-oophoritis are *Neisseria gonorrhoeae*, *Mycoplasma hominis*, *Chlamydia trachomatis* and various anaerobic organisms. The increased number of sexual partners and use of IUD are the common risk factors of the infection. The patients complain of fever, pelvic pain, urinary symptoms and vaginal bleeding. Pelvic examination shows palpable adnexal mass.

*Pathology*

Grossly both ovary and fallopian tube adhered and the shape of ovary is distorted. Microscopically the lesion shows dense acute inflammation and necrotic debris (Figure 11.12). Occasionally, the tubo-ovarian abscess may rupture and may cause peritonitis or fistula formation with the surrounding structure such as colon or bladder.

### Granulomatous Infections

Genital involvement in tuberculosis occurs in 1% cases of tuberculosis.[1] Ovary is involved in 10% cases of tubal tuberculosis. The patients are usually young and mean age of diagnosis is 30 years.

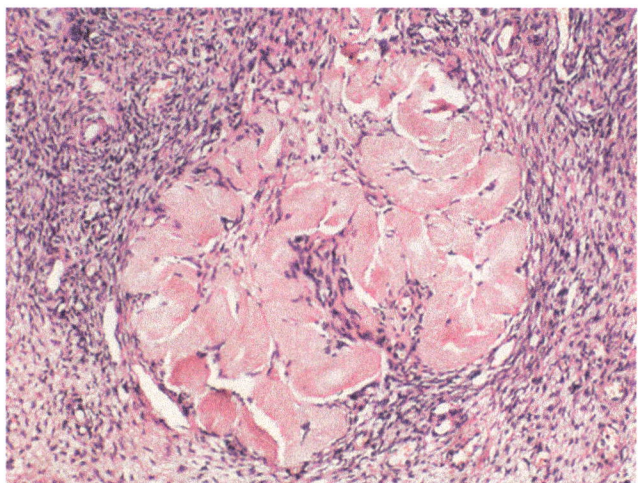

Figure 11.9: Corpus albecans: Deep pink acellular material

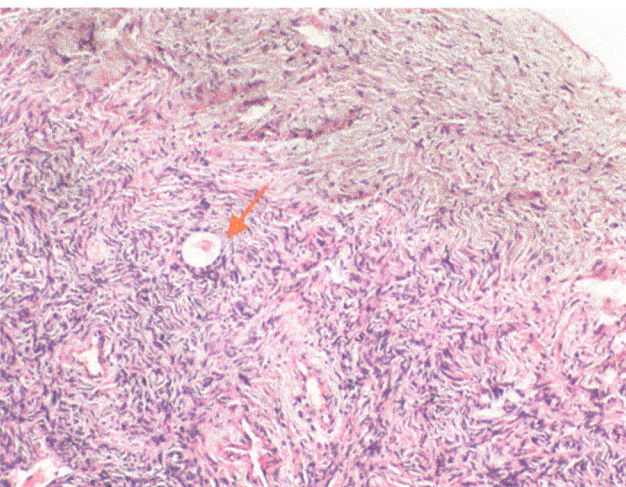

Figure 11.10: Surface inclusion cyst: Small inclusion cyst lined by flattened to cuboidal epithelium

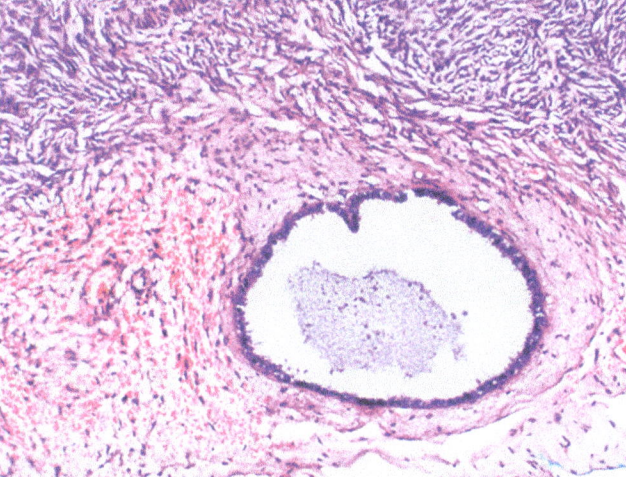

Figure 11.11: Surface inclusion cyst: Higher magnification shows cuboidal lining of the cyst wall

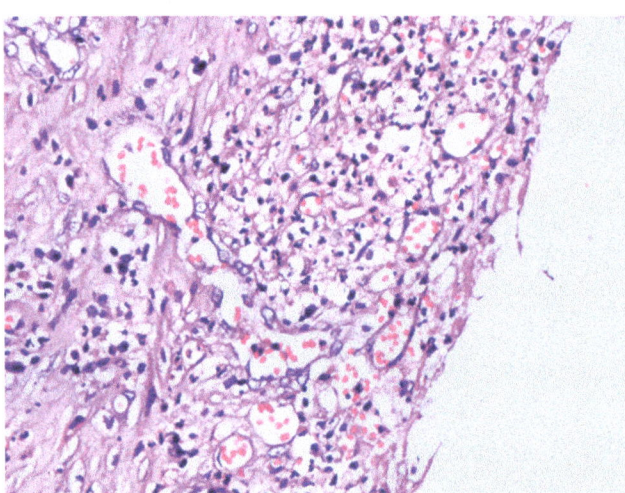

**Figure 11.12:** Inflammation: Predominantly polymorphs and occasional lymphocytes in the stroma of ovary

### Clinical Features

Most of the patients of tuberculosis of ovary are diagnosed at the time of investigation for infertility. Unilateral involvement of ovary along with elevated CA-125 may simulate ovarian cancer.

### Pathology

Histopathology section shows multiple epithelioid cell granulomas with central caseating necrosis. Ziehl-Neelsen stain for acid fast bacilli may show the tubercle bacilli.

## Noninfectious Granulomas

### Foreign Body Granuloma

Foreign body granulomas of the ovary may be due to suture material, starch granules of the gloves or keratin from the ruptured dermoid cyst. Multiple foreign body granulomas of the ovarian surface may mimic ovarian carcinoma.

### Necrobiotic (Palisading) Granulomas

The granulomas are usually multiple with central fibrinoid necrosis encircled by multiple palisading multinucleated histiocytes along with lymphocytes and plasma cells. The histiocytes may contain brown to black carbon pigment.

### Granulomas Secondary to Systemic Diseases

Granulomas may rarely occur in ovary due to sarcoidosis and Crohn's disease. Sarcoidosis of ovary usually affects the para-aortic lymph nodes. The granulomas are compact and non caseating.[2]

### Cortical Granuloma

Cortical granuloma is an incidental finding in the ovary of the postmenopausal patient. The exact etiology of this granuloma is not known. The cortical granuloma typically occurs in the cortex of the ovary as well circumscribed spherical structure composed of multiple multinucleated giant cells, lymphocytes and spindle cells.[3] In course of time, the granuloma becomes fibrotic and remains as spherical round hyaline scar.

## NON-NEOPLASTIC LESIONS OF THE FOLLICULAR AND STROMAL ELEMENTS

### Cysts in Ovary

#### Follicular Cyst

Follicular cyst (FC) is non-neoplastic functional cyst of the ovary with more than 3 cm in diameter.

**Pathogenesis:** The follicular cyst occurs due to abnormalities in the release of gonadotropin releasing hormone from the anterior pituitary and lack of normal LH surge before ovulation. The cyst may also develop due to exogenous gonadotropin administration. The formation of follicle cyst may be part of McCune–Albright syndrome characterized by polyostotic fibrous dysplasia, cutaneous melanin pigmentation, and endocrine organ hyperactivity.

**Clinical features:** The follicular cyst is seen as incidental finding in the women of reproductive age period and mostly around menarche or menopause. The large follicular cysts may present as palpable pelvic mass or with the features of excess estrogen secretion such as amenorrhea, irregular menstrual bleeding, etc. Rarely, the cyst may be large and may rupture in the peritoneum causing hemoperitoneum and acute abdominal pain.

**Gross:** The size of FC varies from 3 cm to 8 cm. The cyst with less than 3 cm is labeled as cystic follicle. The cyst is usually solitary and thin walled with smooth surface. The cyst contains thin watery fluid and blood.

**Histopathology:** The FC is lined by multilayered granulosa cells and theca interna cells (Figures 11.13 and 11.14). The individual cells have abundant cytoplasm with centrally placed round monomorphic nuclei having central nucleoli. The reticulin stain preparation shows condensation of the reticulin fibers around theca interna cells whereas absence of reticulin in the granulosa cells.

**Immunohistochemistry:** The lining cells of the cyst are positive for calretinin and inhibin.

**Differential diagnosis:** (1) Cystic granulosa cell tumor: The tumor is usually large in size and is lined by disorderly arranged granulosa cells. (2) Serous cystadenoma.

**Clinical behavior:** The FC is usually self-regressing and resolves spontaneously within 2 to 3 months. The regression of the cyst can be augmented by the administration of estrogen-progesterone combined preparation. Large cyst may be aspirated by fine needle aspiration cytology under USG guidance. If the cyst persists for several months then there is a chance of neoplasm and the cyst should be excised for histopathological examination,

### Corpus Luteal Cyst

Corpus luteal cyst (CLC) is characterized by cystic corpus luteal structure more than 3 cm diameter. Corpus luteal cyst may occur in corpus luteum of pregnancy or menstruation and morphologically they are indistinguishable.

**Clinical features:** CLC usually occurs in the reproductive age period and is rarely seen in the postmenopausal patient. Most of the cases of CLCs are detected incidentally. The patients occasionally may complain of menstrual disorder and amenorrhea. Rarely the corpus luteal cyst may rupture in the peritoneal cavity causing hemoperitoneum and simulate appendicitis.[4]

**Gross features:** CLC may be of variable in size from 3 cm to several cm (8 to 10 cm) in diameter. The cyst is thick walled with shiny outer surface. Cut surface of the cyst shows yellowish in appearance with central hemorrhagic area.

**Histopathology:** The lining of the cyst shows granulosa cells and theca interna cells which are luteinized (Figures 11.15 and 11.16). These cells have abundant eosinophilic cytoplasm with central round nuclei.

**Clinical behavior:** CLC is spontaneously regressing lesion within a few months.

### Hyperreactio Luteinalis (HL)

HL is a non-neoplastic lesion of ovary that shows bilateral enlargement of ovaries due to multiple luteinized follicular cysts. This lesion is developed mainly due to over secretion of hCG hormone and therefore commonly associated with multiple pregnancies, hydatidiform mole and choriocarcinoma. HL may also occur due to the use of clomiphene.

**Gross:** Both the ovaries are moderately enlarged and are usually more than 5 cm diameter. The surface of the ovary shows multiple variable sized cysts. The cut surface of the lesion shows multiple cysts filled with serosanguinous fluid.

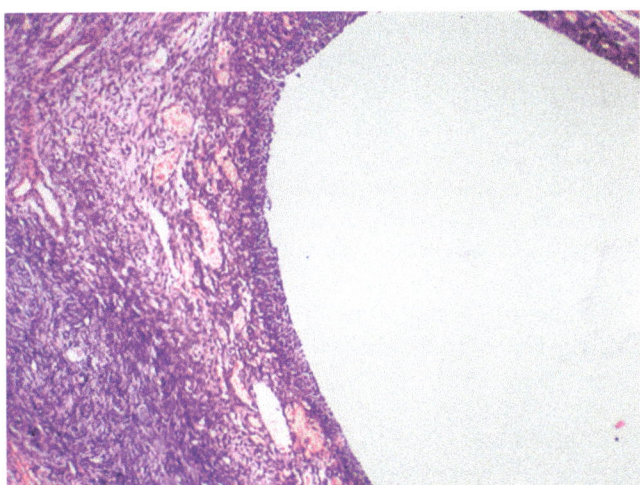

**Figure 11.13:** Follicular cyst: The cyst is more than 3 cm diameter and is lined by multilayered granulosa cells

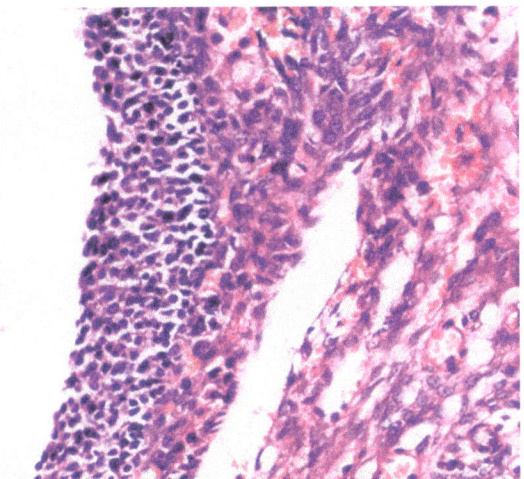

**Figure 11.14:** Follicular cyst: Higher magnification shows multi-layered granulosa cells

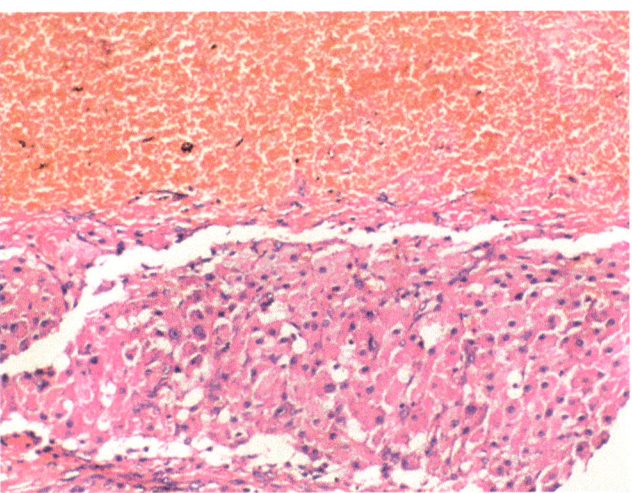

**Figure 11.15:** Corpus luteum: Cystic corpus luteum with large central hemorrhage

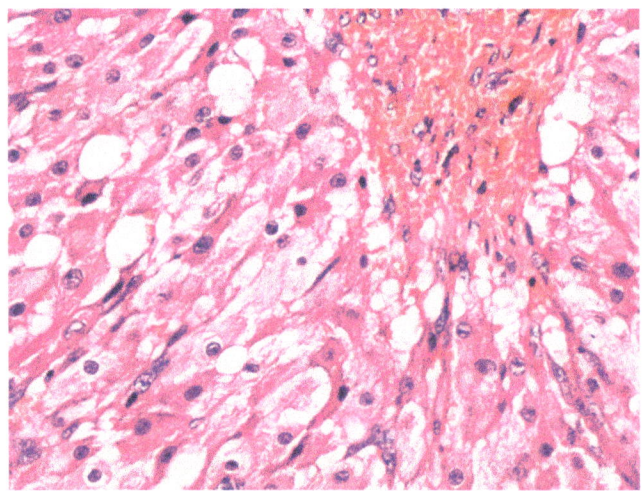

Figure 11.16: Corpus luteal cyst: Higher magnification of the same

**Histopathology:** The lining of the cyst shows several layers of luteinized granulosa and theca cells. The adjacent ovarian stroma is edematous.

**Clinical behavior:** HL regresses within 6 months of the postpartum period. Rarely the cyst may persist for many months. Surgical intervention may be needed in case of torsion or hemorrhage within the HL.

## POLYCYSTIC OVARIAN SYNDROME (PCOS)

Polycystic ovarian syndrome (PCOS) is a disease of unknown etiology and is the commonest endocrine disorder in female of reproductive age. This is one of the commonest cause of infertility. PCOS is characterized by chronic anovulation, enlarged polycystic ovaries and hyperandrogenism (Box 11.1). There is no fixed definition of PCOS. However, Rotterdam ESHRE/ASRM-sponsored PCOS consensus group has proposed any two criteria out of these three for the diagnosis of PCOS: (1) Oligo or anovulation, (2) Clinical or biochemical signs of hyperandrogenism after exclusion of all other etiologies, (3) Polycystic ovaries.[5] Androgenic excess society in 2006 defined PCOS as hyperandrogenism along with either one of the criteria: (1) oligomenorrhea (or amenorrhea), (2) polycystic ovaries by ultrasound examination.[6]

## Clinical Features

PCOS commonly occurs in the women of third to fourth decade of life and 5 to 10% of the female in reproductive age is affected by PCOS. The patient commonly presents with anovulatory bleeding or secondary amenorrhea. The majority of the patients are obese and may often complain of features of hyperandrogenism such as acne, hirsutism, androgenetic alopecia, and acanthosis nigricans (HAIR-AN syndrome means Hyperandrogenic–insulin-resistant-acanthosis syndrome).[7] The patient may also show hyperinsulinemia, insulin resistance, and impaired glucose tolerance test.

### Gross

Both the ovaries are enlarged 3 to 4 times than the normal ovary. The surface of the ovary is smooth with small numerous thin walled translucent areas indicating presence of cysts. The cut section of the ovary shows multiple similar sized cysts usually less than 1 cm diameter. They are arranged in radial manner in the cortex with intervening dense thick fibrous stroma.

### Histopathology[8]

The salient histological features of PCOS are:
1. Dense collagenized tunica of ovary,
2. Cortical and subcortical stroma is thickened three to five times,
3. Number of primordial follicles remain unaltered,
4. Increased number of ripening and subsequent atretic follicles,
5. Numerous cystic follicles that are lined by prominent theca interna cells with marked luteinization. Granulosa cell layers are also present but are less conspicuous,
6. Evidence of prior ovulation such as corpus luteum is commonly absent.

### Pathogenesis

The pathogenesis of PCOS is not clear. However, the major components of pathogenesis of PCOS are: (1) Androgen abnormality (hyperandrogennism), (2) Abnormalities in folliculogenesis, (3) Gonadotropin abnormality (sustained LH level), and (4) Hyperinsulinemia.

1. **Androgen abnormality (hyperandrogenism):** Majority of the patients (80%) of PCOS have high testosterone level in serum and one fourth of the patients have high DHEAS. The excessive androgen hormone is probably derived from the thick theca layer of the cyst.
2. **Gonadotropin abnormality (sustained LH level):** The patients of PCOS secrete excessive LH due to the disorder in hypothalamo-pituitary axis. However FSH level remains normal. Therefore LH: FSH ratio is characteristically high in PCOS cases. The excess LH level stimulates the theca interna cells of the ovarian follicle and subsequently liberation of androstenedione and testosterone. The granulosa cells of the ovarian follicle secrete high level of basal aromatase that converts androgen to estrogen.
3. **Abnormalities in folliculogenesis:** PCOS have excess number of primary, secondary and small antral

**Box 11.1:** Polycystic ovarian syndrome

- Disease of unknown etiology
- The commonest cause of infertility

**Diagnostic criteria:** Any two of
- Oligo or anovulation
- Clinical or biochemical signs of hyperandrogenism after exclusion of all other etiologies
- Polycystic ovaries and exclusion of other causes such as congenital adrenal hyperplasia, androgen-secreting tumors, Cushing's syndrome

**Clinical features:**
- Women in third to fourth decade of life
- Obese
- Anovulatory bleeding or secondary amenorrhea
- Hyperandrogenism : acne, hirsutism, androgenetic alopecia, and acanthosis nigricans
- hyperinsulinemia, insulin resistance, and impaired glucose tolerance test

**Biochemical estimation:** excess serum total testosterone and DHEA sulfate

**USG:** Numerous small cysts less than 1 cm in diameter

**Gross:**
- Both the ovaries are enlarged (3 to 4 times)
- The surface of the ovary: small numerous thin walled translucent areas indicating presence of cysts.
- Cut section: multiple similar sized cysts (<1 cm) arranged in radial manner in the cortex

**Microscopy:**
- Dense collagenized tunica of ovary
- Cortical and subcortical stroma is thickened
- Number of primordial follicles remain unaltered,
- Increased number of ripening and subsequent atretic follicles,
- Numerous cystic follicles that are lined by prominent theca interna cells with marked luteinization
- Evidence of prior ovulation (corpus luteum) commonly absent

**Pathogenesis**
- The exact pathogenesis not clear
- However, the suggested major components of pathogenesis of PCOS are:
  - Androgen abnormality (hyperandrogenism)
  - Abnormalities in folliculogenesis
  - Gonadotropin abnormality (sustained LH level)
  - Hyperinsulinemia
- Differential diagnosis: Cushing's syndrome and congenital adrenal hyperplasia, Primary hypothalamic—pituitary disorders

**Treatment**
- Lifestyle management: Weight loss
- Clomiphene therapy
- Medication: Metformin
- Ovarian puncture by laparoscopic surgery

follicles probably due to excessive androgenic hormone concentration.

4. **Hyperinsulinemia:** PCOS patients show high insulin level and peripheral resistance of insulin. The high concentration of insulin potentiates the action of LH, which is responsible for excess amount of estrogen and progesterone from granulosa cells of ovary.

## Differential Diagnosis

The main differential diagnosis of PCOS include: (1) Cushing's syndrome and congenital adrenal hyperplasia, (2) Primary hypothalamic–pituitary disorders, (3) Ovarian tumors that secrete excessive androgen or estrogen (sex cord stromal tumor and steroid tumors). (4) Autoimmune oophoritis.

## Treatment

1. Lifestyle management: Weight loss is helpful to regain menstruation and getting pregnancy.
2. Clomiphene therapy: The clomiphene therapy is often rewarded with successful ovulation and pregnancy.
3. Medication: Metformin facilitates insulin metabolism and is used to tackle hyperinsulinemia.

4. Ovarian puncture by laparoscopic surgery is also helpful in clomiphene citrate resistant cases.

## STROMAL HYPERPLASIA AND STROMAL HYPERTHECOSIS

Stromal hyperplasia (SH) is characterized by proliferation of the stromal cells in both cortex and medulla of the ovary. Stromal hyperthecosis (HT) is defined as bilateral stromal cell hyperplasia along with luteinized stromal cells. The distinction between SH and HT is mainly based on the basis of the presence of luteinized stromal cells. However, there may be overlapping feature and most likely they are continuous spectrum of the same lesion.

### Clinical Features

The patients of SH are mostly postmenopausal or in the late reproductive life. The cases are usually incidental and are detected in the oophorectomy specimen. Stromal hyperthecosis occurs in the younger patients in the reproductive period. The patient presents with virilization, obesity, hypertension and decreased glucose tolerance test.

### Gross

Macroscopically both the ovaries are 2 to 3 times enlarged and may mimic ovarian neoplasm. The cut section of the ovaries show solid whitish yellow in appearance.

### Histopathology

*SH*

The ovary shows proliferation of stromal cells. The stromal cells may be present in diffusely or in nodular manner. The individual stromal cells are spindle shaped with scanty cytoplasm. The nuclei are oval to elongated with inconspicuous nucleoli.

*HT*

Histopathology of HT shows stromal cell hyperplasia along with multiple small nests or singly arranged luteinized cells. The cells are polygonal with abundant eosinophilic or clear cytoplasm containing lipid material. The nuclei are centrally placed having central small nucleoli. In addition occasionally, atretic follicle, smooth muscle cells and hilus cell hyperplasia may be seen.

### Differential Diagnosis

a. Fibroma: The following features help to distinguish SH from fibroma:
   1. Bilateral ovarian involvement,
   2. Smaller nodules,
   3. Small nodules merge with each other and
   4. Small cells compared to fibroma.
b. Luteinized thecoma: The luteinized thecoma shows grossly tumor like nodular swelling and usually unilateral.
c. Steroid tumor: These tumors are usually unilateral.

### Treatment

SH is diagnosed incidentally and mostly seen postoperatively after oophorectomy. HT is treated with Gonadotropin hormone releasing hormone agonists and oral contraceptive to antagonize androgenic hormone.[9] Bilateral oophorectomy may be needed to treat virilization.

## HILUS CELL HYPERPLASIA

Leydig cell is normally present in the hilum of ovary and is also known as hilus cells. These cells may proliferate to some extent in normal pregnancy due to the effect of hCG. Hilus cell hyperplasia shows nodular or diffuse collection of increased number of Leydig cells in the hilum of ovary. The patients are usually pregnant women. However, the lesion may also be seen in post-menopausal patients. Hilus cell hyperplasia may occur along with other ovarian tumor.

### Pathology

The lesion appears as multiple small yellowish nodule in the hilum of ovary. Microscopical examination shows nodular or diffuse collection of Leydig cells. The individual cells show abundant eosinophilic cytoplasm with centrally placed monomorphic nuclei. The cytoplasm of the cells often contains spherical hyaline globules or crystals of Reinke. The cells may show mild nuclear hyperchromasia and pleomorphism.

## MASSIVE STROMAL EDEMA AND FIBROMATOSIS

Massive ovarian edema shows enlarged single or both ovaries due to accumulation of fluid in the stroma of ovary.[10] Ovarian fibromatosis is also closely related with ovarian edema and shows diffuse proliferation of the fibrous stroma of ovary. They are probably nothing but two ends of the same disease spectrum.[10]

### Clinical Features

The mean age of the patients with massive ovarian edema is 21 years. They usually complain of pain in abdomen or menstrual abnormalities. The patients may also have evidence of hyperandrogenism. Physical examination reveals a pelvic mass with unilateral enlargement of ovary. The torsion of the ovarian pedicle is seen in 50% cases.

The patients of ovarian fibromatosis are also in the reproductive age period with a mean age of 25 years.[10] The patients commonly present with menstrual abnormalities, abdominal pain and occasionally with features of androgen excess.

## Cause

The exact etiology of the massive ovarian edema is unknown. Possibly intermittent torsion of the ovary may cause interference of lymphatic drainage of the ovary. Primary stromal proliferation may also cause edema.

## Pathology

Gross: In ovarian edema, the ovary is enlarged (a range of 5 to 35 cm), soft with shiny whitish and cut surface is gelatinous in appearance. The ovary contains fluid. In case of ovarian fibromatosis the ovary is moderately enlarged (ranges from 8 to 12 cm), whitish with smooth outer surface. The cut section shows solid, firm in appearance.

## Histopathology

In massive edematous ovary, the histopathology section shows massive edema in ovary. The stroma is hypocellular. Foci of ovarian fibromatosis may be noted. Occasionally clusters of lutenized cells may be seen. Normal isolated ovarian follicles are also noted within the edematous ovary.

In fibromatosis, the ovary shows proliferation of spindle cells with intervening dense collagenized material. The cells are organized in small fascicles or storiform pattern. The normal follicles are also seen within the spindle cells. The whole process may be diffuse or may be seen only in cortex giving rise to the cortical fibromatosis.

## Differential Diagnosis

Differential diagnosis of ovarian massive edema includes any neoplasm of ovary with significant edema such as luteinized thecoma, sclerosing stromal tumor, Krukenberg's tumor, and the rare ovarian myxoma. Ovarian fibromatosis may be confused with fibroma of ovary. However identification of the normal ovarian follicle within the spindle cells excludes the possibility of fibroma

## Treatment

Surgical removal of the ovary cures the condition. However, in young patient after confirmation of the non-neoplastic nature of the lesion a conservative approach may be taken.

## PREGNANCY LUTEOMA

Pregnancy luteoma is characterized by the tumor like swelling of the ovary due to proliferation of luteinized cells.[11]

## Clinical Feature

The patients are in the reproductive age period and are asymptomatic. The lesion is detected at the time of caesarian section delivery. One fourth of the patients of pregnancy luteoma cases may also have virilization with high testosterone level.[12]

## Gross

The ovary is enlarged and median diameter is 7 cm (bilateral ovarian enlargement in 33% cases). It is solid and shows single to multiple yellowish well circumscribed nodules.

## Histopathology

The section shows nodular solid collection of cell. The cells are also arranged in loose pseudo acinar like fashion and trabeculae. The individual cells are polygonal having finely vacuolated eosinophilic cytoplasm. The nuclei are central in position with minimal nuclear pleomorphism. Nucleoli are often prominent. Mitotic activities are frequent and 2 to 3 per 10 HPFs may be seen. Foci of interstitial hemorrhage may also be noted.

## Pathogenesis

The exact pathogenesis of luteoma of pregnancy is unknown. Probably it is developed from theca-lutein cells of atretic follicles or the lutenized cells are developed from luteinized follicular granulosa and theca cells.

## Treatment

The luteoma of pregnancy is a benign condition and regresses during puerperal period within 2 weeks after delivery.

## OVARIAN DECIDUA (ECTOPIC DECIDUA)

The presence of ectopic decidual cells is noted in the ovary as early as 9th week of gestation. It is a relatively common feature. The decidual cells may also be present in exogenous progesterone administration, ovarian irradiation and trophoblastic diseases.

## Pathology

Grossly the lesion appears as red nodules on the surface of the ovary. Microscopically the decidual cells are present as confluent sheets in the cortex of ovary.

## OVARIAN TORSION AND INFARCTION

Torsion of ovary is characterized by the twisting of the ovary on its fibrovascular pedicle causing disturbance of the vascular flow and leading to infraction of the ovary. The common causes of ovarian torsion include non-neoplastic cyst, ovarian tumor or ovarian abscess. Ovarian torsion may also be seen in infants and children.

## Clinical Features

The patient commonly complaints of recurrent episodes of acute abdominal pain along with nausea and vomiting. The condition often simulates appendicitis. Physical examination may reveal palpable mass in the lower abdomen.

## Pathology

Grossly the ovary is enlarged and red. The cut surface of the ovary shows areas of hemorrhage and edema. Foci of necrosis may also be seen. Microscopic examination of the ovary shows areas of hemorrhage, edema and foci of necrosis. The ovary should always be examined thoroughly to exclude any evidence of neoplasm.

## OVARIAN FAILURE

### Resistant Ovary Syndrome

This is a rare condition that contributes premature ovarian failure. Resistant ovary syndrome has three important features: (a) High gonadotropin level, (b) Resistant to gonadotropin and (c) Primary or secondary amenorrhea. The exact etiology of this syndrome is unknown. The ovary is grossly normal and histology section of the ovary shows multiple primordial follicles and complete absence of any developing follicle or Graffian follicle.

### Autoimmune Oophoritis

Approximately 10 to 14% of primary ovarian failure cases are associated with autoimmune oophoritis.[13] It is often accompanied with large numbers of autoimmune diseases including Addison's disease, Hashimoto's thyroiditis, myasthenia gravis, rheumatoid arthritis, or systemic lupus erythematosus. Autoantibodies against the steroid forming cells of adrenal gland and ovary suggests the common pathology in these two conditions.[14]

### Clinical Feature

The patients present with irregular menstruation and amenorrhea. They may have prior history of pregnancy and then suddenly develop amenorrhea and infertility.

### Pathology

The ovaries may be normal or enlarged due to multiple follicular cysts. Microscopic examination shows chronic inflammatory cell infiltration in the primary and secondary ovarian follicles. The inflammatory cells are mainly composed of lymphocytes, plasma cells and occasionally eosinophils. Polymorphs are always absent in the infiltrate. Primordial follicles are usually not affected by the inflammation.

### Differential Diagnosis

The differential diagnosis of autoimmune oophoritis includes chronic salpingo-oophoritis. However typical perifollicular inflammation is absent in chronic salpingo-oophoritis.

### Management

Immunosuppression by the corticosteroid therapy.

## CONGENITAL LESIONS OF OVARY

### Absent Ovary

Bilateral ovaries may be absent in gonadal dysgenesis. Both the ovaries may be streak like small. Rarely one ovary may be absent and is detected incidentally during some other operation or in postmortem.

### Lobulated, Accessory, and Supernumerary Ovary

Lobulated ovary is a rare congenital lesion characterized by multiple lobes of ovary separated by fibro-connective tissue. Accessory ovary shows a separate fragment of ovary connected with the main ovary by ligaments. The supernumerary ovary represents completely separate ovary situated away from the main ovary.

### Adrenal Cortical Rest

Adrenal cortical tissue may rarely be present in the wall of the fallopian tube. The presence of such adrenal cortical tissue in the ovary is extremely rare.[15]

## REFERENCES

1. Namavar JB, Parsanezhad ME, Ghane-Shirazi R. Female genital tuberculosis and infertility. Int J Gynaecol Obstet. 2001;75(3):269-72.
2. Parveen AS, Elliott H, Howells R. Sarcoidosis of the ovary. J Obstet Gynaecol. 2004;24(4):465.
3. Hughesdon PE. The endometrial identity of benign stromatosis of the ovary and its relation to other forms of endometriosis. J Pathol. 1976;119:201-9.
4. Hallatt JG, Steele CH Jr, Snyder M. Ruptured corpus luteum with hemoperitoneum: a study of 173 surgical cases. Am J Obstet Gynecol. 1984;149:5-9.
5. Revised 2003 consensus on diagnostic criteria and long-term health risks related to polycystic ovary syndrome. Rotterdam ESHRE/ASRM-Sponsored PCOS Consensus Workshop Group. Fertil Steril. 2004;81(1):19-25.
6. Azziz R, Carmina E, Dewailly D, Diamanti-Kandarakis E, Escobar-Morreale HF, Futterweit W, et al. Positions statement: criteria for defining polycystic ovary syndrome as

a predominantly hyperandrogenic syndrome: an Androgen Excess Society guideline. J Clin Endocrinol Metab. 2006; 91(11):4237-45.
7. Lee AT, Zane LT. Dermatologic manifestations of polycystic ovary syndrome. Am J Clin Dermatol. 2007;8:201-9.
8. Taylor AE .Polycystic ovary syndrome. Endocrinol Metab 1998; Clin N Am. 27:877-902.
9. Steingold KA, Judd HL, Nieberg RK, et al. Treatment of severe androgen excess due to ovarian hyperthecosis with a long-acting gonadotropin-releasing hormone agonist. Am J Obstet Gynecol. 1986;154:1241-48.
10. Young RH, Scully RE. Fibromatosis and massive edema of the ovary, possibly related entities: a report of 14 cases of fibromatosis and 11 cases of massive edema. Int J Gynecol Pathol. 1984;3:153-78.
11. Norris HJ, Taylor HB Nodular theca-lutein hyperplasia of pregnancy (so-called "pregnancy luteoma"). A clinical and pathologic study of 15 cases. Am J Clin Pathol. 1967;47:557-66.
12. Polansky S, dePapp EW, Ogden EB. Virilization associated with bilateral luteomas of pregnancy. Obstet Gynecol. 1975;45(5):516-22.
13. Goswami D, Conway GS. Premature ovarian failure. Hum Reprod Update. 2005;11:391-410.
14. Forges T, Monnier-Barbarino P, Faure GC, Béné MC. Autoimmunity and antigenic targets in ovarian pathology. Hum Reprod Update. 2004;10(2):163-75.
15. Symonds DA, Driscoll SG. An adrenal cortical rest within the fetal ovary: report of a case. Am J Clin Pathol. 1973; 60:562-4.

# Ovarian Tumor: General Aspect

## 12

## CLASSIFICATION OF OVARIAN TUMORS[1]

### Epithelial tumors

Serous tumors
Benign
- Serous cystadenoma
- Serous adenofibroma
- Serous surface papilloma

Borderline
- Serous borderline tumor
  - Atypical proliferative serous tumor
- Serous borderline tumor micropapillary variant/non invasive
- Low-grade serous carcinoma

Malignant
- Low-grade serous carcinoma
- High-grade serous carcinoma

### Mucinous tumors

Benign
- Mucinous cystadenoma
- Mucinous adenofibroma

Borderline
- Mucinous borderline tumous/atypical proliferative mucinous tumor

Malignant
- Mucinous carcinoma

### Endometrioid tumors

Benign
- Endometriotic cyst
- Endometrioid cystadenoma
- Endometrioid adenofibroma

Borderline
- Endometrioid borderline tumor/Atypical proliferative endometrioid tumor

Malignant
- Endometrioid carcinoma

### Clear cell tumors

Benign
- Clear cell cystadenoma
- Clear cell adenofibroma

Borderline
- Clear cell borderline tumor/Atypical proliferative clear cell tumor

Malignant
- Clear cell carcinoma

### Brenner tumor

Benign
- Brenner tumor

Borderline
- Borderline Brenner tumor

Malignant
- Malignant Brenner tumor

### Seromucinous tumors

Benign
- Seromucinous cystadenoma
- Seromucinous cystadenofibroma

Borderline
- Seromucinous borderline tumor

Malignant
- Seromucinous carcinoma

### Undifferentiated carcinoma
### Mesenchymal tumors

- Low-grade endometrioid stromal sarcoma
- High-grade endometrioid stromal sarcoma

### Mixed epithelial and mesenchymal tumors

- Adenosarcoma
- Carcinosarcoma

## Sex cord-stromal tumors

**Pure stromal tumor**
- Fibroma
- Cellular fibroma
- Thecoma
- Luteinized thecoma associated with sclerosing peritonitis
- Fibrosarcoma
- Sclerosing stromal tumor
- Signet-ring stromal tumor
- Microcystic stromal tumor
- Leydig cell tumor
- Steroid cell tumor
- Steroid cell tumor, malignant

**Pure sex cord tumors**
- Adult granulosa cell tumor
- Juvenile granulosa cell tumor
- Sertoli cell tumor
- Sex cord tumor with annular tubules

**Mixed sex cord-stromal tumors**

Sertoli-Leydig cell tumor
- Well-differentiated
- Moderately differentiated
  - With heterologous elements
- Poorly differentiated
  - With heterologous elements
- Retiform
  - With heterologous elements

Sex cord stromal tumors, NOS

## Germ cell tumors

Dysgerminoma
Yolk sac tumors
Embryonal carcinoma
Non-gestational choriocarcinoma
Mature teratoma
Immature teratoma
Mixed germ cell tumor

## Monodermal teratoma and somatic type tumors developed from a dermoid cyst

Struma ovary, benign
Struma ovary, malignant
Carcinoid
- Strumal carcinoid
- Mucinous carcinoid

Neuroectodermal tumors
Sebaceous tumors
- Sebaceous adenoma
- Sebaceous carcinoma

Carcinomas
- Squamous cell carcinoma
- Others

## Germ cell sex cord-stromal tumor

Gonadoblastoma
Mixed germ cell-sex cord stromal tumor, unclassified

## Miscellaneous tumors

Tumors of rete overii
- Adenoma of rete overii
- Adenocarcinoma of rete overii
- Wolffian tumors
- Small cell carcinoma

## Mesothelial tumors

Adenomatoid tumor
Mesothelioma

## Soft tissue tumors

## Tumor-like lesions

- Follicle cyst
- Corpus luteal cyst
- Hyperreactio luteinalis
- Pregnancy luteoma
- Stromal hyperplasia
- Fibromatosis
- Massive edema
- Leydig cell hyperplasia

## Lymphoid and myeloid tumors

Ovarian cancer is the sixth most common cancer in the world and it involves approximately 204,000 women in each year resulting 125,000 lives per year.[2] This tumor represents 4% of cancer in USA and approximately 25% of cancer in the female genital tract.[3] Approximately 2/3rd of the ovarian tumor occurs in the women of reproductive age period and 90% of the tumor is seen in 20–65 year period (Box 12.1). Only 5% of ovarian tumor occurs in children. Majority of the ovarian tumor is benign (80%) and diagnosed under the

---

**Box 12.1:** Ovarian tumor

- Sixth most common cancer in the world
- Ranks 4th in cancer related death in western world
- 90% tumor in 20–60 year
- 5% in children
- 80% benign tumor
- 20% malignant and borderline

age of 40 years. Approximately 90% of the malignant and borderline tumors are seen above the age of 40 year.

## CLASSIFICATION

World Health Organization (WHO) classified ovarian tumor mainly based on the histogenesis of the ovary.[1] There are predominantly three components from which ovarian tumor develops:
a. Surface epithelial cells,
b. Specialized ovarian stromal cells and
c. Germ cell.
   In addition, the cancer may also be seen due to metastasis and a subset of ovarian tumor may be difficult to classify.
Each category of the ovarian tumor has several subtypes. Tumor may be composed of more than one subtype and are known as mixed tumor. The tumor subtypes consist of less than 10% of the total tumor, is ignored for classification purpose.

1. **Surface epithelial cells:** These tumors bear the main bulk of ovarian tumor and they consist of 60% of all ovarian tumors. There are five major subtypes of epithelial tumors according to the predominant cell type: serous, mucinous, endometrioid, clear, and transitional. Each type of surface epithelial tumor is again divided into three broad categories: benign, borderline and malignant.
2. **Sex cord–stromal tumor:** Sex cord–stromal tumor consists of 6% of all ovarian neoplasms. They are derived from the sex cord and specialized stromal component of the gonads. The sex cords of the embryo develop into sertoli cells and granulosa cells in testis and ovary respectively. The stroma develops into Leydig cells of the testis in male and theca cells of the ovary in female. Therefore, the sex cord-stromal cells may be originated from granulosa cells, theca cell, stromal cells, Leydig cells and sertoli cells.
3. **Germ cell tumor:** Germ cell tumor represents 25–30% of all ovarian neoplasms and consist of only 7% of all malignant ovarian tumors. Germ cell tumor is derived from the germ cells of the ovary and as the germ cells are totipotential so a large variety of germ cell tumors may be seen.
4. **Unclassified tumor:** Occasional ovarian tumors are difficult to classify such as tumor of Wolffian origin.
5. **Secondary tumor:** Several tumors may metastasize to ovary from different areas of the body.

## CLINICAL FEATURES

The most of the patients are asymptomatic in early stage and becomes symptomatic when the cancer spreads outside the pelvis. The patients commonly presents with abdominal fullness, early satiety, and abdominal pain. The patients may also have gastrointestinal symptoms such as constipation and diarrhea, and urinary symptoms. Functional ovarian tumor may have excessive vaginal bleeding or virilism. Occasional patients may develop symptoms due to ovarian torsion and rupture. Pelvic examination may show mass in the pelvis due to enlarged ovary. Patients may also initially present with signs of distant metastasis such as pleural effusion, or metastasis of inguinal or axillary lymph nodes. A small subset of patients may present with para-neoplastic syndromes such as hypercalcemia, cerebellar degeneration, chronic intra-vascular coagulation known as Trousseau's syndrome and seborrheic keratosis.

## ETIOLOGY AND RISK FACTORS

a. **Age:** The risk of ovarian cancer increases steadily from lower to higher age group women.
b. **Nulliparity:** It is associated with higher risk of ovarian cancer.
c. **Early menarche and late menopause:** Early menarche and late menopause are significantly associated with higher risk of ovarian cancer. Pregnancy is protective of ovarian endometrioid and clear cell carcinoma.
d. **Oral contraceptive:** Use of oral contraceptive decreases the risk of ovarian cancer.
e. **Ovulation:** Ovulation causes rupture of the surface epithelium of the ovary. This rupture area is healed by the proliferation of the epithelium. Therefore, repeated ovulation stimulates active proliferation of the epithelium and predisposes the epithelial cells to malignant transformation.
f. **Heredity:** Family history of ovarian cancer is a major risk factors of ovarian cancer. In hereditary breast-ovarian cancer syndrome there is an autosomal dominant pattern of inheritance and the patient is predisposed to ovarian and breast cancer. Lynch syndrome II is also another familial ovarian cancer syndrome characterized by autosomal dominant pattern of inheritance and associated with ovarian cancer, endometrial cancer and colonic cancer without any polyposis.
g. **Other risk factors:** The other potential risk factors include obesity, smoking, high starch diet, sedentary life style, delayed age of first child birth, perineal talc use, etc.

## PATHOGENESIS AND PRECURSOR LESIONS OF OVARIAN CARCINOMA WITH MOLECULAR PATHOLOGY

The large amount of evidences now suggest that ovarian carcinoma is not a single disease entity. It is actually a collection of varied entities with variable pathogenesis, molecular alterations and clinical course. Based on morphology and molecular pathology, two types of ovarian epithelial cancer has been proposed: Type I and II tumors.[4]

## Type I Ovarian Tumor

Type I tumor includes low-grade serous carcinoma, low-grade endometrioid, clear cell carcinoma, mucinous carcinoma and Brenner tumors. The characteristics of type I tumors are: (1) Indolent course, (2) Tumors typically confined to ovary at the time of presentation (stage I), (3) Associated with specific mutations that include KRAS, BRAF, ERBB2, CTNB1, PTEN, PIK3CA, ARID1A and PPPR1A and (4) Lack p53 mutation.

## Type II Ovarian Tumor

Type II tumor comprises of high-grade serous carcinoma, high grade endometrioid carcinoma, undifferentiated carcinoma and malignant mixed mesodermal tumors. They bear the following features: (1) Aggressive in behavior, (2) Present in advanced stage, (3) High frequency of p53 mutation, (4) Rarely show mutations that present in type I tumors.

## Fallopian Tube as Source of Epithelial Ovarian Carcinoma

Recent studies indicate that the fallopian tube epithelium is the source of development of the ovarian serous carcinoma.[5] In the late 1990s, salpingo-oophorectomy was carried out as a prophylactic measure in high-risk ovarian cancer cases that showed germ line mutation of BRCA1 and BRCA 2. Instead of getting ovarian carcinoma, occult invasive and non-invasive fallopian tube carcinoma were discovered in such cases.[5] The tubal carcinoma was related more with serous carcinoma and was labeled as "serous tubal intraepithelial carcinoma" (STIC) (Box 12.2). The evidences that suggest the tubal origin of ovarian serous carcinoma are:

1. Serial sections of the fallopian tube showed that STIC was associated with 61% of high-grade serous carcinoma (HGSC).[6]
2. STIC is mainly associated with serous ovarian carcinoma and are not related with other histological types of ovarian carcinoma.
3. Laser capture microdissection studies showed identical TP53 mutation of STIC and HGSC.[7] This evidence strongly indicates the clonal origin of both the lesions. Gene expression profile of HGSC also showed similar profile as that of fallopian tube epithelium.[8]
4. The remote possibility of STIC as metastasis from the HGSC is excluded by the evidence of shortened telomerase of the epithelial cells of STIC compared with ovarian carcinoma.[9] If STIC develops from the metastatic ovarian carcinoma then the cells should have same length of telomere as that of ovarian carcinoma cells.
5. The fimbrial end of the fallopian tube is usually affected by STIC and this area is the close to the ovarian surface to have implantation of tumor cells.

**Box 12.2:** Serous tubal intraepithelial carcinoma (STIC)

**Characteristic histological features:**
- Epithelial stratification and loss of polarity
- Cellular changes:
  - Loss of cilia
  - Nuclear moulding
  - Pleomorphism
  - High nucleocytoplasmic ratio
  - Hyperchromasia
  - Irregular chromatin pattern
  - High mitotic activity
- P53 immunostaining: Strong diffusely positive p53 immunostain
  - Ki-67 index: High Ki-67 index (more than 70%)

**STIC as a source of ovarian serous carcinoma**
- STIC is associated with 61% of high-grade serous carcinoma (HGSC)
- Identical TP53 mutation of STIC and HGSC in laser capture micro dissection
- Identical gene expression profile in tubal and ovarian carcinomas
- STIC is located in the fimbrial end of the fallopian tube close to the ovarian surface to have implantation of tumor cells in ovary.

No STIC lesion is noted in nearly 40% cases of HGSC. It may be possible that STIC lesion is obscured due to extensive growth of HGSC. Alternately, it was postulated that in such cases HGSC is developed from cortical inclusion cyst (CIC) derived from the tubal epithelium.

## STIC Lesion

The characteristic histological features of STIC include (Figures 12.1 to 12.3):

1. **Epithelial stratification and loss of polarity**: The lining epithelium of the fallopian tube shows stratification and loss of cellular polarity. Exfoliated cells may be noted in the lumen of the fallopian tube. Intraepithelial fracture lines may appear.
2. **Cellular changes**: The epithelial cells are composed of both ciliated and secreted cells. The cells show following changes: (a) Loss of cilia, (b) Nuclear moulding, (c) pleomorphism, (d) High nucleocytoplasmic ratio, (e) Hyperchromasia, (f) Irregular chromatin pattern, (g) High mitotic activity.
3. **P53 immunostaining**: STIC usually shows strong diffusely positive p53 immunostain (Figures 12.4 and 12.5). A small subset of cases may be completely negative for p53. This is due to deletion of p53 gene and therefore no expression of p53 protein at all. Therefore p53 is considered abnormal if: (a) More than 75% of

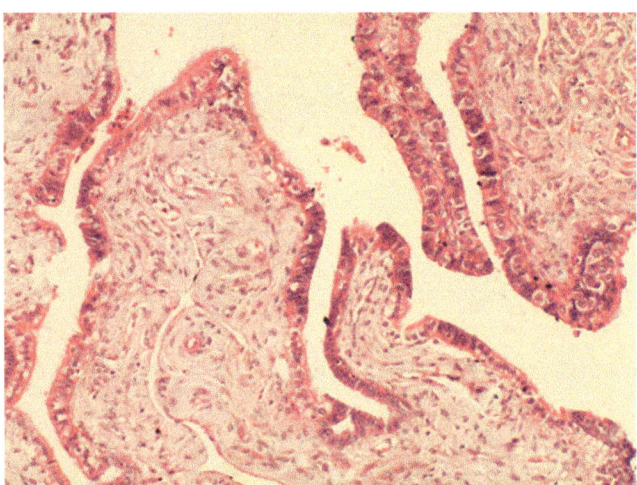

**Figure 12.1:** Serous tubal intraepithelial carcinoma: Nuclear atypia and focal multilayered epithelium

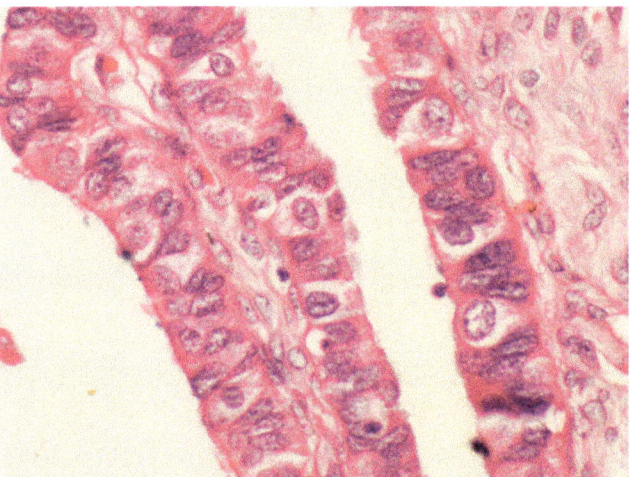

**Figure 12.2:** Serous tubal intraepithelial carcinoma: The cells show loss of cilia and nuclear pleomorphism

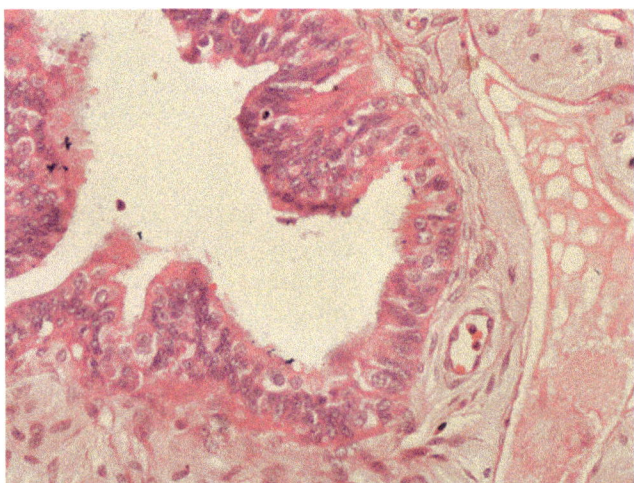

**Figure 12.3:** Serous tubal intraepithelial carcinoma: Mutilayered epithelial lining cells of the fallopian tube

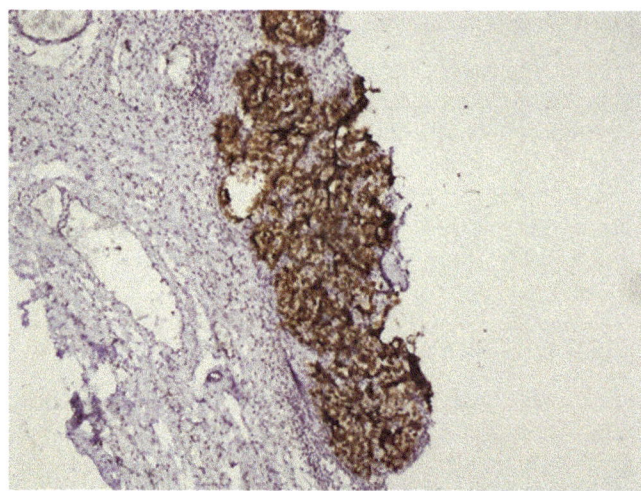

**Figure 12.4:** Serous tubal intraepithelial carcinoma: Strong p53 positivity of the epithelial cells

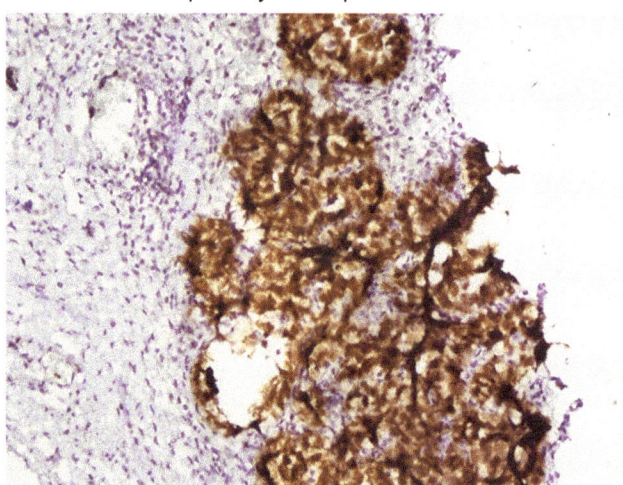

**Figure 12.5:** Serous tubal intraepithelial carcinoma: Higher magnification shows strong nuclear positivity

cells display moderate to strong positivity, (b) Complete absence of expression.

4. Ki-67 index: STIC usually shows high Ki-67 index (more than 70%). More than 10% Ki-67 index is considered as significant and this is the cut off value. This cut-off value is based on the facts that the normal fallopian tube epithelium has 1–3% Ki-67 index, whereas STIC usually shows 36–72% value.[10]

## Secretory Cell Outgrowths

Secretory cell outgrowth (SCOUT) is the recently described entity in the fallopian tube characterized by the discrete linear outgrowth of secretory cells of the fallopian tube epithelium (Box 12.3). The proliferating secretory cells of SCOUT do not show any significant atypia and preserve the pseudostratification of the lining cells. The cells show low Ki-67 index. SCOUT shows altered expression of PTEN and

**Box 12.3: Secretory cell outgrowth**

- Discrete linear outgrowth of secretory cells of the fallopian tube epithelium
- Minimal atypia
- Pseudostratification
- Altered expression of PTEN and PAX2
- Usually negative for p53
- p53 positive SCOUT known as p53 signature

PAX2.[11] SCOUTs usually do not exhibit p53 expression. However certain subset of SCOUTs may be associated with p53 mutation which is also known as p53 signature.

## p53 Signature

p53 signature actually represents p53 positive SCOUT. This lesion is more frequently present in the distal part of the fallopian tube. p53 signature may coexist with STIC lesion and may be noted in continuity or separated by the normal lining mucosa. It is characterized by linear strongly p53 positivity in at least consecutive 12 secretory cell nuclei of the fallopian tube epithelium[12] (Box 12.4). p53 signature shows low Ki-67 index (less than 10%). This lesion exhibits H2AX positivity and thereby shows indirect evidence of DNA damage.[12] p53 signature is noted in the fallopian tube irrespective of BRCA1 positivity in women. The lesion is morphologically indistinguishable from the benign normal epithelial mucosa and is detected only by immunohistochemistry for p53.

**Box 12.4: p53 signature**

- Morphologically normal epithelium
- Often associated with STIC
- Linear strongly p53 positivity in at least consecutive 12 secretory cell nuclei of the fallopian tube epithelium
- γ-H2AX positive
- Low Ki-67 index (<10%)

## Sectioning and Extensive Examination of the Fimbria

Sectioning and extensive examination of the fimbria (SEE-FIM protocol) is needed to detect STIC or SCOUT lesion. The protocol includes (Figure 12.6): (1) The entire tube should be in fixed in formalin for at least 4 hour to preserve the mucosa. (2) The distal 2 cm part of the fimbrial end of the tube is transected. (3) Longitudinal sectioning is done and four pieces are made. (4) Rest of the tube is cut transversely into several pieces at 2 mm interval. (5) These segments and the four longitudinal sections are submitted for histopathological examination.

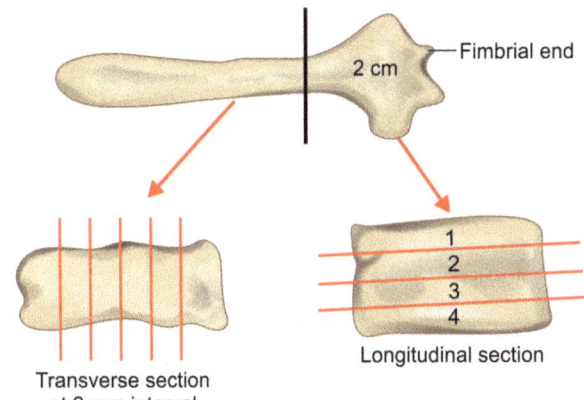

Figure 12.6: Schematic diagram of sectioning and extensive examination of the fimbria (SEE-FIM protocol)

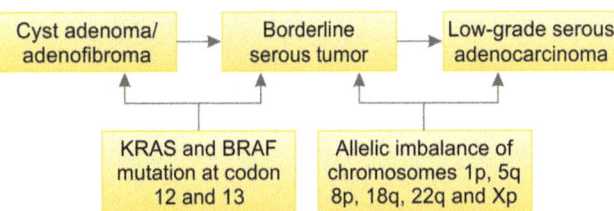

Figure 12.7: Schematic diagram of pathogenesis of ovarian low grade serous carcinoma

## Pathogenesis of Low-Grade Serous Carcinoma

Pathogenesis of ovarian low-grade serous carcinoma (LGSC) is distinctly different and independent from the HGSC. LGSC develops in a stepwise process from cystadenoma/adenofibroma to borderline serous tumor (BST) to carcinoma (Figure 12.7). It is also suggested that micropapillary serous carcinoma (MPSC) may be an intermediate step between BST and LGSC. The evidences of stepwise tumor progression are: (1) KRAS mutation at codon 12 and 13 are noted both in LGSC (35%) and BST (33%).[13] BRAF mutations at codon 599 are seen in both low-grade serous carcinomas (30%) and BST (28%). No such BRAF and KRAS mutation are noted in HGSC.[14] (2) Laser capture microdissection showed similar KRAS and BRAF mutation in BST and neighboring cystadenoma.[15]

### Molecular Pathway

Mutations of KRAS, BRAF and ERBB2 genes cause derangement of the mitogen activated protein kinase (MAPK) pathway. The MAPK pathway is related with cell cycle control and cell survival. Derangement of MAPK pathway due to mutation of the genes may be responsible for tumor initiation and progression. KRAS and BRAF mutation are demonstrated by laser capture microdissection in the serous cyst adenoma and BST element. This finding indicates that the mutation occurs in the early part of carcinogenesis.[15] The pattern of chromosomal change in MPSC is unique from the usual BST and this indicates that LGSC arises stepwise from BST to MPSC. Global epigenetic methylation profile have shown that the methylation profile of LGSC resembles more to BST and serous adenoma compared to HGSC.[16]

### High-Grade Serous Carcinoma (HGSC)

HGSC shows TP53 mutation in 95% of cases[17] and rarely shows KRAS and BRAF mutation. Near about 50% of sporadic HGSC shows inactivation of BRCA due to mutation or by epigenetic change by hypermethylation of the BRCA 1 promoter sequence.

### Clear Cell and Endometrioid Carcinoma

There is strong connection of endometriosis with endometrioid carcinoma and clear cell carcinoma. Near about 50 % of clear cell carcinoma and 30–40% of endometrioid carcinoma and are associated with endometriosis of ovary.[18] It is presumed that both endometrioid and clear cell carcinoma develop from the endometrial tissue implanted in the ovary. The ectopic endometrial tissue shows molecular abnormalities that help the endometrial cells to survive in the extrauterine sites. This activates the initiation of the oncogenic process.[18] The molecular pathology demonstrated similar loss of heterozygosis (LOH) in endometriosis and endometriosis associated cancer.[19] Mutation of PTEN, PIK3CA and CTNNB1 have been demonstrated in endometrioid carcinoma.[20] In clear cell carcinoma mutation of PIK3CA and ARID1A (a tumor-suppressor gene) have been noted.[21]

### Mucinous Tumor

Contrary to the earlier literature, the primary mucinous ovarian carcinomas (particularly gastrointestinal type) are the least common epithelial carcinoma of ovary and represents only 3% of ovarian carcinomas. The probable origins of mucinous tumors of ovary are:
1. **Transitional epithelium: Mucinous tumor** is often associated with Brenner tumor and it is possible that the tumor develops from mucinous metaplasia of the transitional epithelium.
2. **A subset of mucinous tumor** is associated with the mature cystic teratoma of ovary and possibly mucinous tumor develops from the mature teratoma.
3. **Mucinous metaplasia of the surface epithelial inclusion cysts** may be possible. Laser capture microdissection shows similar KRAS mutation in mucinous carcinoma and neighboring benign and borderline areas of mucinous neoplasm suggesting the stepwise progression of mucinous neoplasm and early mutational change in this adenoma–carcinoma sequence.[22]

### Transitional Cell Carcinoma and Malignant Brenner Tumor

Immunophenotype expression of transitional cell carcinoma and Brenner tumor is different indicating divergent pathogenesis.[23] Malignant Brenner tumor expresses uroplakin and thrombomodulin that resembles transitional cell differentiation. Whereas transitional cell carcinomas are positive for WT-1 and negative for uroplakin and thrombomodulin. These changes are similar to HGSC. Transitional cell carcinomas show TP53 and p16 mutation like HGSC.[24] It is suggested that Brenner tumor develops from the Walthard cell rests (transitional epithelial nest) that are present in the tubal-mesothelial junction. However, the cells of the Walthard cell rests do not show uroplakin and these cells are extraovarian. Therefore, there is considerable doubt about the origin of Brenner tumor from Walthard cell rest.

## DIAGNOSIS AND SCREENING

Major goal of ovarian cancer screening should be to pick up the early stage cancer (stage 1). Unfortunately no suitable test is available to detect early ovarian cancer.

### Pelvic Examination

Majority of the palpable ovarian tumors present in advanced stage. Therefore, physical examination may not be helpful to detect such cases.

### Ultrasound

Transvaginal ultrasound (TU) examination may be helpful to detect type I ovarian tumors. Most of the malignancies detected by TU are serous cystadenocarcinomas. It is difficult to detect HGSC in early stage by TU as majority of the cases present in advanced stage and as the tumor rapidly progresses so the screening by TU may not be feasible.

### Biomarker Screening

Near about 80% epithelial ovarian carcinoma show raised CA-125 level in advanced stage. Due to its low sensitivity and specificity, CA-125 is not considered as a good marker in ovarian cancer screening in general population. Mok et al. noted that combination of Prostacin and CA-125 produced a 92% and 94% sensitivity and specificity respectively for detecting ovarian cancer.[25] Visintin et al suggested combination of six biomarkers that include leptin, prolactin, osteopontin, insulin-like growth factor II, macrophage inhibitory factor, and CA-125 for the screening of ovarian cancer.[26] The combined biomarkers improved the sensitivity as 95.3% and specificity 99.4% in cancer detection.

## Symptoms and Signs

Ovarian tumors usually present symptoms in advanced stage. Andersen MR, et al. combined a symptomatic index (based on pain abdomen, bloating, increased abdominal size, difficulty eating, or feeling full quickly) and CA-125 level.[27] This composite index identified more than 80% of women with early stage disease.

## STAGING

Ovarian tumor staging is one of the most important prognostic factors. The Federation of Gynecologists and Obstetricians (FIGO) staging system is the most popular and widely used in the staging of ovarian cancer[28] (Box 12.5). For successful implementation of FIGO staging, the surgeon should properly examine the surface of the peritoneum, the undersurface of liver and any enlargement of pelvic or para-aortic lymph nodes. The FIGO staging is surgico-pathological staging system and both the surgical information and complete histopathological findings are needed for the exact staging.

**Box 12.5:** FIGO staging of ovarian cancer

**Stage I:** Tumor confined to the ovaries: one or both ovaries

**Stage IA:** Tumor limited to one ovary; no malignant cells in ascites or peritoneal washing. No tumor on the outer surface of ovary; capsule preserved

**Stage IB:** Tumor limited to both ovaries; no ascites. No tumor on the outer surface of ovary; capsules preserved

**Stage IC:** Tumor confined to one or both ovaries with capsule ruptured, or tumor on the surface of ovary or with ascites containing malignant cells, or with positive peritoneal washings

**Stage II:** Tumor containing one or both ovaries with pelvic extension

**Stage IIA:** Spread and/or metastases to the uterus and/or tubes and absence of malignant cells in ascitic fluid, or peritoneal washings

**Stage IIB:** Spread to other pelvic tissues and no malignant cells in ascities, or peritoneal washings

**Stage IIC:** Tumor either stage IIA or IIB with malignant cells in ascitic fluid, or peritoneal washings

**Stage III:** Tumor involves one or both ovaries with implants in the peritoneum outside the pelvis and/or metastatic retroperitoneal or inguinal nodes.

**Stage IIIA:** Tumor grossly confined to the true pelvis with negative nodes but with microscopic deposits of abdominal peritoneal surfaces.

**Stage IIIB:** Tumor of one or both ovaries with macroscopic peritoneal deposit 2 cm or less in diameter.

**Stage IIIC:** Abdominal metastatic deposit larger than 2 cm in diameter and/or positive retroperitoneal or inguinal nodes

**Stage IV:** Distant metastasis. Positive pleural effusion may be present, Liver parenchymal involvement

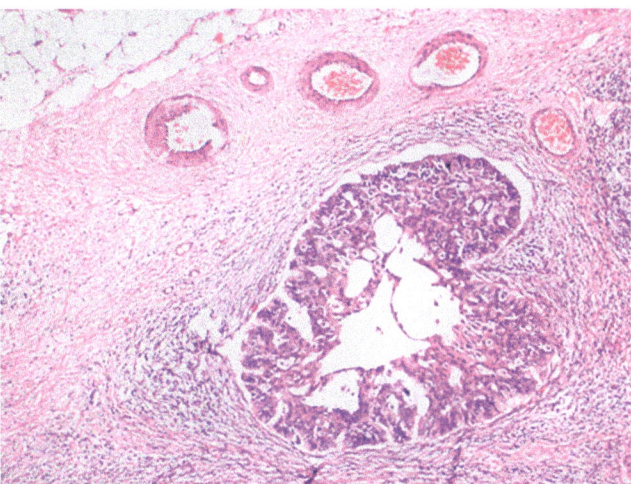

**Figure 12.8:** Omental deposit: Microscopic foci of omental deposit in the omentectomy specimen

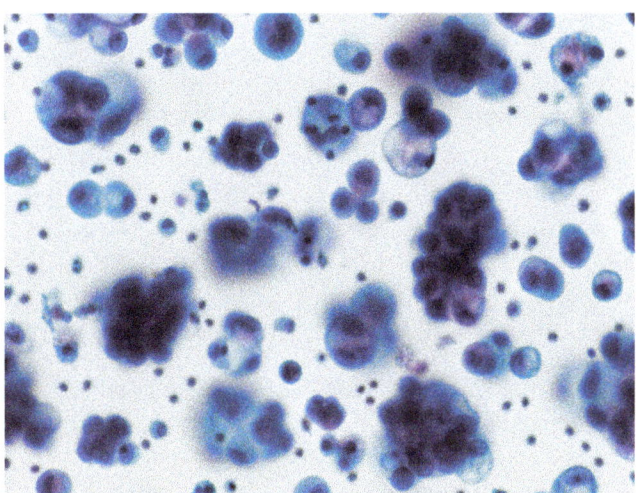

**Figure 12.9:** Malignant cells in ascetic fluid: Multiple ball-like tight clusters in the pleural effusion of ovarian carcinoma patient

## PROGNOSTIC FACTORS

a. Staging: FIGO staging of the ovarian cancer is the most important and well accepted prognostic factor (Figures 12.8 and 12.9). The overall 5 year survival rate of ovarian cancer is 86, 71, 34 and 19% in stage I, stage II, stage III and stage IV respectively.[29]

b. Age: The older patients has poor survival than the younger patients.

c. Histological type of tumor: Possibly there is no prognostic relevance of histological type and prognosis of the patients.

d. Histological grading: Histological grading have been described as relevant prognostic factor in some studies.[30] Histological grading is not well-reproducible. FIGO grading system stresses on the amount of solid areas in the tumor. Grade I tumor shows less than 5% solid area, grade II equivalent to 5–50% solid area and grade III represents more than 50% solid areas.[31] Silverberg SG[32] proposed a score-based grading system of the ovarian carcinoma (Table 12.1).

Table 12.1: Proposed grading of ovarian cancer

| Score | Predominant architectural pattern | Cytological atypia | Mitosis per 10 high power field |
|---|---|---|---|
| 1 | Glandular | Mild | 0–9 |
| 2 | Papillary | Moderate | 10–24 |
| 3 | Solid | Marked | 25 or more |

Total score: 3 to 5 = grade I, 6 to 7= grade II, 8 to 9 = grade III

e. Oncogene: Over expression of epidermal growth factor receptor (EGFR) is related with a poor prognosis in ovarian cancer.[33]
f. Mitotic activity index: Mitotic activity index and volume corrected mitotic index have proven prognostic value in ovarian cancer.[34]

## TREATMENT

In confirmed case of ovarian carcinoma, total abdominal hysterectomy, bilateral salpingo-oophorectomy, along with omentectomy is performed. During operation, following things should be done:
1. Peritoneal surface examination,
2. Undersurface of the liver and diaphragm to examine,
3. Sampling of palpable retroperitoneal lymph node,
4. Cytological examination of ascitic fluid, and
5. Peritoneal washing for cytological examination.

### Postoperative Therapy

Systemic chemotherapy including platinum-based chemotherapy cisplatin and carboplatin is given in postoperative patients with residual disease or chances of risk of recurrence.

## REFERENCES

1. Kurman RJ, Carcangiu ML, Herrington S, Young RH. WHO classification of tumors of female genital reproductive organs. 4th Edition, International agency for research on Cancer, Lyon; 2014.
2. Boyle P, Levin B (Eds). World Cancer Report 2008. World Health Organization, Lyon, 2008.
3. Jemal A, Thomas A, Murray T, et al. Cancer Statistics. 2002. Ca-Cancer I Clin. 2002;52:23-47.
4. Kurman RJ, Shih I. Molecular pathogenesis and extraovarian origin of epithelial ovarian cancer–shifting the paradigm. Hum Pathol. 2011;42:918-31.
5. Piek JM, van Diest PJ, Zweemer RP, et al. Dysplastic changes in prophylactically removed fallopian tubes of women predisposed to developing ovarian cancer. J Pathol. 2001;195:451-6.
6. Przybycin CG, Kurman RJ, Ronnett BM, et al. Are all pelvic (nonuterine) serous carcinomas of tubal origin? Am J Surg Pathol. 2010;34:1407-16.
7. Kuhn E, Kurman RJ, Vang R, et al. TP53 mutations in serous tubal intraepithelial carcinoma and concurrent pelvic high-grade serous carcinoma-evidence supporting the clonal relationship of the two lesions. J Pathol. 2012;226:421-6.
8. Tone AA, Begley H, Sharma M, et al. Gene expression profiles of luteal phase fallopian tube epithelium from BRCA mutation carriers resemble high-grade serous carcinoma. Clin Cancer Res. 2008;14:4067-78.
9. Kuhn E, Meeker A, Wang TL, et al. Shortened telomeres in serous tubal intraepithelial carcinoma. An early event in ovarian high-grade serous carcinogenesis. Am J Surg Pathol. 2010;34:829-36.
10. Kuhn E, Kurman RJ, Sehdev AS, Shih I. Ki-67 labeling index as an adjunct in the diagnosis of serous tubal intraepithelial carcinoma. Int J Gynecol Pathol. 2012;31;416-22.
11. Roh MH, Yassin Y, Miron A, Mehra KK, Mehrad M, Monte NM, et al. High-grade fimbrial-ovarian carcinomas are unified by altered p53, PTEN and PAX2 expression. Mod Pathol. 2010;23(10):1316-24.
12. Lee Y, Miron A, Drapkin R, et al. A candidate precursor to serous carcinoma that originates in the distal fallopian tube. J Pathol. 2007;211:26-35.
13. Singer G, Kurman RJ, Chang H-W, Cho SKR, Shih I-M. Diverse tumorigenic pathways in ovarian serous carcinoma. Am J Pathol. 2002;160:1223-8.
14. Singer G, Oldt III R, Cohen Y, Wang BG, Sidransky D, Kurman RJ, et al. Mutations in BRAF and KRAS characterize the development of low-grade ovarian serous carcinoma. J Natl Cancer Inst. 2003;95:484-6.
15. Ho CL, Kurman RJ, Dehari R, et al. Mutations of BRAF and KRAS precede the development of ovarian serous borderline tumors. Cancer Res. 2004;64:6915-8.
16. Dehari R, Kurman RJ, Logani S, Shih IM. The development of high-grade serous carcinoma from atypical proliferative (Borderline) serous tumors and low-grade micropapillary serous carcinoma: A morphologic and molecular genetic analysis. Am J Surg Pathol. 2007;31:1007-12.
17. Senturk E, Cohen S, Dottino PR, Martignetti JA. A critical re-appraisal of BRCA1 methylation studies in ovarian cancer. Gynecol Oncol. 2010;119:376-83.
18. Bulun SE. Endometriosis. N Engl J Med. 2009;360:268-79.
19. Treloar SA, Wicks J, Nyholt DR, et al. Genomewide linkage study in 1,176 affected sister pair families identifies a significant susceptibility locus for endometriosis on chromosome 10q26. Am J Hum Genet. 2005;77:365-76.
20. Campbell IG, Russell SE, Choong DY, Montgomery KG, Ciavarella ML, Hooi CS, et al. Mutation of the PIK3CA gene in ovarian and breast cancer. Cancer Res. 2004;64:7678-81.
21. Kuo KT, Mao TL, Jones S, et al. Frequent activating mutations of PIK3CA in ovarian clear cell carcinoma. Am J Pathol. 2009;74:1597-601.

22. Mok SC, Bell DA, Knapp RC, et al. Mutation of K-ras protooncogene in human ovarian epithelial tumors of borderline malignancy. Cancer Res. 1993;53:1489-92.
23. Riedel I, Czernobilsky B, Lifschitz-Mercer B, et al. Brenner tumors but not transitional cell carcinomas of the ovary show urothelial differentiation: immunohistochemical staining of urothelial markers, including cytokeratins and uroplakins. Virchows Archiv. 2001;438:181-91.
24. Cuatrecasas M, Catasus L, Palacios J, et al. Transitional cell tumors of the ovary: a comparative clinicopathologic, immunohistochemical, and molecular genetic analysis of Brenner tumors and transitional cell carcinomas. Am J Surg Pathol. 2009;33:556-67.
25. Mok SC, Chao J, Skates S, Wong K, Yiu GK, Muto MG, Berkowitz RS, Cramer DW. Prostasin, a potential serum marker for ovarian cancer: identification through microarray technology. J Natl Cancer Inst. 2001;93(19):1458-64.
26. Visintin I, Feng Z, Longton G, Ward DC, Alvero AB, Lai Y, et al. Diagnostic markers for early detection of ovarian cancer. Clin Cancer Res. 2008;14(4):1065-72.
27. Andersen MR, Goff BA, Lowe KA, et al. Combining a symptoms index with CA 125 to improve detection of ovarian cancer. Cancer. 2008;113:484-9.
28. Prat J. FIGO Committee on Gynecologic Oncology. Staging classification for cancer of the ovary, fallopian tube, and peritoneum. Int J Gynaecol Obstet. 2014;124(1):1-5.
29. Heintz APM, Odicino F, Maisonneuve P. Carcinoma of the ovary. In: 26th annual report on the results of treatment in gynecological cancer. Int J Gynecol Obstet. 2006;95(Suppl 1):S161-S192.
30. Friedlander ML, Dembo AJ. Prognostic factors in ovarian cancer. Semin Oncol. 1991;18(3):205-12.
31. International Federation of Gynecology and Obstetrics. Classification and staging of malignant tumors in the female pelvis. Acta Obstet Gynecol Scand. 1971;50:1-7.
32. Silverberg SG. Histopathologic grading of ovarian carcinoma: a review and proposal. Int J Gynecol Pathol. 2000; 19(1):7-15.
33. Berchuck A, Rodriguez GC, Kamel A, et al. Epidermal growth factor receptor expression in normal ovarian epithelium and ovarian cancer. I. Correlation of receptor expression with prognostic factors in patients with ovarian cancer. Am J Obstet Gynecol. 1991;164:669-74.
34. Baak JPA, Fox H, Langley FA, Buckley CH. The prognostic value of morphometry in ovarian epithelial tumors of borderline malignancy, lnt J Gynecol Pathol. 1985;4:186-91.

# Epithelial Carcinoma of Ovary

The surface epithelial tumor of the ovary is broadly classified as: (a) Serous tumors, (b) Mucinous tumors, (c) Endometrioid tumors, (d) Clear cell tumors, (e) Transitional cell tumors, (f) Squamous cell tumors, (g) Mixed epithelial tumors, (h) Undifferentiated carcinoma.

## SEROUS TUMOR

Serous tumor represents nearly 46% of all ovarian tumors. These tumors constitute 50% of all malignant tumors. Near about 50% of the serous tumors are benign, 35% are malignant and 15% are borderline tumors.

The serous tumors are sub-classified as benign, borderline and malignant.

### Benign Serous Tumor: Serous Cystadenoma, Cystadenofibroma, Serous Adenofibroma

The benign serous tumors represent 50% of all serous tumors.

*Clinical Features*

Benign serous tumors may occur in any age; however they are most common in reproductive age period. The tumor is usually asymptomatic. The patient may occasionally present with abdominal swelling, pain or vaginal bleeding.

*Gross Pathology*

Serous cystadenomas are cystic and may be either unilocular or multilocular with thin translucent wall (Figure 13.1). The cyst usually contains clear fluid. The interior or exterior surface of the cyst may be smooth or may show small papillary excrescence. Adenofibroma is solid and firm and cut section shows white fibrous in appearance with small cysts (Figure 13.2). Cystadenofibroma is more common and contain both cystic areas and solid fibrous component.

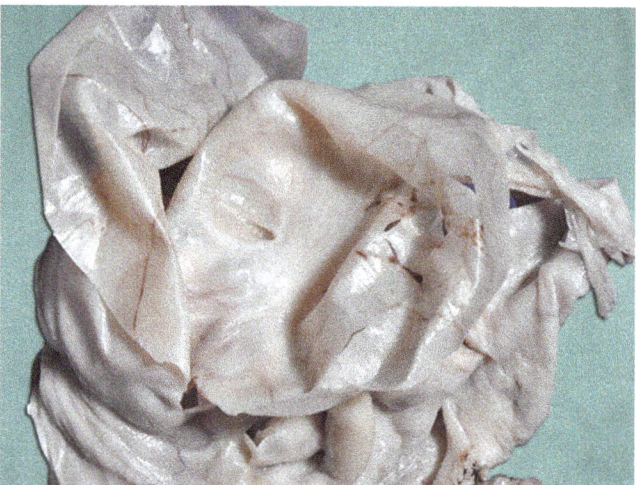

**Figure 13.1:** Serous cyst cystadenoma: Thin translucent wall

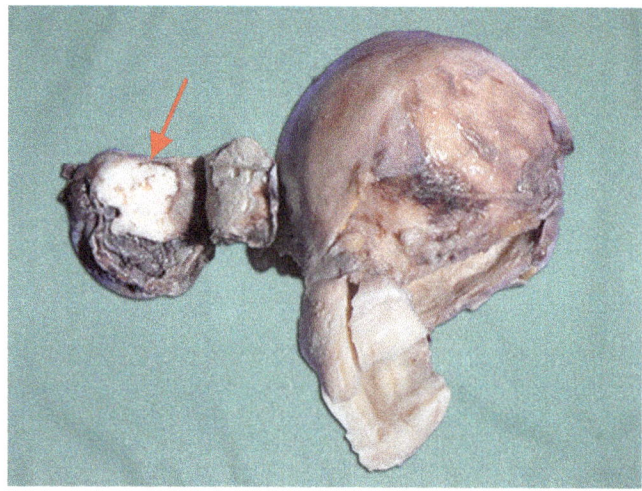

**Figure 13.2:** Cystadenofibroma ovary: Solid firm growth of the ovary

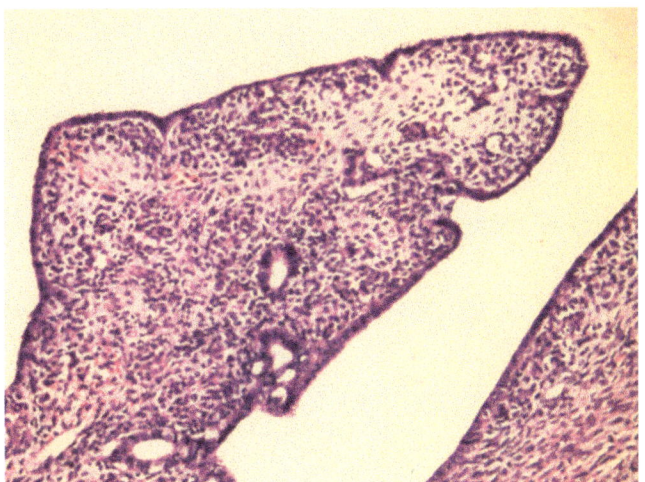

Figure 13.3: Serous cystadenoma: Cyst is lined by single layer of cuboidal to flattened epithelial cells

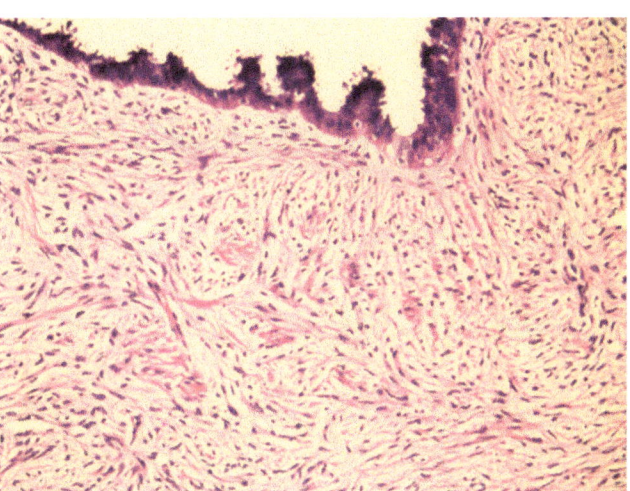

Figure 13.4: Cystadenofibroma: Thick fibrocollagenous wall is lined by cuboidal to columnar cells

### Histopathology

The terminology of "cyst" is applied when grossly visible cyst is present. Depending on the relative amount of fibrous stroma the terminology of "fibroma" is applied. The lining epithelium of the cyst is cuboidal to columnar cells that often show cilia (Figure 13.3). The individual cells show scanty cytoplasm and monomorphic round nuclei having small nucleoli. In case of papillary cystadenofibroma, the core of the papillae is composed of thick fibrocollagenous stroma. The lining cells are single layer of cuboidal cells. The cystadenoma may show psammoma bodies. The cases of adenofibroma or cystadenofibroma show collagenous stroma with many slit like glands (Figure 13.4). In serous cytsadenoma small foci may show papillary excrescences lined by mildly pleomorphic cells. The serous cystadenomas with small foci (less than 10%) of proliferative activity clinically behave as benign lesion and they should not be categorized as borderline tumor. Immunohistochemistry: Serous cystadenomas are positive for CK 7 and negative for CK20. In addition the tumor also shows WT-1 and BER-EP4 positivity.

### Differential Diagnosis

a. **Surface inclusion cyst**: Surface inclusion cysts are less than 1 cm in diameter.
b. **Mesonephric cyst**: Mesonephric cyst is lined by cuboidal epithelial cells and the wall is surrounded by smooth muscle cells.
c. **Endometriotic cyst**: The endometriotic cyst is differentiated from the serous cystadenoma by the presence of endometrial stroma and/or glands in the former.
d. **Hydrosalpinx**: Detailed history of the operative findings is helpful to reveal the origin of the cystic swelling as fallopian tube.
e. **Borderline tumor**: This lesion is differentiated from the serous cystadenoma by focal proliferation of lining epithelium and pseudostratification, the presence of nuclear atypia and hierarchical branching papillae.

### Treatment

This is a benign lesion and therefore simple cystectomy or unilateral salpingo-oophorectomy is sufficient for its treatment.

## Serous Borderline Tumor of Ovary/ (Atypical Proliferative Serous Tumor (APST)

In 1973, World Health Organization (WHO) applied the term "tumor of borderline malignancy" to the group of tumor that show atypia in epithelial cells without any stromal invasion. The terminology was used in all the histological types of epithelial tumors.[1] This terminology is still retained in the current classification of ovarian epithelial tumor by WHO.[2]

### Clinical Features

Serous borderline tumor (SBT) of ovary represents 10% of all ovarian tumors and near about 25% of all malignant serous tumors. The tumor is bilateral in 25–30% cases. The tumor occurs in 4th to 5th decade of life. The average age of the patient is 46 year which is less than the cases of serous carcinoma (65 year). Most of the patients are asymptomatic and occasionally they may present with abdominal enlargement and pain.

### Gross Pathology

Serous borderline tumor is usually large with predominantly cystic and partly solid. The tumor may show papillary excrescences in the outer surface. The tumor with papillary

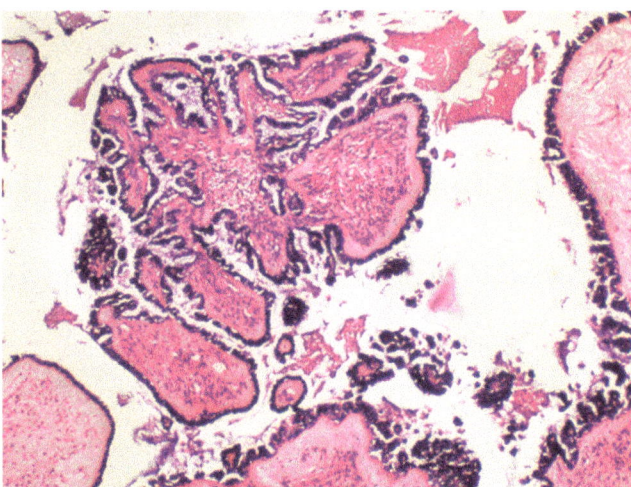

Figure 13.5: Serous borderline tumor of ovary: Multiple papillae that show characteristic hierarchical branching pattern

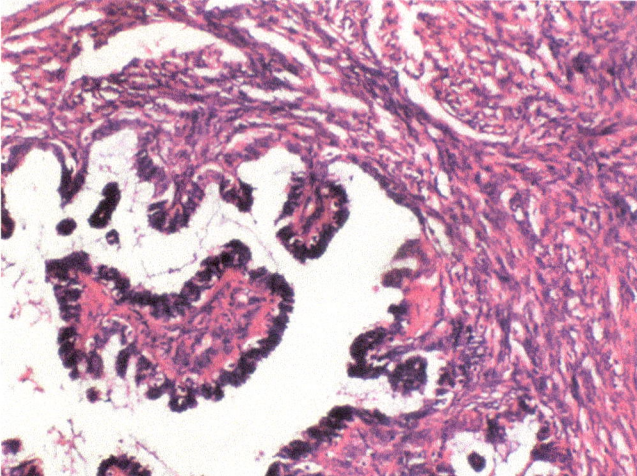

Figure 13.7: Serous borderline tumor of ovary: Cuboidal to columnar lining of the cells with nuclear atypia

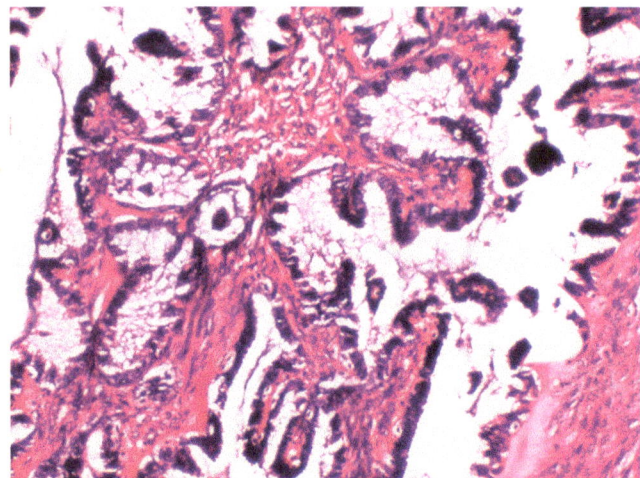

Figure 13.6: Serous borderline tumor of ovary: Papillae divide into larger to smaller branch with fibrovascular core

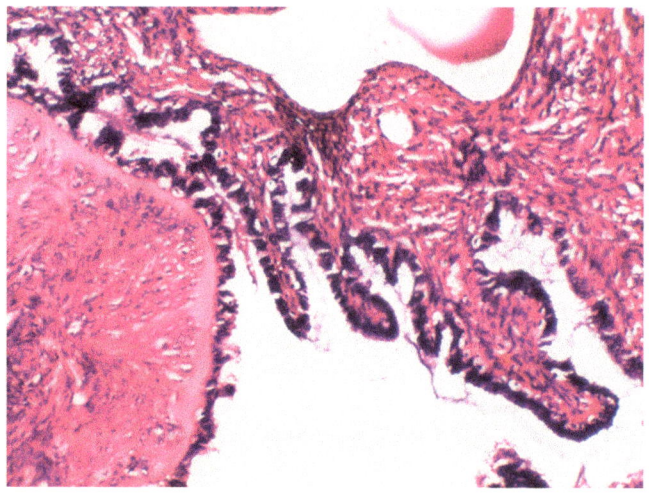

Figure 13.8: Serous borderline tumor of ovary: Nuclear atypia of the lining cells

growth in the outer surface shows frequent peritoneal implants. Borderline serous cystadenofibroma cases show solid firm whitish area. Areas of hemorrhage and necrosis is usually absent in borderline tumors.

### Microscopic Features (Figures 13.5 to 13.8)

The three main characteristic features of SBT are:
1. Hierarchical branching pattern of papillae,
2. Nuclear atypia and
3. Lack of stromal invasion.

SBT is composed of multiple papillary excrescences and glands. The papillae show characteristic hierarchical branching pattern and larger papillae divide into smaller and the smallest papillae. Infrequently only 5–10% cases show non-hierarchical branching pattern where the smaller papillae arise directly from the central large papillae. The lining epithelium often shows stratification. The epithelial cells are cuboidal to columnar with basally placed nuclei. Nuclei show variable atypia and pleomorphism may be mild to moderate. The cells may show cilia. Occasionally, cells with abundant eosinophilic cytoplasm having round nuclei are seen. These cells resemble mesothelial cells and they are often located at the tip of the papillae. These cells are known as indifferent cell or metaplastic cell. Occasionally, there may be tuft of cells in the lining epithelium. Clusters and isolated cells may be detached into the cyst lumen. Mitotic activity of the cell is low. Psammoma bodies are seen in 25% cases. At times tip of the papillae may show infraction.[5]

The papillae may often cut tangentially and may simulate stromal invasion. However, lack of stromal fibroblastic and inflammatory response distinguishes them from invasion.

### Stromal Microinvasion in Borderline Tumor

The various patterns of microinvasion in SBT include:[3]

**Individual eosinophilic cells and cell clusters:** The tumor shows small cords or cluster of cells within the fibrous stroma. These cells show moderate amount of eosinophilic cytoplasm and centrally placed round nuclei with prominent nucleoli. The cells simulate squamoid or mesothelial cells. The cluster of cells is surrounded typically by clear cleft like space.

**Cribriform pattern:** This pattern is characterized by glands with bridging structures and small interglandular papillae resembling cribriform appearance. The epithelial cells are serous type with mild to moderate atypia.

**Simple and noncomplex branching papillae:** This pattern is characterized by discrete and small papillae with a central fibrovascular core. There are no anastomosing or complex papillary structures.

**Inverted macropapillae:** Inverted macropapillae show inverted or endophytic papillae. There are large intrastromal papillae with central fibrovascular core.

**Complex branching micropapillae:** There are multiple branching micropapillae with cribriform pattern. Unlike cribriform variant, these micropapillae are surrounded by retraction like spaces.

### Peritoneal and Omental Implants

Peritoneal and omental implants are noted in 15–40% of ovarian borderline serous tumors.[4] They present as small macroscopic foci of 2–3 mm in diameter or microscopic area (Figures 13.9 and 13.10). The implant may be of following types:
1. **Non-invasive epithelial type:** Non-invasive epithelial type is characterized by the well-circumscribed and superficial papillary proliferation of the atypical cells on the surface of the peritoneum. The papillary growth does not invade the underlying stromal tissue. Psammoma bodies are frequently seen in the implant.
2. **Non-invasive desmoplastic type:** This is characterized by the presence of isolated clusters of epithelial cells or glands over the peritoneal surface. The tumor cells look like plastered on the peritoneal surface and form a plaque-like thickening of the peritoneum. There is marked proliferation of the fibroblastic stroma around the epithelial cells. The desmoplastic stromal implant often shows psammoma body.
3. **Invasive implant:** Invasive implant is seen in 9-12% patients of SBT. This is characterized by: (1) Invasion of the glands in the underlying tissue with irregular margin, (2) Micropapillary architecture and (3) Cleft-like clear space around the nest of epithelial cells.

Table 13.1 highlighted the important distinguishing features of invasive and non-invasive implants.

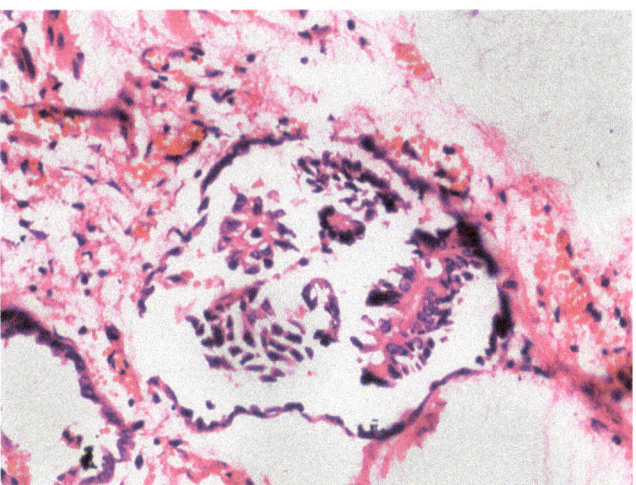

Figure 13.9: Peritoneal implant from serous borderline tumor of ovary: The tumor surrounded by clear space. No stromal reaction is seen

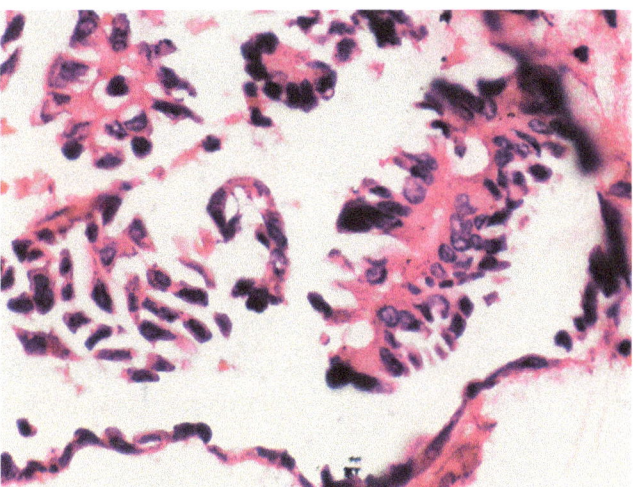

Figure 13.10: Peritoneal implant from serous borderline tumor of ovary: Higher magnification of the same

### Serous Borderline Tumor in Lymph Node

Pelvic or para-aortic lymph node involvement is seen in about 23% cases of SBT.[5] The metastasis is usually seen in the sinusoidal space. The two common pattern of metastasis

Table 13.1: Invasive versus non-invasive implant

| Features | Invasive implant | Noninvasive implant |
|---|---|---|
| Arrangement of glands | Disorderly arranged | Orderly arranged |
| Epithelial cells | Abundant with less stroma | Less with more stroma |
| Margin | Irregular | Regular |
| Stromal fibroblastic reaction | Less | Marked in desmoplastic non-invasive implant |
| Inflammatory reaction | Minimal | Moderate |
| Psammoma body | Infrequent | Frequent |

include: (1) Papillary clusters of tumor cells within the lymph node, (2) Small nests of the cells within the subcapsular sinus.

## Serous Borderline Tumor with Micropapillary Pattern

Serous borderline tumor with micropapillary pattern (SBT-MP) was also designated as micropapillary serous carcinoma (MPSC) due to their aggressive behavioral pattern. The mean age of the patients of SBT-MP is 42 year. The patients are usually asymptomatic and may have abdominal swelling, pain and fullness. SBT-MP represents 14–26% of SBT.[6] Majority of SBT-MP are bilateral.

### Gross

The tumor is usually cystic with solid component and 8–9 cm in diameter. The papillae are noted within the cyst and also over the surface of the ovary.

### Histopathology (Figures 13.11 and 13.12)

The tumor shows focal or diffuse proliferation of the epithelial cells arranged in papillae with no evidence of invasion. The papillae are highly complex and with non-hierarchical branching. They are slender with almost no fibrous stalk and the length of the papillae is more than five times of its width. In low power examination, the micropapillary structures are seen as 'Medusa head-like appearance'. The papillae are lined by cuboidal, hobnail and columnar cells. The cells show round nuclei with uniform nuclear atypia. Ciliated cells are less frequent than that of usual SBT. Mitotic activity is rare, and no atypical mitosis is seen. Occasionally, the tumor may show predominant cribriform appearance or solid pattern of growth.

### Immunohistochemistry

SBT-MPs are negative for p53 and positive for WT-1, ER, PR, and CK-7.

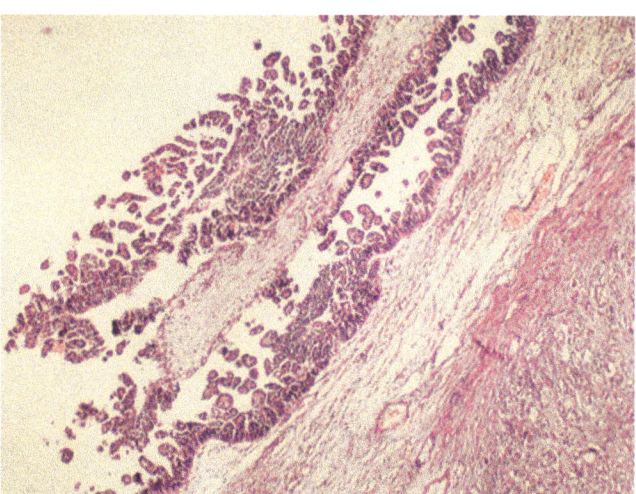

Figure 13.11: Serous borderline tumor with micropapillary pattern: Epithelial cells arranged in papillae with no evidence of invasion

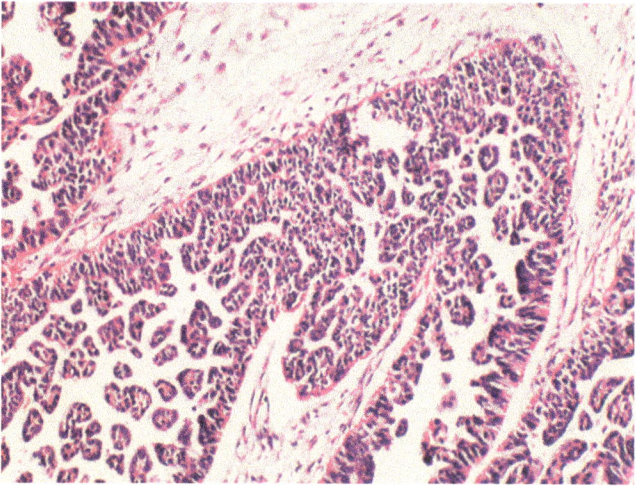

Figure 13.12: Serous borderline tumor with micropapillary pattern: Complex papillary structures with non-hierarchical branching

### Prognosis and Treatment

SBT has very good favorable outcome. Overall 10 year survival rate of SBT is 96–100%.[7] The prognosis of non-invasive peritoneal implant and lymph node involvement are good (95–98% at 6 year follow-up). Invasive peritoneal implant is prognostically bad. It was noted that the survival rate of invasive implants is 66% in comparison to 95.3% in noninvasive peritoneal implants after 7.5 year follow-up.[8]

Surgery is the main treatment of SBT. Total abdominal hysterectomy with bilateral salpingo-oophorectomy is the standard treatment in postmenopausal patients or those patients who have completed their family. Conservative treatment such as unilateral salpingo-oophorectomy or cystectomy is done in young patient who wants to maintain fertility. No additional chemo or radiotherapy is recommended is SBT. Postoperative chemotherapy is recommended in those patients with invasive implant.

## SEROUS CARCINOMA

Serous carcinoma represents 40–62% of all epithelial carcinoma of ovary. Approximately 79% of the serous tumors present in advanced stage (stage III and stage IV) and only 15% cases initially show stage I disease. The tumor is rare under 20 year of age and average age of the patient is 56 year. The patient usually presents with vague symptoms such as fullness of abdomen, early satiety, bloating, urinary complaints, etc. On physical examination, the pelvic mass is found. CA-125 level is raised in 80% of the serous carcinoma. Near about 70% of serous adenocarcinomas are bilateral. Grossly, the serous carcinomas are of variable size from microscopically small to as large as 20 cm in diameter. The tumor is cystic and solid (Figure 13.13). The cut section may show papillary excrescences. Areas of hemorrhage and necrosis are also seen. The surface of the tumor is usually smooth. However, there may be superficial growth over the surface giving an irregular appearance.

### Low-Grade Serous Carcinoma

Low-grade serous carcinoma (LGSC) is uncommon and represents less than 10% of serous carcinomas. The tumor shows glands, micropapillae, cribriform appearance and solid areas (Figures 13.14 to 13.18). The epithelial cells

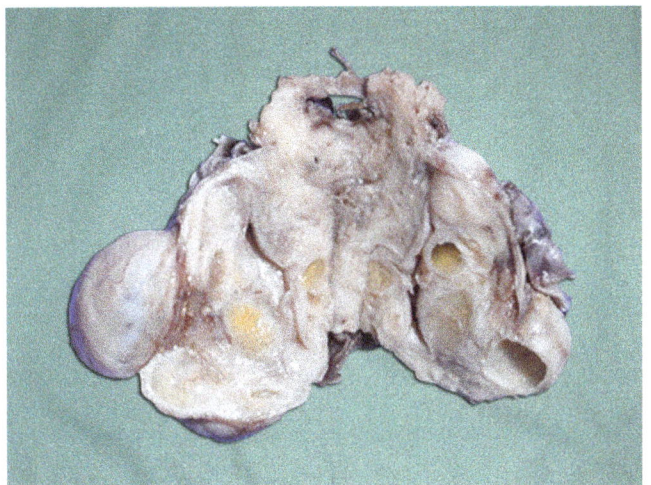

Figure 13.13: Serous adenocarcinoma of ovary: Solid and cystic grey white lesion

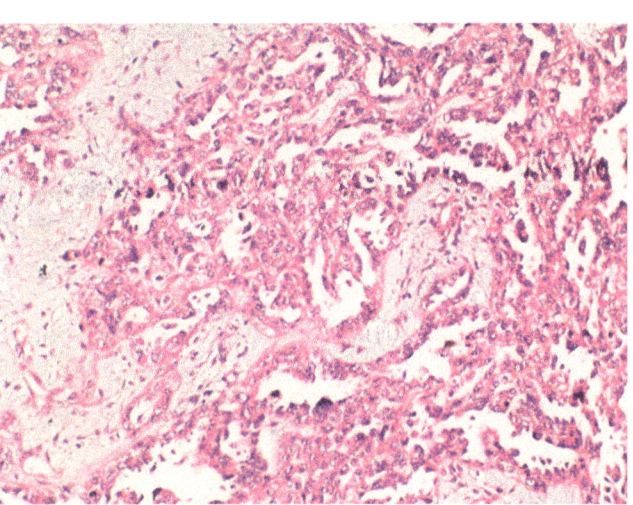

Figure 13.15: Low-grade serous carcinoma: The glands and papillary structures

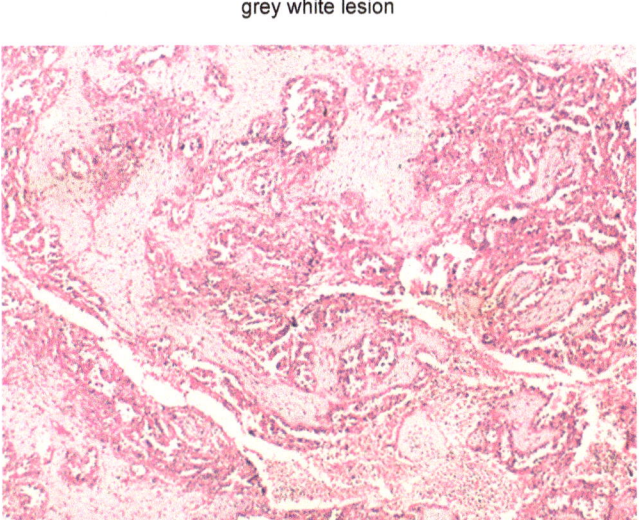

Figure 13.14: Low-grade serous carcinoma: Multiple glands with stromal invasion

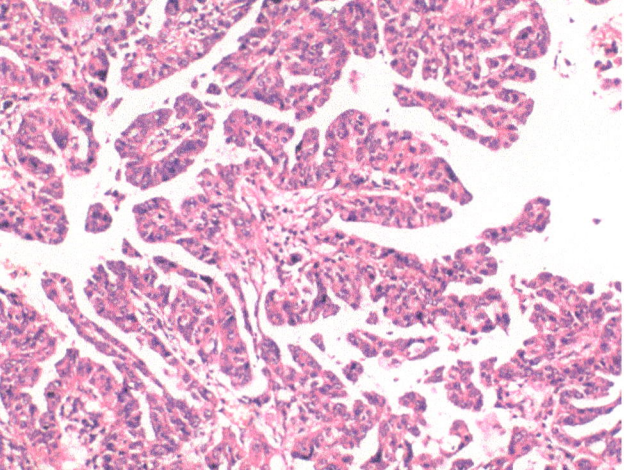

Figure 13.16: Low-grade serous carcinoma: The papillae with fibrovascular core lined by cuboidal to columnar cells with relatively uniform nuclei

show low nuclear grade. The cells are cuboidal to columnar with relatively uniform nuclei having small nucleoli and evenly dispersed chromatin. Definite stromal invasion is present and the glands or papillae or nests of tumor cells are embedded deep in the fibrous stroma. The infiltrating tumor cells or papillae are usually surrounded by a clear space. The areas of invasive carcinoma are often intermingled with areas of borderline serous tumor specially micropapillary carcinoma. In rare psammomatous variant of LGSC there may be abundant psammoma bodies in the tumor obscuring the epithelial cells. This carcinoma has favorable prognosis. The main criteria of psammomatous carcinoma are:[9] (a) At least 75% of papillary structures or nests should be associated with psammoma body, (b) Stromal invasion, (c) Mild to moderate nuclear atypia, (d) Tumor epithelial cell nest consist more than 15 cells.

## High-Grade Serous Carcinoma

High-grade serous carcinoma (HGSC) is characterized by cells with high nuclear grade. The epithelial cells show enlarged nuclei with moderate to marked atypia (Figures 13.19 to 13.21). The nuclei are hyperchromatic with large prominent nucleoli. Mitotic activity is high and often exceeds more than 30 per 10 high power fields. The tumor shows marked architectural variability having large slender papillae, small papillae, and solid nests of cells. The papillae may be slender and long with less fibrous stroma and the epithelial cells may be piled up on the surface. Micropapillary structures with thin papillae projected into the cystic spaces are seen. There

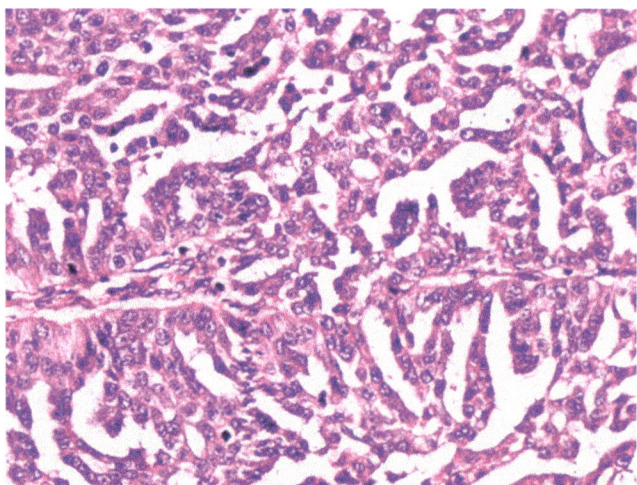

Figure 13.17: Low-grade serous carcinoma: Higher magnification shows cells with mild nuclear pleomorphism

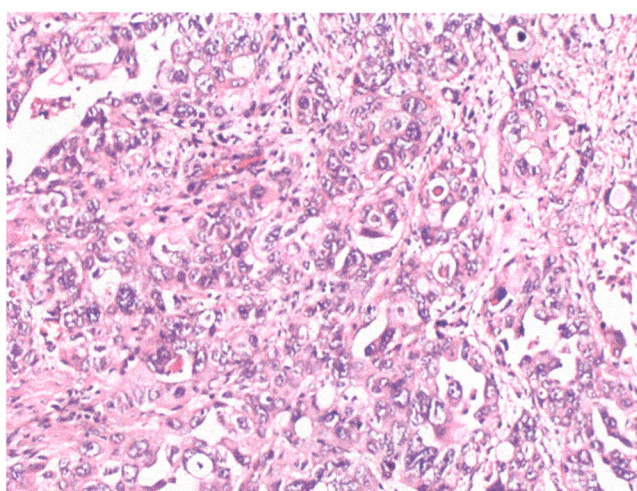

Figure 13.19: High-grade serous carcinoma: The epithelial cells show enlarged nuclei with moderate to marked atypia

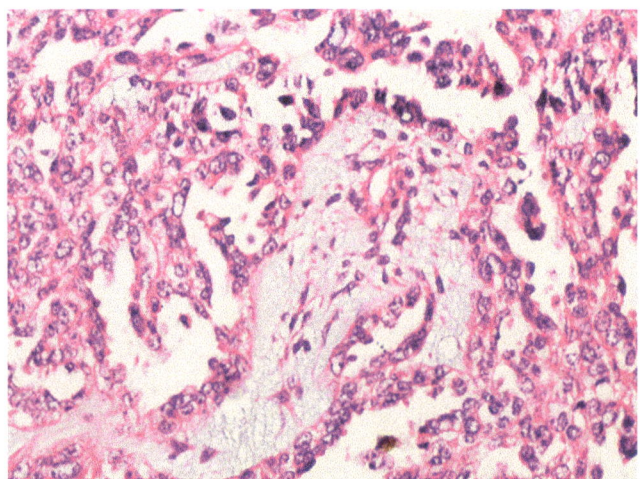

Figure 13.18: Low-grade serous carcinoma: Higher magnification of papillae

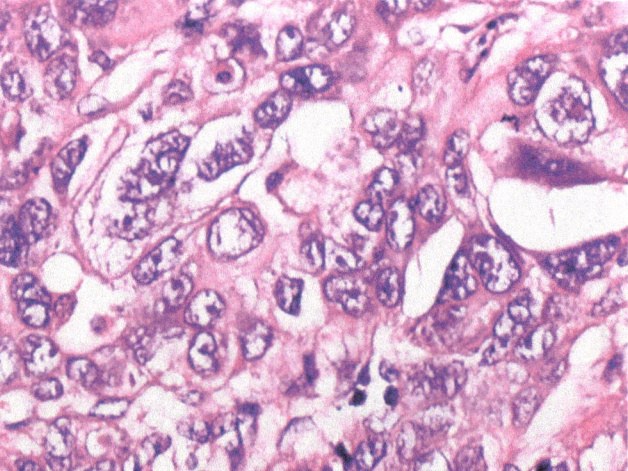

Figure 13.20: High-grade serous carcinoma: Higher magnification shows cells with moderately enlarged pleomorphic nuclei having large prominent nucleoli

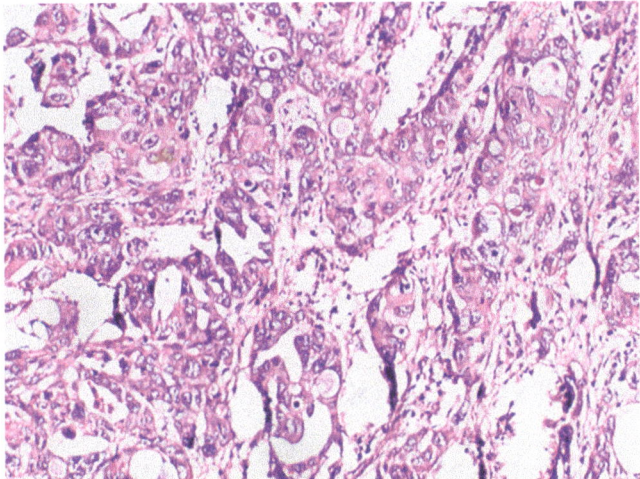

Figure 13.21. High-grade serous carcinoma: Predominant solid areas with occasional glandular component

Table 13.2: Immunostaining in HGSC and endometrioid carcinoma

| Immunostain | Serous carcinoma | Endometrioid carcinoma |
|---|---|---|
| WT-1 | Strong positive | Negative |
| P53 | Strong positive in HGSC | Negative |
| P16 | Strong positive in HGSC | Negative |
| ER/PR | Negative positive | Strong positive |

may be extensive bridging and confluence of papillae and this may give rise to characteristic slit-like spaces. The tumor may have solid nests of cells. Psammoma bodies may be variably present and may be scanty to abundant. The stroma of the tumor is fibrous and often edematous or desmoplastic.

## Immunohistochemistry of Serous Carcinomas

All serous carcinomas are positive for CK 7, EMA, BerEP4, Leu M1 and negative for CK 20, CDX-2, calretinin (Box 13.1). The serous epithelial tumors show nuclear positivity of WT-1 which is helpful to differentiating this tumor from endometrioid and clear cell carcinomas. HGSC shows strong and diffuse nuclear stain for p53 and strong nuclear positivity of p16 immunostain. LGSC and SBT show strong PAX-2 positivity and in comparison HGSC rarely show PAX-2 positive cells.[10]

Box 13.1: Immunohistochemistry of serous carcinoma

All serous carcinomas
Positive: CK 7, EMA, BerEP4, Leu M1, WT-1
Negative: CK 20, CDX-2, calretinin
HGSC: Positive for p53, p16, negative PAX-2
LGSC: Negative for P53 and positive for PAX-2

## Differential Diagnosis

Endometrioid carcinoma: Table 13.2 highlights the differentiating features of serous carcinoma from endometrioid carcinoma.

## MUCINOUS TUMOR OF OVARY

Mucinous tumor of ovary represents 12–15% of all ovarian neoplasm. The large majority of mucinous tumors are benign (75–80%), followed by carcinoma (15%) and borderline tumors (10%).[11] Mucinous adenocarcinoma comprised 10–13% of all malignant epithelial ovarian tumors. However, Seidman JD et al. have shown that exact incidence of mucinous carcinoma of ovary is only 2.4% primary mucinous carcinoma.[12]

## Benign Mucinous Tumor (Mucinous Adenoma and Adenofibroma)

### Gross

Mucinous cystadenomas are mainly unilateral tumor. The tumor is usually large and cystic with average 10 cm in diameter. The cut section of the tumor is unilocular to multilocular and often filled with mucinous material (Figures 13.22 and 13.23). The content of the material does not indicate the nature of the tumor. Solid fibrous component are seen in mucinous adenofibroma cases.

### Histopathology

Depending on the amount of stromal material and glands the tumor is labeled as cystadenoma, cystadenofibroma and adenofibroma. The mucinous cyst adenoma is composed of predominantly cysts and multiple glands that are lined by tall columnar mucus secreting cells (Figure 13.24). The

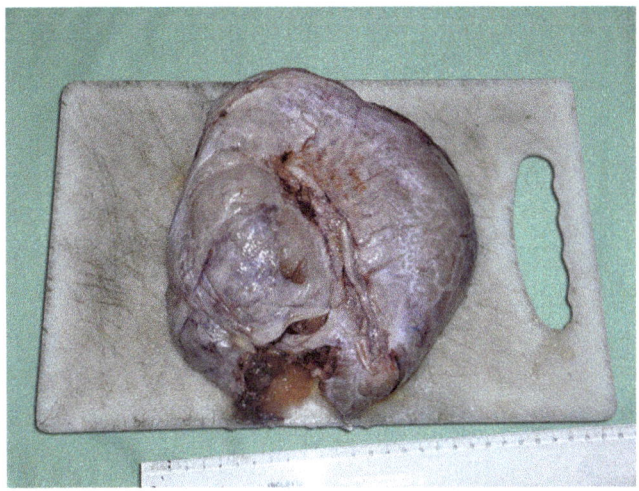

Figure 13.22: Mucinous cystadenoma: Solid well-encapsulated tumor

cells show basally located nuclei having mild atypia. The mucous cells either resemble cervical or intestinal mucosa. Goblet cells or paneth cells may also be seen. Occasionally, small foci of the tumor may show nuclear enlargement and pleomorphism. If this area consists of less than 10% of the tumor then the behavior of such tumor is benign. In cystadenofibroma and adenofibroma cases the tumor shows considerable amount of fibrous stroma. The stroma surrounds the benign glands.

## Borderline Mucinous Tumors

Mucinous borderline tumor (MBT) is characterized by proliferation of the mucin containing epithelial cells more than the benign mucinous cystadenoma, with lack of any invasive stromal component. There are two types of MBT: (1) intestinal like and, (2) endocervical like.

### Intestinal Type of Mucinous Borderline Tumor

**Intestinal type of mucinous borderline tumor (IMBT)** is much common and accounts for almost 85–90% of MBT. The patients are elderly female and average age of the patient is 52 years. Majority of the patients present in stage IA and the tumor remains within the same ovary. Only 5% of IMBTs are bilateral. Most of the patients are asymptomatic and occasionally may present with abdominal swelling and pain.

**Gross:** IMBTs are usually large in size and average diameter is 15 cm. The tumor is usually unilateral and cystic with smooth surface. Cut section shows multiloculated cyst filled with mucin (Figures 13.25 and 13.26).

**Microscopy (Figures 13.27 to 13.31):** The tumor is composed of multiple glands and cystic spaces lined by mucin secreting columnar epithelial cells. Stratification of

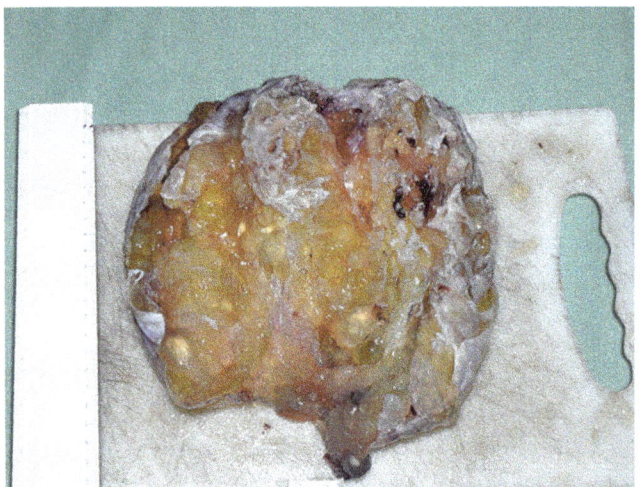

Figure 13.23: Mucinous cystadenoma: The cut section shows mucinous material

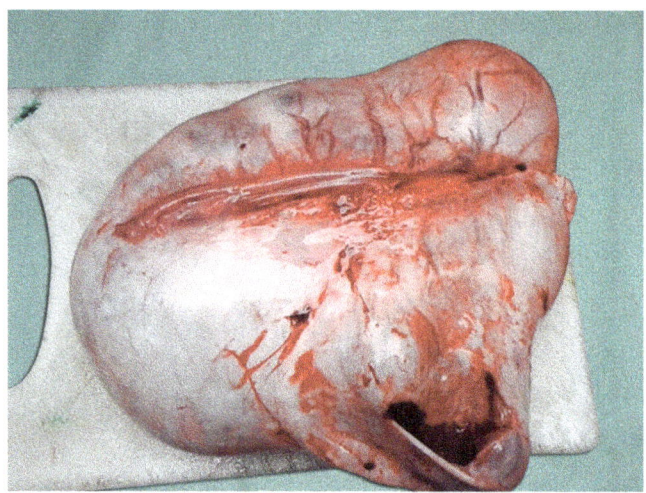

Figure 13.25: Mucinous borderline tumor: Well-encapsulated tumor with shiny capsule

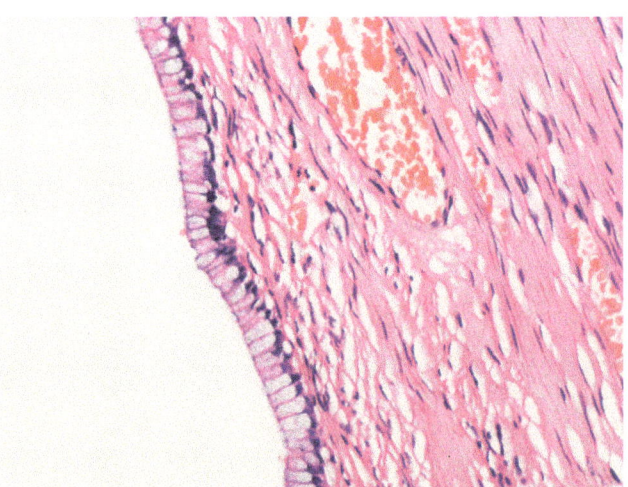

Figure 13.24: Mucinous cystadenomas: The cyst is lined by tall mucin secreting cells

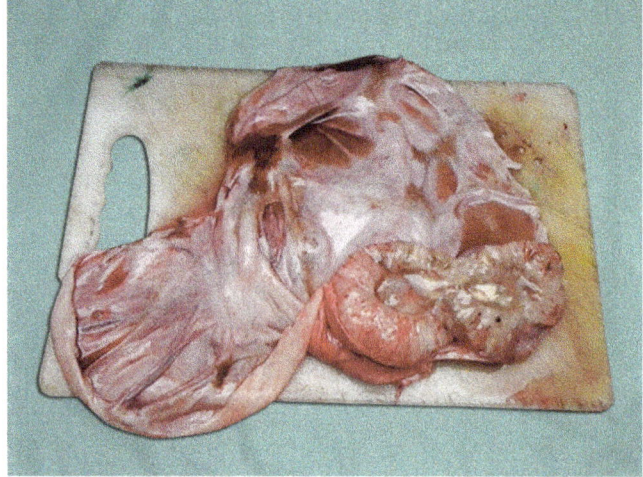

Figure 13.26: Mucinous borderline tumor: Cut section shows both solid and cystic areas

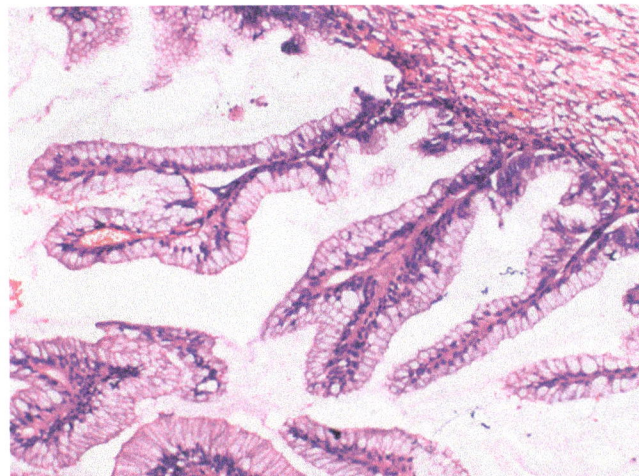

Figure 13.27: Mucinous borderline tumor: Multiple filiform papillae without any stromal tissue

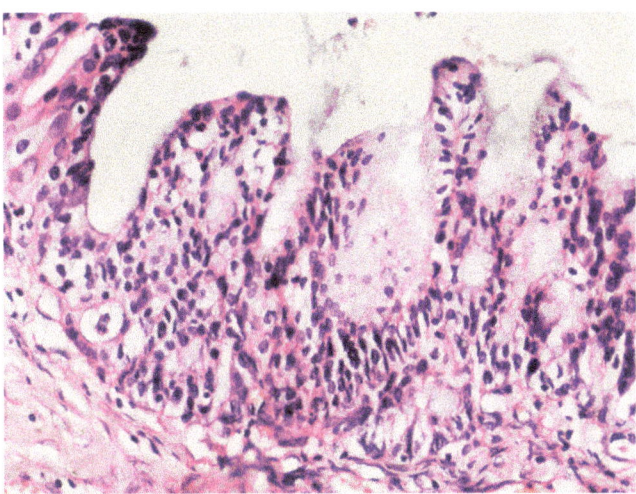

Figure 13.30: Mucinous borderline tumor: The papillae are lined by mucus secreting cells with mild nuclear pleomorphism

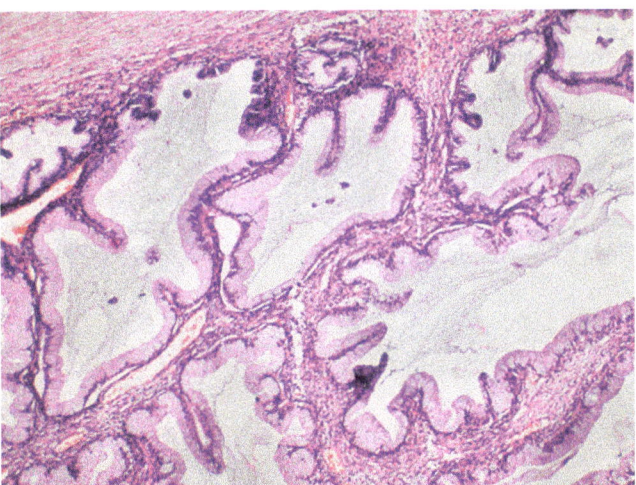

Figure 13.28: Mucinous borderline tumor: Both glands and papillary structures

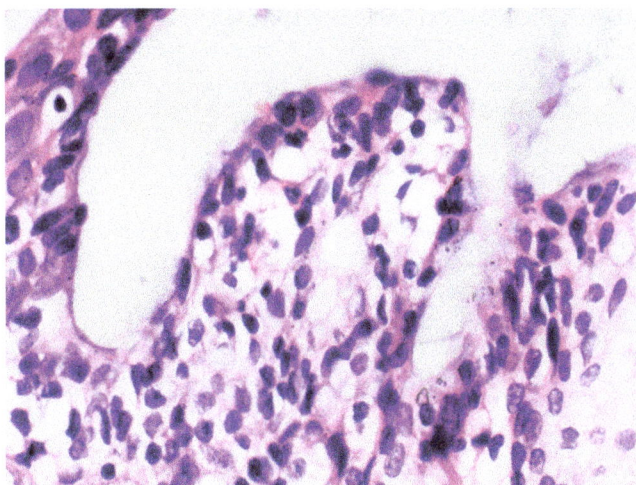

Figure 13.31: Mucinous borderline tumor: Higher magnification shows nuclear atypia

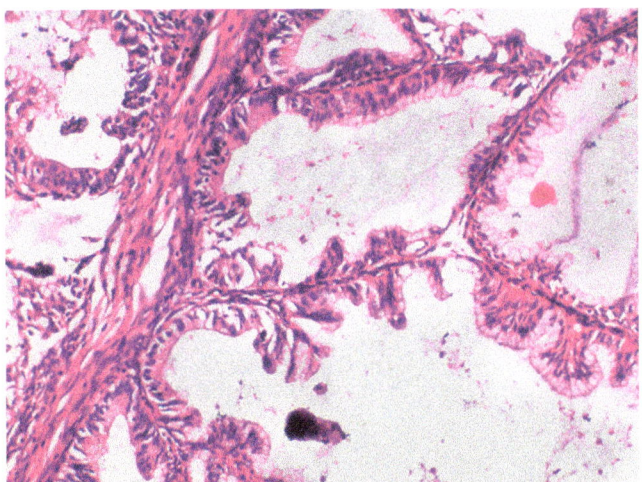

Figure 13.29: Mucinous borderline tumor: Papillae with fibrovascular core

the epithelial lining is seen. However, the epithelial cell layer does not exceed more than 3 layers. Multiple filiform papillae without any stromal tissue may be seen. These tuft of epithelial cells show mild nuclear enlargement and mild to moderate nuclear pleomorphism. The nuclei are round to oval vesicular with prominent nucleoli. Mitotic activity is usually more than benign mucinous adenoma. In addition many goblet cells and occasionally Paneth's cells are seen. Occasionally, the thickness of the epithelial layer may be four or more and the cells may show marked nuclear enlargement and pleomorphism. This tumor should be labeled as borderline tumors with intraepithelial carcinoma.[13]

**Stromal microinvasion:** Small foci of microinvasion may be noted in 30% of BMT of ovary. The microinvasion is defined as the foci of invasion that must not exceed 3 mm linear dimension or 10 mm$^2$ area. To determine the size of the microinvasive foci only the measurement of the largest foci should be considered and the sum of the measurement of all the small foci should not be done. Two types of microinvasion are seen: (1) Small nests of cells or isolated individual cells within the stroma having low nuclear atypia and similar morphology as that of borderline tumor cells in the other area of tumor. (2) Nests of cells or glands within the stroma with marked nuclear atypia resembling high-grade carcinoma. This pattern is more commonly seen in microinvasive carcinoma of MBT.

### Endocervical Type of Mucinous Borderline Tumor

Endocervical type of mucinous borderline tumor accounts for only 10–15% of all MBT. The age range of the patient of EMBT is 20–60 year and mean age of the patient is 34 year. EMBT is often associated with endometriosis. Nearly 13–40% of EMBT are bilateral in distribution.

**Gross:** The tumor varies in size and the average diameter of the tumor is 8 cm. The tumor is predominantly unilocular and occasionally multilocular. The content of the cyst is thick mucinous fluid. Intracystic papillary excrescences may be seen grossly. In small number of cases superficial papillary growth may also be seen.

**Microscopy (Figures 13.32 and 13.33):** EMBT shows multiple arborizing complex papillary structures lined by cuboidal to columnar mucus secreting endocervical like cells. The cells show mild nuclear atypia. Mitotic figures are sparse. No goblet cells or Paneth cell is seen. The tumor also shows large round to polygonal cells with abundant eosinophilic cytoplasm. These cells are known as "indifferent cell" and are typically located in the tip of the papillae. In addition, the tumor also shows endometrioid cells, squamous cells and ciliated serous cells. Near about 30–40% of EMBTs are associated with endometriosis.

**Treatment and prognosis:** Approximately 90% of EMBTs are detected in stage I FIGO staging and simple oophorectomy is adequate for the treatment. The prognosis of EMBT is excellent and no death has been reported in the literature.

### Mucinous Tumor with Pesudomyxoma Peritonei

Mucinous cystic tumor with associated pesudomyxoma peritonei (PMP) is a distinct entity. Most of such cases are associated with primary tumor of appendix and ovary is secondarily involved. These cases should not be labeled as stage II or III mucinous tumor of ovary. PMP is most often associated with appendiceal mucinous tumor such as cyst adenoma, adenoma and villous adenoma or it may be seen with mucinous adenocarcinoma of appendix. It is characterized by abundant thick gelatinous mucoid material within the abdominal and pelvic cavity. The mucinous material may be acellular or may contain epithelial cells (Figures 13.34 and 13.35). Thin strands of fibrous tissues may dissect the material. Pseudomyxoma peritonei may show scanty benign looking epithelial cells or moderate to marked pleomorphic malignant looking epithelial cells. Ronnett et al. classified PMP as "disseminated peritoneal adenomucinosis" (DPAM) and "peritoneal mucinous carcinomatosis" (PMCA).[14] In DPAM cases the epithelial cells are scanty in number and show mild nuclear pleomorphism. These cases have indolent course and they have better prognosis. In PMCA cases, the cells are usually much more in number and show significant nuclear enlargement and pleomorphism. These cases are bad in prognosis. Majority of such cases have tumor in

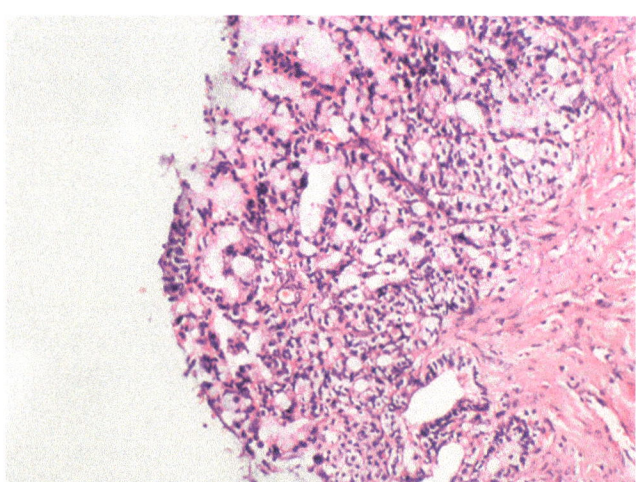

**Figure 13.32:** Mucinous borderline tumor of cervical type: Focal cribriform appearance

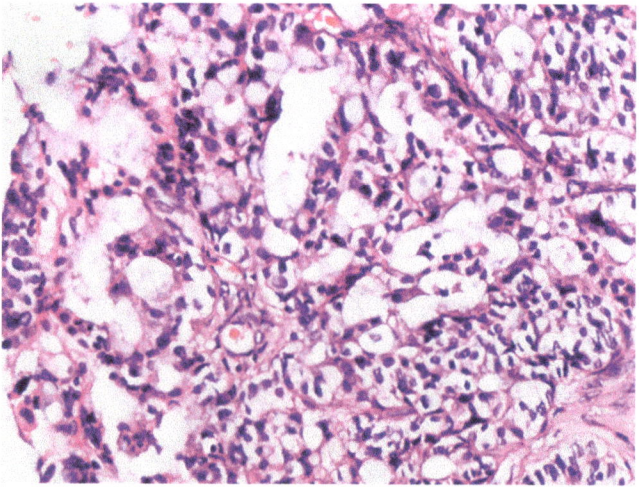

**Figure 13.33:** Mucinous borderline tumor of cervical type: Higher magnification of the same

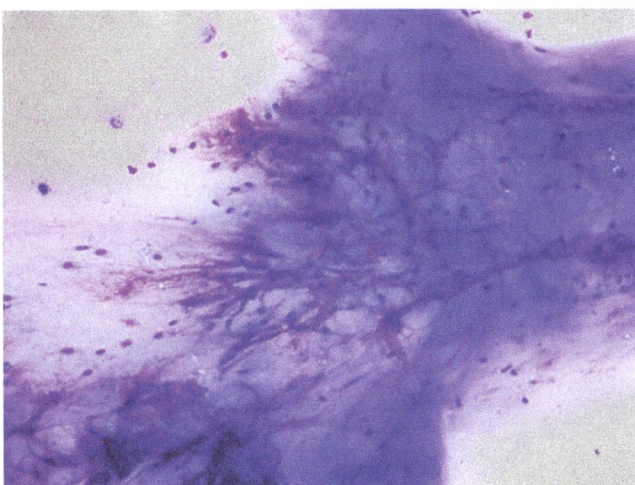

**Figure 13.34:** Pseudomyxoma peritonei: Abdominal aspirate shows abundant thick mucinous material (May Grunwald Giemsa stain)

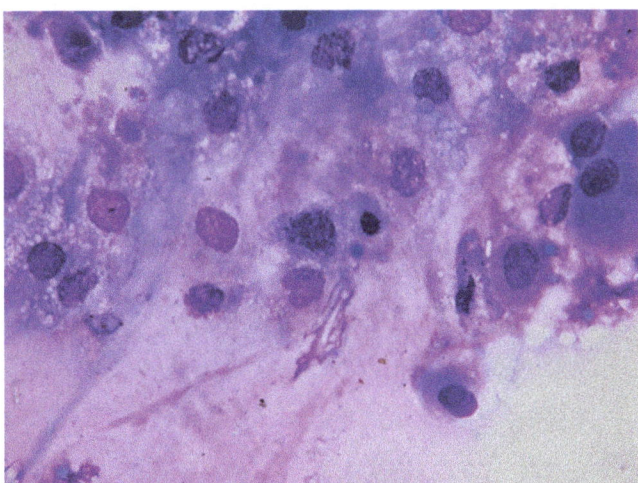

**Figure 13.35:** Pseudomyxoma peritonei: Abdominal aspirate shows epithelial cells within the mucinous material (May Grunwald Giemsa stain)

the appendix or other part of the intestine. The cases with simultaneous presence of ovarian and appendicular tumor were considered as primary appendicular tumor with secondary involvement of ovary.

The ovarian cyst associated with PMP is usually bilateral and large. The large size of the ovarian cyst and small or almost visibly unrecognizable tumor in the appendix may give false impression that the tumor is primarily developed from the ovary. The mucinous material and tumor cells of the peritoneum penetrate the ovarian cortex and the cells proliferate to produce a large mucinous ovarian cyst. Overall the ovarian cyst may resemble borderline mucinous tumor. As the appendicular tumor may not be grossly visible so a careful microscopic examination of the appendix is mandatory in all such cases. Thorough examination of the appendix reveals tumor in the appendix.

### Mural Nodule

Uncommonly mucinous tumor of ovary shows mural nodule. These nodules are common in intestinal type of mucinous tumor. These nodules are firm and few mm to few cm in diameter and reddish-brown in color. The nodules are of three types, which are as follows:

**Sarcoma-like nodule:** Three types of sarcoma like nodules have been described: (a) Epulis like: This lesion consists of multinucleated giant cells and mononuclear histiocytes, (b) Pleomorphic type: It consists of pleomorphic spindle cells and multinucleated giant cells, (c) Histiocyte type.[15] These reactive nodules are strongly positive for vimentin and CD 68 and weakly positive for CK.

**Sarcomatous nodule:** This is composed of spindle cells with moderate nuclear enlargement and pleomorphism. The tumor cells are strongly positive for vimentin and weakly positive for CK.

**Carcinomatous nodule:** The lesion shows sheets of polygonal cells or spindle cells arranged in fascicles. The cells show moderately pleomorphic nuclei with variable degree of mitotic activity usually more than 4 per 10 HPFs. The lesion may show rhabdoid like cells or spindle cells.[16] The rhabdoid cell have abundant eosinophilic cytoplasm with eccentric nuclei having prominent nucleoli. Whereas the spindle cells have elongated spindle shaped nuclei with moderate pleomorphism. The tumor cells are strongly positive for CK and EMA.

## Mucinous Adenocarcinoma

### Clinical Features

The patients are usually elderly female with mean age 45 years. Most of the patients are asymptomatic. CA-125 level of the patients are usually not much elevated as that of serous carcinoma.

### Gross

Mucinous carcinomas are mostly unilateral (95%), large, solid cystic, multiloculated cyst containing mucinous fluid (Figures 13.36 and 13.37). The tumor size varies from 10–40 cm and average size is 16 cm diameter. The cut section of the cyst may show whitish firm fleshy solid areas with hemorrhage and necrosis. Approximately 4% of the tumor may be completely solid. The capsular surface is smooth and shiny. However, the tumor may often show rupture of capsule or adhesion due to its large size and thick mucinous content.

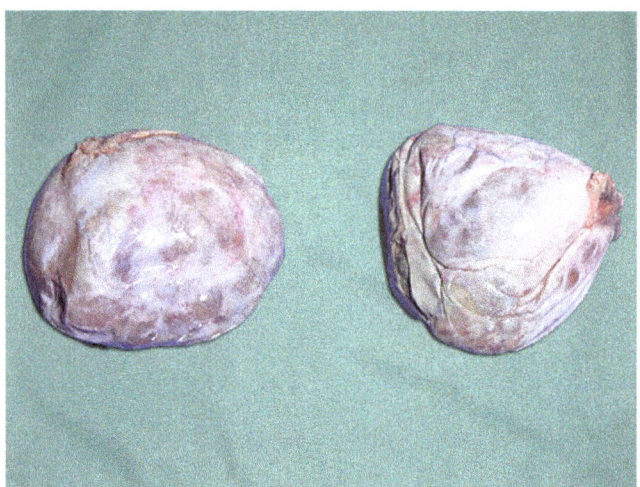

Figure 13.36: Mucinous carcinomas: Solid encapsulated tumor with shiny outer surface in a bilateral carcinoma

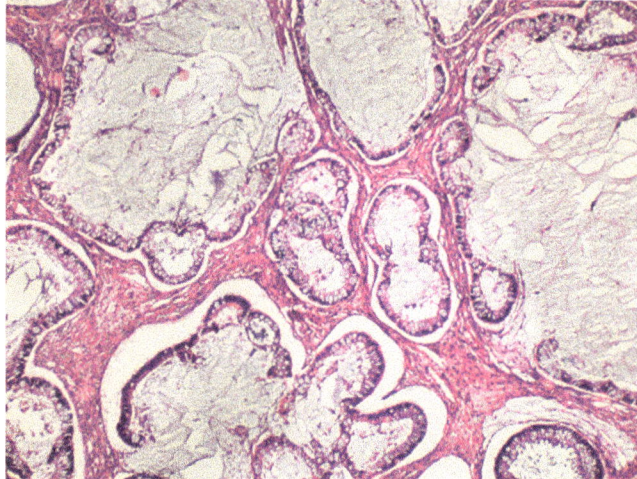

Figure 13.38: Mucinous carcinomas: Multiple varying sized glands deep within the stroma

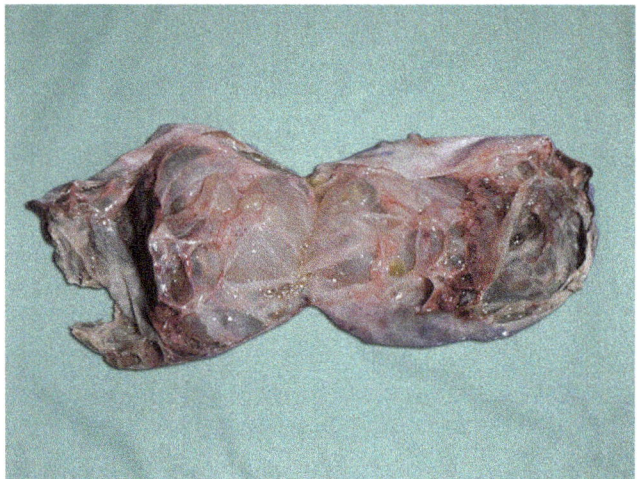

Figure 13.37: Mucinous carcinomas: Cut section shows solid cystic areas

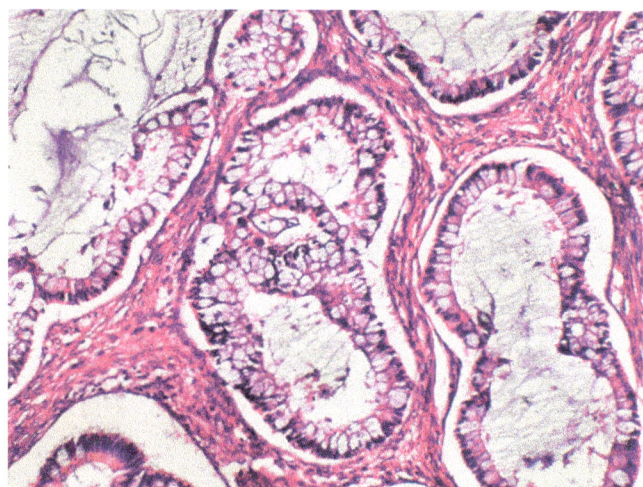

Figure 13.39: Mucinous carcinomas: Higher magnification shows tall mucin secreting glands

### Histopathology (Figures 13.38 to 13.42)

It is always preferable to take section from the solid area of the ovarian cyst and at least one section should be taken from each cm area of the tumor. The most of the mucinous carcinomas show intestinal type of cells and 80% mucinous carcinoma shows IMBT.[17]

Microscopical examination of the mucinous adenocarcinoma shows multiple glands and cysts. The glands show crowding and complex architectural pattern. The glands or cyst wall is lined by single to multiple layers of epithelial cells. The cells are tall columnar with moderate amount of eosinophilic cytoplasm. The nuclei are enlarged with moderate pleomorphism. Nuclear chromatin is coarse with prominent nucleoli. Goblet cells are often seen within the epithelial cells. The cells show frequent mitotic activity. Rarely signet ring type of cells may be noted, however, the

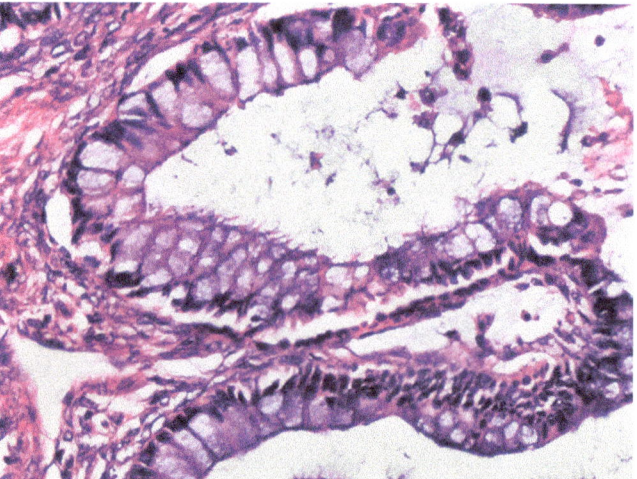

Figure 13.40: Mucinous carcinomas: Papillary structure lined by mucus secreting cells

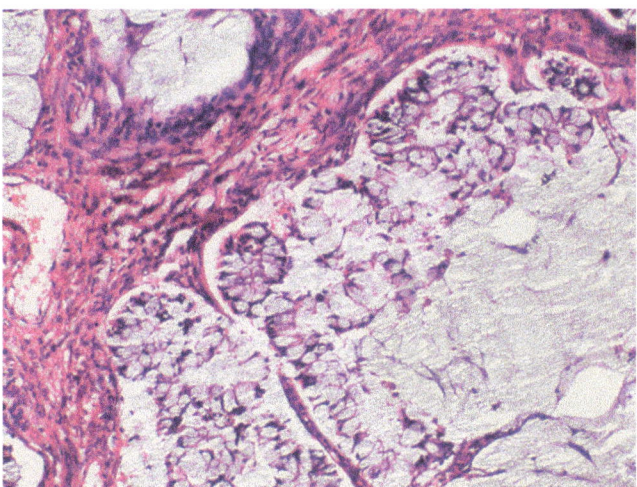

Figure 13.41: Mucinous carcinomas: Pool of mucin within the tumor

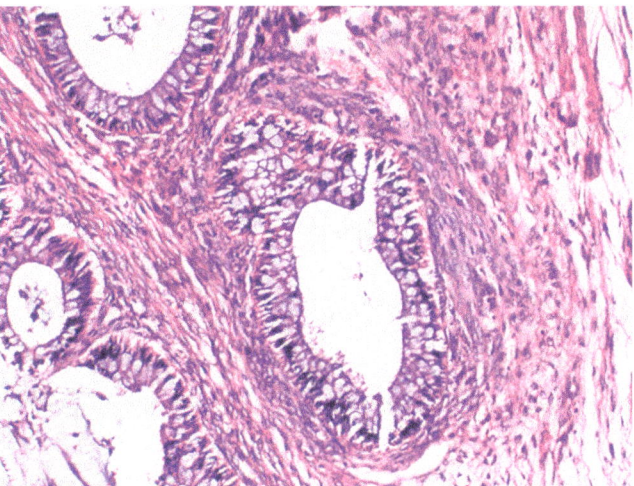

Figure 13.42: Mucinous carcinomas: Desmoplasia around the invasive foci

presence of signet ring cells generally indicate metastatic carcinoma from non-ovarian source.

Two categories of mucinous carcinoma have been described:
1. **Infiltrating type**: It is characterized by the stromal invasion by glands, nests of cells or individual cells with an associated stromal desmoplastic reaction. The tumor cells may be in small clusters within the stroma surrounded by clear space.
2. **Expansile growth pattern**: The expansile type of growth pattern is much more common and is characterized by confluent architecturally complex glands with scanty intervening stroma that gives a labyrinthine appearance. There are multiple well-circumscribed glands or cystic spaces lined by mucin secreting cells with moderate to marked nuclear atypia.

Table 13.3: Immunostaining in primary mucinous adenocarcinoma versus metastatic from gastrointestinal adenocarcinoma

| Immunostain | Primary mucinous adenocarcinoma | Metastatic from gastrointestinal adenocarcinoma |
| --- | --- | --- |
| CK7 | Strong positive | Negative |
| CK20 | Weak patchy positive | Strong diffuse |
| CDX2 | Weak positive | Strong diffuse |
| Beta catenin | Negative | Positive |
| MUC5AC | Positive | Negative |
| MUC2 | Positive in intestinal type (70%) | Positive |

*Immunohistochemistry*

Approximately 80% of primary ovarian carcinoma shows strong CK7 positivity and also MUC5AC and MUC2 positivity.[18-20] The tumor is negative for CK20, beta catenin and CDX2. These immunostaining is helpful to differentiate primary ovarian mucinous carcinoma from metastatic colorectal carcinoma (Table 13.3).

## Molecular Pathology

Mucinous carcinoma is not related with BRCA mutation and the tumor commonly shows KRAS mutation.[21]

*Differential Diagnosis*

Metastatic adenocarcinoma in ovary: Table 13.4 highlights the differentiating features between primary ovarian mucinous carcinoma from metastatic colorectal carcinoma.

*Treatment and Prognosis*

The prognosis of such stage I mucinous adenocarcinoma is excellent and after surgical excision the five year survival rate is near about 98%. In this stage I mucinous carcinoma with confluent pattern of growth the chance of recurrence is less and no postoperative chemotherapy is required. Mucinous carcinoma with infiltrative pattern of growth recurs frequently. Five year survival rate of stage II, III and IV mucinous tumor are 55%, 21% and 9% respectively.

## ENDOMETRIOID CARCINOMA OF OVARY

Endometrioid tumor of ovary accounts for 2–4% of all ovarian tumors. The benign and borderline variants of endometrioid tumors are exceedingly uncommon and comprise less than 1% and 3% of ovarian tumors. The large majority of endometrioid tumors are endometrioid carcinomas and it represents 10–20% of all ovarian carcinomas.[22] Endometrioid tumors are much more frequently associated with endometriosis than other types of epithelial tumors of ovary and up to 42% of

Table 13.4: Differentiating primary mucinous carcinoma from Metastatic ovarian carcinoma

| Features | Primary mucinous carcinoma | Metastatic ovarian carcinoma |
|---|---|---|
| Size | More than 10–13 cm | Less than 10–13 cm |
| Laterality | Unilateral | Bilateral |
| Type of growth | Confluent growth pattern | Infiltrative growth |
| Hilar growth | Absent | Present |
| Signet ring cells | Usually absent | May be present |
| Stromal extravasation of mucin | Uncommon | More frequent |
| Dirty necrosis | Absent | More frequent |
| Vascular invasion | Less frequent | More frequent |
| Peritoneal or lymph node involvement | Absent, Stage I | Present, advanced stage |
| Coexisting Brenner tumor or cystic teratoma | Present | Absent |
| Immunostaining panel | Strong positive CK7; weak, patchy positive CK20/CDX2; negative beta catenin/strong positive MUC5AC | Negative CK7; strong positive CK20/CDX2/ beta catenin; negative MUC5AC |

endometrioid carcinomas are associated with endometriosis of the ovary.[22]

## Clinical Features

The endometrioid tumors usually occur in perimenopausal and postmenopausal patients. The mean age of the patient is 56 years. The majority of the patients are asymptomatic and occasionally they may present with abdominopelvic mass.

## Gross Features

Macroscopical appearance of endometrioid tumors is similar to other surface epithelial tumors. Endometrioid carcinomas are bilateral in 17% cases. The tumors are solid–cystic. The cut section shows firm areas along with hemorrhage and necrosis.

## Benign Tumors

The tumor consists of multiple glands and cysts lined by cuboidal to columnar epithelial cells.

## Borderline Tumors

Borderline tumor is characterized by the presence of endometrioid glands or cysts lined by endometrial type of cells showing nuclear atypia without any evidence of stromal invasion. Three types of borderline tumors are seen:

1. Adenofibromatous: The tumor is composed of multiple crowded endometrioid glands with mild to moderate nuclear atypia within adenofibromatous stroma.
2. Villoglandular: The tumor is composed of villoglandular or papillary hyperplasia of the glands lined by atypical cells in a fibromatous stroma.
3. Mixed: The tumor consists of both adenofibromatous and villoglandular type.

### Endometrioid Carcinoma (Figures 13.43 to 13.48)

Endometrioid carcinomas shows features of stromal invasion characterized by irregular glands, nests of tumor cells with irregular margin and infiltration of the tumor cells in the deeper stroma.[23] The tumor shows various patterns that include glands, tubules, insular, microglandular, villoglandular, adenoid basal, adenoid cystic, and cribriform appearances. The glands are lined by single to multilayered nonmucus secreting cuboidal to columnar cells with round nuclei. Metaplastic squamous cells in the form of morules are seen in 30–40% of endometrioid carcinoma. Low-grade endometrioid carcinoma shows crowded glands with back to back appearance having scanty to absent intervening stromal material. The tumor may often show villous papillary pattern. The glandular lining cells in low-grade endometrioid carcinoma show mild pleomorphism. However, high grade nuclei may also be seen focally in architecturally well-differentiated endometrioid carcinoma. In case of less well-differentiated endometrioid carcinoma variable amount of solid areas are seen along with glandular areas. The nuclei may also show moderate to marked pleomorphism. Endometrioid carcinoma is graded similarly as we grade endometrial carcinoma of endometrium: (a) Grade 1: Less than 5% solid growth, (b) Grade 2:[24] 5 to 50% solid growth, (c) Grade 3: More than 50% solid growth.

Areas of squamous or spindle cell differentiation should not be counted as solid growth. In case of grade 3 nuclear changes, the grade of tumor should be increased by one.

Variable cytological features are seen in endometrial carcinoma that include: (a) Mucin rich cells: Mucin in the apical part of the cell and in the glandular lumen. (b) Secretory cells: Prominent secretory changes in the glandular lining epithelial cells (c) Oxyphil cells: Cells with polygonal cells with abundant eosinophilic cytoplasm. The nuclei are central in position with large prominent nucleoli. (d) Ciliated cells: The glandular lining cells show cilia. (e) Spindle cells: The spindle cell variant may simulate carcinosarcoma or high-grade endometrioid carcinoma.

Various morphological variant of endometrioid carcinomas have been described. These include: (1) Microglandular pattern that simulate granulosa cell tumor: The solid areas of

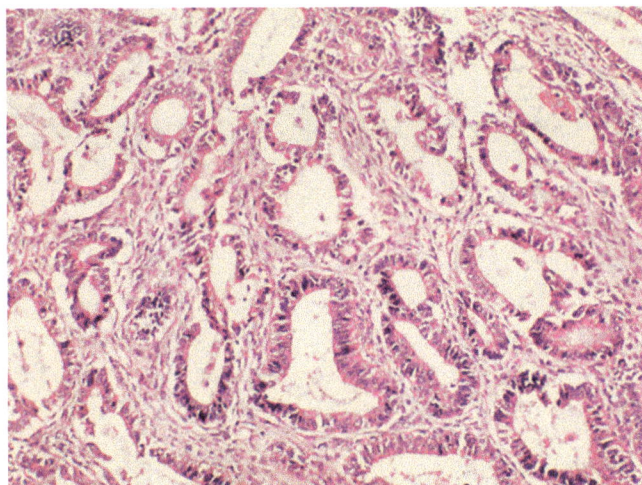

**Figure 13.43:** Endometrioid carcinoma: The tumor simulating endometrial glands

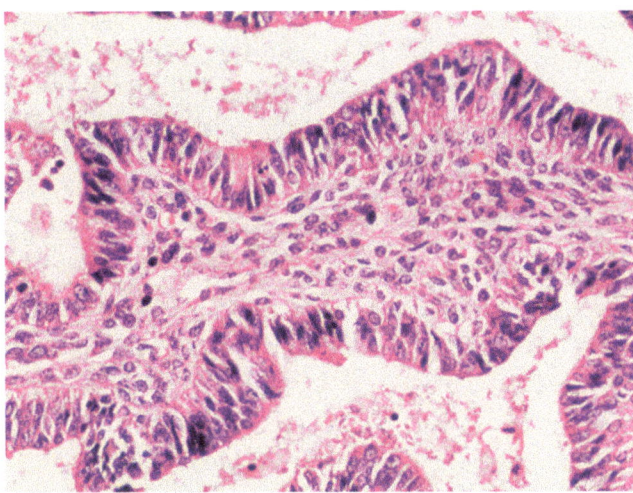

**Figure 13.46:** Endometrioid carcinoma: The glandular epithelium shows moderate nuclear pleomorphism

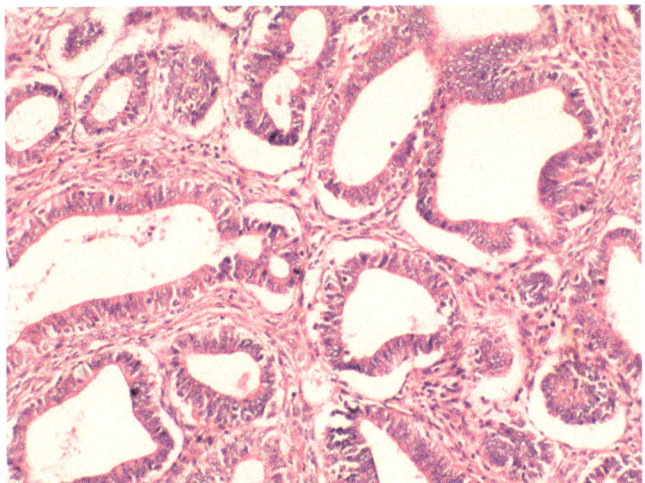

**Figure 13.44:** Endometrioid carcinoma: The glands lined by single to multilayered nonmucus secreting cuboidal to columnar cells with round nuclei

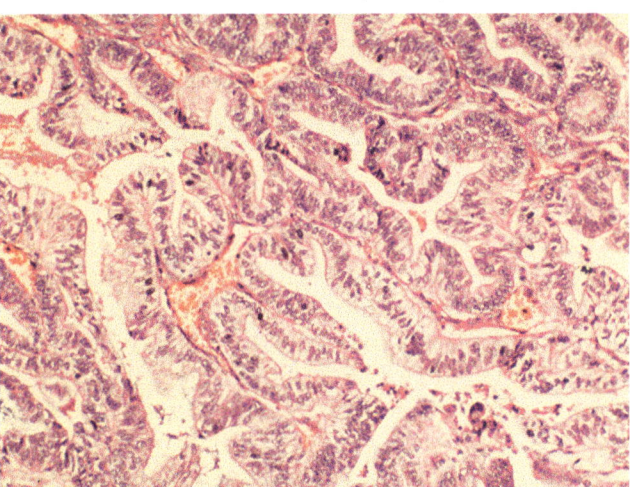

**Figure 13.47:** Endometrioid carcinoma: The glands show secretory change

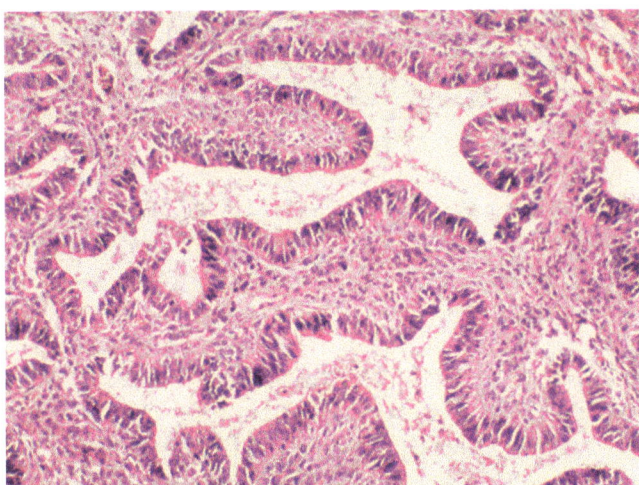

**Figure 13.45:** Endometrioid carcinoma: Closely packed malignant glands

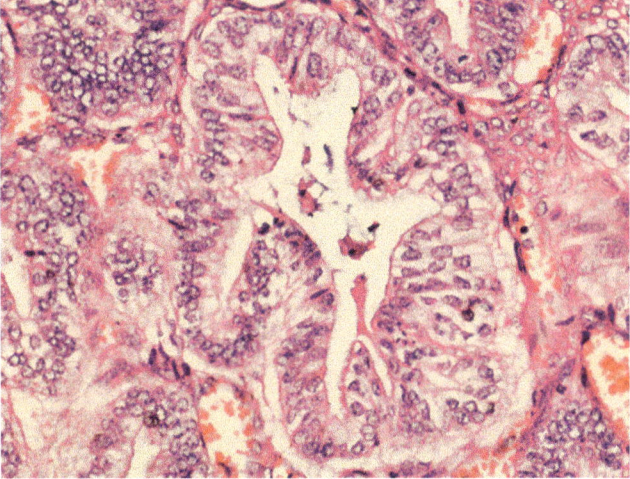

**Figure 13.48:** Endometrioid carcinoma: Higher magnification with secretory change in the gland

endometrioid carcinoma often show tubular or round glands and small rosette-like glands and resembles Call-Exner bodies. (2) Sertoli cell or Sertoli-Leydig cell pattern: The tumor shows multiple hollow tubules, solid tubules with small openings and small glands in a fibromatous stroma. The stroma may show luteinized cells. The epithelial cells are often arranged as thin cords and mimic sex cord.

### Immunohistochemistry

Endometrioid carcinomas are positive for CK7, EMA, B72.3, ER and PR. The cells may also vimentin positivity in 30% cases. The tumor cells are negative for inhibin, WT1 and p16.

### Molecular Genetics

Endometrioid carcinomas show somatic mutations of beta-catenin (CTNB1) and PTEN gene (20%). The CTNB1 mutation of endometrioid carcinoma show good prognosis.[24] PTEN mutation probably occurs in early stage of endometrioid carcinomas. Microsatellite instability (MI) is seen in 12–19% cases of endometrioid carcinomas. MI occurs due to MLH1 promoter methylation.[25]

### Differential Diagnosis

a. **Metastatic colonic carcinoma**: The metastatic colonic carcinoma shows garland-like pattern of the glands lined by tall columnar epithelial cells. Dirty necrosis is also seen in the background. Colonic carcinomas are always strongly positive for CK 20 and negative for CK7.
b. **Sex cord-stromal tumor**: The differentiating features are highlighted in Table 13.5.
c. **Clear cell carcinoma**: The following features are helpful; (1) Hobnail appearance in clear cell carcinoma, (2) High grade nuclei in clear cell carcinoma, (3) Both basal and supranuclear vacuoles in endometrioid carcinoma.

Table 13.5: Endometrioid carcinoma of sex cord variant versus Sertoli-Leydig cell tumor

| Features | Endometrioid carcinoma of sex cord variant | Sertoli-Leydig cell tumor |
|---|---|---|
| Age | Pre and post-menopausal | Younger patient |
| Virilizing features | Absent | Present |
| Squamous metaplasia | Present | Absent |
| Adenofibromatous component | Present | Absent |
| Endometriotic foci | May be present | Absent |
| Immunohistochemistry | | |
| EMA | Positive | Negative |
| Inhibin | Negative | Positive |

### Treatment and Prognosis

Endometrioid carcinoma is treated like other surface epithelial malignancy of ovary. The prognosis of endometrioid carcinoma depends on the FIGO staging. Five year survival of stage I carcinoma confined to ovary is 78% compared to 63%, 24% and 6% in stage II, III and IV respectively.[26]

## MALIGNANT MÜLLERIAN MIXED TUMOR (CARCINOSARCOMA)

Malignant Müllerian mixed tumor (MMMT) is rare and represents less than 1% of all ovarian carcinomas. This tumor is also known as carcinosarcoma and metaplastic carcinoma.

### Clinical Features

Malignant Müllerian mixed tumor occurs in elderly females from 6th to 8th decade and mean age of the patient is 66 years. The clinical presentation of the MMMT is similar to other ovarian tumors.

### Histogenesis

Malignant Müllerian mixed tumor is developed from the ovarian surface epithelium or from endometriotic foci. As mentioned in the Chapter of uterus, both the epithelial and mesenchymal tumor components are monoclonal in origin. The gene mutational analysis and LOH studies have shown similar genetic changes in both the epithelial and mesenchymal components of MMMT.[27] MMMT is primarily an epithelial tumor that secondarily develops mesenchymal component by metaplastic changes.

### Macroscopy

MMMT is usually bulky and fleshy tumor with large solid areas. Foci of hemorrhage and necrosis are also seen. The tumor is bilateral in 33% cases.

### Histopathology (Figures 13.49 to 13.56)

Similar to uterine tumor mentioned in previous Chapter, MMMT is composed of both adenocarcinoma and sarcoma elements. The adenocarcinoma element is commonly endometrioid carcinoma and high-grade serous carcinoma. Occasionally, clear cell carcinoma, mucinous carcinoma and squamous cell carcinoma elements are also seen. The sarcomatous component is usually divided into homologous or heterologous elements. The homologous component may show leiomyosarcoma, endometrial stromal sarcoma, undifferentiated sarcoma, and malignant fibrous histiocytoma. The heterologous component commonly consists of rhabdomyosarcoma and occasionally chondrosarcoma. Rarely, the heterologous element shows osteosarcoma or liposarcoma.

## 196 Essentials of Gynecologic Pathology

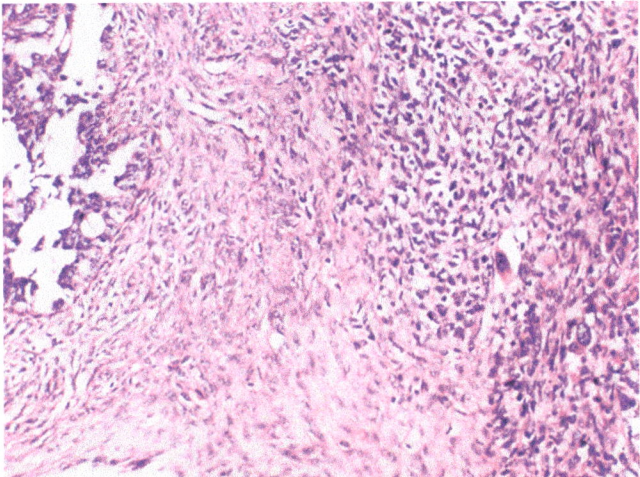

**Figure 13.49:** Malignant Müllerian mixed tumor: Tumor shows both carcinoma and sarcoma elements

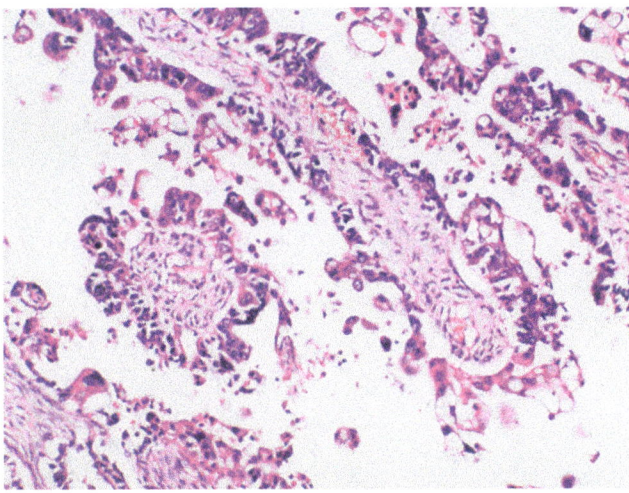

**Figure 13.52:** Malignant Müllerian mixed tumor: High-grade serous carcinoma area showing papillae-like structures with fibrovascular core

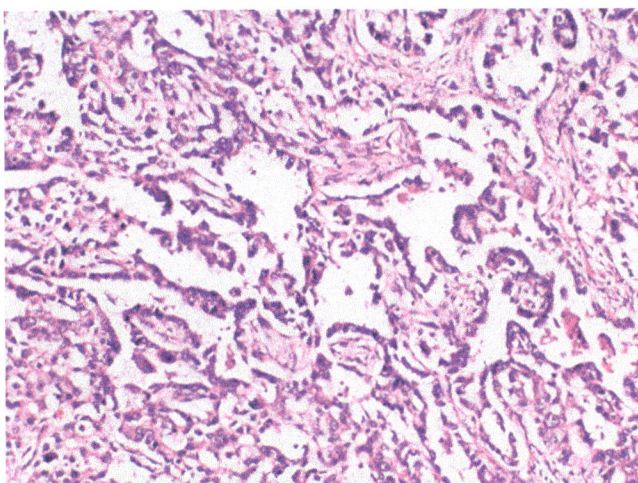

**Figure 13.50:** Malignant Müllerian mixed tumor: High-grade serous carcinoma area

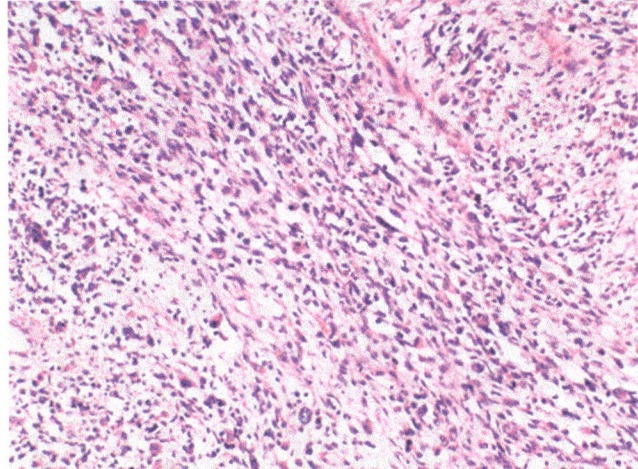

**Figure 13.53:** Malignant Müllerian mixed tumor: Sarcomatous area showing oval to spindle cells

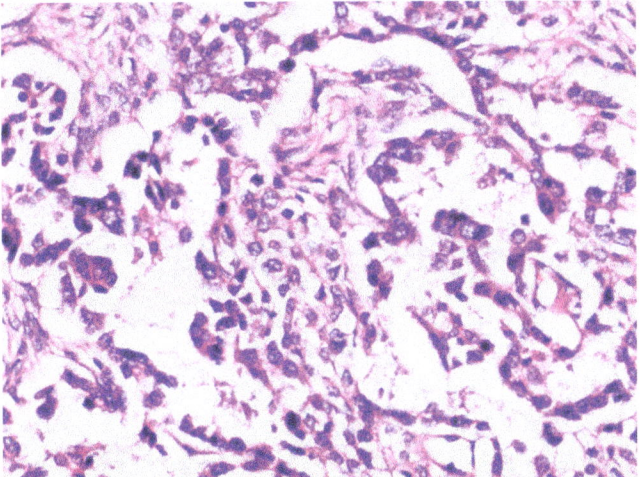

**Figure 13.51:** Malignant Müllerian mixed tumor: High-grade serous carcinoma area show glands lined by moderately pleomorphic cells

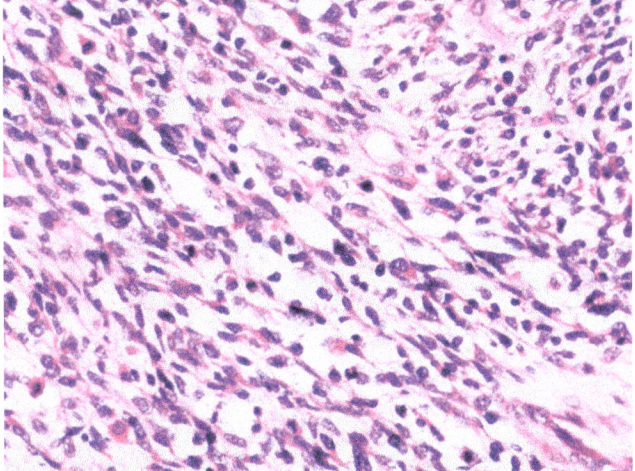

**Figure 13.54:** Malignant Müllerian mixed tumor: Higher magnification shows oval to spindle cells with moderate nuclear pleomorphism

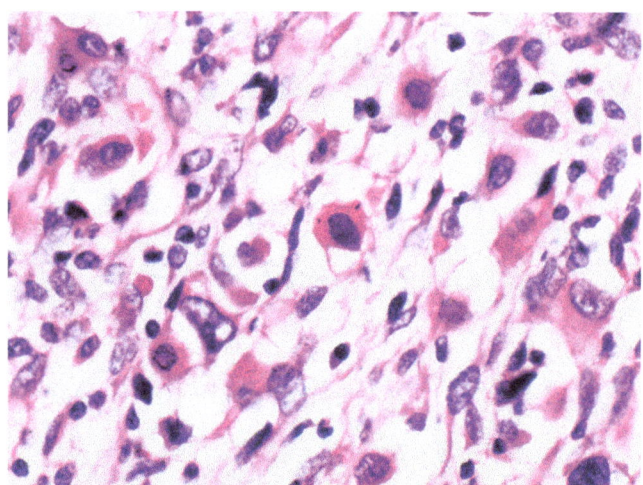

Figure 13.55: Malignant Müllerian mixed tumor: Rhabdoid differentiation in the sarcomatous area

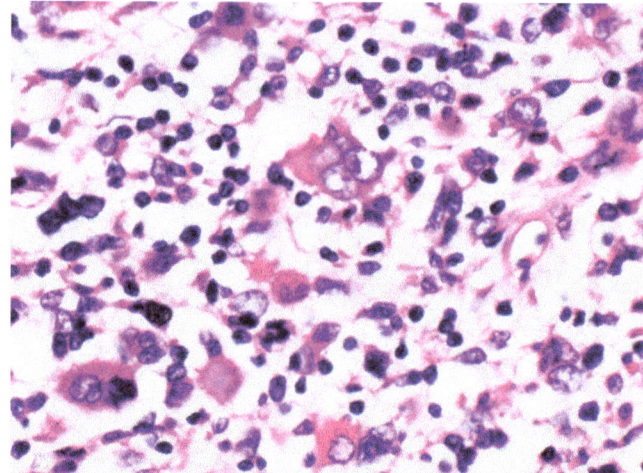

Figure 13.56: Malignant Müllerian mixed tumor with rhabdoid differentiation: The cells with abundant eosinophilic cytoplasm and large pleomorphic nuclei

### Immunohistochemistry

The carcinoma component is positive for cytokeratin, and epithelial membrane antigen. Mesenchymal element is positive for vimentin. The sarcomatous component often shows CK and EMA positivity. Homologous sarcomatous components are positive for CD10 and CD34. In addition, leiomyosarcoma is positive for smooth muscle actin. Rhabdomyosarcoma shows desmin and myogenin positivity. Chondrosarcoma element is positive for S-100.

### Differential Diagnosis

Immature teratoma: Immature teratoma may simulate MMMT. However, the following features suggest immature teratoma: (1) Younger age of the patient, (2) All three germ layers, (3) Immature neural elements.

### Prognosis

Majority of MMMT (>70%) presents in stage III or stage IV. The tumor has poor prognosis and overall 5 year survival is 18–27 months. The median survival is 19 months.

## ENDOMETRIOID STROMAL SARCOMA

Endometrioid stromal sarcoma (ESS) is a rare tumor and is the counterpart of the uterine endometrioid stromal sarcoma. The tumor may occur from 10 to 75 years of age, however it commonly occurs around 50–60 years. The clinical symptoms of ESS is similar to any other ovarian carcinoma.

### Gross

The tumor is usually unilateral (more than 75% cases), large and more than 15 cm in diameter. It is mostly solid, firm with foci of variable sized cysts containing mucoid material or blood.

### Histopathology (Figures 13.57 to 13.59)

Near about 50% cases of ESS show features of endometriosis. The tumor is mainly composed of small round to oval cells or occasionally spindle shaped cells. The cells have scanty pale cytoplasm and relatively monomorphic nuclei. The tumor contains multiple small thick walled vessels that simulate spiral arterioles of the uterus. The individual cells are arranged around the vessels in a concentric manner. The reticulin stain shows group of tumor cells surrounded by reticulin fibers.

### Immunohistochemistry

Endometrioid stromal sarcoma is positive for vimentin and CD10. The tumor shows focal positivity of CK and muscle associated protein.

### Differential Diagnosis

a. Adenosarcoma,
b. Granulosa cell tumor: The following features favor ESS:
   1. Lack of nuclear grooving,
   2. Typical reticulin stain around individual cells,
   3. Presence of endometriosis,
   4. Negative inhibin and calretinin immunostain.

### Prognosis

More than 50% of the ESS presents with extraovarian spread at the time of diagnosis. Therefore, the stage of the tumor is an important prognostic factor. Undifferentiated tumors have adverse prognosis.

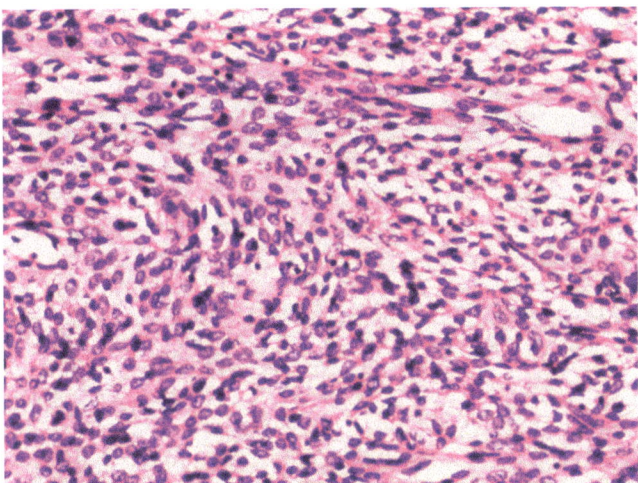

Figure 13.57: Endometrioid stromal sarcoma of ovary: Diffuse sheet of round to spindly cells

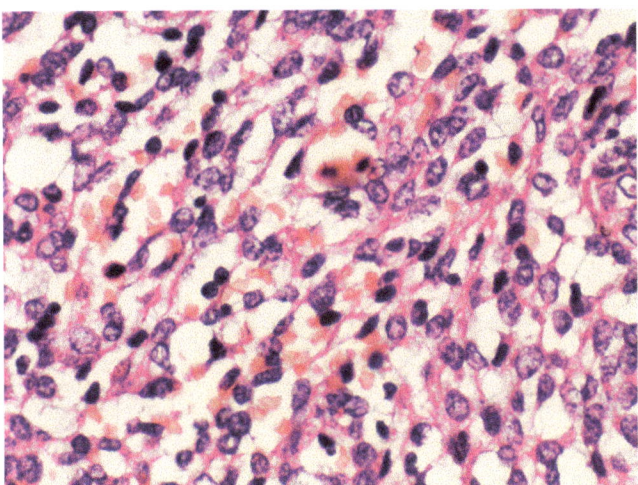

Figure 13.58: Endometrioid stromal sarcoma of ovary: Higher magnification of the same

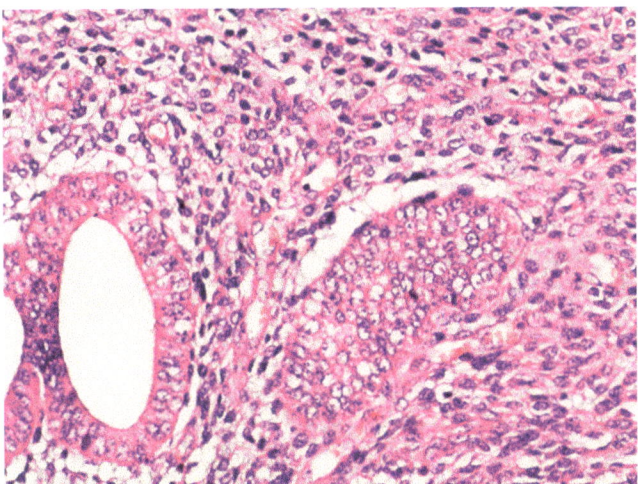

Figure 13.59: Endometrioid stromal sarcoma of ovary: Endometriotic foci along with the tumor

### Treatment

Total abdominal hysterectomy with bilateral salpingo-oophorectomy is the treatment of choice. In recurrent or residual cases progesterone therapy and radiotherapy have been used.

## CLEAR CELL TUMORS OF OVARY

Clear cell tumors are the group of surface epithelial tumors that contain predominantly clear cells or hobnail cells. However, the other types of cells such as oxyphil cells, flat cell and cuboidal cells are also admixed with clear cell tumors. The majority of clear cell tumors are clear cell carcinoma (CCC) that represents 8.5% of all ovarian carcinomas. Benign variety of clear cell tumors is exceptionally rare and borderline clear cell tumors represent only 1% of ovarian tumors.

### Clear Cell Adenofibroma

Clear cell adenofibroma is composed of benign glands or cysts that are lined by cells with clear cytoplasm and hobnail cells in dense connective tissue stroma. This tumor is very rare.

*Gross*

Grossly clear cell adenofibroma is solid cystic tumor with median diameter 12 cm. Cut section shows honey combed appearance with rubbery stroma.

*Microscopy*

The tumor shows multiple tubular glands in a fibrocollagenous stroma. The glands are lined by single to multiple layers of hobnail cells. The individual cells are oval to polygonal with abundant eosinophilic or granular cytoplasm. The nuclei show mild atypia. Mitotic activity is rare.

### Borderline Clear Cell Tumor

This is also very uncommon tumor and represents less than 1% of all ovarian tumors. The mean age of borderline clear cell tumor is 60–70 year.

*Gross*

Gross appearance of borderline clear cell tumor is similar to that of its benign counterpart. However, this tumor may be much fleshier in appearance.

*Microscopy*

The tumor shows similar morphological appearance as that of clear cell adenofibroma. In addition, the lining epithelial cells show much more proliferation of cells along with moderate nuclear enlargement and pleomorphism.

*Prognosis*

Following removal of the ovary the tumor behaves in a benign fashion.

## Clear Cell Carcinoma

Clear cell carcinoma (CCC) comprises the vast majority of clear cell tumors of ovary (more than 90%). The mean age of CCC is 57 year. The patients present with pelvic or abdominal mass. This tumor has the highest association with ovarian and pelvic endometriosis. The patients often have paraneoplastic syndrome and hypercalcemia. Near about 18–46% patients of CCC show thromboembolic events in the form of deep venous thrombosis and pulmonary emboli.[28]

*Macroscopy*

The size of the CCC varies from few cm to 30 cm and the mean diameter is 15 cm. The tumor is predominantly solid and partly cystic. The surface of CCC is nodular. The cut section shows solid grey white to tan areas (Figure 13.60). The tumor may show unilocular or occasionally multilocular cysts filled with watery to mucinous fluid. Soft fleshy polypoidal mass often protrudes from the lumen.

*Histopathology (Figures 13.61 to 13.65)*

Clear cell carcinoma shows tubulocystic, papillary or solid pattern. There may be admixture of these patterns in a same tumor. Papillary and tubulocystic patterns are the commonest pattern of CCC and solid pattern is uncommon.

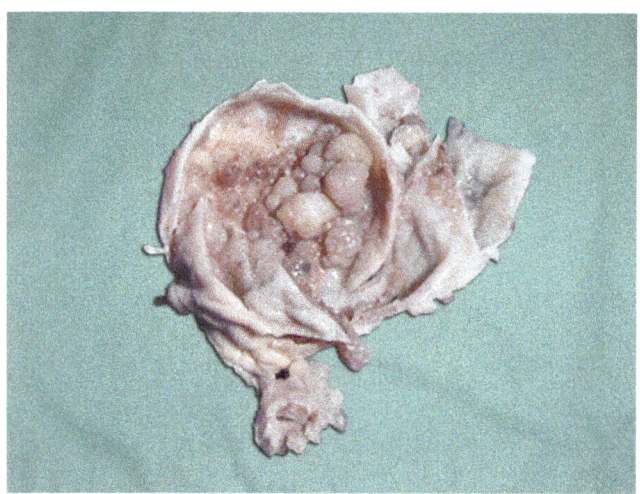

Figure 13.60: Clear cell carcinoma of ovary: Solid cystic growth on cut section

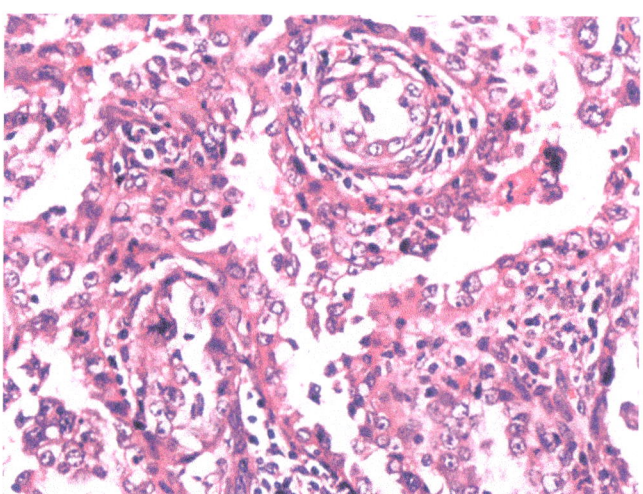

Figure 13.62: Clear cell carcinoma: Tubular and cystic pattern

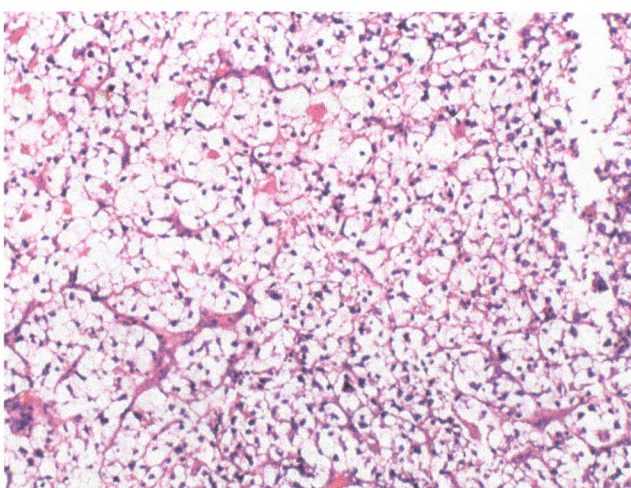

Figure 13.61: Clear cell carcinoma: Solid sheet of cells with clear vacuolated cytoplasm

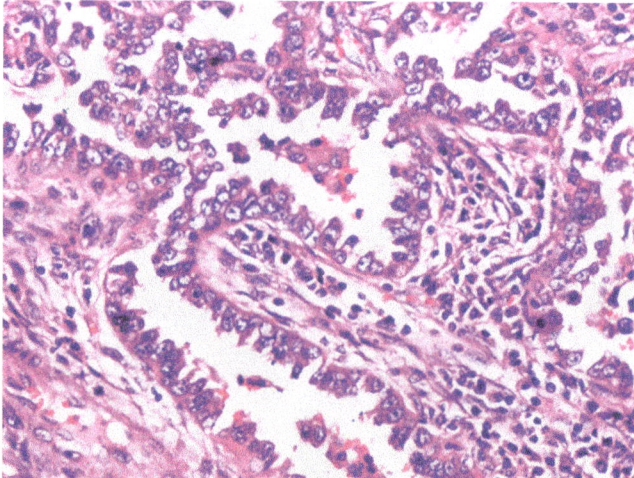

Figure 13.63: Clear cell carcinoma: Tubular pattern of cells with hobnail appearance

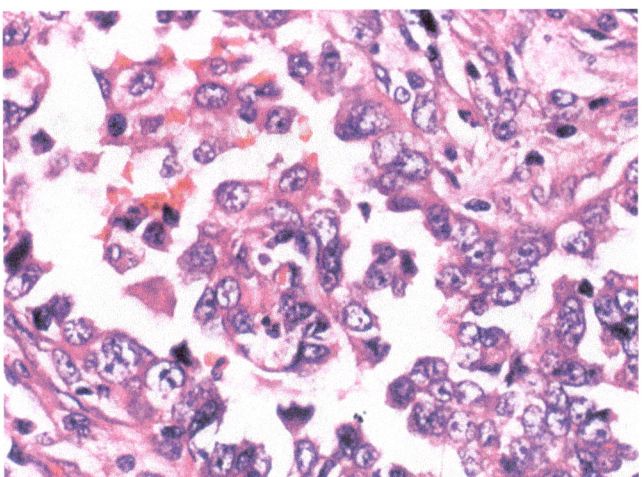

Figure 13.64: Clear cell carcinoma: Higher magnification of the same

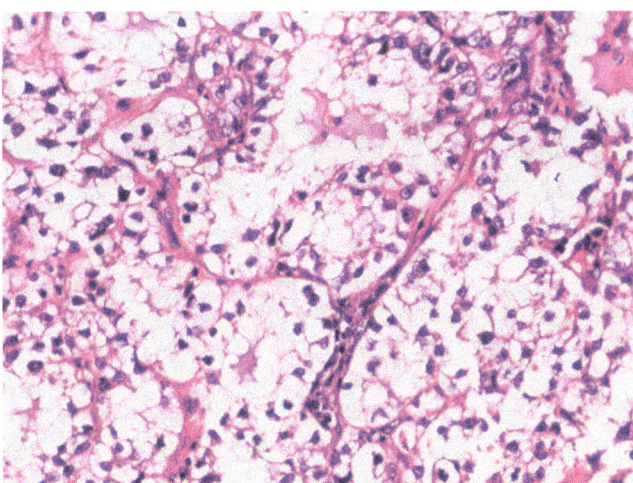

Figure 13.65: Clear cell carcinoma: Solid nests of cells composed of clear cells with central nuclei

The papillary pattern shows thick or thin complex branching papillary structures with fibrovascular stroma or abundant hyalinized material. The papillae are lined by clear cell or hobnail cells. The tubulocystic pattern shows multiple tubular glands or cysts with variable size that are lined by cuboidal cells or hobnail cells. The solid pattern shows diffuse sheets of polygonal cells with clear cytoplasm separated by thick fibrous or hyalinized stroma. Rarely, the tumor may show reticular pattern that simulates yolk sac tumor. Clear cell carcinomas predominantly show clear cell and hobnail cells. The clear cells are cuboidal or polyhedral cells with abundant clear cytoplasm. The nuclei are central in position with vesicular chromatin and prominent nucleoli. The cytoplasm of the clear cells show abundant glycogen demonstrated by PAS stain. Hobnail cells are cuboidal in shape and contain granular eosinophilic or clear cytoplasm. The nuclei of the cells are hyperchromatic and protrude into the lumen crossing the cytoplasmic limits. In addition the tumor may also contain other cells such as oxyphil cells, cuboidal cells, flat cells and rarely signet ring cells. Amorphous eosinophilic hyaline globules are often noted in CCC. They are frequently seen within the stroma and also in the core of the papillae. These globules are PAS positive. The hyaline globule is probably derived from the basement membrane as they are positive for type IV collagen and laminin. CCC is frequently associated with endometriosis in more than 50% cases.[29]

The association of CCC and endometriosis may be as high as 88% particularly in cystic variant of CCC. CCC is subdivided into three groups:

1. **Cystic clear cell carcinomas**: This group of tumor is thought to originate from endometriosis
2. **Adenofibromatous clear cell carcinomas**: This tumor is originated from adenofibroma
3. **Indeterminate**: The probable origin is obscured. It was noted that cystic clear cell carcinomas had better prognosis and most of the tumors were related with endometriosis.

*Immunocytochemistry*

Clear cell carcinoma is positive for CK, EMA, B 72.3 and Leu M1. The tumor is negative for alpha fetoprotein, CK20, p53, and CD 10.

*Somatic Genetics*

The genetic alterations of CCC are similar to that of endometrioid carcinoma. CCC often shows KRAS, BRAF, and TP53 mutation.[30] Near about 20% of CCC shows PTEN mutation. The inactivation of PTEN gene due to mutation is probably an early event of carcinogenesis.

*Differential Diagnosis*

a. **Yolk sac tumor**: Following feature are helpful to diagnose yolk sac tumor: (1) Young age, (2) High alpha fetoprotein, (3) Presence of Schiller-Duval bodies, (4) Lack of hyalinized core in papillae.
b. **Dysgerminoma**: The following feature favor dysgerminoma: (1) Young age, (2) Round cells rather polyhedral cells in CCC, (3) Central nuclei with multiple prominent nucleoli, (4) Sprinkling of lymphocytes, (5) Positive placental alkaline phosphatase.
c. **Krukenberg's tumor**: Rarely, CCC may show predominantly signet ring type of cells containing mucin. This type of CCC may be confused with Krukenberg's tumor. The following features are helpful in diagnosis of Krukenberg's tumor: (1) In 80% cases, Krukenberg's

tumors are bilateral, (2) "Targetoid" appearance of CCC is not seen in Krukenberg's tumor, (3) Tubular or tubulocystic pattern is lacking in Krukenberg's tumor.
d. **Endometrioid carcinomas with secretory changes** may mimic CCC. The following features favors endometrioid carcinoma: (1) Lack of any hobnail appearance, (2) Both basal and supranuclear vacuoles in endometrioid carcinoma, (3) The presence of hyaline globules.

*Prognosis*

Near about 43% of CCC presents in FIGO stage I. Compared to serous adenocarcinoma, the prognosis of CCC is mildly lower. The 5 year survival of CCC is 69%, 55%, 14% and 4% in stage I, II, III and IV tumor respectively.

## TRANSITIONAL CELL TUMOR

Transitional cell tumors of ovary are the group of surface epithelial tumors that are composed of epithelial cells resembling transitional cells of urinary bladder. The transitional cell tumor of ovary represents 1–2% of all ovarian tumors. The cytokeratin profile of transitional cell tumor favors Müllerian (CK7 positive, CK20 negative) rather than urothelial tumor (CK20 positive).

### Benign Brenner Tumor

Benign Brenner tumor represents 4–5% of all benign epithelial tumors. The patients are usually 30–60 years old and the mean age is 56 years. The majority of the patients are asymptomatic and the tumor is detected incidentally. The size of the tumor varies macroscopical to several cm. More than 50% of Brenner tumors are less than 2 cm in diameter at the time of detection.

*Gross*

Brenner tumor is usually solid well-circumscribed with bosselated lesion with smooth outer surface. The cut section of the tumor is solid, gray white, nodular and fibrous mass. The tumor may show small cysts and rarely the tumor is predominantly cystic. Approximately, one-fourth of Brenner tumor is associated with mucinous neoplasm.

*Histopathology (Figures 13.66 to 13.70)*

Brenner tumor shows nests, islands and cords of transitional epithelial cells in fibrous stroma. The individual cells show abundant clear cytoplasm with well-defined cell border. The nuclei of the cells are round with small nucleoli and central longitudinal groove giving characteristic "coffee bean" appearance. The nests of cells may show central lumen-like structure with mucinous material. The tumor may be cystic and the cysts may be lined by transitional cells or mucin

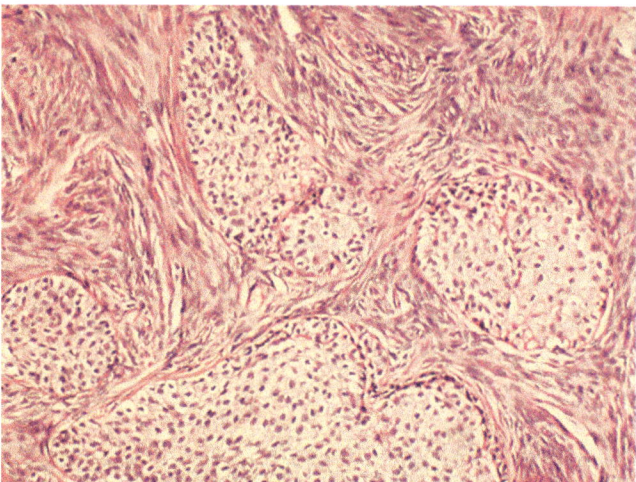
**Figure 13.66:** Brenner tumor: Nests, islands and cords of transitional epithelial cells in fibrous stroma

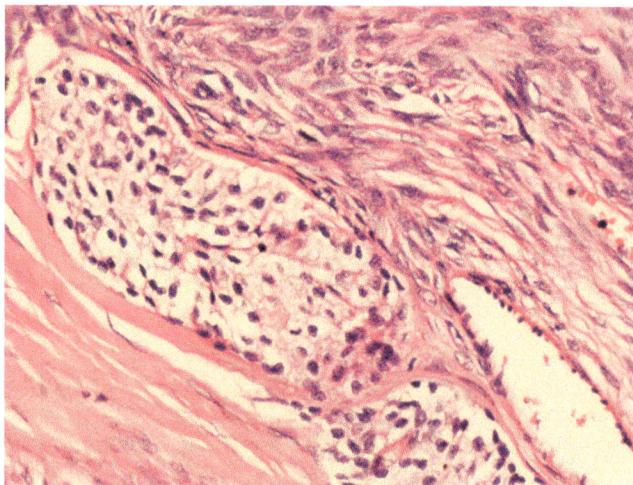
**Figure 13.67:** Brenner tumor: Higher magnification shows nests of transitional cells

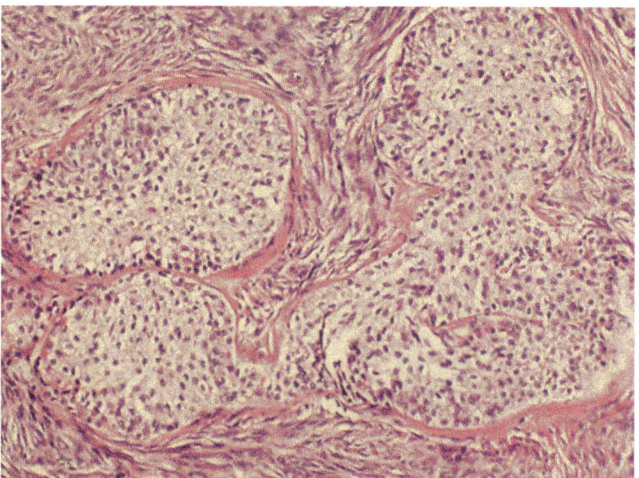
**Figure 13.68:** Brenner tumor: Higher magnification shows nests of transitional cells

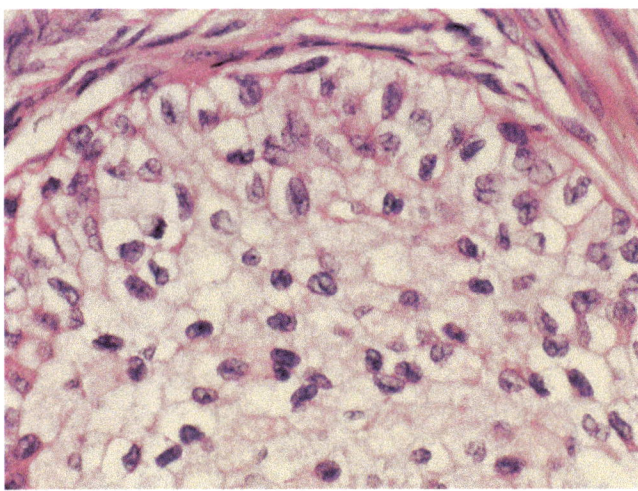

**Figure 13.69:** Brenner tumor: The cells show abundant clear cytoplasm with well-defined cell border. Nuclei are round with longitudinal groove

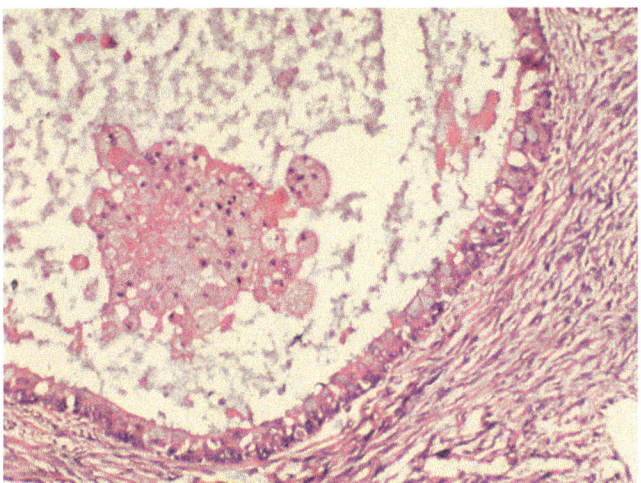

**Figure 13.70:** Brenner tumor: Brenner with mucinous element

secreting columnar cells. In case of extensive mucinous changes in the epithelial lining, the tumor may be designated as "metaplastic Brenner tumor". This tumor should not be labeled as mixed epithelial tumor as the two types of epithelium are intimately admixed rather than separate.

*Immunohistochemistry*

Benign Brenner tumor is positive for uroplakin. However, this tumor is negative for CK20 and thrombomodulin.

## Borderline Brenner Tumor

The borderline Brenner tumor (BBT) is also known as proliferating Brenner tumor and Brenner tumor of low malignant potential. Borderline Brenner tumor represents only 3–5% of Brenner tumor. The patients are usually elderly women and the mean age of the patient is 59 year. The patients present with mass abdomen and pain.

*Gross*

The Borderline Brenner tumor is mostly unilateral tumor. The tumor is well-circumscribed and larger than benign Brenner tumor. The average size of the tumor is 14 cm in diameter. The tumor is solid and partly cystic. The cut section shows friable polypoid mass projecting from the cyst wall.

*Histopathology*

The tumor shows complex architectural pattern compared to Brenner tumor. The branching papillae arise from the cyst wall lined by transitional epithelial cells resembling low-grade transitional carcinoma of bladder. The other part of the cyst wall is lined by transitional epithelium. The tumor cells show mild increased of nucleocytoplasmic ratio. The nuclei show mild atypia. The mitotic activity of the tumor cells is variable. The wall of the cyst invariably shows nests of benign transitional epithelial cells.

*Prognosis*

The borderline Brenner tumor without any stromal invasion behaves like a benign ovarian tumor.

## Malignant Brenner Tumor

Malignant Brenner tumor represents only 5% of all Brenner tumors. The patients are 50 to 70 years of age and the mean age of the patient is 63 years. The patient presents with vague abdominal pain and swelling.

*Gross*

Approximately, 16% of malignant Brenner tumor is bilateral. The tumor shows both solid and cystic component. The cyst shows solid friable polypoid areas.

*Histopathology (Figures 13.71 to 13.74)*

For the diagnosis of malignant Brenner tumor there should be foci of benign or borderline Brenner tumor. The malignant Brenner tumor simulates high-grade transitional cell carcinoma. The branching papillae and cords of cells invade the deeper stroma of the tumor. The cells are polygonal with moderate amount of cytoplasm. The nuclei are round, regular with moderately pleomorphic. Mitotic figures are numerous. Small and large cysts with foci of hemorrhage are also seen.

*Prognosis*

The malignant Brenner tumor has excellent prognosis and 5-year survival rate is 88% in stage IA tumor.

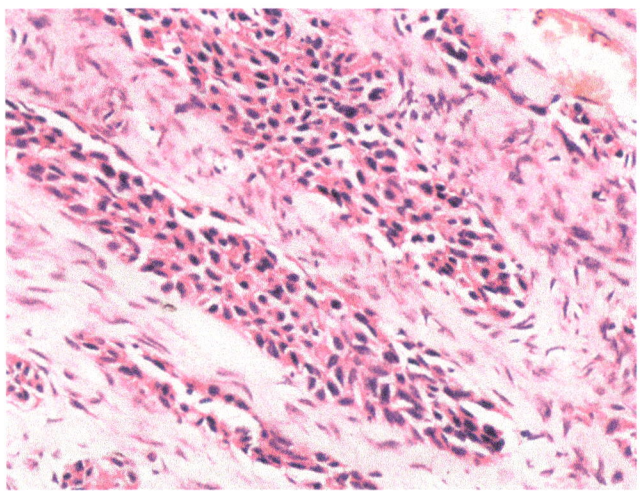

Figure 13.71: Malignant Brenner tumor: Nests of malignant cells within the stroma

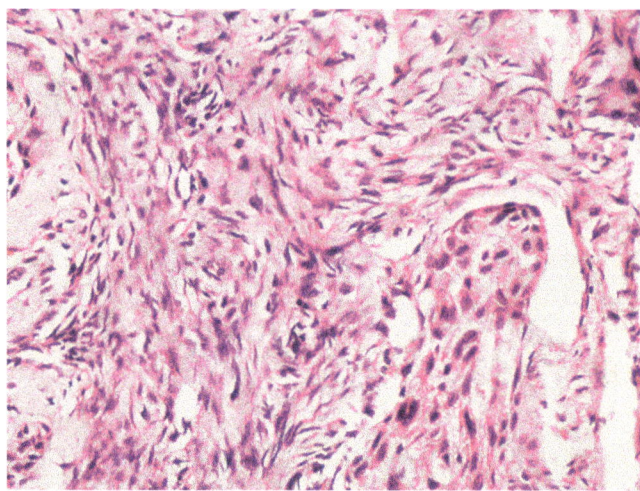

Figure 13.73: Malignant Brenner tumor: Tumor cells infiltrating in the stroma

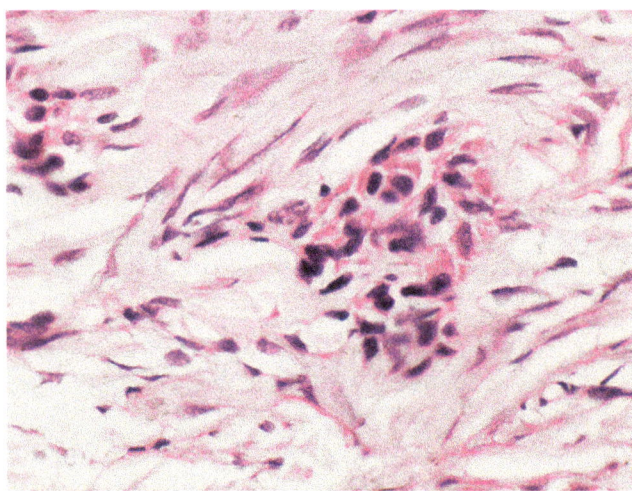

Figure 13.72: Malignant Brenner tumor: Tumor cells are polygonal with moderate amount of cytoplasm having pleomorphic nuclei

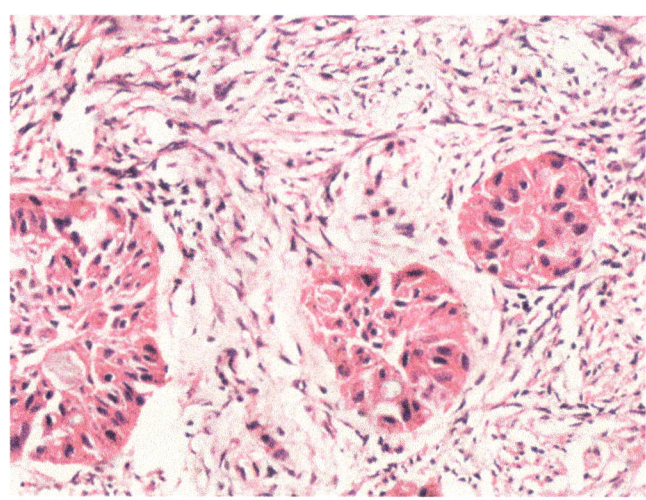

Figure 13.74: Malignant Brenner tumor: Higher magnification shows transitional cells with moderate nuclear atypia

## Transitional Cell Carcinoma

The transitional cell carcinoma (TCC) represents 6% of all ovarian carcinomas. The mean age of TCC is 56 year. The clinical presentation of the tumor is similar to that of other surface epithelial tumors of ovary. Approximately 15% TCCs are bilateral. The tumor is partly solid and partly cystic. The average diameter of the tumor is 10 cm. Grossly, the cyst resembles serous cyst adenocarcinoma.

### Histopathology (Figures 13.75 to 13.78)

Transitional cell carcinoma resembles high-grade urothelial carcinomas; however, it lacks any benign or borderline component of Brenner tumor. Two types of histological pattern of TCC are seen.[31] In the first type, TCC shows multiple papillary clusters lined by multilayered epithelial cells. The papillae shows fibrovascular core. The luminal surface of such papillae is smooth. The individual cells show moderately abundant cytoplasm with marked nuclear atypia. The nuclei show multiple prominent nucleoli. Mitotic activity is high. The tumors shows obvious invasion as nests and sheets of cells invade the deeper stromal tissue. The papillary pattern is commonly seen. The second type of TCC shows solid Brenner-like growth pattern. Here the tumor shows solid sheets of cells that invade the adjacent stroma.

### Immunohistochemistry

Ovarian TCC shows positive CK7, vimentin and CA 125. Unlike urothelial carcinoma of bladder, ovarian TCC is negative for uroplakin, CK20 and thrombomodulin.

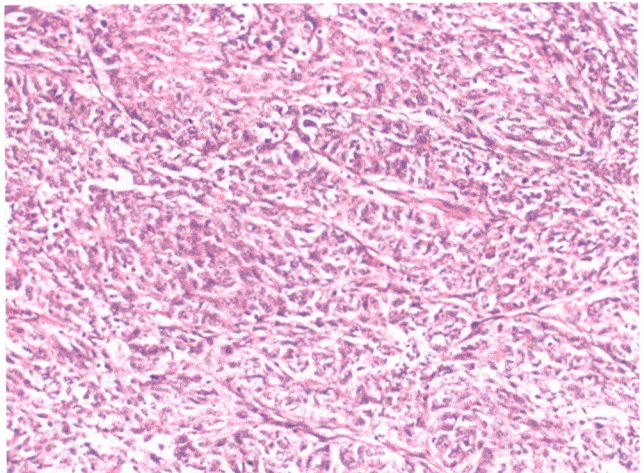

**Figure 13.75:** Transitional cell carcinoma of ovary: Solid nests of malignant transitional cells

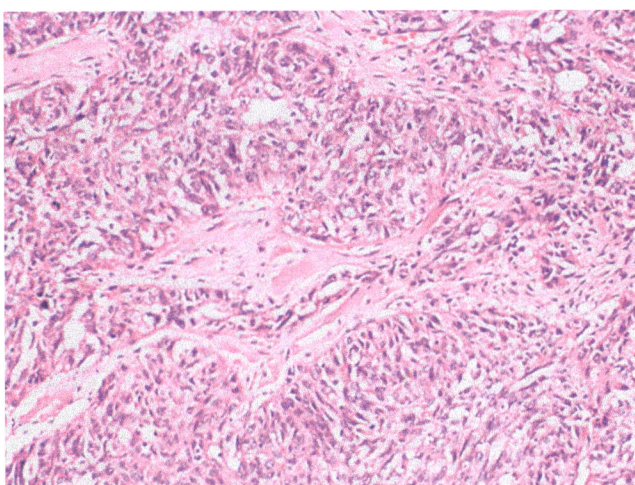

**Figure 13.77:** Transitional cell carcinoma of ovary: Nests of transitional cells invading in the stroma

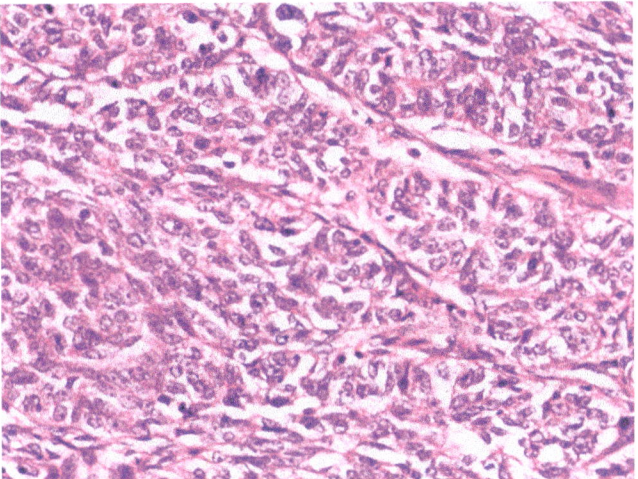

**Figure 13.76:** Transitional cell carcinoma of ovary: Higher magnification of the transitional cells

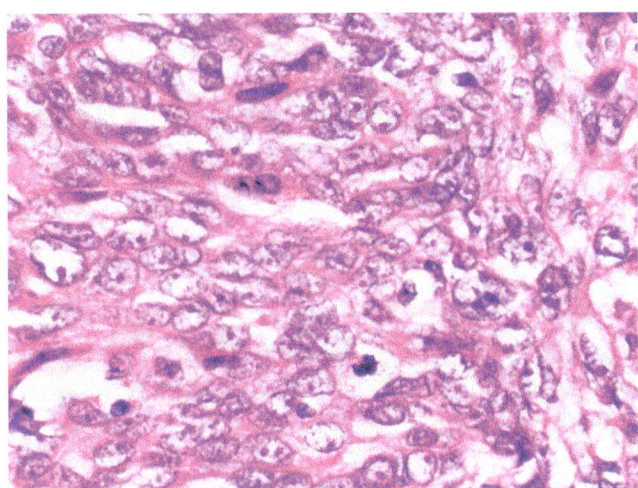

**Figure 13.78:** Transitional cell carcinoma of ovary: Higher magnifications shows moderate atypia and frequent mitosis

*Differential Diagnosis*

a. Undifferentiated carcinoma: Secondary to tumor necrosis pseudopapillae may be formed in undifferentiated carcinomas that may simulate TCC.
b. Adult type of granulosa cell tumor (AGCT): Occasionally, microspaces in TCC may simulate AGCT. The microspaces of TCC are larger and of variable sized than that of Call–Exner bodies. Moreover nuclei of TCC show prominent nucleoli. The mitotic activity in TCC is also higher compared to AGCT.

*Prognosis*

TCC responds better than high-grade serous adenocarcinoma and the overall 5-year survival rate of TCC is 35%.

## MIXED EPITHELIAL TUMOR

Mixed epithelial tumor is characterized by the presence of two or more types of epithelium consisting of at least more than 10% of the tumor mass out of the main five types of epithelium that include serous, mucinous transitional, clear and endometrioid. Endometrioid tumor with squamous differentiation and neuroendocrine tumors in association with other surface epithelial tumors are not considered as mixed epithelial tumor. The mixed epithelial tumor may be benign, borderline or malignant in nature.

### Histology

Most common mixed epithelial tumor is serous with mucinous epithelium. The mucinous epithelial cells show abundant mucinous material. Brenner tumor often shows associated mucinous tumor. The Brenner component may be benign or borderline. Brenner tumor with foci of mucinous metaplasia should not be designated as mixed epithelial tumor. The other combinations of mixed epithelial tumors are serous-endometrioid, endometrioid clear cell, and serous clear cell combination.

### Prognosis

The prognostic behavior of mixed epithelial tumor depends on the behavior of the dominant cell types and FIGO staging of the ovarian tumor.

## SQUAMOUS CELL CARCINOMA

Pure squamous cell carcinoma of ovary is extremely rare and comprises only 0.5% of all ovarian cancer. Majority of squamous cell carcinoma of ovary is developed from mature teratoma and they should be grouped in germ cell tumors. In case of squamous cell carcinoma of ovary, a careful search should be undertaken to exclude any evidence of metastasis from the cervical squamous cell carcinoma or malignant squamous cell component in metaplastic element of endometrioid carcinoma. The tumor may be solid or solid-cystic. The malignant squamous cells are arranged in diffuse sheets infiltrating within the adjacent stroma (Figures 13.79 and 13.80). Most of the patients of squamous cell carcinoma of ovary present in advanced stage and have poor prognosis.

## UNDIFFERENTIATED CARCINOMA

Undifferentiated carcinomas represent less than 5% of all ovarian carcinomas. Probably the number of such cases is much less if appropriate immunocytochemistry panel is used.[32]

Macroscopically, the tumor is large and solid mass with areas of hemorrhage and necrosis. On histology section the tumor shows diffuse sheets of large cells (Figures 13.81 and 13.82). The individual cells show scanty cytoplasm with large vesicular nuclei having prominent nucleoli. Large pleomorphic cells with bizarre nuclei may also be seen. Areas of high-grade serous carcinoma or foci of transitional cell carcinoma may also be seen.

### Immunohistochemistry

The undifferentiated carcinomas show CK and EMA positivity. These epithelial markers are often weakly positive. Tumors also show B72.3 positivity.

### Differential Diagnosis

a. Diffuse granulosa cell tumor: The following features favor granulosa cell tumor:
   (1) Prominent nuclear groove and fine chromatin,
   (2) Relatively low nuclear grade and low mitosis in comparison to undifferentiated carcinoma,
   (3) Positive inhibin and negative EMA immunostain.
b. Small cell carcinoma
c. Metastatic carcinoma.

### Prognosis

The prognosis of undifferentiated carcinoma is worse than other serous and transitional cell carcinomas of ovary. The overall 5-year survival is only 6%.

## NEUROENDOCRINE CARCINOMA OF THE OVARY

Neuroendocrine carcinoma of the ovary has similar clinical presentation as that of other surface epithelial carcinoma

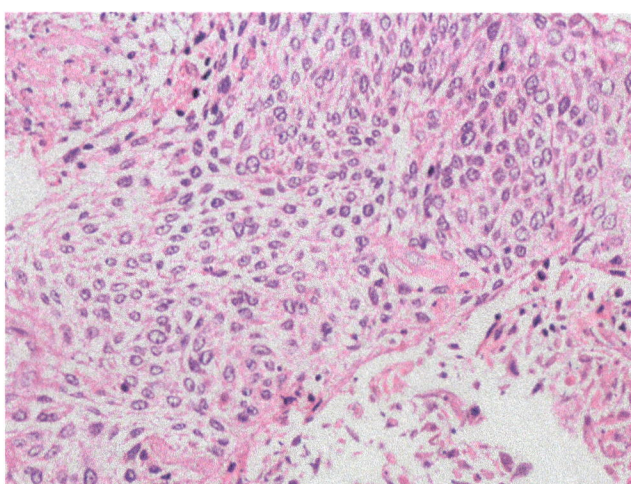

Figure 13.79: Squamous cell carcinoma of ovary: Diffuse sheet of polyhedral squamoid cells with moderate nuclear atypia

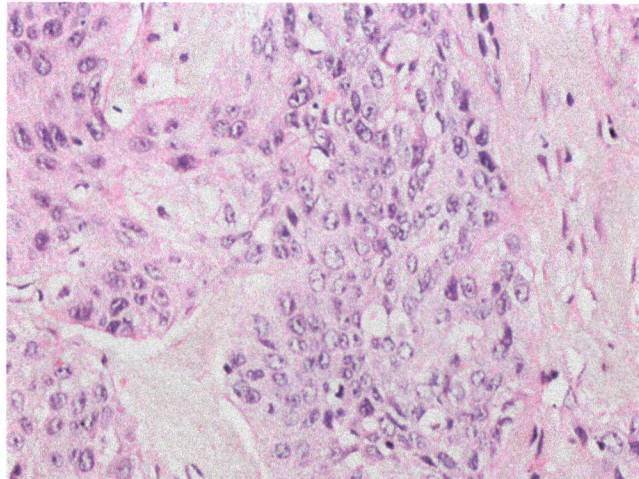

Figure 13.80: Squamous cell carcinoma of ovary: Malignant cells with squamoid differentiation

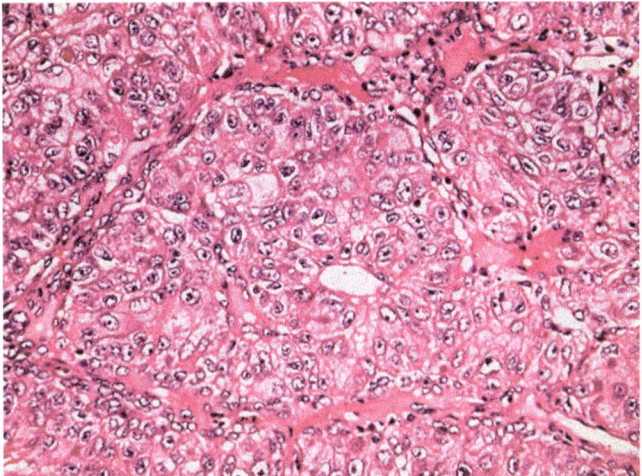

**Figure 13.81:** Undifferentiated carcinoma of ovary: Diffuse sheets of large cells

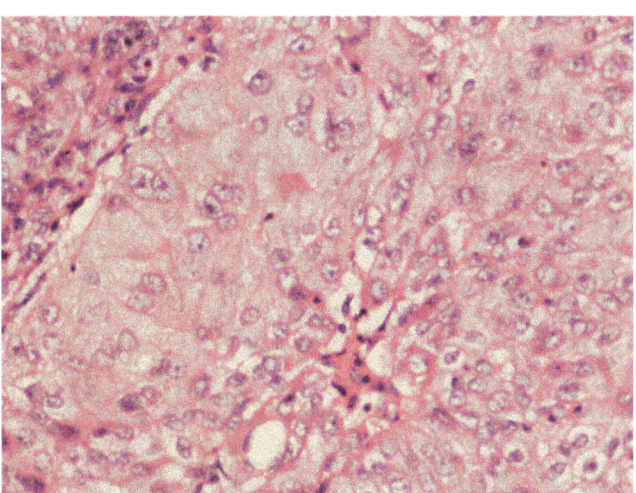

**Figure 13.84:** Large cell type of neuroendocrine carcinoma: Large cells with abundant cytoplasm and centrally placed pleomorphic nuclei with prominent nucleoli

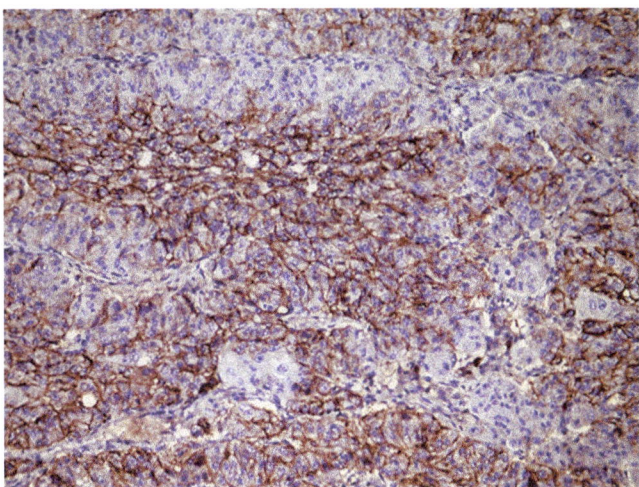

**Figure 13.82:** Undifferentiated carcinoma of ovary: Strong CK7 positive cells

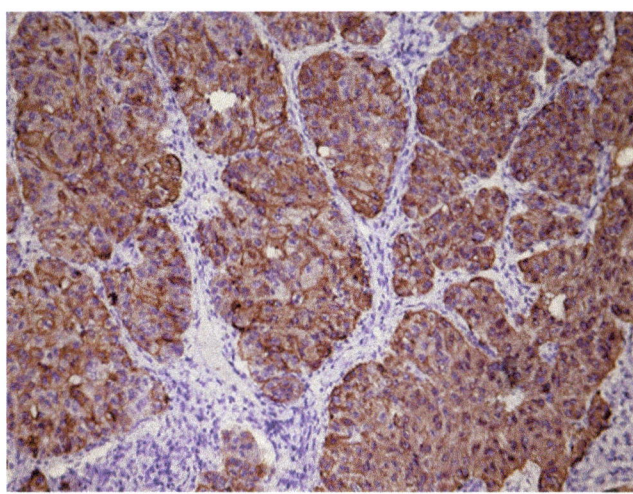

**Figure 13.85:** Large cell type of neuroendocrine carcinoma: Strong CD 56 positive tumor

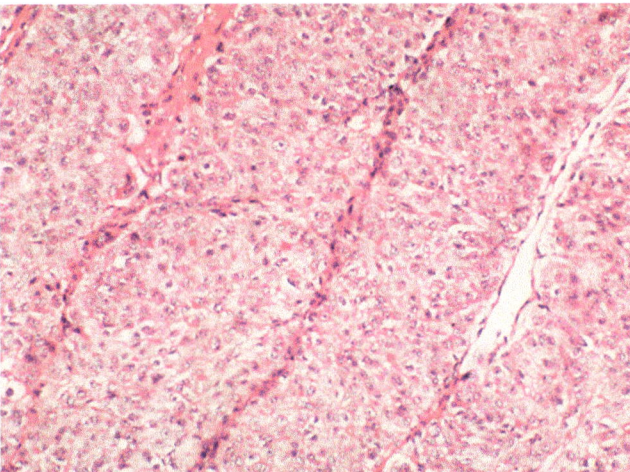

**Figure 13.83:** Large cell type of neuroendocrine carcinoma: Diffuse sheets of malignant cells

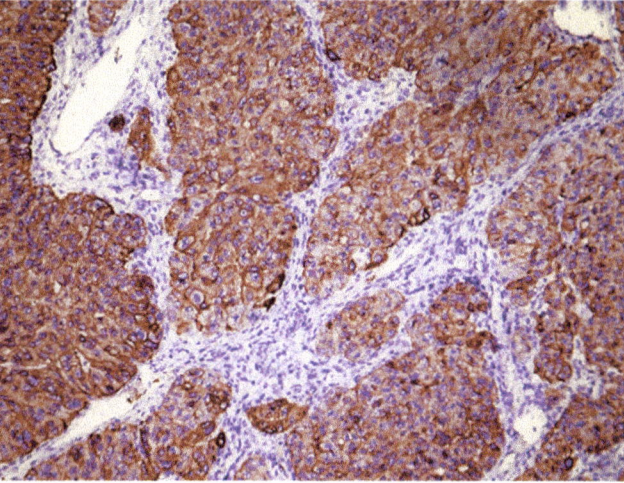

**Figure 13.86:** Large cell type of neuroendocrine carcinoma: Strong CK7 positive tumor

of ovary. The patients often have associated paraneoplastic syndrome particularly hypercalcemia due to secretion of PTH by the tumor cells.[33] The neuroendocrine carcinomas of ovaries are two types:

a. **Small cell type**: It is the most common type and the tumor is identical to small cell carcinoma of lung. The tumor shows nests and diffuse sheets of cells. The individual cells are small round with scanty cytoplasm and dark hyperchromatic nuclei. The nuclei show fine granular chromatin and inconspicuous nucleoli. Nuclear moulding is often seen. The tumor is positive for NSE and CD 56. However, the tumor cells are often negative for chromogranin and synaptophysin. Almost 50% of tumor shows positive CK and EMA.

b. **Large cell type:** Large cell type of neuroendocrine carcinoma shows nests, trabeculae, and sheets of large cells. The individual cells are large with moderate to abundant cytoplasm (Figures 13.83 to 13.86). The nuclei are large with coarse chromatin having prominent large nucleoli. The cells are positive for neuroendocrine and epithelial markers.

## REFERENCES

1. Serov SE, Scully RE, Sobin LH. International histology of tumors (no. 9). Histological typing of ovarian tumors. Geneva, Switzerland: World Health Organization: 1973:9.
2. Kurman RJ, Carcangiu ML, Herrington S, Young RH. WHO classification of tumours of female genital reproductive organs. 4th Edition, International agency for research on Cancer, Lyon; 2014.
3. McKenney JK, Balzer BL, Longacre TA. Patterns of stromal invasion in ovarian serous tumors of low malignant potential (borderline tumors): a reevaluation of the concept of stromal microinvasion. Am J Surg Pathol. 2006;30:1209-21.
4. Michael H, Roth LM. Invasive and noninvasive implants in ovarian serous tumors of low malignant potential. Cancer. 1986;57(6):1240-7.
5. McKenney JK, Balzer BL, Longacre TA. Lymph node involvement in ovarian serous tumors of low malignant potential (borderline tumors): pathology, prognosis, and proposed classification.Am J Surg Pathol. 2006;30:614-24.
6. Burks RT, Sherman ME, Kurman RJ. Micropapillary serous carcinoma of the ovary. A distinctive low-grade carcinoma related to serous borderline tumors. Am J Surg Pathol. 1996;20(11):1319-30.
7. Akeson M, Zetterqvist BM, Dahllof K, et al. Population-based cohort follow-up study of all patients operated for borderline ovarian tumor in western Sweden during an 11-year period. Int J Gynecol Cancer. 2008;18:453-59.
8. Seidman JD, Kurman RJ. Ovarian serous borderline tumors:a critical review of the literature with emphasis on prognostic indicators. Hum Pathol. 2000;31:539-57.
9. Gilks CB, Bell DA, Scully RE. Serous psammocarcinoma of the ovary and peritoneum Int J Gynecol Pathol. 1990;9(2):110-2.
10. Tung CS, Mok SC, Tsang YT, et al. PAX2 expression in low malignant potential ovarian tumors and low-grade ovarian serous carcinomas. Mod Pathol. 2009;22:1243-50.
11. Katsube Y, Berg JW, Silverberg SG. Epidemiologic pathology of ovarian tumors: a histopathologic review of primary ovarian neoplasms diagnosed in the Denver Standard Metropolitan Statistical Area, 1 July-31 December 1969 and 1 July-31 December 1979. Int J Gynecol Pathol. 1982;1(1):3-16.
12. Seidman JD, Kurman RJ, Ronnett BM. Primary and metastatic mucinous adenocarcinomas in the ovaries: incidence in routine practice with a new approach to improve intraoperative diagnosis. Am J Surg Pathol. 2003;27(7):985-93.
13. Khunamornpong S, Settakorn J, Sukpan K, et al. Mucinous tumor of low malignant potential ("borderline" or "atypical proliferative" tumor) of the ovary: a study of 171 cases with the assessment of intraepithelial carcinoma and microinvasion. Int J Gynecol Pathol. 2011;30:18-230.
14. Ronnett BM, Zahn CM, Kurman RJ, et al. Disseminated peritoneal adenomucinosis and peritoneal mucinous carcinomatosis. A clinicopathologic analysis of 109 cases with emphasis on distinguishing pathologic features, site of origin, prognosis, and relationship to "pseudomyxoma peritonei". Am J Surg Pathol. 1995;19:1390-1408.
15. Bague S, Rodriguez I M, Prat J. Sarcoma-like mural nodules in mucinous cystic tumors of the ovary revisited: a clinicopathologic analysis of 10 additional cases. Am J Surg Pathol. 2002;26:1467-76.
16. Provenza C, Young R H, Prat J. Anaplastic carcinoma in mucinous ovarian tumors: a clinicopathologic study of 34 cases emphasizing the crucial impact of stage on prognosis, their histologic spectrum, and overlap with sarcomalike mural nodules. Am J Surg Pathol. 2008;32:383-9.
17. Lee KR, Scully RE. Mucinous tumors of the ovary: a clinico-pathologic study of 196 borderline tumors (of intestinal type) and carcinomas,including an evaluation of 11 cases with ''pseudomyxoma peritonei.'' Am J Surg Pathol. 2000;24:1447-64.
18. Chu PG, Weiss LM. Keratin expression in human tissues and neoplasms. Histopathology. 2002;40:403-39.
19. Fraggetta F, Pelosi G, Cafici A, et al. CDX2 immunoreactivity in primary and metastatic ovarian mucinous tumours. Virchows Arch. 2003;443:782-6.
20. Albarracin CT, Jafri J, Montag AG, et al. Differential expression of MUC2 and MUC5AC mucin genes in primary ovarian and metastatic colonic carcinoma. Hum Pathol. 2000; 31:672-7.
21. Enomoto T, Weghorst CM, Inoue M, et al. K-ras activation occurs frequently in mucinous adenocarcinomas and rarely in other common epithelial tumors of the human ovary. Am J Pathol. 1991;139:777-85.
22. DePriest PD, Banks ER, Powell DE, van Nagell JR Jr, Gallion HH, Puls LE, et al. Endometrioid carcinoma of the ovary and endometriosis: the association in postmenopausal women. Gynecol Oncol. 1992;47(1):71-5.
23. Chen S, Leitao MM, Tornos C, et al. Invasion patterns in stage I endometrioid and mucinous ovarian carcinomas:a clinicopathologic analysis emphasizing favorable outcomes in carcinomas without destructive stromal invasion and the

occasional malignant course of carcinomas with limited destructive stromal invasion. Modern Pathol. 2005;18:903-11.
24. Moreno-Bueno G, Gamallo C, Pérez-Gallego L, de Mora JC, Suárez A, Palacios J. beta-Catenin expression pattern, beta-catenin gene mutations, and microsatellite instability in endometrioid ovarian carcinomas and synchronous endometrial carcinomas. Diagn Mol Pathol. 2001;10(2):116-22.
25. Gras E, Catasus L, Argüelles R, Moreno-Bueno G, Palacios J, Gamallo C, et al. Microsatellite instability, MLH-1 promoter hypermethylation, and frameshift mutations at coding mononucleotide repeat microsatellites in ovarian tumors. Cancer. 2001;92(11):2829-36.
26. Pettersson F. Annual report of the results of treatment in Gynecological cancer. Stockholm: International Federation of Gynecology and Obstetrics. 1991.
27. Fujii H, Yoshida M, Gong ZX, et al. Frequent genetic heterogeneity in the clonal evolution of gynecological carcinosarcoma and its influence on phenotypic diversity. Cancer Res. 2000;60:114-20.
28. Duska L R, Garrett L, Henretta M, et al. When "neverevents" occur despite adherence to clinical guidelines: the case of venous thromboembolism in clear cell cancer of the ovary compared with other epithelial histologic subtypes. Gynecol Oncol. 2010;116:374-7.
29. Stern RC, Dash R, Bentley RC, et al . Malignancy in endometriosis: frequency and comparison of ovarian and extraovarian types. Int J Gynecol Pathol. 2001;20:133-9.
30. Mayr D, Hirschmann A, Lohrs U, et al. KRAS and BRAF mutations in ovarian tumors: a comprehensive study of invasive carcinomas, borderline tumors and extraovarian implants. Gynecol Oncol. 2006;103:883-7.
31. Prat J. Ovarian carcinomas, including secondary tumors: diagnostically challenging areas. Mod Pathol. 2005;18(Suppl 2):S99-S111.
32. Köbel M, Kalloger S E, Huntsman D G, et al. Differences in tumor type in low-stage versus high-stage ovarian carcinomas. Int J Gynecol Pathol. 2010;2:203-11.
33. Ohira S, Itoh K, Shiozawa T, et al. Ovarian non-small cell neuroendocrine carcinoma with paraneoplastic parathyroid hormone-related hypercalcemia. Int J Gynecol Pathol. 2004;23:393-7.

# Sex Cord Tumors of Ovary

# 14

Sex cord stromal tumor is derived from sex cord and specialized stromal cells of ovary. The tumor comprises of granulosa cells, fibroblasts, theca cells, Sertoli cells and Leydig cells. Sex cord stromal tumor represents 10% of all ovarian tumors.[1] The tumor that are composed of ovarian cell types are estrogenic, whereas, the tumors that are composed of testicular cell type are androgenic in nature. Both types may be non-functioning.

## GRANULOSA CELL TUMOR

Granulosa cell tumor (GCT) accounts for 1 to 2% of all ovarian neoplasms.[1] GCT occurs in all ages from child to postmenopausal women. Granulosa cell tumor is of two types: Adult and juvenile GCT.

### Adult Granulosa Cell Tumor (AGCT)

AGCT represents more than 95% of GCT and 1% of all ovarian tumors.

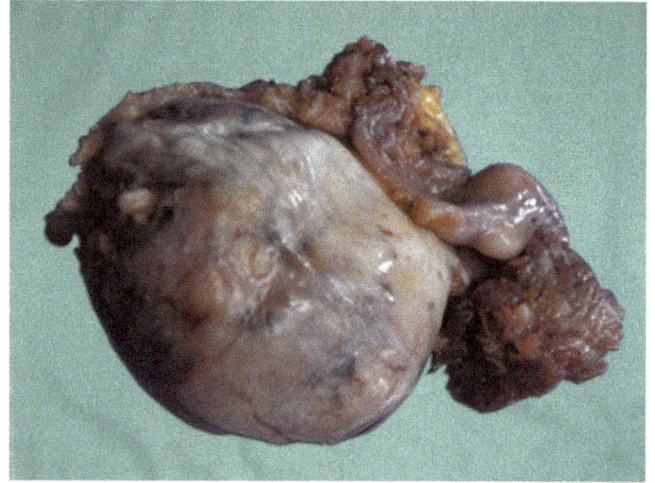

Figure 14.1: Granulosa cell tumor: Solid well encapsulated tumor

*Clinical Features*

AGCT may occur from the teen agers to postmenopausal women. The tumor is commonly seen in elderly female and the mean age of the patient is 45 to 50 years.[2] The patients commonly presents with post-menopausal bleeding in postmenopausal patient and menorrhagia or metrorrhagia in the premenopausal patients. In functioning tumor endometrial hyperplasia occurs and well differentiated carcinoma of endometrium is seen in approximately 5% cases of AGCT. Rarely the tumor may secrete androgen resulting in virilization characterized by hirsutism, enlarged clitoris and deepening of voice.

*Gross*

The tumor is unilateral in 95% cases. AGCT may be small microscopic size to as large as 30 cm in size. The mean diameter of the tumor is 10 cm. The tumor may be totally

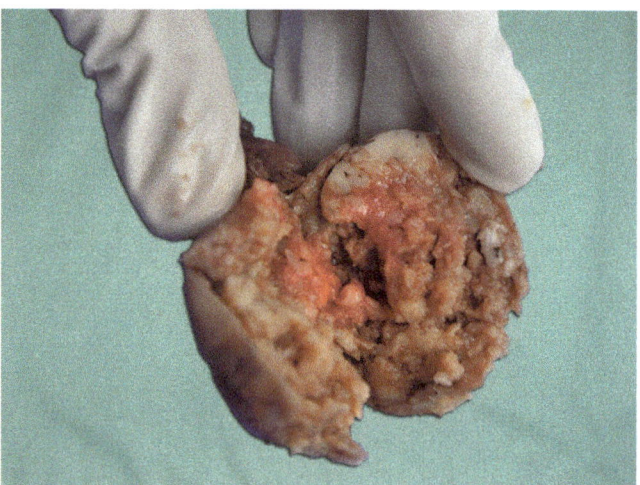

Figure 14.2: Granulosa cell tumor: Cut section is gray white, solid

solid or solid cystic (Figures 14.1 and 14.2). Rarely the whole tumor is cystic. The solid area is yellowish to white depending on the amount of lipid within the cells.

## Histopathology (Figures 14.3 to 14.24)

The tumor is usually composed of only granulosa cells and occasionally is admixed with theca cell or fibroblasts. The tumor cells simulate the normal granulosa cells. The individual cells are round, or spindle-shaped with scanty pale cytoplasm. The nuclei of the cells show characteristic central longitudinal groove. Nuclear chromatin is fine with inconspicuous nucleoli. Mitotic figures are scanty. Occasionally, the tumor cell show significant luteinization. The luteinized granulosa cells contain abundant eosinophilic cytoplasm with centrally-located nuclei. In addition, foci of bizarre cells may be seen and the presence of such cells have no adverse prognostic effect. The common histological patterns in GCT include: microfollicular, macrofollicular, insular, trabecular, ribbon like, and solid tubular. These patterns have no prognostic significance.

**Microfollicular pattern:** Microfollicular pattern is characterized by small cavity like spaces within the sheet or nests of granulosa cells that contains degenerated nuclei, basement membrane like material or secretory material. These small spaces resemble Call Exner bodies of the Graffian follicle. The small spaces are surrounded by typical well-differentiated granulosa cells.

**Macrofollicular pattern:** Macrofollicular pattern shows multiple large variable sized follicles lined by granulosa cells.

**Tubular:** Tumor shows multiple small tubules with central lumen surrounded by peripheral arrangement of cells.

**Insular and trabecular:** These patterns are characterized by large nests and trabecular cells separated by fibrous stroma.

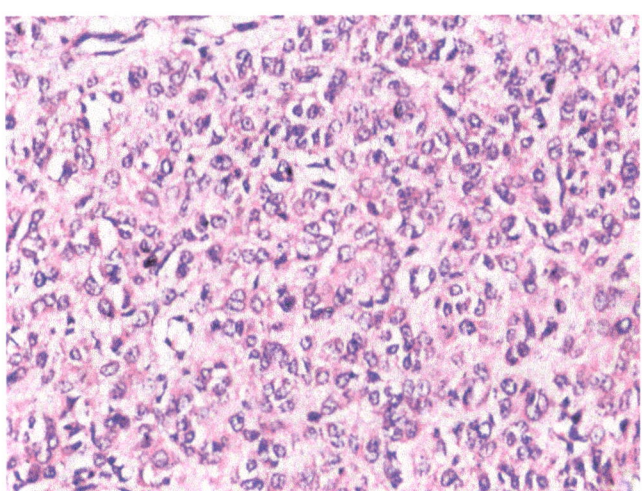

Figure 14.3: Granulosa cell tumor: Diffuse sheet of tumor cells

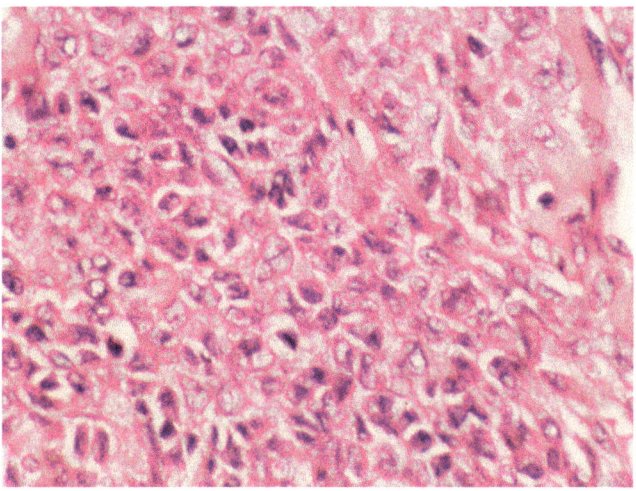

Figure 14.5: Granulosa cell tumor: Round to oval cells with deep longitudinal groove

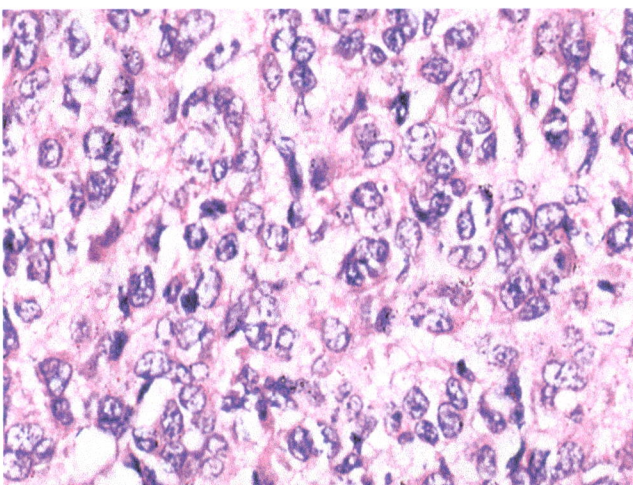

Figure 14.4: Granulosa cell tumor: Higher magnification of diffuse sheet of tumor cells

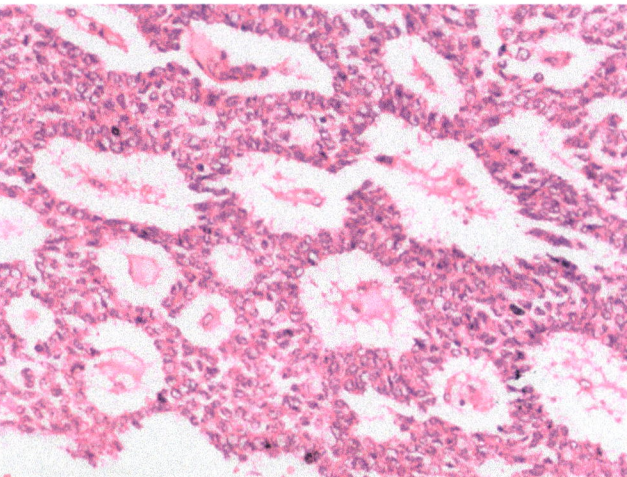

Figure 14.6: Granulosa cell tumor: Microfollicular pattern

Sex Cord Tumors of Ovary 211

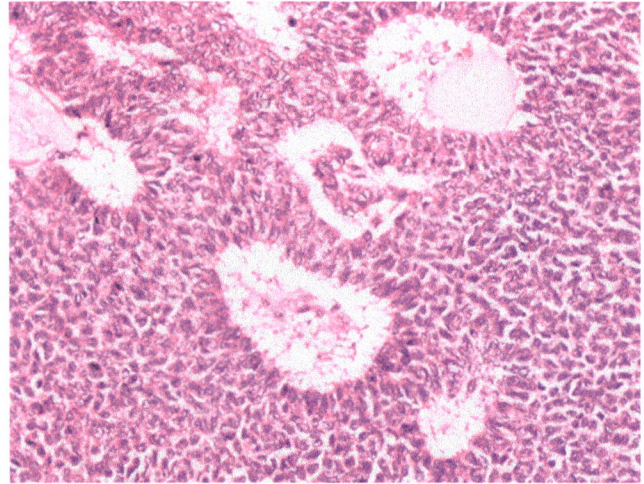

**Figure 14.7:** Granulosa cell tumor: Microfollicule lined by tumor cells

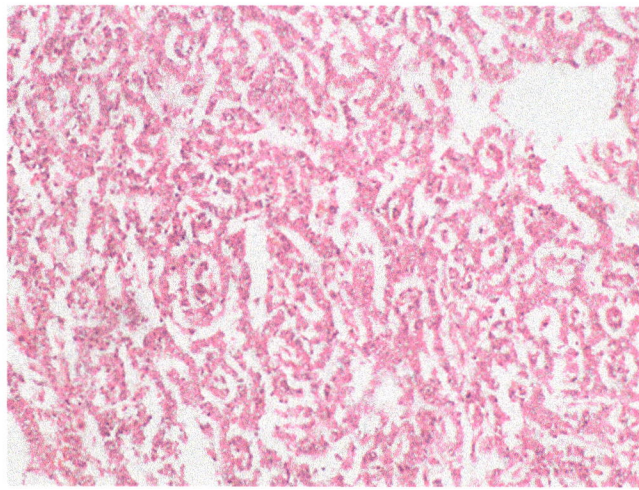

**Figure 14.10:** Granulosa cell tumor: Reticular pattern

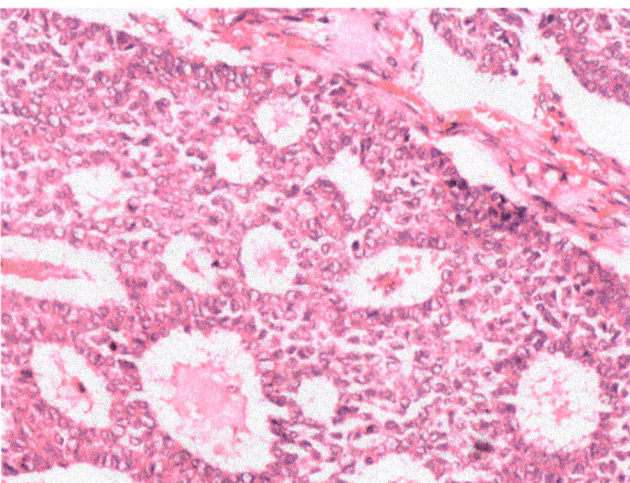

**Figure 14.8:** Granulosa cell tumor: Call Exner bodies

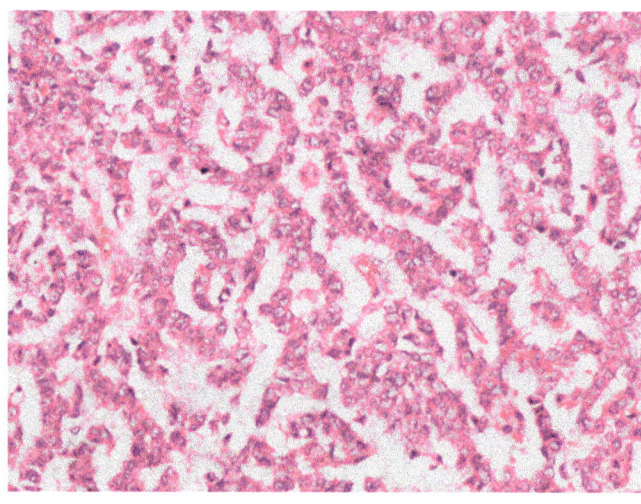

**Figure 14.11:** Granulosa cell tumor: Higher magnification of the same

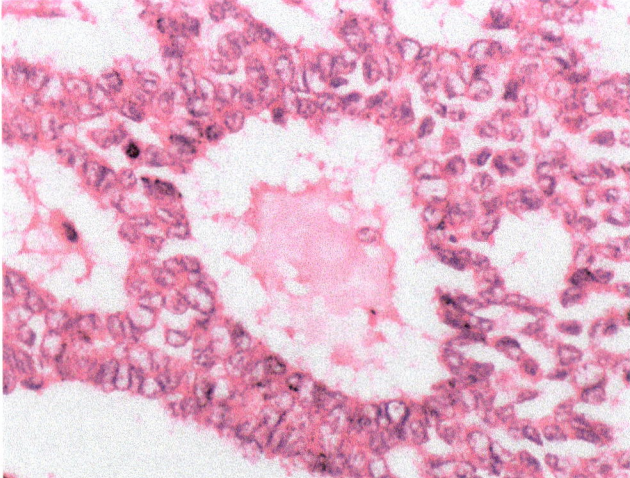

**Figure 14.9:** Granulosa cell tumor: Higher magnification of Call Exner body

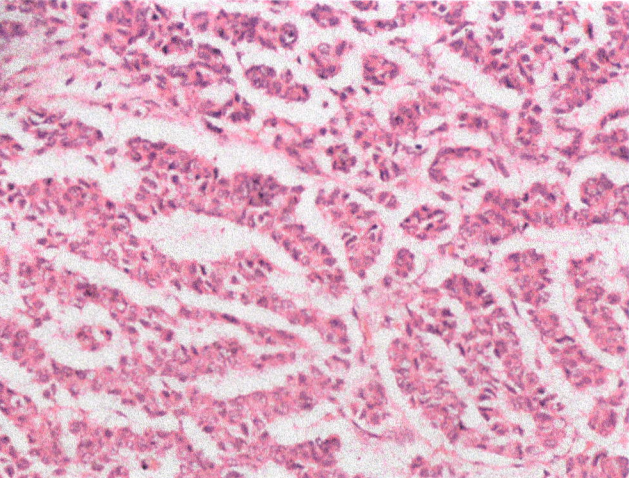

**Figure 14.12:** Granulosa cell tumor: Granulosa cell tumor: higher magnification of the reticular pattern

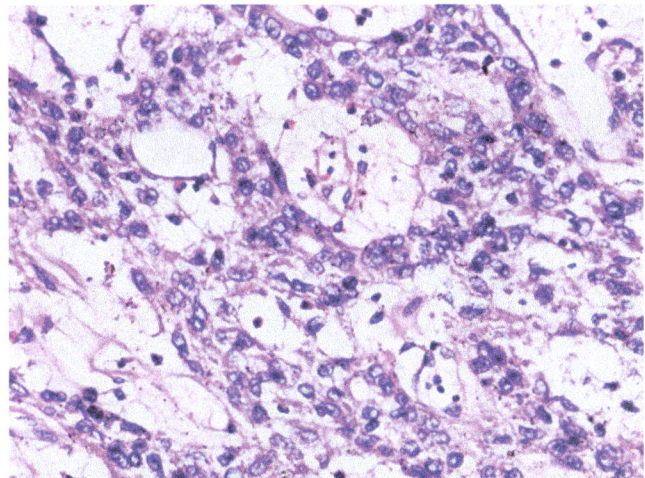

**Figure 14.13:** Granulosa cell tumor: Macrofollicular pattern

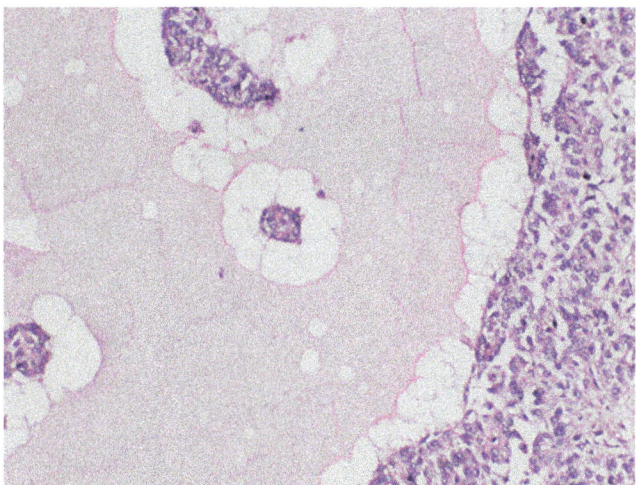

**Figure 14.16:** Granulosa cell tumor: Higher magnification of the macrocyst

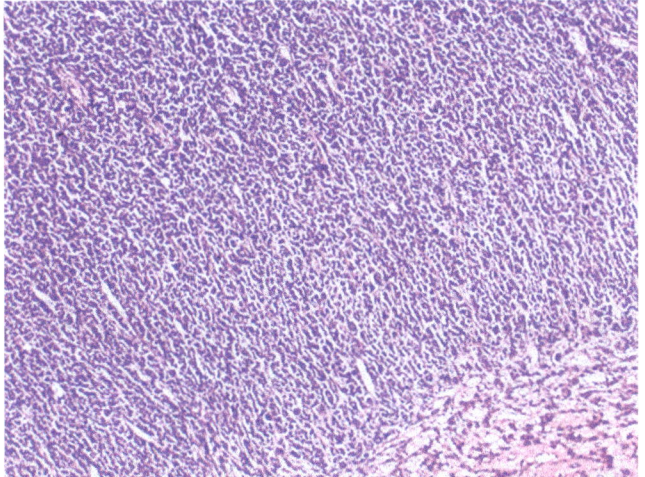

**Figure 14.14:** Granulosa cell tumor: Solid sheet of the tumor cells

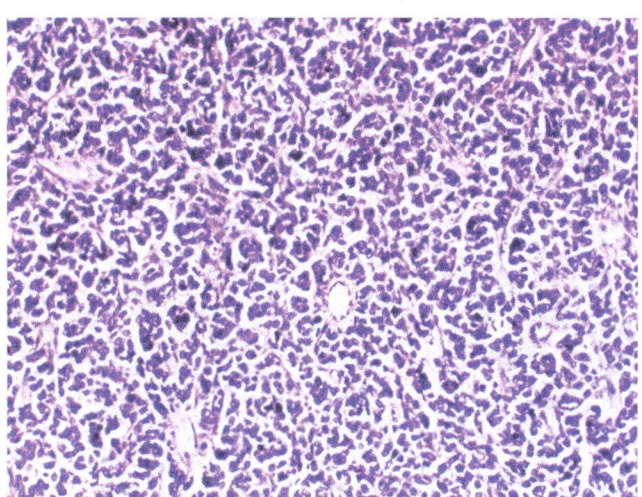

**Figure 14.17:** Granulosa cell tumor: Insular pattern

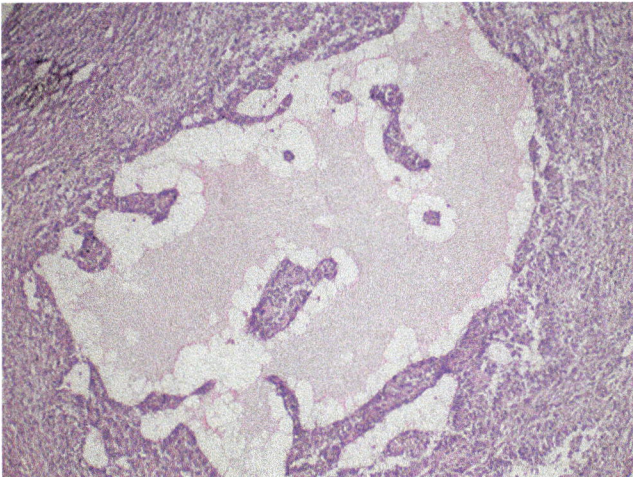

**Figure 14.15:** Granulosa cell tumor: Macrocyst in tumor

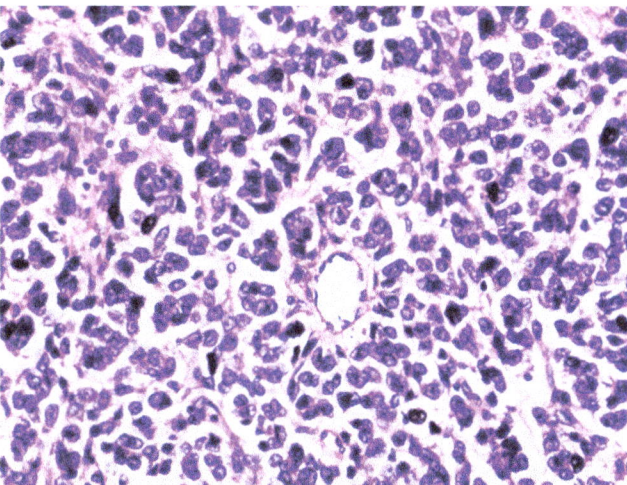

**Figure 14.18:** Granulosa cell tumor: Higher magnification of insular pattern

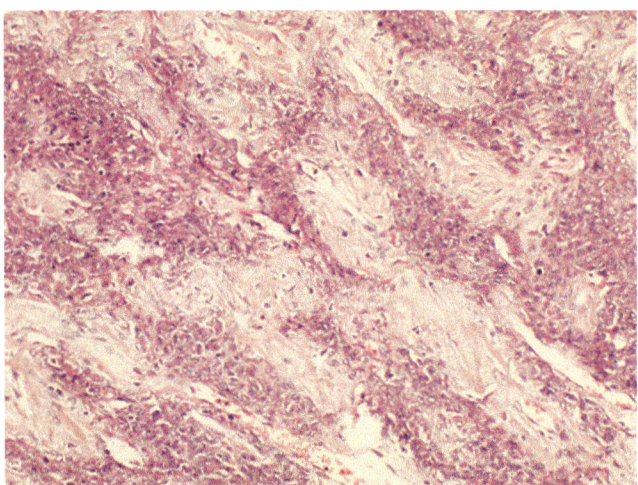

**Figure 14.19:** Granulosa cell tumor: Solid sheet of cells with intervening fibrocollagenous tissue

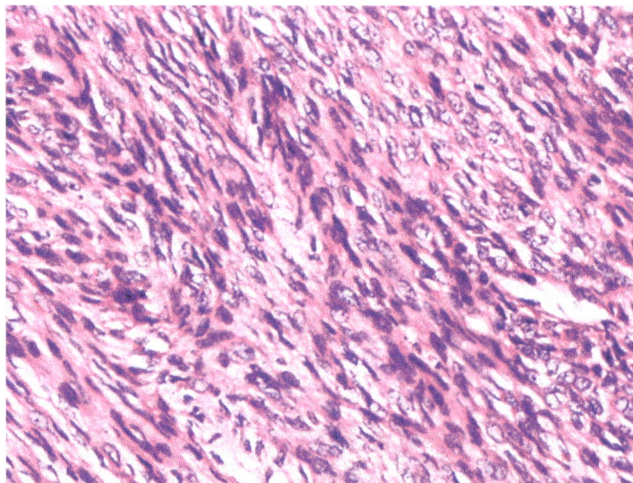

**Figure 14.22:** Granulosa cell tumor: Sarcomatoid tumor showing oval to spindle cells

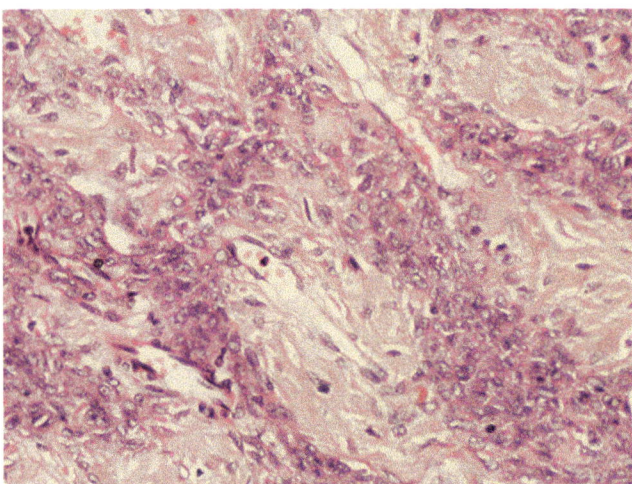

**Figure 14.20:** Granulosa cell tumor: Higher magnification of the same

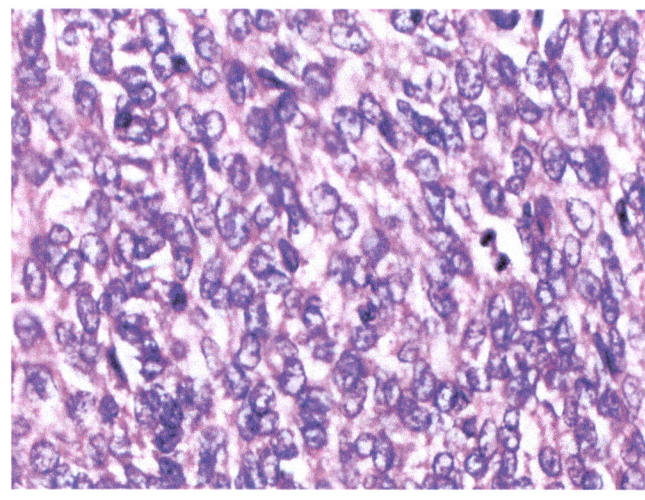

**Figure 14.23:** Granulosa cell tumor: Higher magnification of the sarcomatoid variety

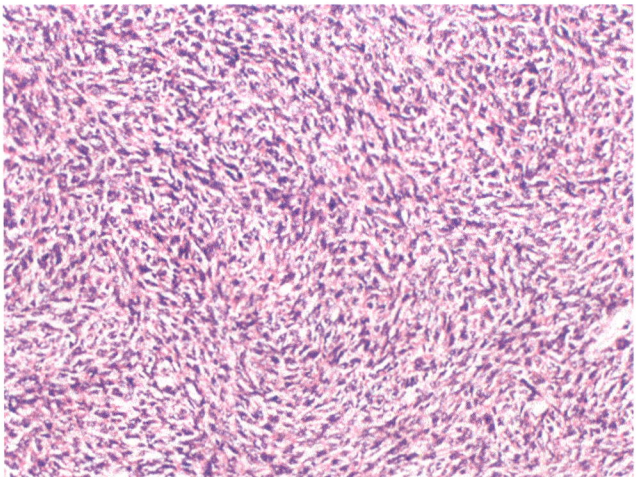

**Figure 14.21:** Granulosa cell tumor: Sarcomatoid GCT

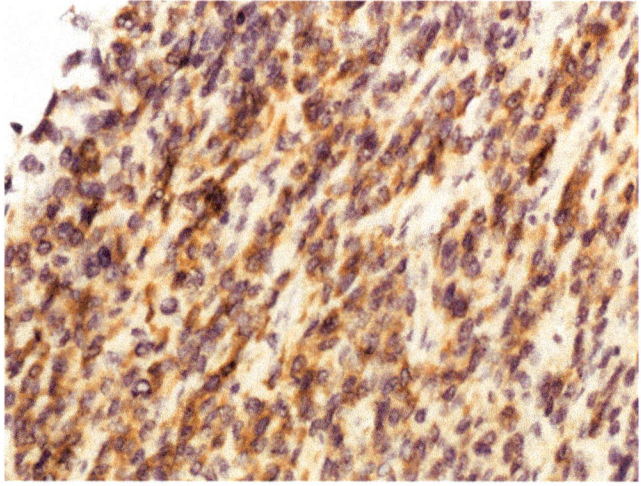

**Figure 14.24:** Granulosa cell tumor: Strong inhibin positive cells

**Cystic pattern:** In case of cystic pattern, the tumor shows large cysts filled with blood or hemosiderin laden macrophages. The cyst is lined by granulosa cells.

**Other cells:** Occasionally GCT may show other cellular components such as fibrothecomatous, and mucinous epithelium.

*Immunohistochemistry*

Most of the GCTs are positive for inhibin and calretinin. Steroidogenic factor-1 (SF-1) and FOXL2 are always positive for GCT.[3] All GCTs are positive for vimentin, CK8 and CK18 (30 to 60%). The tumor also show variable positivity of S100 (50%) and CD 99 (70%).

*Differential Diagnosis*

a. Undifferentiated carcinoma: The following features favor granulosa cell tumor over undifferentiated carcinoma: (1) Prominent nuclear groove, (2) lower nuclear grade and low mitosis, (3) positive inhibin and negative EMA immunostain.
b. Small cell carcinoma: Hypercalcemia, lack of estrogenic symptoms, presence of nuclear moulding and grooving, and positive neuroendocrine markers (CD 56, chromogranin, NSE, synaptophysin) are helpful in diagnosis of small cell carcinoma.
c. Cellular thecoma and fibroma: Thecoma and fibromas are rich in reticulin stain, compared to AGCT.
d. Endometrial stromal sarcoma: Endometrial stromal sarcoma shows: (1) Numerous small arterioles, (2) reticulin stain around the individual tumor cells, (3) negative for inhibin and calretinin.
e. Follicular cysts: Occasionally large solitary AGCT may resemble follicular cyst particularly large luteinized cyst in the pregnant women. The luteinized follicular cyst is lined by large luteinized cells whereas the cyst in GCT is lined by granulosa cells.
f. Endometrioid carcinoma: Foci of squamous cells is often seen in endometrioid carcinoma.

*Treatment and Prognosis*

Bilateral salpingo-oophorectomy is the treatment of choice in case of postmenopausal patient or the women who have completed her family. In young patient with stage I tumor, conservative surgery such as unilateral salpingo-oophorectomy could be done. AGCT is a potentially aggressive tumor and may have recurrence in long run even as late as 20 years. Almost 90% of AGCT presents as stage I tumor. The 10 years survival of stage I tumor is 86% compared to 49% survival in advanced stage.[4] The bad prognostic markers of stage I tumors are: (1) Lower age, (2) Bilateral tumor, (3) More than 5 cm diameter of tumor, (4) High mitotic figures and atypia.

### Juvenile Granulosa Cell Tumor (JGCT)

Juvenile granulosa cell tumor (JGCT) represents 5% of all GCT and it predominantly occurs below the age of 30 years.

*Clinical Features*

Near about 80% of the child before puberty presents with isosexual pseudoprecocity. The patients develop secondary sex characters such as development of breast along with pubic and axillary hair. The patients after puberty present with pain abdomen, abdominal swelling and menstrual disorders.

*Macroscopy*

The grossly JGCT is similar to that of AGCT.

*Microscopic Features (Figures 14.25 to 14.28)*

JGCT shows diffuse solid sheets or nodules and cystic structures. The sheets of cells are punctuated by macrofollicles. The follicles are round to oval and of variable sized. These follicles are slightly smaller than that of AGCT. The central part of the follicular lumen contains eosinophilic or basophilic secretion that is positive for mucicarmine stain. These macrofollicles are surrounded by single to many layers of granulosa cells. The tumor may be variably admixed with spindle shaped theca cells or fibroblastic stromal cell. Rarely hyaline bands are seen. The microfollicular and insular pattern are usually absent in JGCT. The cells of granulosa cell tumors also differ from AGCT (Table 14.1). The cells are large polygonal to spindle shaped and show abundant cytoplasm with central large hyperchromatic nuclei. Nuclear margin is regular and no nuclear groove is noted. Mitotic activity is numerous in JGCT (more than 6 per 10 HPFs).

*Immunohistochemistry*

Immunohistochemistry of JGCT is almost same as AGCT except intense positivity of CD99.

*Differential Diagnosis*

a. AGCT: JGCT lacks typical Call Exner bodies, microfollicles and insular pattern (Table 14.1).
b. Yolk sac tumor: Yolk sac tumors lack typical macrofollicular pattern and show high alpha feto protein level in serum.
c. Theca cell tumor: The following features favor theca cell tumor: (1) Elderly patients, (2) predominant theca cells, (3) lack of follicles, (4) reticulin rich theca cell.

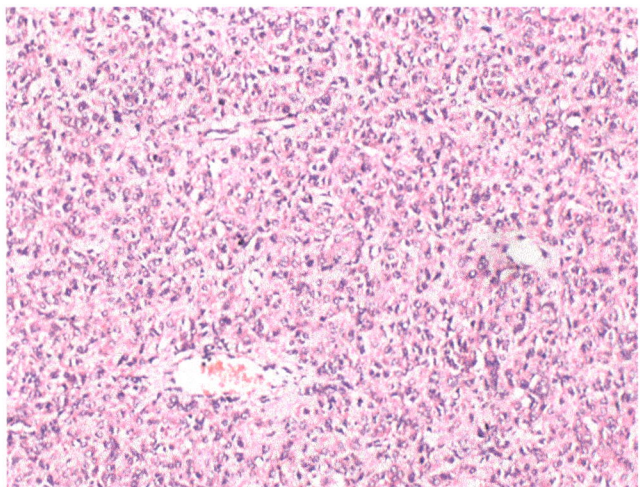

**Figure 14.25:** Juvenile granulosa cell tumor: Diffuse sheet of tumor cells

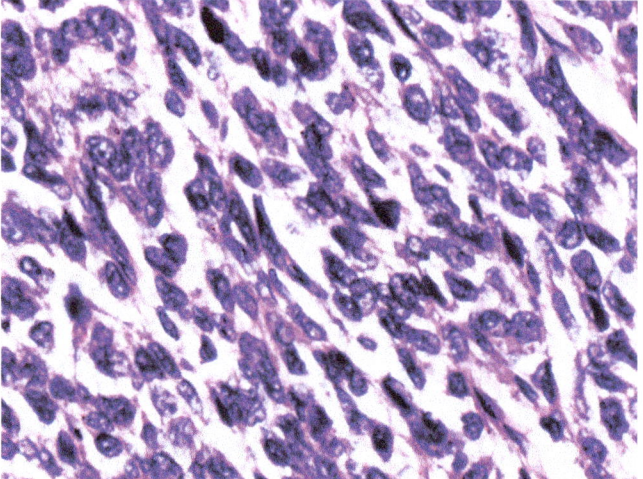

**Figure 14.27:** Juvenile granulosa cell tumor: Diffuse sheet of tumor cells

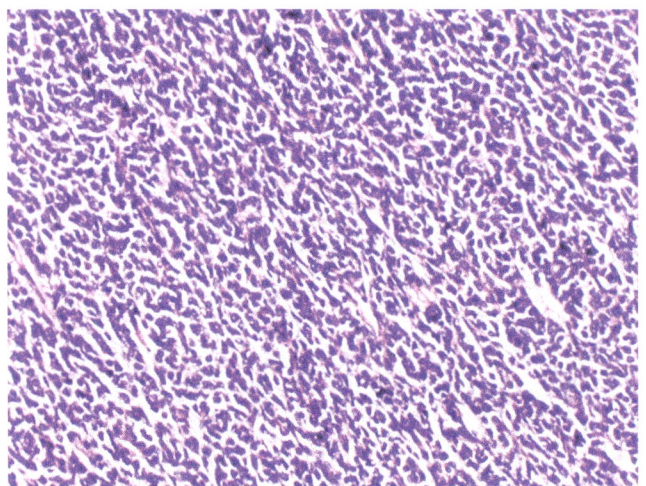

**Figure 14.26:** Juvenile granulosa cell tumor: Diffuse sheet of tumor cells

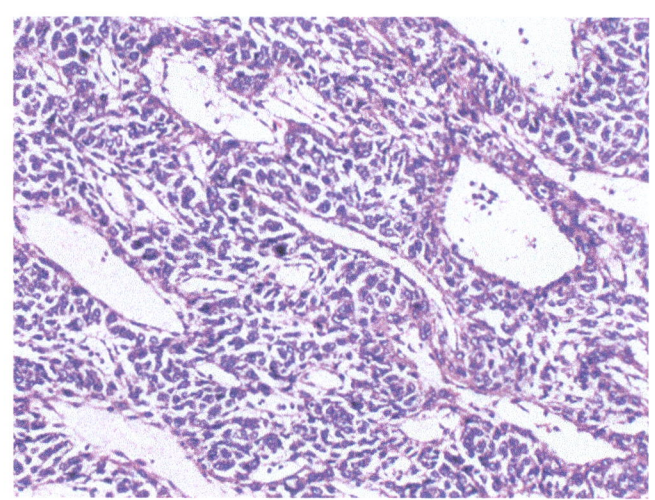

**Figure 14.28:** Juvenile granulosa cell tumor: Macrofollicle

**Table 14.1:** Distinguishing features between adult and juvenile granulosa cell tumor

| Features | AGCT | JGCT |
|---|---|---|
| Age | Elderly patient | Young, before 30 years |
| Microfollicles and insular pattern | Present | Absent |
| Macrofollicles | Large | Smaller |
| Cells<br>Cytoplasm<br>Nuclei<br>Nuclear groove | Scanty<br>Fine chromatin<br>Present | Abundant<br>Coarse chromatin<br>Absent |
| Mitosis | Less | Abundant |

d. Surface epithelial tumor: JGCT may be confused with clear cell carcinoma, undifferentiated carcinoma or transitional cell carcinoma.

*Prognosis*

Prognosis of JGCT is relatively better than AGCT. FIGO staging of tumor is the most important prognostic factor. Stage I tumor shows only 1.5% mortality rate.

## Thecoma

Thecoma is the stromal tumor that is characterized by lipid containing cells simulating theca interna cells of the developing follicles and the less than 10% granulosa cells. It accounts for less than 1% of all ovarian neoplasms.

*Clinical Features*

Thecoma predominantly occurs in elderly women and mean age of the patient is 59 years. Thecomas are usually asymptomatic and detected incidentally. The elderly postmenopausal patients often present with vaginal bleeding (60%) and nearly 21% of them showed associated endometrial carcinoma.[5] Approximately 10% of luteinized thecomas may show features of over secretion of androgenic hormone.[6]

*Gross*

Thecomas are mostly unilateral tumor (97%). They are firm, smooth surfaced solid mass. The size of the tumor varies from non-palpable microscopic to several cm. The cut section of the tumor is typically solid yellowish appearance.

*Histopathology (Figures 14.29 and 14.30)*

Thecoma shows diffuse sheets of round to spindle cells containing abundant pale vacuolated cytoplasm. The lipid filled cytoplasmic vacuoles are best demonstrated by fat stain in frozen section specimen. The nuclei of the cells are round to elongated with fine chromatin. No nuclear atypia or mitosis is seen. Occasionally thecoma may show focal large atypical cells that do not have any prognostic significance. Band of fibromatous component often intersects the sheets of thecoma cells. Hyalinized connective tissue plaques and microcalcifications may also be seen in thecoma. The reticulin stain shows reticulin fibrils around the tumor cells. Nests of luteinized cells in a fibromatous stroma are seen in case of luteinized thecoma. Almost all androgenic thecomas are luteinized thecoma.

*Immunohistochemistry*

Thecoma shows vimentin, calretinin and inhibin positivity.

*Differential Diagnosis*

a. Adult granulosa cell tumor (AGCT): Thecoma is reticulin rich and reticulin invests individual tumor cells in thecoma.
b. Smooth muscle cell neoplasm: Leiomyomas show classic interlacing fascicles. They are also positive for SMA and negative for inhibin.
c. Fibroma: There is considerable overlap between fibroma and thecoma. The tumor with predominant population of lipid rich vacuolated cells should be designated as thecoma.
d. Sclerosing stromal tumor: Younger age, lack of any hormonal manifestation and characteristic hemangioma like vascular pattern favor the diagnosis of Sclerosing stromal tumor.

*Prognosis*

Thecomas are benign tumor. Rarely luteinized thecoma with atypia may metastasize.[7]

## Fibroma

Fibromas are group of stromal tumor consist of spindle cells producing collagen. They account for less than 4% of all ovarian tumors.

*Clinical Features*

Fibroma commonly occurs in 50 to 60 years age with mean age 48 years. Fibroma may be asymptomatic and is noted incidentally or it may present as pelvic mass. This tumor is characteristically associated with Meigs' syndrome (1%) and the basal cell nevus syndrome. Meigs' syndrome is characterized by ascites, pleural effusion and fibroma of ovary.[8] The Ascites and pleural effusion vanishes after removal of the ovarian tumor. Basal cell nevus syndrome is characterized by any one or more features that include the presence of basal cell carcinomas, keratocysts of the jaw, calcification of the dura and mesenteric cysts.[9]

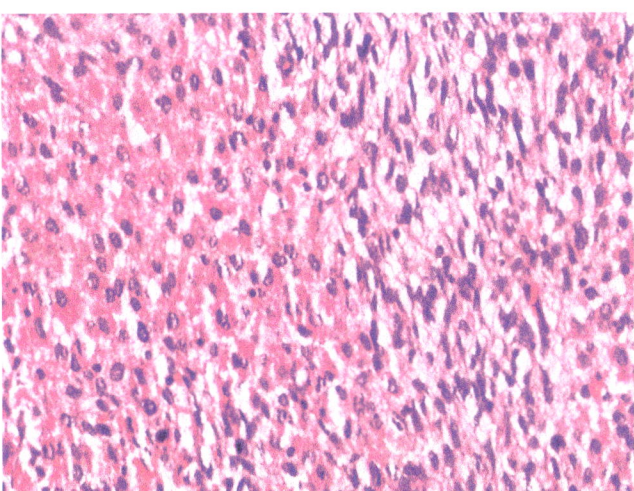

**Figure 14.29:** Thecoma: Diffuse sheets of round to spindle cells

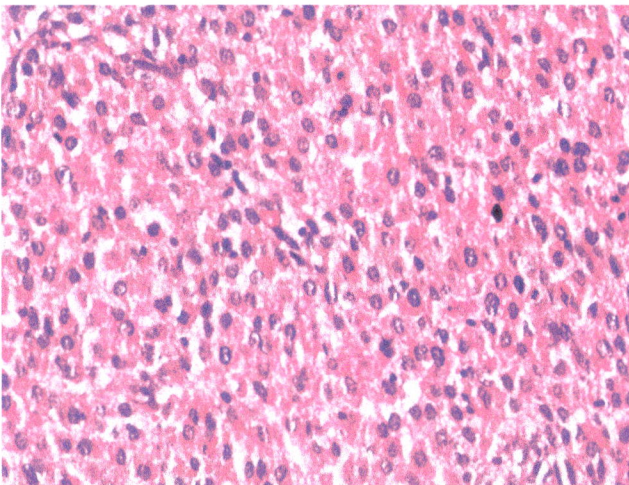

**Figure 14.30:** Thecoma: The tumor cells contain abundant pale vacuolated cytoplasm having centrally placed round nuclei

*Gross*

Fibromas are usually unilateral (more than 90%). The tumor is solid firm with average diameter 6 cm. The cut section shows gray white solid tissue (Figure 14.31). Occasionally cut surface may show whorled appearance.

*Histopathology (Figures 14.32 and 14.33)*

The fibromas are sparse to moderately cellular tumors. They show anastomosing bundles and storiform pattern of cells. The individual cells are oval to spindle-shaped with scanty indistinct cytoplasm that often contain lipid droplets. The nuclei of the cells are hyperchromatic spindle-shaped with mild to moderate atypia. Mitotic figures are usually sparse to absent. Approximately 10% fibroma are hypercellular with little intervening collagen and is labeled as cellular fibromas. The cellular fibromas may show mild nuclear atypia and mitotic activity from one to three per 10 high power fields. Hyaline globules may also be seen in cellular fibroma. Mitotic activity of the cellular fibroma may be as high as 4 to 19 per 10 HPFs. Cellular fibromas with bland nuclei and high mitotic activity should be designated as mitotically active cellular fibromas (MACF) as the long-term follow-up of such cases show favorable outcome.

*Treatment*

Fibroma is a benign tumor with no malignant potential. Therefore, unilateral salpingo-oophorectomy is the treatment of choice.

## Fibrosarcoma

Fibrosarcomas are rare stromal tumors of ovary. However, it is the common form of sarcoma of ovary.[10] They are usually noted in elderly women and average age of the patient is 58 years

*Macroscopy*

Grossly the tumor is large and average size is 17 cm. The tumor is soft with lobulated surface. The cut section is solid, gray white with areas of hemorrhage and necrosis.

*Histopathology (Figures 14.34 to 14.36)*

The tumor is composed of spindle-shaped cells organized in herringbone pattern. The cells show scanty eosinophilic cytoplasm with hyperchromatic spindle-shaped nuclei. The nuclei show moderate to marked pleomorphism. Fibrosarcoma should only be diagnosed in the presence of following features:
1. Marked nuclear atypia
2. Mitosis more than 4 per 10 high power fields

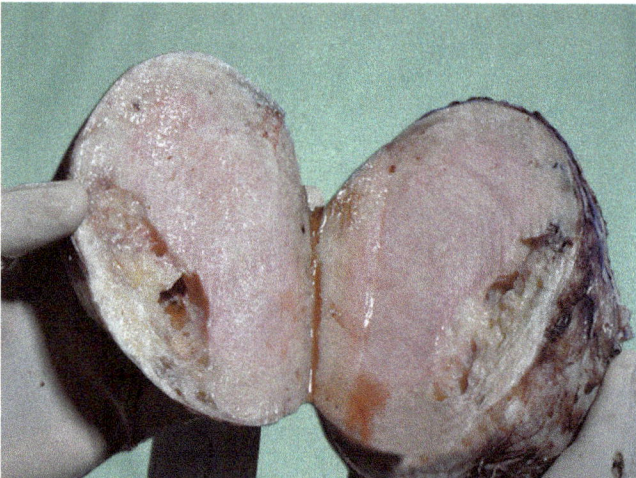

**Figure 14.31:** Fibroma: Solid firm grey white tumor

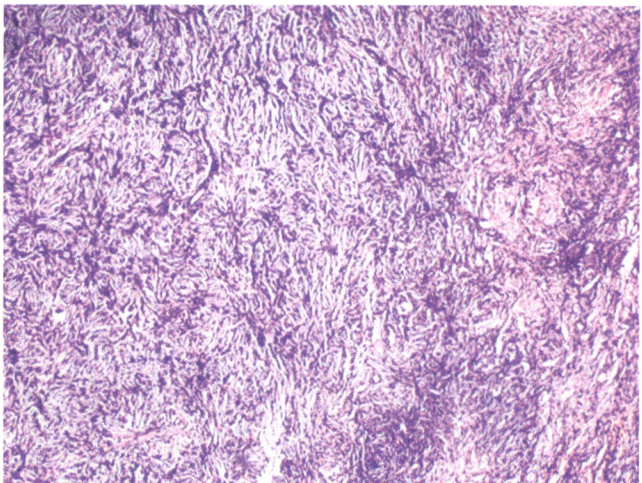

**Figure 14.32:** Fibroma: Anastomosing bundles and storiform pattern of cells

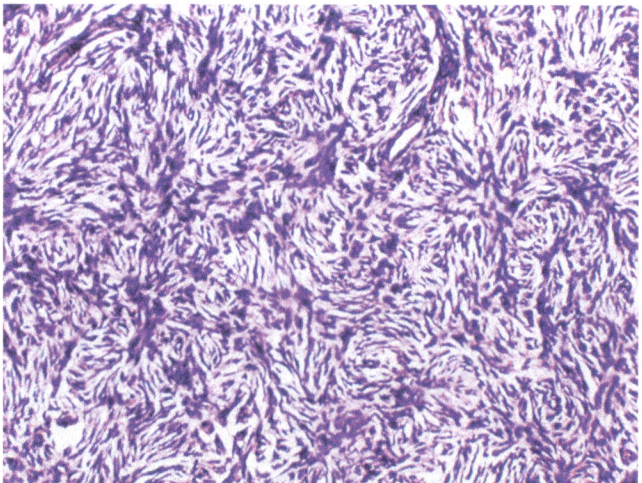

**Figure 14.33:** Fibroma: Higher magnification shows cells with spindle-shaped nuclei

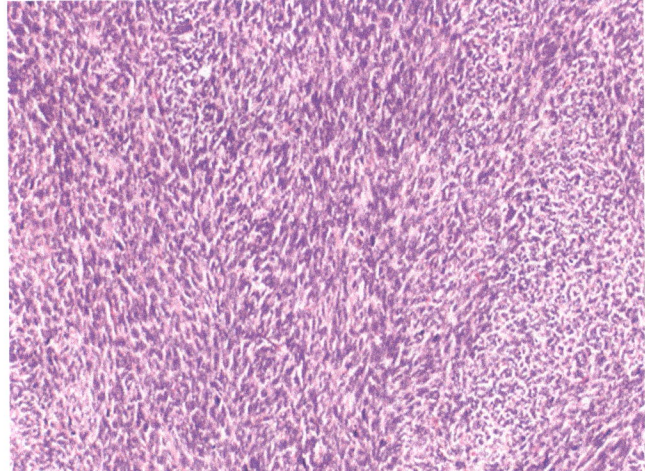

Figure 14.34: Fibrosarcoma of ovary: Spindle-shaped cells arranged in herringbone pattern

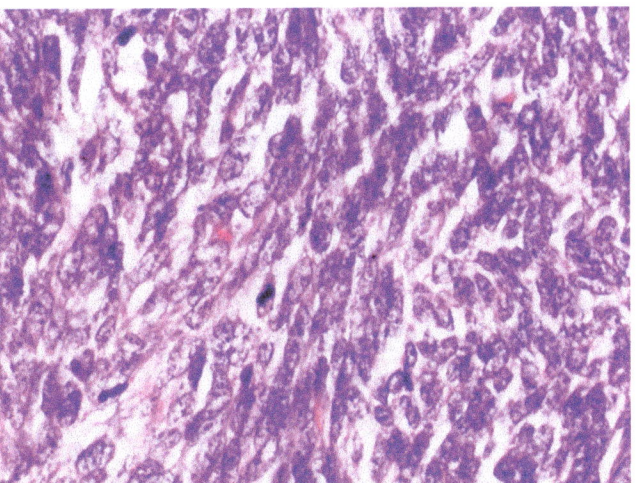

Figure 14.36: Fibrosarcoma: Higher magnification shows detailed cell morphology

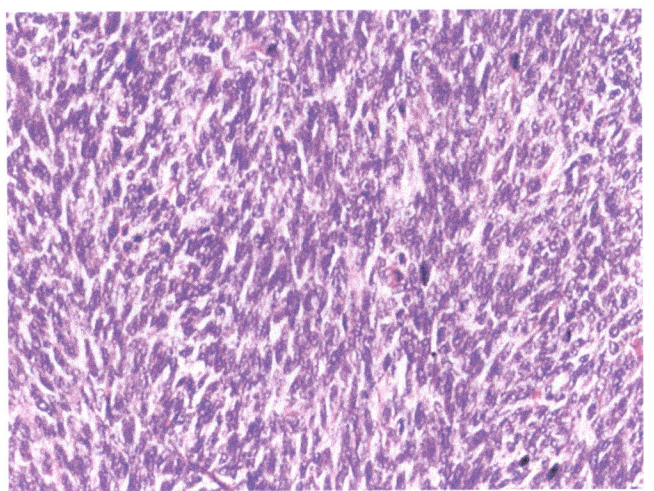

Figure 14.35: Fibrosarcoma of ovary: Oval to spindle cells with frequent mitotic activity

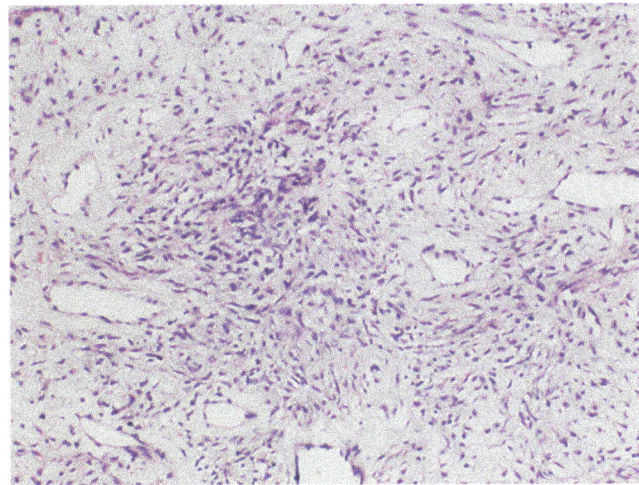

Figure 14.37: Sclerosing stromal tumor: Pseudolobular pattern with alternating cellular and hypocellular areas

3. Tumor cell necrosis, and
4. Atypical mitotic figures.

## Sclerosing Stromal Tumor

Sclerosing stromal tumor is a rare stromal tumor and represents less than 2% of sex-cord stromal tumor of ovary.

### Clinical Features

The tumor occurs in the 2nd and 3rd decade of life and 80% of sclerosing stromal tumor is noted under the age of 30 years. The patients usually present with menstrual abnormalities, abdominal discomfort, pelvic pain and rarely with virilization.

### Gross

The tumor varies in size from 2 to 17 cm in diameter. The tumors are characteristically solid and yellowish to gray white in appearance.

### Histopathology (Figures 14.37 to 14.40)

The tumor shows characteristic pseudolobular pattern with alternating cellular and hypocellular areas. The tumor cells are composed of spindle-shaped cells, luteinized cells with vacuolated cytoplasm and myoid cells. Occasional signet ring like cells may be present that may create confusion with Krukenberg's tumor. The tumor shows characteristic "stag horn" or "hemangiopericytoma-like" thin-walled blood vessels.

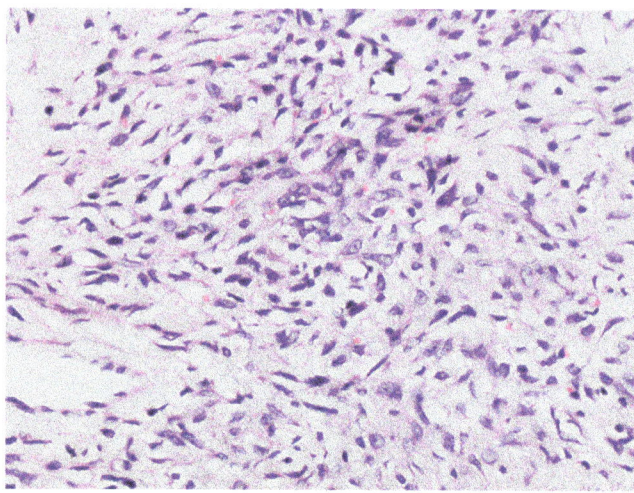

**Figure 14.38:** Sclerosing stromal tumor: Spindle-shaped cells with elongated nuclei

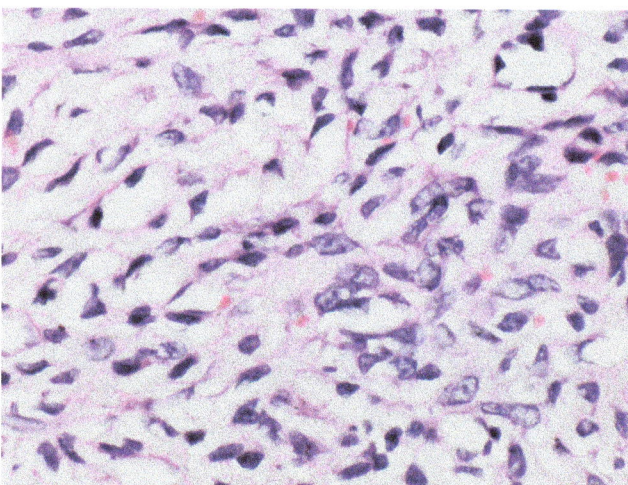

**Figure 14.39:** Sclerosing stromal tumor: Higher magnification shows better cell morphology

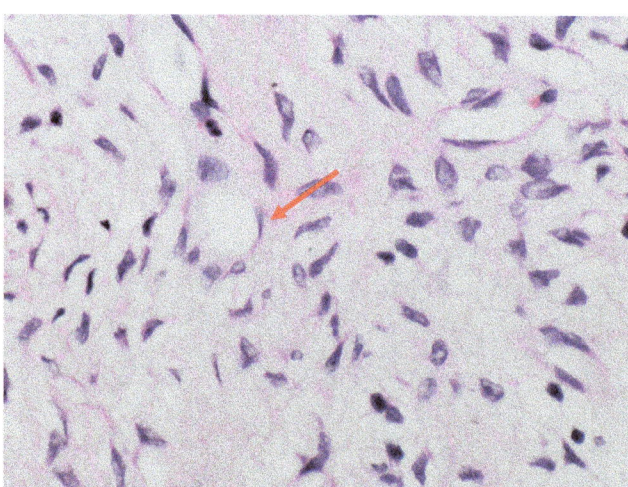

**Figure 14.40:** Sclerosing stromal tumor: Signet ring type of cells

*Immunohistochemistry*

Sclerosing stromal tumors are positive for alpha-inhibin, calretinin, vimentin, melan A, and CD 34 immunostain.[11] In addition, the myoid cells are positive for desmin.

*Prognosis*

The sclerosing stromal tumor has a benign out come and tumor does not recur.

## Signet Ring Stromal Tumor

Signet ring stromal tumor is a rare stromal cell tumor of ovary.[12] These are benign and non-functioning tumor. The tumor occurs in adult female. Grossly, the tumor is solid-cystic. The clinical and macroscopic features of the tumor are similar to that of fibromas of ovary.

*Histopathology*

The tumor shows diffuse sheets of spindle cells admixed with round to oval signet ring type of cells. The signet ring cells have moderate amount of cytoplasm with single large vacuoles. The nuclei are round with eccentric in position. Hyaline bodies are also present in signet ring cell stromal tumor. Occasionally, the tumor contains predominant population of signet ring cells only. Unlike Krukenberg's tumor, the cells of signet ring cell stromal tumors are negative for mucin.

*Prognosis*

This tumor is benign.

## SERTOLI–LEYDIG CELL TUMOR

Sertoli–Leydig cell tumor (SLCT) shows variable proportion of sertoli cells, Leydig cells, primitive gonadal cells and heterologous elements. SLCT is rare and represents less than 0.5% of all ovarian tumors.

## Clinical Features

SLCT commonly occurs in young female and the mean age of the patient is 25 years. Majority of the patients (75%) are under 30 years of age at the time of presentation. However, the patients of well-differentiated SLCT are usually 10 to 15 years older and average age of such patient is 40 years. More than 50% patient complaints of nonspecific symptoms such as abdominal swelling and pain. About 40% patients have excess androgenic hormone secretion present with virilizing symptoms that include hirsutism, acne, hypertrophic clitoris and amenorrhea.[13] A small fraction of SLCT may have estrogenic effect.

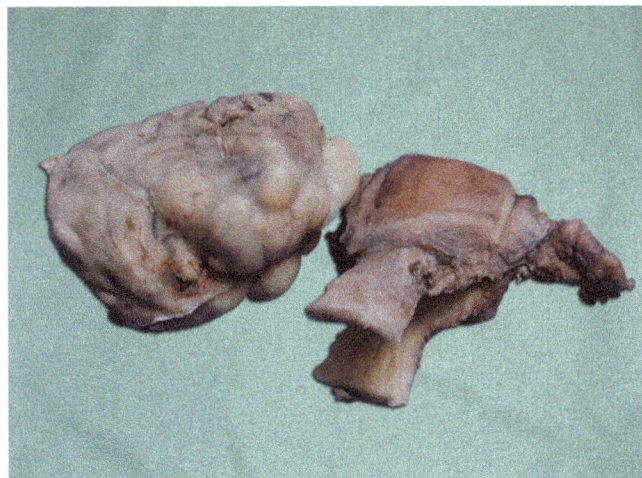

Figure 14.41: Sertoli–Leydig cell tumor: Solid well-encapsulated tumor

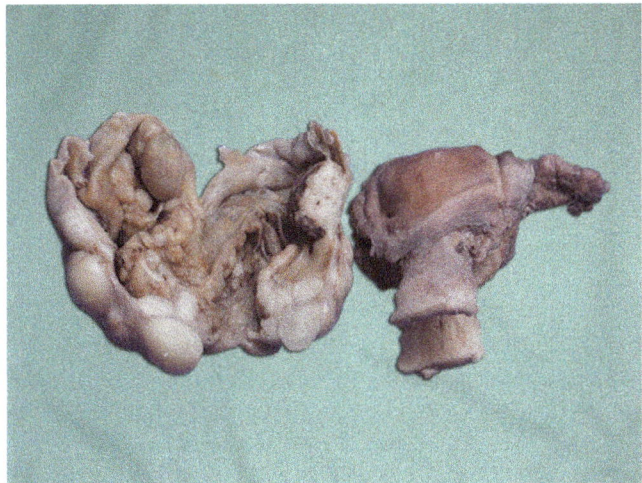

Figure 14.42: Sertoli–Leydig cell tumor: Solid, gray to yellowish tumor on cut section

## Gross

The tumor is solid or partly cystic and average diameter is 13 cm. The cut section of the tumor is yellow or brown (Figures 14.41 and 14.42). Poorly differentiated SLCT shows areas of hemorrhage and necrosis. Retiform differentiation of SLCT often shows papillary structures.

## Histopathological Features (Figures 14.43 to 14.61)

SLCT is divided into five histological types: (1) Well-differentiated, (2) Intermediately differentiated, (3) Poorly differentiated, (4) Retiform and (5) SLCT with heterologous elements

1. **Well-differentiated SLCT:** The tumor predominantly shows multiple lobules separated by fibrous stroma. The lobules are composed of multiple tubules formed by sertoli cells. The tubules are lined by cuboidal cells with scanty to moderate amount of cytoplasm and round monomorphic nuclei. No atypia or mitosis is seen. The clusters of leydig cells are also identified in between the tubules. The Leydig cells contain abundant eosinophilic cytoplasm containing lipochrome pigments. Rarely crystalloids of Reinke may also be identified within the Leydig cells.
2. **Intermediately-differentiated SLCT:** The tumor shows multiple lobular growth with cellular areas interspersed by hypocellular edematous stroma. The lobulated cellular areas show solid sheets of immature sertoli cells, nests of cells, small tubules or trabeculae. The immature sertoli cells have scanty cytoplasm and round to angulated nuclei. Occasionally bizarre looking nuclei may be seen. The sertoli cells may be admixed with Leydig cells. Abortive tubular structures simulating early sex cord of embryonic testis are also seen. Small to large cysts may be seen with central eosinophilic material. These cystic structure often resemble thyroid tissue.
3. **Poorly-differentiated SLCT:** Poorly-differentiated SLCT shows spindle cells arranged in small fascicles. The tumor resembles fibrosarcoma of ovary. The tumor cell shows scanty cytoplasm and spindle-shaped nuclei with moderate to marked nuclear pleomorphism. Numerous mitotic activities are seen. Foci of areas may show occasional tubules or cords of sertoli cells.
4. **Retiform SLCT:** Retiform SLCT represents 15% of SLCT. The tumor shows growth pattern that simulates rete testis. The tumor is composed of: (1) multiple slit like elongated tubules, (2) cystic structure, and (3) short blunted papillae with hyalinized core. These structures are lined by small cuboidal cells with scanty cytoplasm. The cells have monomorphic round nuclei.
5. **SLCT with heterologous elements:** This accounts for 20% of all SLCT. The tumor generally has androgenic effect. The SLCT with heterologous elements are separated into two groups on the basis of prognosis: (1) the presence of gastrointestinal epithelium with goblet cells and argentaffin cells: favorable prognosis.[14] (2) SLCT with immature cartilaginous and skeletal muscle differentiation (5% of SLCT): adverse prognosis.

## Immunohistochemistry

SLCTs show positive immunostaining for alpha inhibin, calretinin. Minor fraction of cases are positive for progesterone and androgen receptor.

## Differential Diagnosis

a. **Endometrioid carcinoma:** The following features favor the diagnosis of endometrioid carcinoma: (1) Higher age,

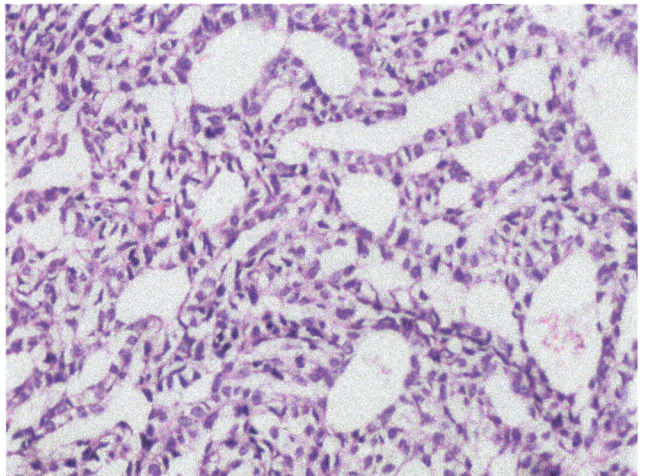

**Figure 14.43:** Sertoli-Leydig cell tumor, well differentiated: Tumor is composed of multiple tubules

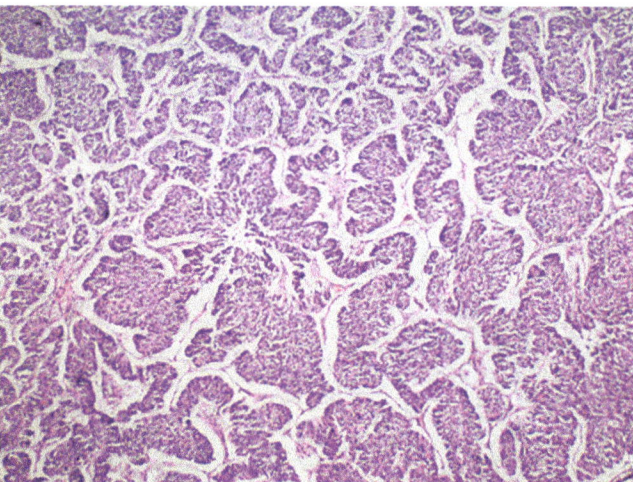

**Figure 14.46:** Sertoli-Leydig cell tumor: Nest pattern of the tumor

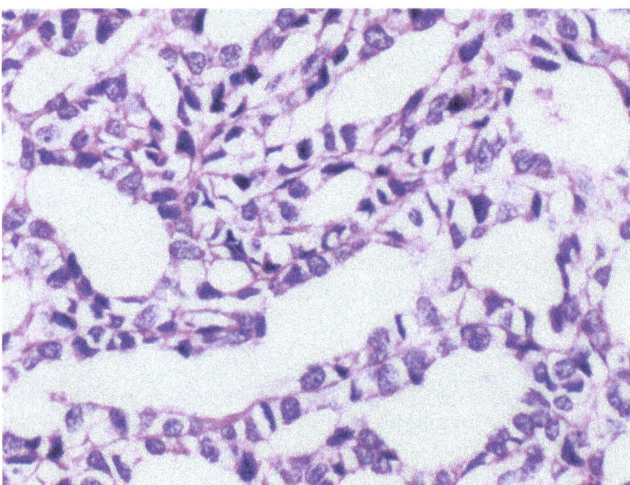

**Figure 14.44:** Sertoli-Leydig cell tumor, well differentiated: Tubules are lined by sertoli cells

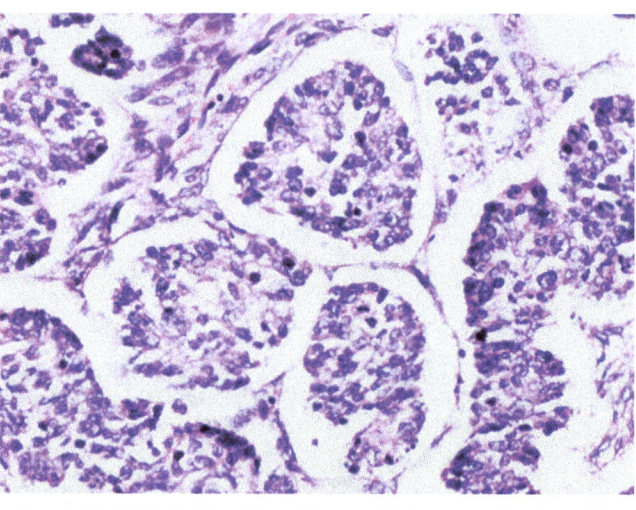

**Figure 14.47:** Sertoli-Leydig cell tumor: Higher magnification of the nest pattern

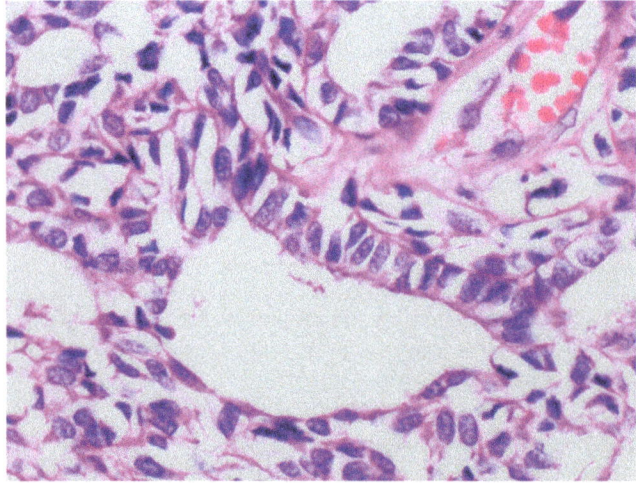

**Figure 14.45:** Sertoli-Leydig cell tumor, well differentiated: Higher magnification of the tubules show cuboidal cells with scanty to moderate amount of cytoplasm and round monomorphic nuclei

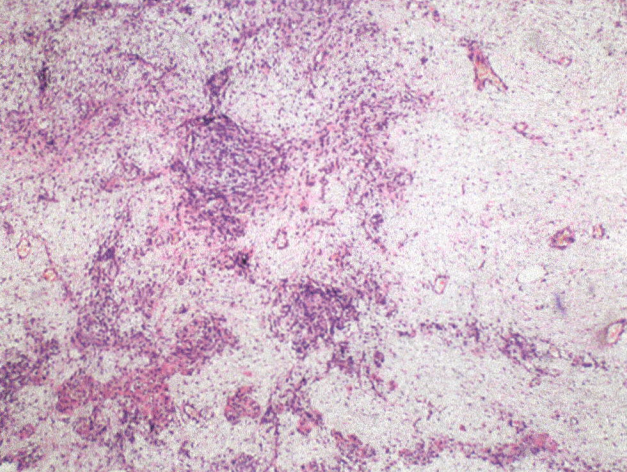

**Figure 14.48:** Sertoli-Leydig cell tumor: Significant edema within the tumor

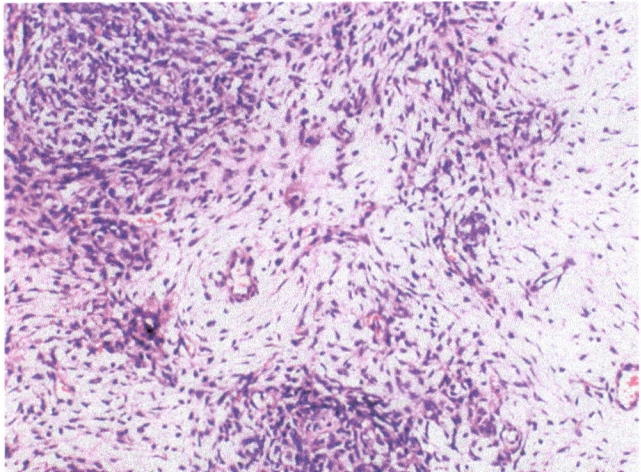

Figure 14.49: Sertoli-Leydig cell tumor: Higher magnification of the same

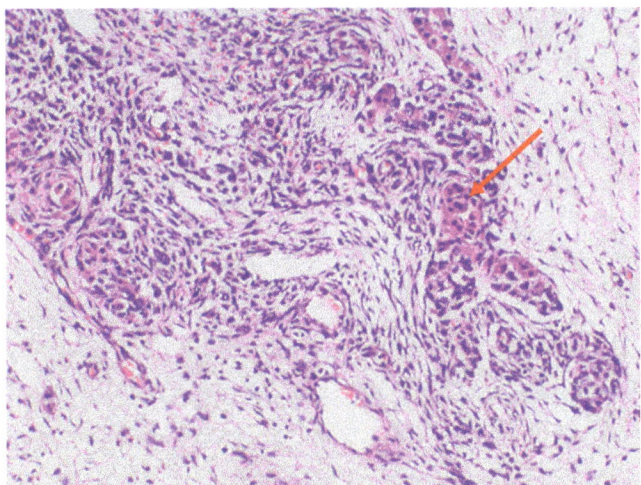

Figure 14.50: Sertoli-Leydig cell tumor: Occasional foci of Leydig cells

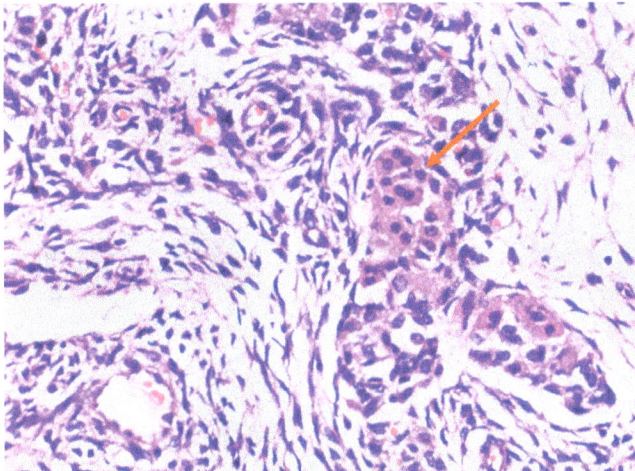

Figure 14.51: Sertoli-Leydig cell tumor: Higher magnification shows better morphology of the Leydig cells

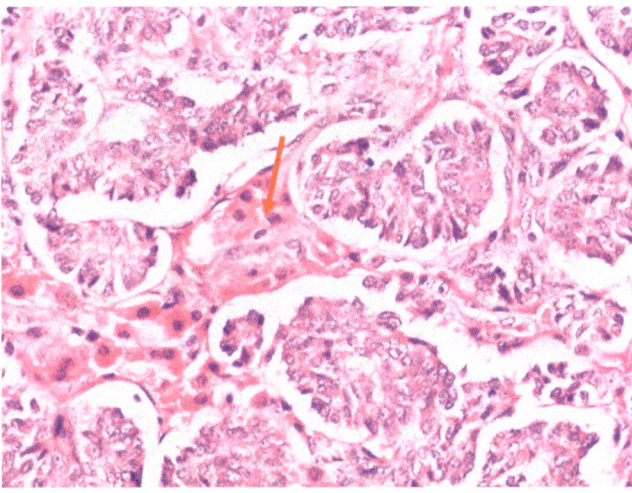

Figure 14.52: Sertoli-Leydig cell tumor, intermediately differentiated: Multiple lobulated cellular areas. Leydig cells are also present focally (arrow)

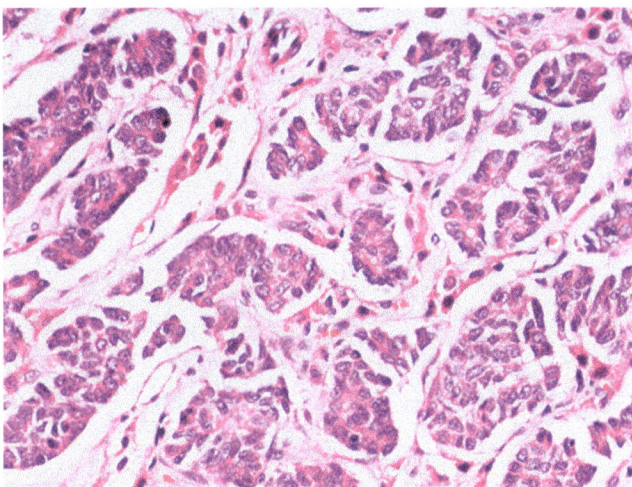

Figure 14.53: Sertoli-Leydig cell tumor, intermediately differentiated: Lobules with intervening stroma

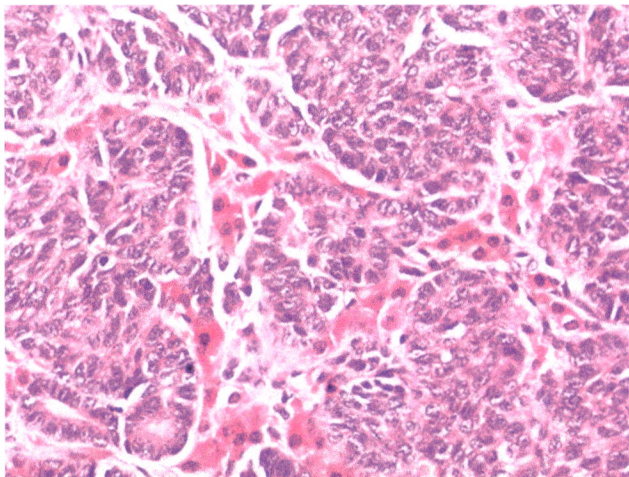

Figure 14.54: Sertoli-Leydig cell tumor, intermediately differentiated: Cellular areas show round cells with scanty cytoplasm and round angulated nuclei. Occasional tubules are seen

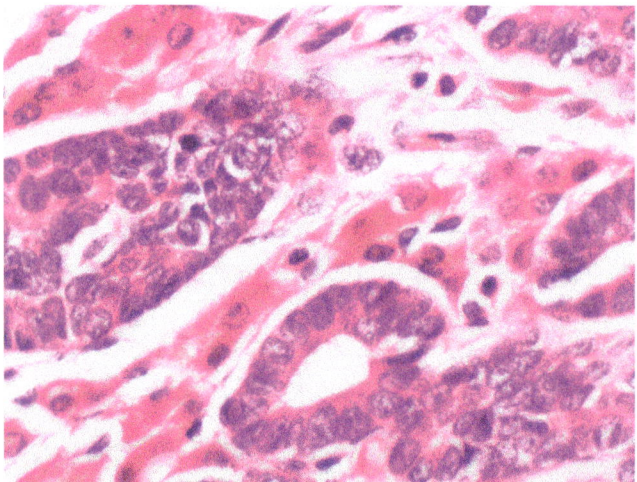

**Figure 14.55:** Sertoli-Leydig cell tumor, intermediately differentiated: Tubules are interspersed along with Leydig cells

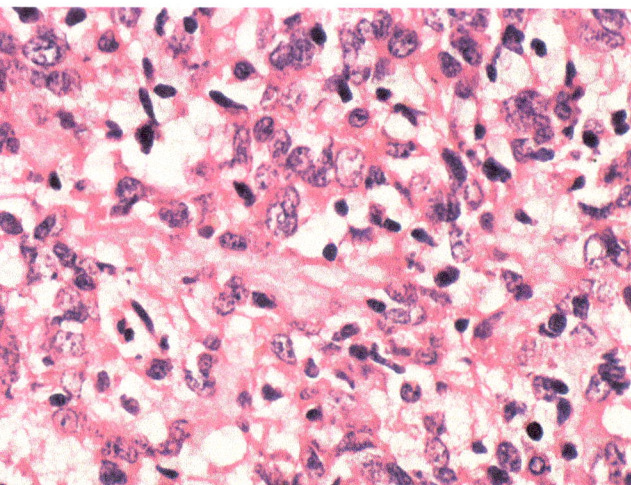

**Figure 14.58:** Sertoli-Leydig cell tumor, poorly differentiated: Cells with moderately pleomorphic nuclei

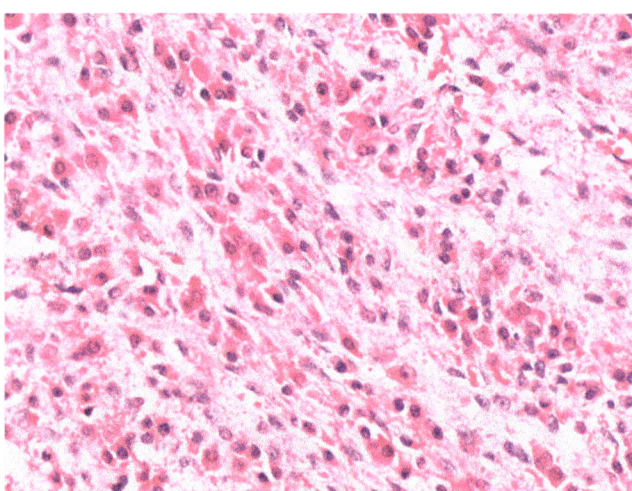

**Figure 14.56:** Sertoli-Leydig cell tumor, intermediately differentiated: Large areas of Leydig cells

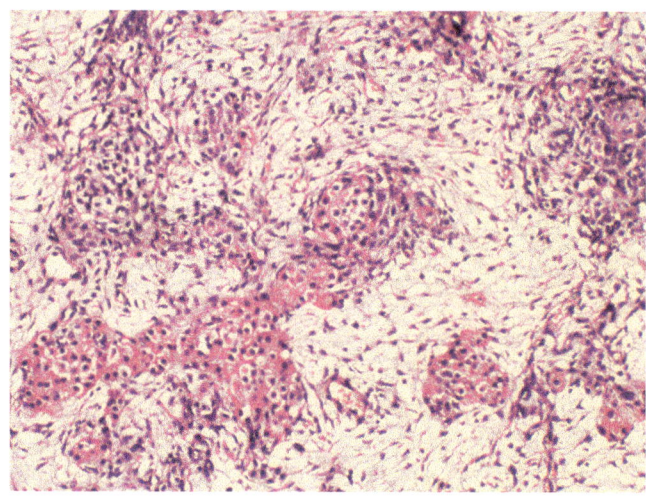

**Figure 14.59:** Sertoli-Leydig cell tumor, poorly differentiated: Occasional foci of Leydig cells in the stroma

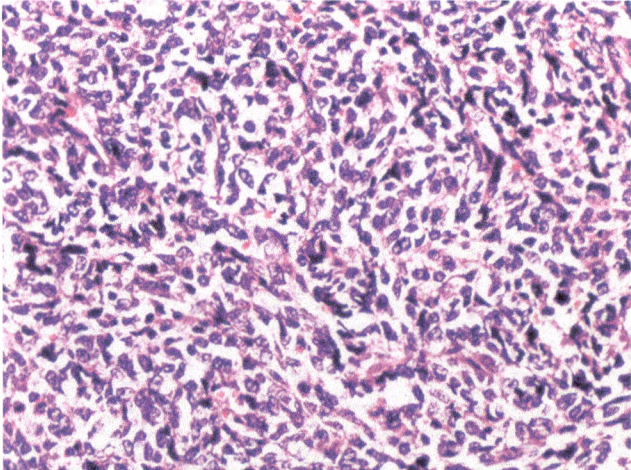

**Figure 14.57:** Sertoli-Leydig cell tumor, poorly differentiated: Solid sheets of cells with moderately pleomorphic nuclei

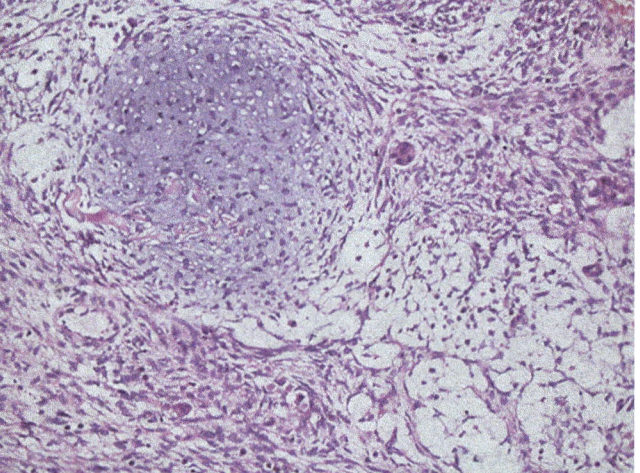

**Figure 14.60:** Sertoli-Leydig cell tumor with heterologous element: Foci of cartilaginous differentiation

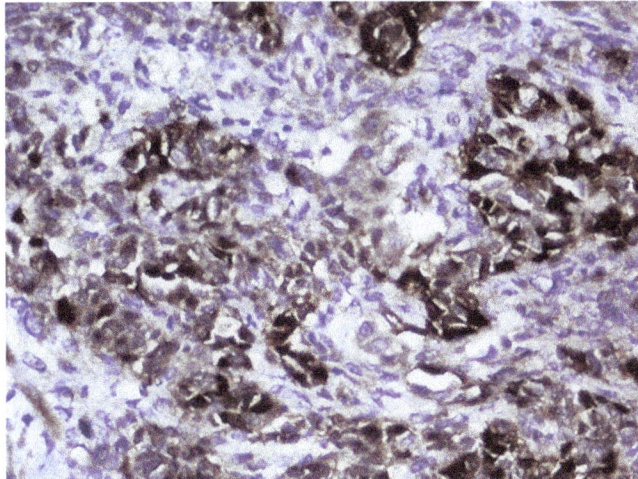

Figure 14.61: Sertoli-Leydig cell tumor: Strong calretinin positive cells

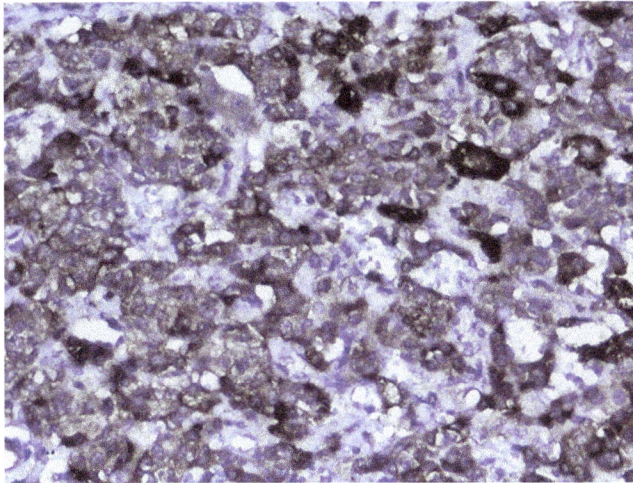

Figure 14.62: Sertoli-Leydig cell tumor: Strong inhibin positive cells

(2) Lack of androgenic activity, (3) Presence of squamous element, (4) Fibromatous stroma, and (5) Negative inhibin immunostain.
b. **Carcinoid tumor:** Trabecular arrangement of cells in SLCT may mimic carcinoid tumor. However differentiating points are: (1) Much longer ribbon of cells in carcinoid, (2) Less cellular stroma in carcinoid, (3) About 70% carcinoid tumor shows associated teratoma elements.
c. **Struma ovarii:** The following features favor struma ovarii: (1) Typical thyroid follicles, (2) Thyroglobulin positivity.
d. **Krukenberg's tumor:** The following features favor Krukenberg's tumor: (1) Bilateral tumor, (2) Typical signet ring cells, (3) Positive mucin stain, (4) Clinical history.
e. **Malignant Mullerian mixed tumor (MMMT):** The presence of heterologous elements in SLCT may mimic MMMT. The following features favor the diagnosis of MMMT: (1) Higher age of the patient, (2) No androgenic effect, (3) High-grade epithelial carcinoma, (4) The cartilage is malignant in MMMT.
f. **Yolk sac tumor:** Retiform type of SLCT may simulate yolk sac tumor. However, the following features are helpful in diagnosis of yolk sac tumors: (1) No androgenic effect, (2) High serum alpha feto-protein level, (3) the retiform structure appears more malignant than that of SLCT.
g. **Teratoma:** Heterologous elements of SLCT may mimic teratoma. However, the other teratomatous component such as ectodermal or endodermal components are also seen in teratoma.

### Treatment and Prognosis

The prognosis of SLCT mainly depends on the degree of differentiation and stage of tumor. Well-differentiated stage I SLCT behaves completely benign. Malignant SLCTs are mostly poorly differentiated, retiform type or contain heterologous mesenchymal elements. In young patients, simple unilateral salpingo-oophorectomy is the treatment of choice. Removal of the tumor is followed by recovery of menstruation and disappearance of virilizing symptoms with one month. In advanced cases, radical surgery along with chemotherapy may be needed.

## SERTOLI CELL TUMOR

Sertoli cell tumors are rare and represent less than 5% of sex cord stromal tumor.

### Clinical Features

Sertoli cell tumors are commonly seen in reproductive age period with an average age of 30 years. The patient may have abdominal swelling, pain or menstrual abnormalities. The tumor is predominantly nonfunctioning, but the patients may show estrogenic (30%) or uncommonly androgenic effect.

### Macroscopy

Grossly, the tumor is unilateral with variable in size from 1 to 30 cm. Average size of the tumor is 9 cm. They are well circumscribed with smooth surface and cut section show solid yellow to brown color appearance.

### Microscopic Features

The tumor is composed of well-formed tubules, cords, trabeculae and diffuse sheets of cells. The tubules may be hollow or solid type lined by small cuboidal to columnar cells having moderate amount of pale eosinophilic cytoplasm. The nuclei are round and monomorphic. Mitosis is scanty to absent. The solid tubules are crowded with elongated or round in shape.

### Differential Diagnosis

a. Struma ovarii: Discussed with Sertoli-Leydig cell tumor.
b. Endometrioid carcinoma: Discussed with Sertoli-Leydig cell tumor.
c. Carcinoid: Discussed with Sertoli-Leydig Cell Tumor. Prognosis: The majority of the Sertoli cell tumors are benign and unilateral salpingo-oophorectomy is sufficient for treatment.

## GYNANDROBLASTOMA

Gynandroblastomas are very rare type of sex cord stromal tumor.[15] This tumor is characterized by admixture of both granulosa cell tumor and sex-cord stromal tumors. The minor component of the tumor should contain at least 10% of the tumor. Gynandroblastomas mostly present in stage I and are benign in outcome.

## SEX CORD TUMOR WITH ANNULAR TUBULES

The tumor occurs in the third to fourth decade of life. The average one-third of the patients may also have Peutz-Jegher syndrome (PJS) which is characterized by gastrointestinal hamartomatous poly, mucocutaneous pigmentation and adenoma malignum.[16] The age range of the patient widely varies from 4 to 70 years. However mean age of the patient is 27 years. The tumor is mostly detected as incidental finding.

### Gross

This tumor is associated with PJS are often bilateral and those tumors unassociated with PJS are unilateral. The tumors are small microscopic size to several cm in diameter. The cut section of the tumor is solid yellowish in appearance.

### Microscopy

The tumor is composed of multiple ring like simple or complex tubules. The simple tubules are lined by basement membrane with central hyalinized material. The lining cells of the tubules are Sertoli cells with pale cytoplasm. The complex tubules are formed by large tubules with multiple small tubules at the periphery of the large tubules. The tumors associated with PJS show discrete annular tubules throughout the stroma. Whereas, the tumors unassociated with PJS show mass like collection of tubules within the stroma.

### Prognosis

The tumor associated with PJS behaves as benign tumor. However those tumors unrelated with PJS are often malignant (25%). The tumors with more than 3–4 mitotic figures per 10 HPFs and infiltrative pattern of growth show aggressive behavior. In younger patients, unilateral salpingo-oophorectomy with staging is the treatment of choice.

## STEROID CELL TUMORS

Steroid cell tumors are composed of cells that resemble steroid secreting cells and this type of cells should be present in more than 90% of the tumor mass. Steroid cell tumor represents only 1% of all sex cord stromal tumors. There are three types of steroid cell tumor: (1) stromal luteoma, (2) Leydig cell tumor and (3) steroid cell tumor, not otherwise specified.

## Stromal Luteoma

This is a benign neoplastic lesion of stromal origin and represents almost 21% of steroid cell tumor.[17]

### Clinical Feature

The tumor commonly occurs in the post-menopausal patients. The most patients complain of vaginal bleeding due to the manifestation of excess estrogen and 12% patients may have androgenic manifestation.

### Gross

The tumors is usually unilateral and is seen in the center of the ovary. The tumor is small and varies from 0.5 to 2 cm in diameter. It is well-circumscribed gray-white or yellow-brown in appearance.

### Histology

The tumor is well circumscribed and is composed of diffuse sheets, nests or cords of uniform population of cells. The cells are polygonal with abundant vacuolated pale to eosinophilic cytoplasm. The nuclei are central in position and round monomorphic in shape having prominent nucleoli. The surrounding normal ovarian stroma of the same side or opposite side ovary shows stromal hyperthecosis.

### Immunohistochemistry

The tumor cells are positive for calretinin and inhibin.

### Differential Diagnosis

1. Pregnancy luteoma: Pregnancy luteoma gives the history of pregnancy and are multifocal.

2. Leydig cell tumor of the nonhilar type: Leydig cell tumor of the nonhilar type are androgenic. This tumor shows Reinke crystals.

*Prognosis*

This is a benign tumor and no recurrence or metastasis has been reported after removal of the tumor.

## Leydig Cell Tumor

This tumor represents 15% of ovarian steroid cell tumors. This tumor is derived from the Leydig cells of ovary and therefore mainly present in the hilum of ovary. The tumor is divided into two types: Hilus cell tumor and Leydig cell tumor, nonhilar cell type.

*Hilus Cell Tumor*

This is the most common type of Leydig cell tumor. This tumor is developed from the hilar cells of the ovary located in the hilum of ovary.

**Gross:** The tumor is unilateral and located in the hilum of ovary. It is usually small in size and is well circumscribed. The cut section is firm and yellow in appearance.

**Histology:** The tumor is well circumscribed and shows lobulated or diffuse sheets of cells. The intervening stroma is edematous or hyalinized. The individual cells show abundant eosinophilic cytoplasm. The cells often show lipofuscin pigment or Reinke crystals. Intranuclear cytoplasmic inclusions are also seen. The nuclei are round with small nucleoli. At times, the tumor shows nuclear rich area with crowding of nuclei followed by adjacent nuclear free area. Mitotic activity is rarely seen. Reinke crystals are seen in half of Leydig cell tumor. These crystals are rod shaped structures and are better visualized by PTAH stain.

**Prognosis:** This is a benign tumor and unilateral salpingo-oophorectomy is the treatment of choice.

*Leydig Cell Tumor, Nonhilar Cell Type*

This tumor develops from the hilus cell of the stroma of ovary. The tumor is present in the medulla of ovary. It is usually small and well circumscribed. The histology of the tumor is similar to that of hilus type Leydig cell tumor.

## Steroid Cell Tumor, Not Otherwise Specified

Steroid cell tumor, not otherwise specified represents 60% of steroid cell tumor.

*Clinical Feature*

The tumor commonly occurs in younger patients than the other steroid cell tumors. The average age of the patient is 43 years. The majority of the patients present either androgenic manifestation as virilizing symptoms or estrogenic manifestation as postmenopausal bleeding or menorrhagia. Patients may be asymptomatic or may have non-specific symptoms.

*Gross*

The tumors are mostly unilateral and with variable size (1 to 30 cm). The tumor is solid and cut section shows yellow to brown appearance.

*Histology*

The tumor is composed of diffuse sheets, solid aggregates and trabeculae of cells separated by thin fibrous septae. The cells are polygonal with eosinophilic cytoplasm or vacuolated cytoplasm. The nuclei are round in shape with prominent nucleoli. Nuclear atypia is minimal to nil. Occasional tumors may show significant nuclear atypia and mitosis. In small fraction of patient areas of hemorrhage and necrosis are also noted.

## Differential Diagnosis

a. Stromal luteoma and Leydig cell tumor: Stromal cell tumor shows associated ovarian hyperthecosis. Leydig cell is located characteristically in hilum of ovary and contains Reinke crystal.
b. Luteinized thecoma: This tumor is reticulin rich and reticulin fibers invest individual tumor cells.
c. Luteinized granulosa cell tumor: Characteristic morphological pattern of granulosa cell tumor helps to distinguish it from steroid cell tumor.
d. Oxyphilic endometrioid carcinoma: Typical glandular pattern and the presence of squamous cell component are helpful to identify oxyphilic endometrioid carcinoma tumor.

## Prognosis

The biological behavior of the tumor is unpredictable and about 43% of the steroid cell tumor may be malignant.[18] The tumor may recur even 5 years after surgery. The features suggestive of malignant behavior of the tumor are: (a) Large size, (>7 cm in diameter), (b) areas of hemorrhage and necrosis, (c) mitotic count 2 or more per 10 HPFs and (d) Moderate to marked nuclear atypia.

## REFERENCES

1. Koonings PP, Campbell K, Mishell DR Jr, et al. Relative frequency of primary ovarian neoplasms: a 10-year review. Obstet Gynecol. 1989;74:921-6.
2. Bjorkholm E. Granulosa cell tumors: a comparison of survival in patients and matched controls. Am J Obstet Gynecol. 1980; 138:329-31.

3. Al-Agha OM, Huwait HF, Chow C, et al. FOXL2 is a sensitive and specific marker for sex cord-stromal tumors of the ovary. Am J Surg Pathol. 2011;35:484-94.
4. Björkholm E, Silfverswärd C. Prognostic factors in granulosa-cell tumors. Gynecol Oncol. 1981;11(3):261-74.
5. Bjorkholm E, Silfversward C. Theca-cell tumors. Clinical features and prognosis. Acta Radiol Oncol Radiat Phys Biol. 1980;19:241-4.
6. Zhang J, Young RH, Arseneau J, Scully RE. Ovarian stromal tumors containing lutein or Leydig cells (luteinized thecomas and stromal Leydig cell tumors)--a clinicopathological analysis of fifty cases. Int J Gynecol Pathol. 1982;1(3):270-85.
7. McCluggage WG, Sloan JM, Boyle DD, Toner PG. Malignant fibrothecomatous tumour of the ovary: diagnostic value of anti-inhibin immunostaining. J Clin Pathol. 1998;51(11):868-71.
8. Meigs JV. Fibroma of the ovary with ascites and hydrothorax. Meigs' syndrome. Am J Obstet Gynecol. 1954;67:962-87.
9. Gorlin RJ. Nevoid basal-cell carcinoma syndrome. Medicine (Baltim). 1987;66:98-113.
10. Shakfeh S M, Woodruff J D. Primary ovarian sarcomas: report of 46 cases and review of the literature. Obstet Gynecol Surv. 1987;42:331-49.
11. Tiltman A J, Haffajee Z. Sclerosing stromal tumors, thecomas, and fibromas of the ovary: an immunohistochemical profile. Int J Gynecol Pathol. 1999;18:254-8.
12. Vang R, Vague S, Tavassoli F, Prat J .Signet-ring stromal tumor of the ovary: clinicopathologic analysis and comparison with Krukenberg tumor. Int J Gynecol Pathol. 2003;23:45-51.
13. Roth LM, Anderson MC, Govan ADT, et al. Sertoli-Leydig cell tumors: a clinicopathologic study of 34 cases. Cancer. 1981;48:187-97.
14. Young RH, Prat J, Scully RE. Cancer. Ovarian Sertoli-Leydig cell tumors with heterologous elements. I. Gastrointestinal epithelium and carcinoid: a clinicopathologic analysis of thirty-six cases. 1982;50(11):2448-56.
15. Anderson MC, Rees DA. Gynandroblastoma of the ovary.Br J Obstet Gynaecol. 1975;82:68-73.
16. Scully RE. Sex cord tumor with annular tubules. A distinctive ovarian tumor of the Peutz–Jeghers syndrome. Cancer (Phila) 1970;25:1107-21.
17. Hayes MC, Scully RE. Stromal luteoma of the ovary: a clinicopathological analysis of 25 cases. Int J Gynecol Pathol. 1987;6:313-21.
18. Hayes MC, Scully RE. Ovarian steroid cell tumor (not otherwise specified): a clinicopathological analysis of 63 cases. Am J Surg Pathol. 1987;11:835-45.

# Germ Cell Tumor of Ovary

The germ cell tumors of ovary are histologically different heterogeneous group of tumors that are derived from the primitive germ cells. They represent 30% of all ovarian neoplasms. About 95% germ cell tumors are benign cystic teratoma. Malignant germ cell tumors consists of only 3% of all ovarian malignancies. Majority of the malignant germ cell tumors are seen in children and young women. WHO classified germ cell tumors as mentioned in Table 15.1.[1]

**Table 15.1:** Germ cell tumor

| |
|---|
| 1. Dysgerminoma: variant-with syncytiotrophoblast cells |
| 2. Yolk sac tumors (endodermal sinus tumors): |
|    – Polyvesicular vitelline tumor |
|    – Hepatoid |
|    – Glandular |
| 3. Embryonal carcinoma |
| 4. Polyembryoma |
| 5. Choriocarcinoma |
| 6. Teratomas |
|    – Immature |
|    – Mature |
|       - Cystic |
|       - Solid |
|    – Monodermal |
|    – Struma ovary |
|    – Carcinoid |
|    – Neuroectodermal tumors |
| 7. Mixed germ cell |

## DYSGERMINOMA

Dysgerminoma is the commonest germ cell tumor of ovary and represents 1% of all ovarian malignancies (Box 15.1).[2]

## Clinical Features

The tumor commonly occurs in second and third decades of life with a median age of 22 years. About 20 to 30% dysgerminoma may occur during pregnancy. The patient commonly presents with rapidly growing mass in the abdomen along with pain and pressure symptoms. It may also be detected incidentally during investigations of primary amenorrhea. Rarely the patients may show excess estrogenic effect such as menstrual irregularities, vaginal bleeding, isosexual pseudoprecocity and pseudopregnancy. These endocrine symptoms are mainly due to beta hCG secretion from the tumor. Most of the patients of dysgerminoma have high LDH level. Elevated hCG or AFP level in serum indicates the presence of other germ cell elements in dysgerminoma.

## Gross

Dysgerminoma often affects the right ovary (50%) and 10% of the tumor is bilateral. The tumor is of variable size with an average diameter of 15 cm. Dysgerminomas are commonly solid, firm and well-circumscribed tumor (Figures 15.1 and 15.2). The cut section is lobulated, soft pale tan to gray-pink in appearance. Foci of hemorrhage, necrosis and small cystic spaces may be seen.

## Histopathology (Figures 15.3 to 15.5)

The tumor is composed of monotonous population of round cells with polygonal in shape having distinct cytoplasmic margin. The cytoplasm is abundant and pale or eosinophilic to clear that contains glycogen. The nuclei are large round with central prominent nucleoli. The cells are also arranged in diffuse sheets, insular pattern, trabeculae, cords or small nests. Loss of intercellular cohesion may show the formation of pseudoglandular space. The large clusters of tumor cells are frequently separated by fibrous septa. These fibrous septa are usually infiltrated by lymphocytes that are T cell

**Box 15.1:** Dysgerminoma

→ It represents 1% of all ovarian malignancies

**Clinical features:**
- Commonly occurs in second and third decades of life
- Median age of 22 years
- Rapidly growing mass in the abdomen along with pain and pressure symptoms
- High LDH level

**Gross:**
- 10% of the tumor is bilateral
- Size: variable with mean diameter of 15 cm
- Solid, firm and well-circumscribed tumor
- The cut section:
  - Lobulated, soft pale tan to gray-pink in appearance
  - Foci of hemorrhage, necrosis and small cystic spaces may be seen

**Microscopy**
- Monotonous population of round cells
- Arrangement of cell: Diffuse sheets, insular pattern, trabeculae, cords or small nests
- Cells
  - Polygonal in shape with distinct cytoplasmic margin
  - Cytoplasm abundant and pale or eosinophilic to clear
- Large clusters of tumor cells are often separated by fibro-collagenous tissue
- Fibrous septa are usually infiltrated by lymphocytes

**Immunohistochemistry:**
- Positive for PLAP, CD117 and D2-40

**Molecular pathology:**
- Chromosome 12p abnormalities
- c-KIT mutation in 25% cases

**Differential diagnosis:** Solid EST, embryonal carcinoma, clear cell carcinoma, large cell lymphoma

**Prognosis and treatment**
- Surgery is the treatment of choice: Unilateral salpingo-oophorectomy with frequent follow-up
- Very good prognosis
- The five year survival rate is more than 90% in stage I tumor

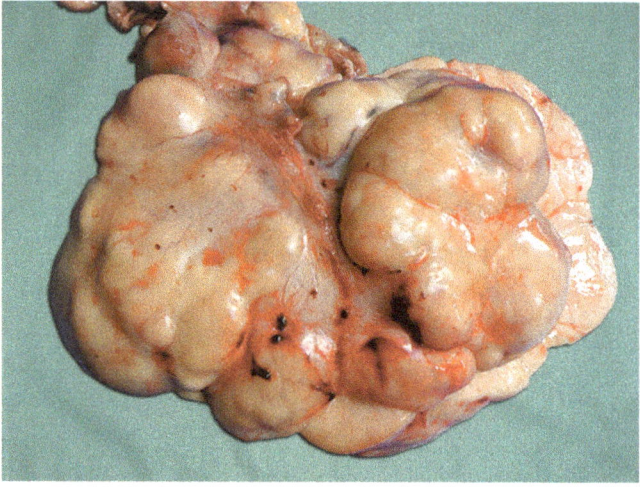

Figure 15.1: Dysgerminoma: Solid gray-white nodular tumor

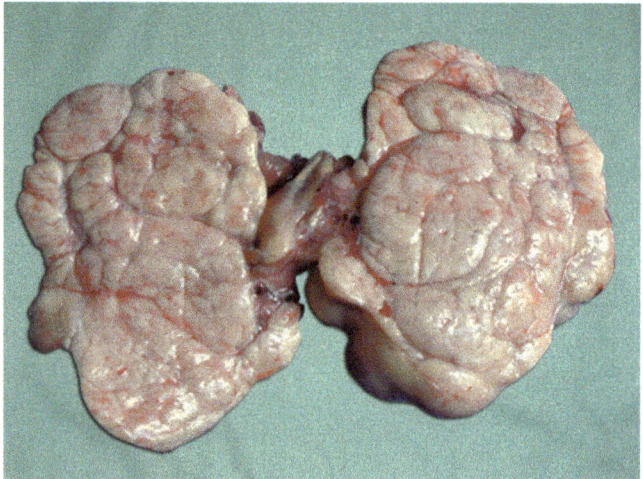

Figure 15.2: Dysgerminoma: Soft to firm lobulated grayish cut section

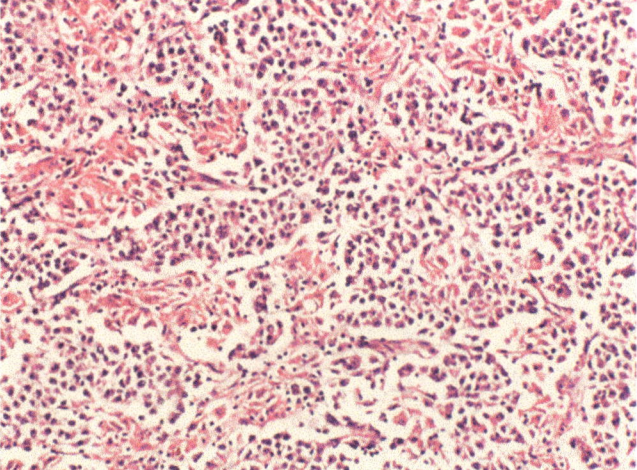

Figure 15.3: Dysgerminoma: Large clusters of tumor cells separated by fibrocollagenous tissue

in nature. Lymphocytes may also sprinkle within the tumor cells. Occasionally germinal center formation may be seen numerous mitotic figures are seen. Multinucleated giant cells with epithelioid granulomas are seen in 20% cases of dysgerminoma. About 5% cases of dysgerminomas show syncytiotrophoblastic giant cells without any evidence of other non-germinomatous elements.

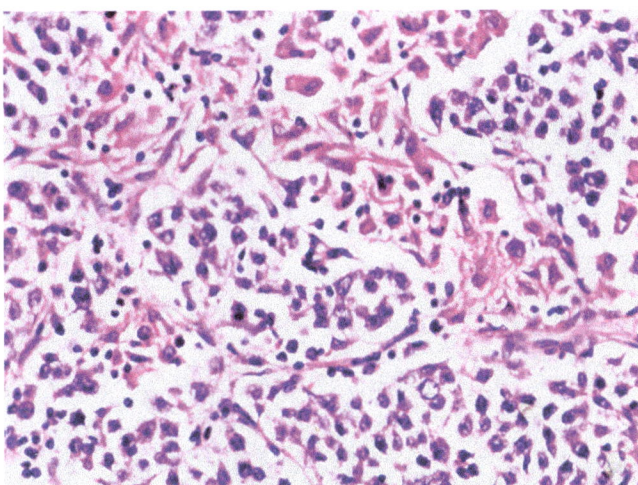

**Figure 15.4:** Dysgerminoma: Tumor cells in clusters along with lymphocytes in the intervening stroma

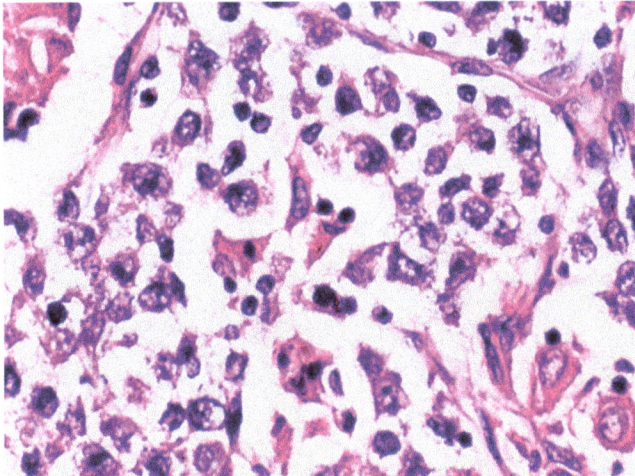

**Figure 15.5:** Dysgerminoma: Tumor cells with moderate cytoplasm having round regular nuclei with prominent nucleoli

### Immunohistochemistry

Dysgerminomas are positive for PLAP, CD117 and D2-40. CD 117 positivity in dysgerminoma cases is independent of mutation of c-kit gene. In addition, the tumor is also positive for NSE, CK, desmin and inhibin.

### Molecular Pathology

Dysgerminomas show characteristic Chromosome 12p abnormalities. c-KIT mutation is noted in 25% cases of dysgerminoma.[3]

### Differential Diagnosis

a. **Solid EST:** Following features favor EST: (1) Marked nuclear variation, (2) Absent lymphocytic infiltration, (3) Presence of hyaline bodies, and (4) High AFP.

b. **Embryonal carcinoma:** The presence of large cells with moderate amount of cytoplasm and CK positivity help in the diagnosis of rare embryonal carcinoma.

c. **Clear cell carcinoma:** Discussed before with clear cell carcinoma.

d. **Large cell lymphoma:** The following features help in the diagnosis of lymphoma: (1) Bilateral involvement, (2) Positive CD45, (3) Negative PLAP.

### Prognosis and Treatment

Unilateral salpingo-oophorectomy with frequent follow-up is the treatment of choice for the women who want to preserve the fertility. In advanced or recurrent disease combination chemotherapy including cisplatin, etoposide, and bleomycin combination have been used successfully.[4]

Dysgerminoma has very good prognosis. The five year survival rate is more than 90% in stage I tumor. The tumor shows unfavorable prognosis if the patient presents with bilateral tumor, large size of tumor, or adhesion with the surrounding tissues or metastasis.[5] The follow-up of the patients should be done by repeated estimation of serum AFP, HCG, chest X-ray and CT scan of abdomen. Recurrence may occur in 15% cases within 24 months. The recurrent cases are treated with combination chemotherapy and radiotherapy.[6]

## YOLK SAC TUMORS

Yolk sac tumor (YST) is also known as endodermal sinus tumor (EST). YST represents 20% of all malignant germ cell tumors of ovary (Box 15.2).

**Box 15.2:** Yolk sac tumor (YST)

- YST represents 20% of all malignant germ cell tumors of ovary
- It accounts for 1% of all ovarian malignancies

**Clinical features**
- YST mainly occurs in children and young adults
- Median age of the patient is 18 years
- Rapidly growing abdominal mass with pelvic pain

**Gross**
- Unilateral
- Size: large with a mean diameter 15 cm.
- Well encapsulated solid mass with smooth and glistening surface
- Cut section:
  - Tan white to gray.
  - Areas of hemorrhage and necrosis are frequently seen

**Histopathology:** histological patterns:
- Reticular or microcystic: The most common pattern, multiple mesh like microcystic spaces in a loose myxoid stroma

*Contd...*

*Contd...*

- Endodermal sinus:
  - Tumor shows labyrinthine anastomosing glands and papillae
  - The papillae are lined by columnar cells with hyperchromatic atypical nuclei
  - Schiller Duval bodies
- Polyvesicular vitelline:
  - Large cystic spaces and vesicles within dense spindle cell stroma
- Alveolar–glandular
  - Multiple alveolar and gland like structure within a myxomatous stroma
- Macrocystic: multiple large cystic spaces are seen
- Papillary
  - Multiple papillary structures with central fibrovascular core
  - Lining: moderate to highly pleomorphic epithelial cells
- Solid
  - Solid aggregates of tumor cells
  - The cells are polygonal in shape with clear cytoplasm
- Hepatoid
  - Clusters or cords of cells having hepatoid look
  - The cells are polygonal with abundant eosinophilic cytoplasm
- Hyaline globules
  - A characteristic finding of YST
  - Small round eosinophilic bodies
  - PAS positive and diastase resistant
  - Composed of laminin and type IV collagen material.

**Immunohistochemistry:**
- Positive: alpha fetoprotein, cytokeratin, PLAP, CD 117
- Negative for EMA

**Differential diagnosis:** Clear cell carcinoma, endometrioid carcinomas, embryonal carcinoma, dysgerminoma, Sertoli-Leydig cell tumor, hepatocellular carcinoma

**Prognosis and treatment:**
- Highly malignant tumor with aggressive behavior
- The treatment of choice: Unilateral salpingo-oophorectomy with combination chemotherapy (cisplatinum, etoposide, and bleomycin)

## Clinical Features

YST mainly occurs in children and young adults and the median age of the patient is 18 years. The patients usually present as rapidly growing abdominal mass with pelvic pain. Occasionally, the tumor may have torsion and rupture and the patients may have acute abdomen simulating appendicitis or rupture ectopic pregnancy. YST shows high AFP level and usually the level is more than 1000 ng/ml.[7]

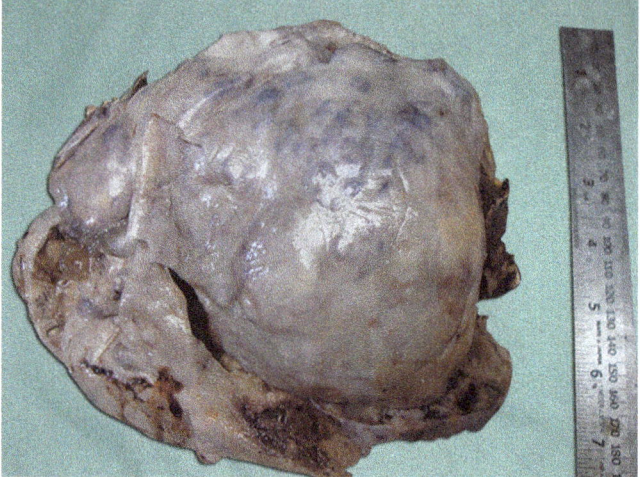

**Figure 15.6:** Endodermal sinus tumor: Large tumor with areas of hemorrhage over the surface

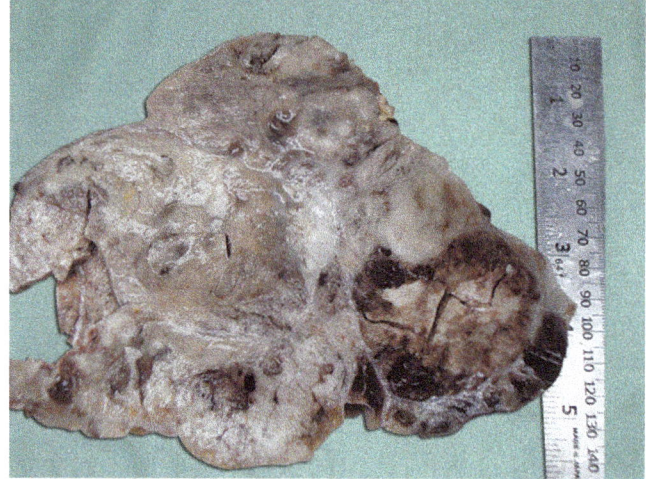

**Figure 15.7:** Endodermal sinus tumor: Cut section shows solid areas with necrosis

## Gross

YST is always unilateral and bilateral tumor indicates metastasis from other ovary. The size of the tumor is large with an average diameter 15 cm. The tumor is well-encapsulated solid mass with smooth and glistening surface. The cut section of the tumor is tan white to gray. Areas of hemorrhage and necrosis are frequently seen (Figures 15.6 and 15.7).

## Histopathology (Figures 15.8 to 15.16)

YST shows marked variation of histological patterns that are described below:

a. **Reticular or microcystic:** This is the most common pattern of YST. In this pattern, the tumor shows multiple mesh like microcystic spaces in a loose myxoid stroma.

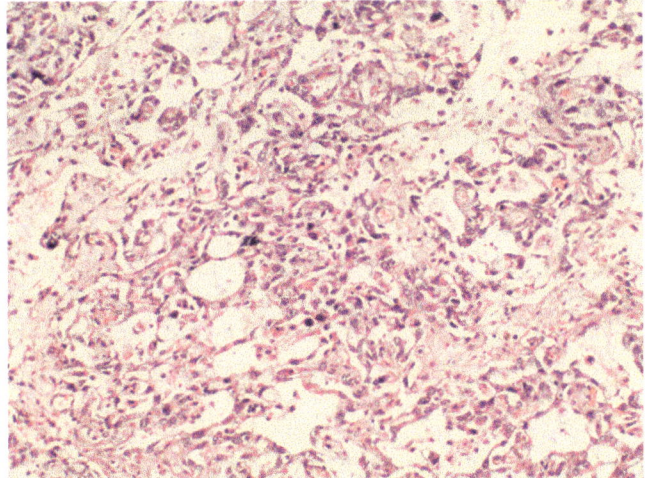

Figure 15.8: Endodermal sinus tumor: Small cystic spaces

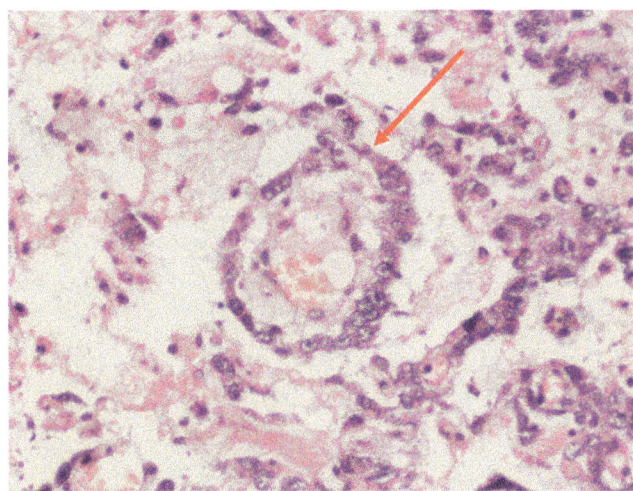

Figure 15.11: Endodermal sinus tumor: Classical Schiller-Duval body characterized by central capillary space surrounded by loose primitive stroma with a peripheral mantle of cuboidal tumor cells

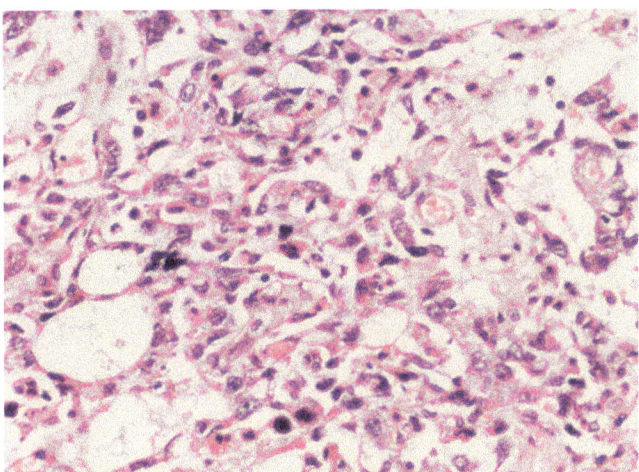

Figure 15.9: Endodermal sinus tumor: Cystic structures are lined by malignant cells

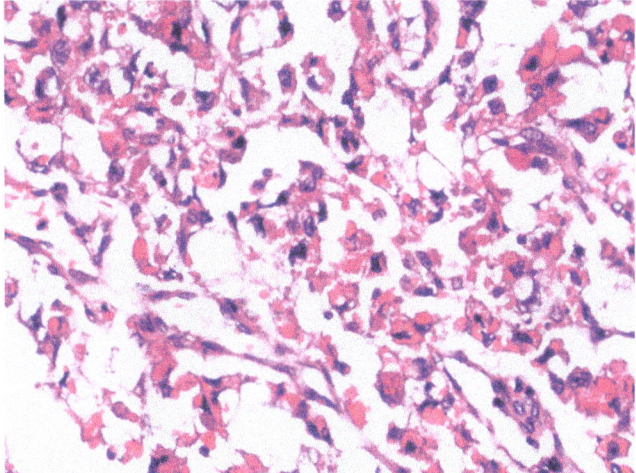

Figure 15.12: Endodermal sinus tumor: Hyaline globules in the tumor

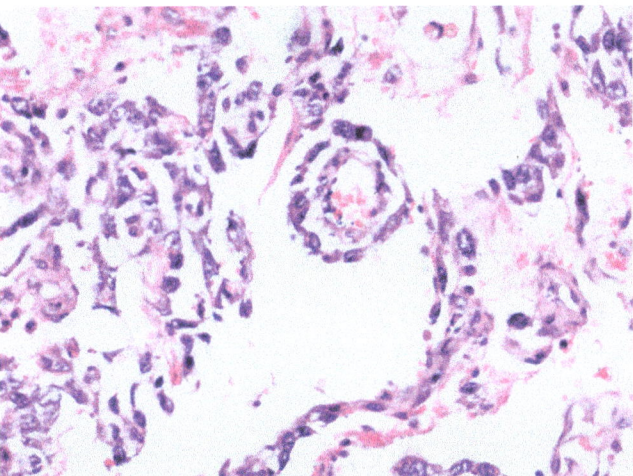

Figure 15.10: Endodermal sinus tumor: Multiple cystic spaces and Schiller-Duval body

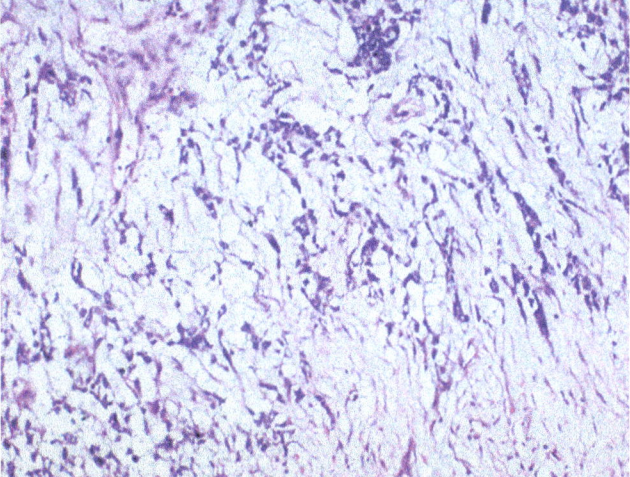

Figure 15.13: Endodermal sinus tumor: Myxomatous area with rows of tumor cells

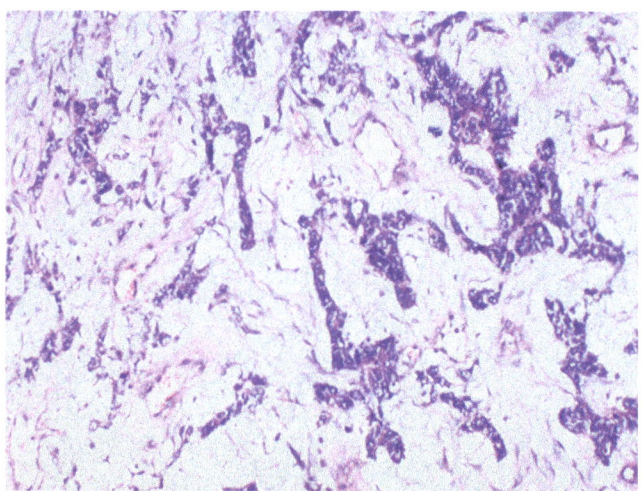

Figure 15.14: Endodermal sinus tumor: Higher magnification of the rows of tumor cells

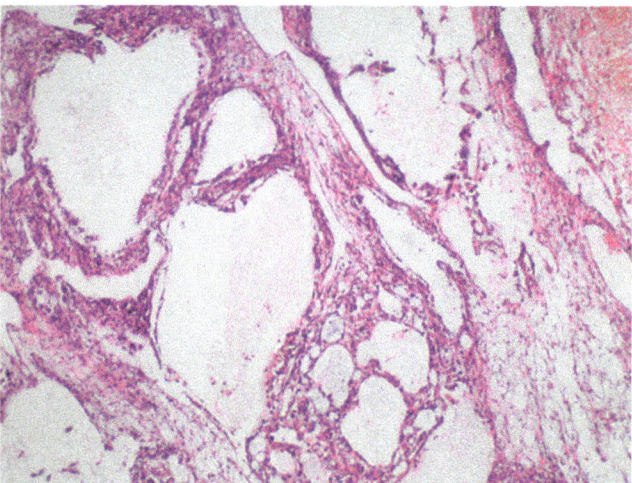

Figure 15.15: Endodermal sinus tumor: Macrocystic pattern shows multiple large cystic spaces

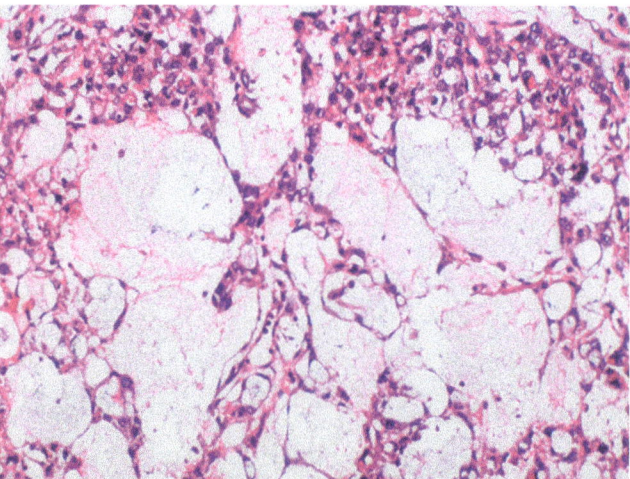

Figure 15.16: Endodermal sinus tumor: Solid clusters of cells along with large cysts in macrocystic pattern

This gives a characteristic honeycomb like pattern. The microcystic spaces are lined by single layer of flat to cuboidal tumor cells. The cells have clear cytoplasm with moderately pleomorphic hyperchromatic nuclei.

b. **Endodermal sinus:** Here the tumor shows anastomosing glands and papillae. The papillae are lined by columnar cells with hyperchromatic atypical nuclei. The endodermal sinus pattern shows distinctive perivascular formation known as Schiller-Duval bodies. The Schiller-Duval body is characterized by central capillary space surrounded by loose primitive stroma with a peripheral mantle of cuboidal tumor cells. Schiller-Duval body is seen in almost 20% cases of YST.[8]

c. **Polyvesicular vitelline pattern:** This pattern is characterized by large cystic spaces and vesicles within dense spindle cell stroma. The cystic spaces and vesicles are lined by flat cells, columnar cells or mucinous epithelial cells. The cysts resemble the yolk sac vesicles.

d. **Alveolar–glandular pattern:** Alveolar–glandular pattern shows multiple alveolar and gland like structure within a myxomatous stroma. The glands are lined by single to multiple layers of cuboidal or columnar epithelial cells with enlarged nuclei. The lining epithelial cells may be focally multilayered and may show small papillary like structure.

e. **Macrocystic pattern:** In this pattern, multiple large cystic spaces are seen.

f. **Papillary pattern:** This pattern is characterized by multiple papillary structures with central fibrovascular core lined by moderate to highly pleomorphic epithelial cells. High mitotic activities are also seen.

g. **Solid pattern:** Solid pattern shows solid aggregates of tumor cells. The individual cells are polygonal in shape with clear cytoplasm. The nuclei are large vesicular having prominent nucleoli. Mitotic activity is high.

h. **Hepatoid pattern:** This pattern is characterized by clusters or cords of cells having hepatoid look. The individual cells are polygonal with abundant eosinophilic cytoplasm. The hepatoid cells are seen in 33 to 50% of YST. However if the tumor shows dominant hepatoid pattern then only it should be designated as hepatoid yolk sac tumor.

The presence of hyaline globules is a characteristic finding of YST. These are small round eosinophilic bodies. They are present both intracellular and extracellular location. Hyaline globules may be noted in all the variants of YST. The hyaline bodies are PAS positive and diastase resistant and are composed of laminin and type IV collagen material.

## Immunohistochemistry

AFP immunostaining shows dense granular cytoplasmic positivity in all cases of YST. The tumor cells are also positive for cytokeratin and negative for EMA. YST is positive for PLAP and negative for CD117.

## Differential Diagnosis

a. **Clear cell carcinoma (CCC):** Following feature are helpful to diagnose CCC: (1) Elderly patients, (2) normal level of alpha fetoprotein level, (3) Lack of Schiller-Duval bodies, (4) The presence of hyalinized core in papillae, (5) The presence of endometriotic foci that are frequently seen in CCC, (6) CCCs are positive for CK 7 and EMA, and are mostly negative for AFP.
b. **Endometrioid carcinomas:** YST with endometrioid-like pattern may mimic secretory endometrioid carcinoma. The following features favor the diagnosis of EST over endometrioid carcinoma: (1) Younger age, (2) Lack of squamous cells, (3) Lack of endometriosis, (4) High nuclear grade of the cells with high mitosis, (5) Positive AFP and negative EMA.
c. **Embryonal carcinoma:** The following features are helpful to diagnose embryonal carcinoma over YST: (1) The cells are larger with more granular cytoplasm, (2) Nuclei show marked pleomorphism with large prominent nucleoli, (3) specific pattern of YST absent.
d. **Dysgerminoma:** The solid variant of YST may often be confused with dysgerminoma. The following features favor YST: (1) The presence of hyaline globules, (2) The absence of lymphocytes, (3) The positive AFP and CK, and negative CD117.
e. **Sertoli-Leydig cell tumor:** Retiform variant of Sertoli-Leydig cell tumor (SLCT) may be confused with YST. The following features favor the diagnosis of SLCT: (1) Androgenic manifestation is often seen in SLCT, (2) Typical Schiller-Duval bodies are absent, (3) The absence of various patterns of YST, (4) The presence of inhibin positive and AFP negative cells.
f. **Hepatocellular carcinoma:** The presence of hepatoid cells may be confused with metastatic hepatocellular carcinoma.

## Prognosis and Treatment

YST is a highly malignant tumor with aggressive behavior. Unilateral salpingo-oophorectomy with combination chemotherapy (cisplatinum, etoposide, and bleomycin) is the treatment of choice. Presently complete cure is possible in more than 80% cases in stage I tumor.[9]

Serum AFP is a useful marker both for diagnosis and monitor the response of therapy. The serum level of AFP falls rapidly after removal of tumor and it becomes normal within 6 weeks unless metastasis or residual tumor mass.

## EMBRYONAL CARCINOMA

Embryonal carcinoma is a very rare tumor and represents 3% of all germ cell tumors of ovary (Box 15.3).

**Box 15.3:** Embryonal carcinoma

- It represents 3% of all germ cell tumors of ovary

**Clinical features**
- The age varies from 4 to 28 years
- Mean age 12 years
- Commonly presents with rapidly developing pelvic mass

**Gross**
- Unilateral large tumor
- Median size of 17 cm
- Solid and well circumscribed
- Cut section: gray to yellow in color with areas of hemorrhage and necrosis

**Histopathology**
- Composed of diffuse solid sheets or nests of undifferentiated cells
- Cells: large with amphophilic to clear cytoplasm
- Nuclei:
  - Large
  - Highly pleomorphic
  - Irregular nuclear membrane having coarse chromatin
  - Large prominent nucleoli
- Occasional gland-like spaces and papillae
- Areas eosinophilic hyaline globules may also be noted

**Immunohistochemistry:**
- Positive: PLAP, AFP, CK, CD30 and hCG

**Differential diagnosis:** Yolk sac tumor, dysgerminoma, juvenile granulosa cell tumor, and undifferentiated carcinoma

**Treatment:**
- Highly malignant tumor
- Unilateral salpingo-oophorectomy along with combination chemotherapy is the treatment of choice

## Clinical Features

The age of the patient ranges from 4 to 28 years with a mean age 12 years. The patient commonly presents with rapidly developing pelvic mass.

## Gross

Embryonal carcinomas are unilateral large tumor with a median size of 17 cm. The tumor is solid and well circumscribed. The cut section shows gray to yellow in color with areas of hemorrhage and necrosis.

## Histopathology

The tumor is composed of diffuse solid sheets or nests of undifferentiated cells. The cells are large with amphophilic to clear cytoplasm. The nuclei are large, markedly pleomorphic with irregular nuclear membrane and coarse chromatin. The cells show large prominent nucleoli. The tumor may show occasional gland like spaces and papillae. Areas of necrosis and high mitotic activity are also seen. Eosinophilic hyaline globules may also be noted. In addition, the tumor also shows many syncytiotrophoblastic cells that are positive for hCG.

## Immunohistochemistry

The tumor is positive for PLAP, AFP, CK, CD30 and hCG.

## Differential Diagnosis

Embryonal carcinoma may be confused with YST, dysgerminoma, Juvenile granulosa cell tumor (JGCT), and undifferentiated carcinoma.

## Treatment

This is a highly malignant tumor. Unilateral salpingo-oophorectomy along with combination chemotherapy is the treatment of choice. With the advent of combination chemotherapy long-term survival is now possible.[10]

## POLYEMBRYOMA

This is a very rare tumor. Polyembryoma resembles morphologically normal embryonic disk.[11] The patients show elevated serum hCG and AFP. The patients usually present with vaginal bleeding in adult women and precocious puberty in young child.

## Gross

Polyembryoma is unilateral and usually large tumor. The tumor is solid and cut section shows multiple small cysts.

## Histopathology

The tumor shows large number of embryoid bodies within an extraembryonic mesenchymal matrix. This so called embryonic body contains embryonic disk, yolk sac, amniotic cavity and chorionic element. These embryonic bodies may be malformed and never develop beyond 18 days stage. The yolk sac elements and fetal hepatic tissue are responsible for the secretion of AFP.

## Prognosis and Treatment

Polyembryoma is a highly malignant tumor. The surgical removal of ovary along with combination chemotherapy is the treatment of choice.

## CHORIOCARCINOMA

Pure primary choriocarcinoma of the ovary is an exceptionally rare tumor and represents less than 1% of malignant germ cell tumor of ovary. Choriocarcinoma of ovary is usually seen as a part of mixed germ cell tumor of ovary or metastasis from uterine choriocarcinoma.

## Clinical Features

The tumor commonly occurs in children and young female. The presenting symptoms of the patient are similar to that of other malignant germ cell tumors. The patients may have isosexual pseudoprecocity and menstrual irregularities due to high hCG level.

## Gross

The tumor is commonly large and unilateral. The cut section is solid gray white. Areas of hemorrhage and necrosis is frequently seen.

## Histopathology (Figures 15.17 and 15.18)

The tumor is composed of uniform admixture of syncytio- and cytotrophoblastic cells. Chorionic villi are characteristically absent. The tumor shows large areas of hemorrhage and necrosis. The cytotrophoblastic cells are large polygonal cells with abundant clear cytoplasm having well-defined border and single large nuclei. The syncytiotrophoblast show large cells with abundant basophilic to vacuolated cytoplasm. The nuclei are multiple, and large pleomorphic. The tumor cells often show vascular invasion.

## Immunohistochemistry

The tumor cells are positive for hCG, keratin, HPL, AFP, PLAP and inhibin.

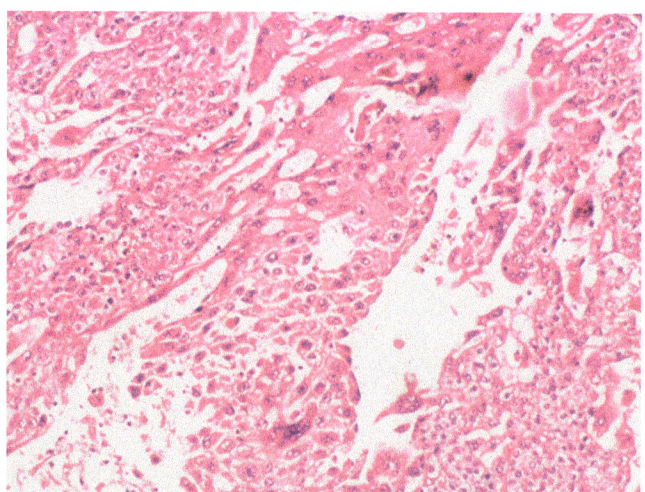

**Figure 15.17:** Choriocarcinoma of ovary: Tumor composed of both cyto and syncytiotrophoblastic cells

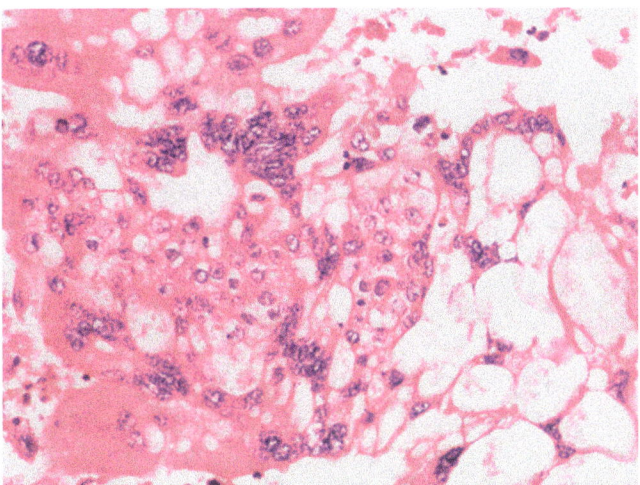

Figure 15.18: Choriocarcinoma of ovary: Large multinucleated syncytiotrophoblastic cells

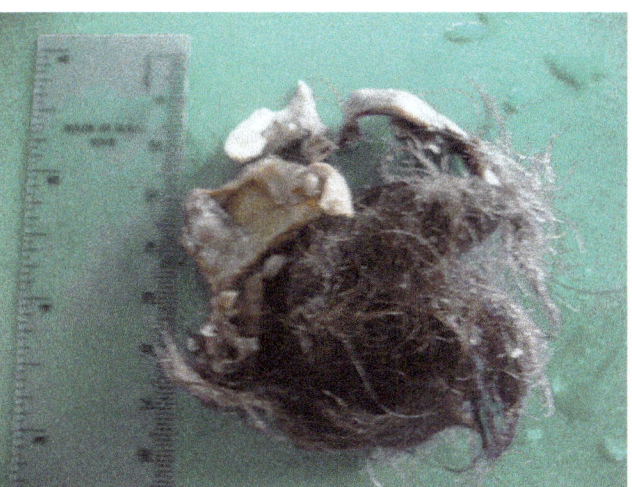

Figure 15.19: Mature teratoma: Bunch of hair and pultaceous material within the tumor

## Differential Diagnosis

The tumor should be distinguished from undifferentiated carcinoma, dysgerminoma, YST, and embryonal carcinoma.

## Treatment and Prognosis

Non-gestational choriocarcinoma of ovary is an aggressive tumor. The tumor frequently involves the adjacent structures and invades the blood vessel to have distant metastasis. Removal of the tumor mass followed by combination chemotherapy (Cisplatin, etoposide, and bleomycin) is the treatment of choice.[12]

## TERATOMA

Teratoma is composed of three germ cell layers: ectoderm, endoderm and mesoderm. Majority of the teratomas are benign cystic teratomas that represent about 25% of all ovarian tumors. The teratomas are mainly classified as: Immature teratoma, mature teratoma and monodermal teratoma.

## Mature Teratoma

Mature teratoma is the most common tumor and represents the major bulk of teratomas. It is also known as dermoid cyst.

### Clinical Features

The dermoid cyst commonly occurs between 20 to 50 years and rarely occurs in post-menopausal patients. The patients commonly present with pelvic mass and pain in the abdomen. Occasionally, there may be complications such as torsion, rupture or superadded infection. In 1–2% cases of teratoma cases, there may be malignant transformation. Majority of cases are squamous cell carcinoma (80%).

### Gross

Mature teratomas are mostly cystic and 15% cases are bilateral. The size of the tumor varies from 1 to 40 cm diameter with an average 15 cm diameter. The tumor is ovoid with gray white outer surface. The cut section of the tumor shows commonly uniloculated and occasionally multiloculated cysts. The cysts contain sebaceous material and hair (Figure 15.19). The bone, cartilage or teeth are also seen. The prominent solid areas from which the mesenchymal elements are attached is known as Rokitansky's protuberance. Solid areas of the tumor may also show soft brain tissue and thyroid tissue.

### Histopathology (Figures 15.20 and 15.21)

The mature cystic teratoma shows all three elements: ectodermal, endodermal and mesenchymal. The ectodermal derivatives include epidermis, sweat gland, hair follicles, sebaceous glands, glial tissue, cerebrum, retina, etc. The endodermal derivatives include gastrointestinal epithelium, respiratory epithelium and thyroid tissue. The mesenchymal elements show bone, cartilage, adipose tissue and muscle. These various tissues are arranged in organoid pattern.

### Treatment

Dermoid cyst is a benign tumor and surgical removal of the tumor is optimal treatment.

## Immature Teratoma

Immature teratoma (IT) represents more than 80% of all germ cell tumors of ovary and represents less than 1% of all ovarian malignancies.[13]

# Germ Cell Tumor of Ovary

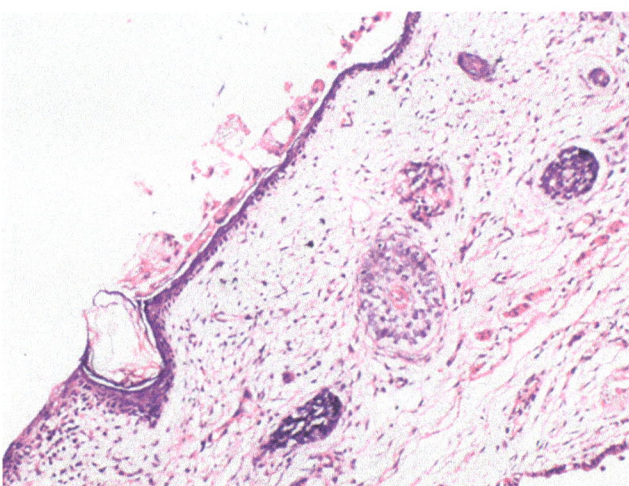

Figure 15.20: Mature teratoma: The cyst contains hair follicles and squamous epithelium

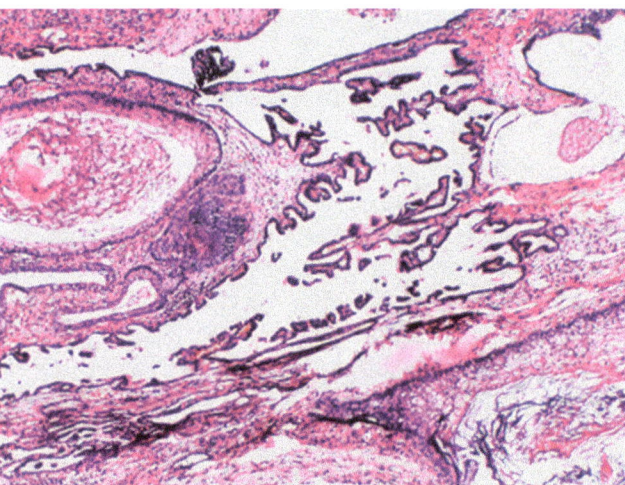

Figure 15.21: Mature teratoma: The cyst contains both squamous epithelial and glandular elements

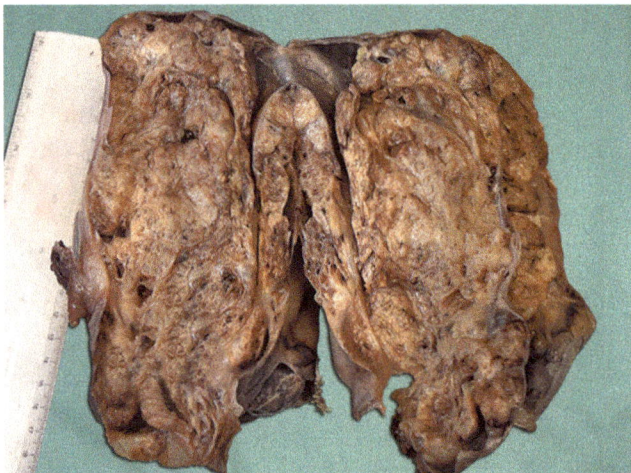

Figure 15.22: Immature teratoma: Solid tumor with cut section shows soft, fleshy grayish area

## Clinical Features

IT commonly occurs in children and young adults with a mean age of 19 years. Only 10% of ITs are seen after 30 years. The patient presents with pelvic mass, pain abdomen, and vaginal bleeding. Gross: ITs are mostly unilateral, but in 10% cases. There may be dermoid cyst in the contralateral ovary. The tumor is usually large with a mean diameter of 18 cm. The mass is mostly solid and cut section shows soft, fleshy grayish area with variegated appearance (Figure 15.22). Areas of hemorrhage and necrosis are also seen.

## Histopathology (Figures 15.23 to 15.32)

The tumor is composed of both mature elements and immature elements. These elements are admixed in a haphazard manner and no organoid arrangement is noted. The immature element is mostly composed of immature neuroepithelium (neuroepithelial rosettes) and tubules. The neuroepithelial rosettes show central lumen with fibrillary material surrounded by columnar basophilic cells that show brisk mitosis. Surrounding tissues may show immature glial tissue, and primitive retina with melanin pigmentation. The immature mesenchymal elements show loose myxomatous stroma along with immature cartilage and bone. The embryonal endodermal elements in the form of hepatic tissue and intestinal epithelium may also be seen. Most of the cases of IT are admixed with variable proportion of mature teratomatous elements. Therefore, in every cases of teratoma multiple sections from different parts of the tumor should be taken to eliminate the possibility of an IT. The tumor may often be admixed with other malignant germ cell elements such as yolk sac tumor, dysgerminoma, and choriocarcinoma. This tumor should be designated as mixed germ cell tumor. In occasional cases, immature teratoma may contain mucinous carcinoma component.

## Grading

ITs are graded on the basis of amount of immature neuroepithelial tissue. Three tier grading system from grade 1 to grade 3 is applied to grade the tumor (Box 15.4). In case of grade I tumor, immature neural tissue is seen in less than one low power field of microscope (4 X objective), in grade 2, the number of immature neural tissue is seen in more than 1 and less than 4 low power field. In grade III tumor, the

**Box 15.4:** Grading of immature teratoma

| Immature neural tissue |
|---|
| Grade I: Rare foci in <1 per LPF (4 X objective) per slide |
| Grade 2: >1 and <4 per LPF (4 X objective) per slide |
| Grade 3: ≥4 per LPF (4 X objective) per slide |

LPF= Low power field

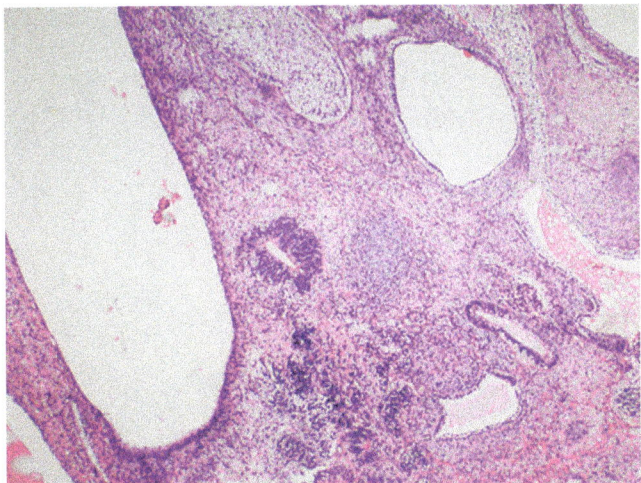

**Figure 15.23:** Immature teratoma: Immature neuroepithelium in the form of neuroepithelial rosettes and tubules

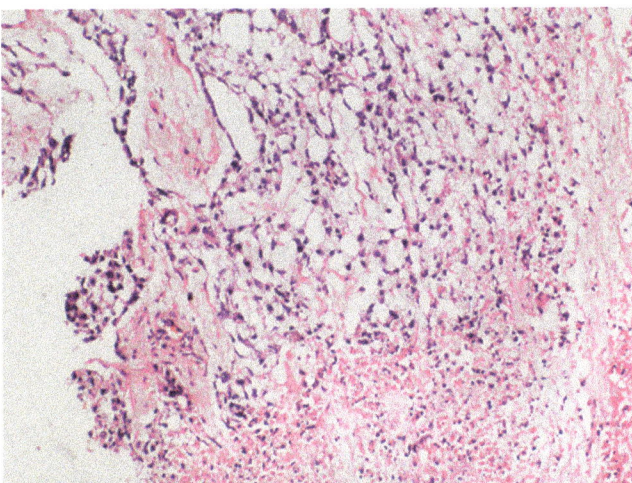

**Figure 15.26:** Immature teratoma with endodermal sinus tumor: Cystic spaces lined by malignant cells

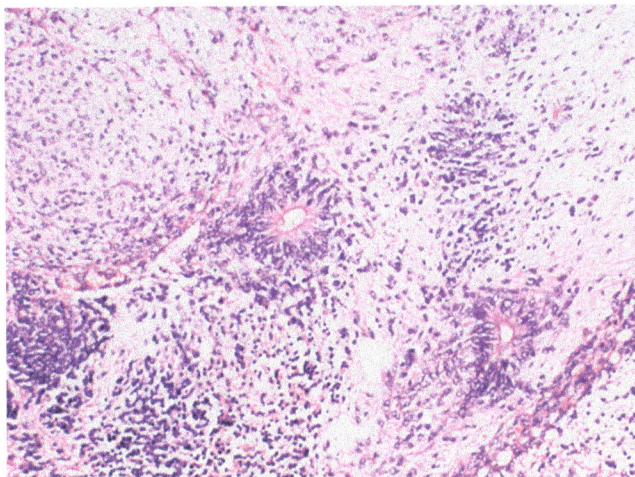

**Figure 15.24:** Immature teratoma: Multiple neuroepithelial rosettes

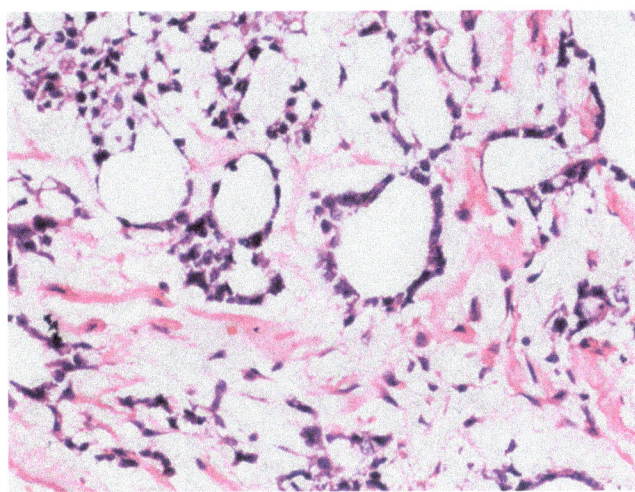

**Figure 15.27:** Immature teratoma with endodermal sinus tumor: The cystic spaces lined by malignant cells with scanty cytoplasm and pleomorphic nuclei

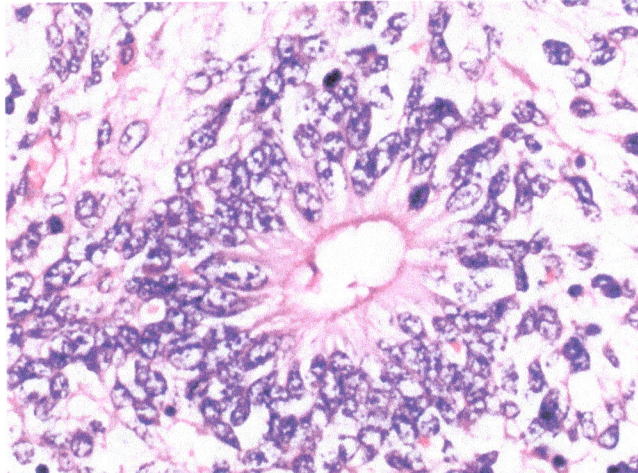

**Figure 15.25:** Immature teratoma: Higher magnification of the neuroepithelial rosette

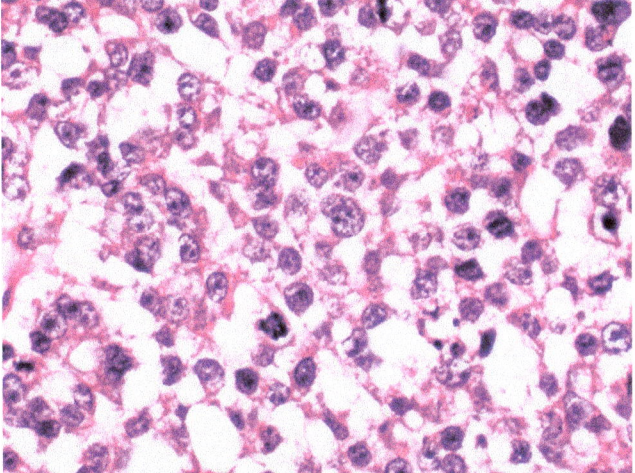

**Figure 15.28:** Immature teratoma with endodermal sinus tumor: Higher magnification of the malignant cells

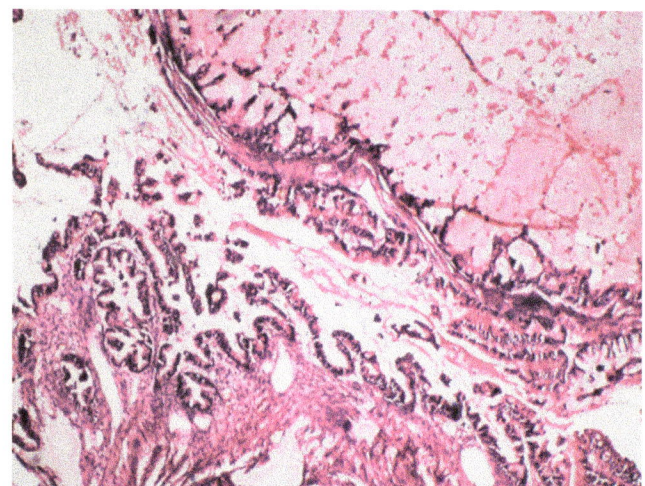

Figure 15.29: Immature teratoma with mucinous component: Mucinous carcinoma in the right upper corner

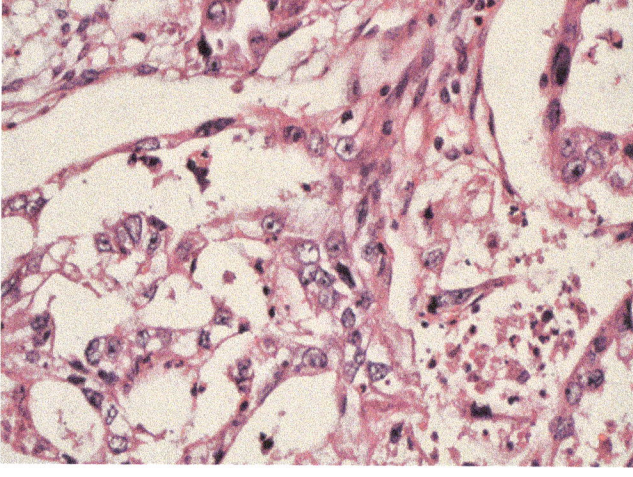

Figure 15.31: Immature teratoma with mucinous component: Marked nuclear atypia of the mucinous cells

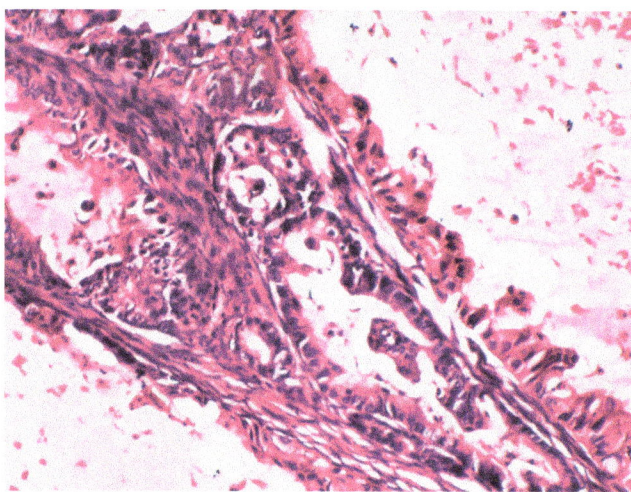

Figure 15.30: Immature teratoma with mucinous component: Mucinous cells with moderate nuclear pleomorphism

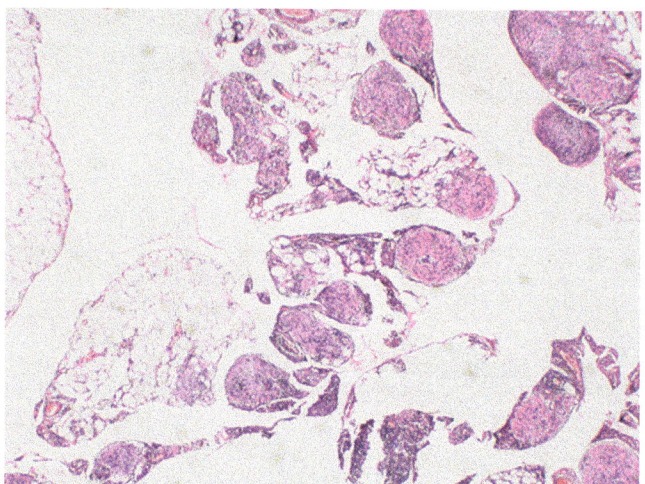

Figure 15.32: Immature teratoma: Omental gliomatosis

number of immature neural tissue is seen in more than 4 low power field of microscope.

### Immunohistochemistry

Immunohistochemistry plays no significant role in ITs. The tumor cells are positive for GFAP, S100, NSE. Intestinal type epithelium and hepatic tissue stains strongly positive for AFP.

### Differential Diagnosis

a. Mature solid teratoma: The simple presence of immature embryonal tissue such as cartilage, cerebrum, etc. may not indicate IT. The presence of immature neuroepithelium is needed for the diagnosis of IT.
b. Malignancy in dermoid: Malignant dermoid cyst usually shows squamous cell carcinoma and no immature neuro-epithelium is seen.
c. Malignant mixed Mullerian tumor (MMMT): The following features favor MMMT: (1) elderly patient, (2) lack of the immature neural tissue, (3) lack of the various other ectodermal, endodermal and mesenchymal elements.

### Prognosis and Treatment

The treatment of choice in a young female with stage I tumor is unilateral salpingo-oophorectomy and staging of tumor. In case of involvement of contralateral ovary or the patients who does not need child, total abdominal hysterectomy is the preferred choice of treatment. The prognosis of the patient largely depends on grade and stage of tumor. Grade 1 and stage I cases of IT has excellent prognosis. The grade 2 or 3 IT needs postoperative combination chemotherapy that include either vincristine, dactinomycin, and cyclophosphamide (VAC) regimen or cisplatin, etoposide, and bleomycin (BEP) regimens. The 5 year survival in grade 2 and 3 ITs after combination chemotherapy is more than 80%.

## Monodermal Teratomas

### Struma Ovarii

Struma ovarii is a type of mature teratoma that consists of more than 50% thyroid tissue. It consists only 1 to 3% of all benign ovarian teratomas. Malignancy in this tumor is rare and is seen in 5 to 10% of struma ovarii.

### Clinical Features

The patients are usually in their reproductive age period, however, it is most frequently seen around 40 years of age. The patients usually do not have any specific symptoms and commonly presents with pelvic mass. Occasional patients may have Meigs syndrome or thyroid enlargement and features of hyperthyroidism. Rarely the patient may have thyrotoxic crisis after removal of struma ovarii.

### Gross

The tumor varies in size from 0.5 cm to 10 cm in diameter. The tumor is unilateral and solid. The cut section shows grayish brown or greenish brown with a meaty appearance. The tumor may have small cysts with gelatinous material. Occasional tumors are cystic. In some cases, the struma ovarii is accompanied with mature teratoma in contralateral ovary.

### Histopathology (Figures 15.33 to 15.35)

The tumor is composed of benign thyroid tissue. The thyroid elements show variable pattern that include microfollicular, macrofollicular, trabecular or solid. The follicles contain colloid material. The lining of follicular cells is cuboidal to columnar in shape with round monomorphic nuclei. Cystic variant of struma ovarii is lined by thyroid follicular epithelial cells and this variant is difficult to recognize. The tumor often shows calcification, fibrosis and hemosiderin laden macrophages. Occasionally, there may be focal crowding of microfollicles that may give rise to the appearance of follicular adenoma of thyroid. This tumor should be better designated as 'proliferative struma ovarii'.[14]

### Carcinomas in Struma Ovarii (Figures 15.36 to 15.39)

Rarely struma ovarii may show carcinoma. Papillary thyroid carcinoma is the commonest carcinoma and it bears similar morphology as that of main thyroid gland.[15] Follicular carcinomas in struma ovarii may also occur, but they are difficult to recognize as the struma ovarii has no true capsule. The presence of nuclear atypia, high mitosis and vascular invasion indicate the diagnosis of follicular carcinoma.

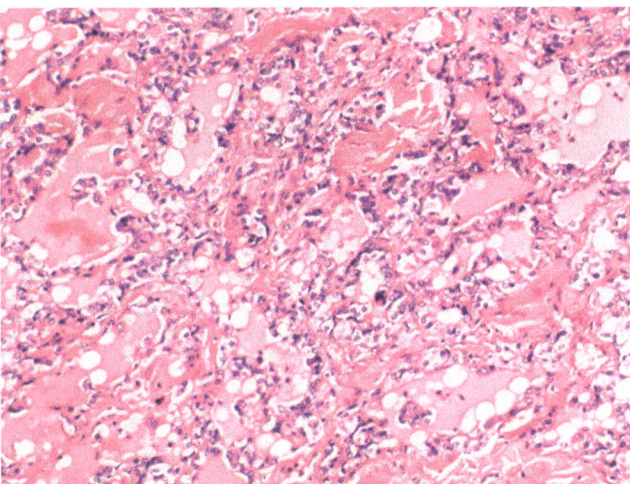

**Figure 15.33:** Struma ovarii: Tumor is mainly composed of thyroid follicles

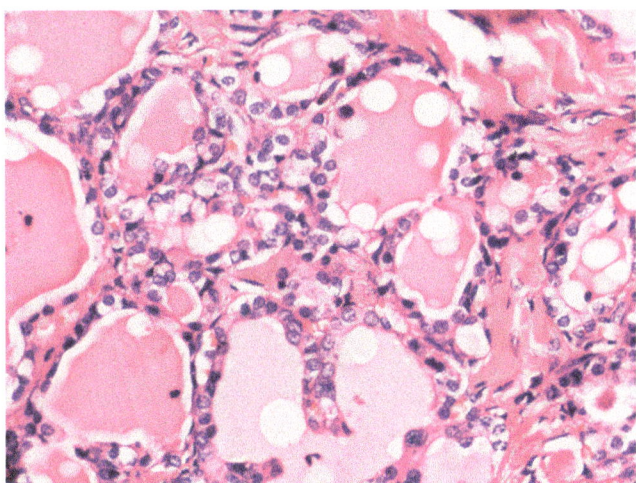

**Figure 15.34:** Struma ovarii: Variable-sized thyroid follicles filled with colloid

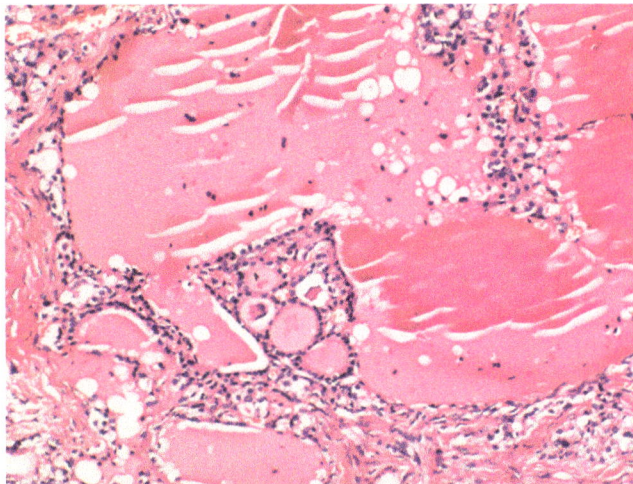

**Figure 15.35:** Struma ovarii: Higher magnification

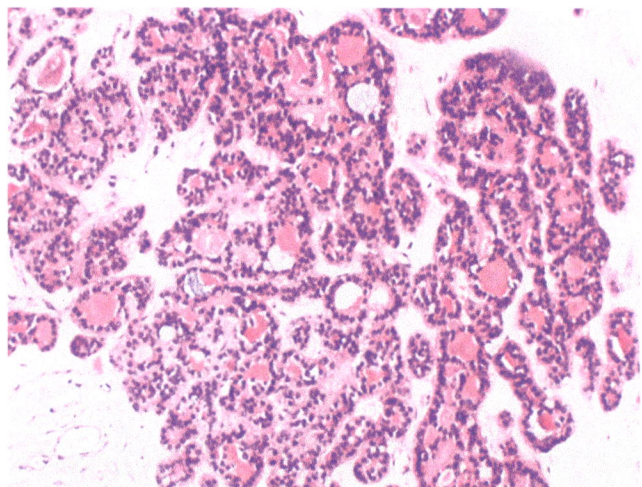

**Figure 15.36:** Follicular carcinomas in struma ovarii: Abundant microfollicles

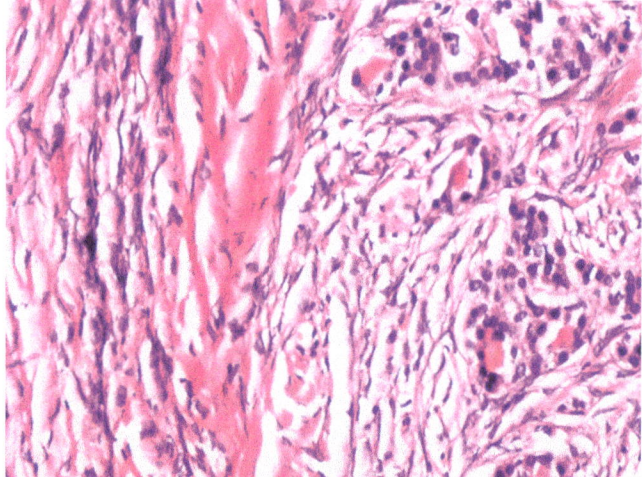

**Figure 15.38:** Follicular carcinomas in struma ovarii: Ovarian capsule is infiltrated by the microfollicles

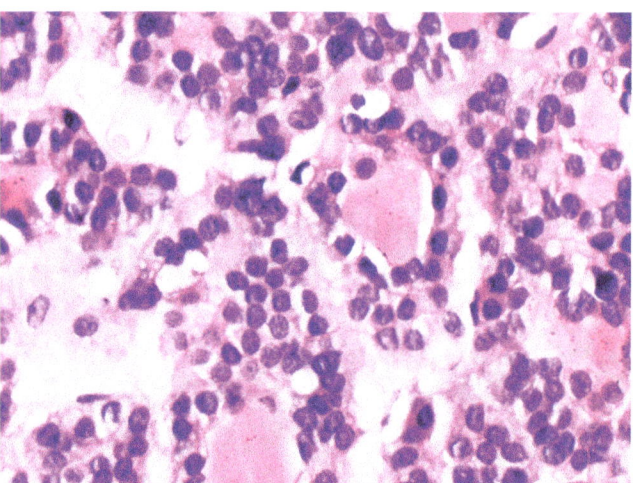

**Figure 15.37:** Follicular carcinomas in struma ovarii: The lining cells of the follicles show moderate nuclear atypia

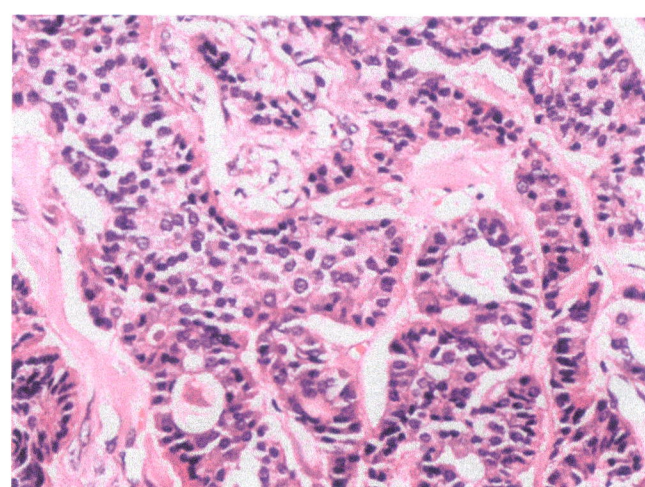

**Figure 15.39:** Follicular carcinomas in struma ovarii: Moderate nuclear atypia of the follicular cells

*Immunohistochemistry*

The cells of struma ovarii are positive for TTF1 and thyroglobulin.

*Differential Diagnosis*

a. Granulosa cell tumor (GCT): Call-Exner bodies in GCT may simulate thyroid follicles of struma ovarii.
b. Sertoli-Leydig cell tumor (SLCT): Pseudotubular pattern of struma ovarii can mimic SLCT. Immunohistochemical stains such as TTF 1 and thyroglobulin positivity and negative inhibin confirm the diagnosis of struma ovarii.
c. Endometrioid carcinoma: Follicles in struma ovarii may mimic glands of endometrioid carcinoma.
d. Metastatic thyroid carcinoma: Rarely metastatic thyroid carcinoma may be confused with struma ovarii. Appropriate clinical history is helpful in such cases.

*Prognosis and Treatment*

Struma ovarii is a benign tumor and simple unilateral salpingo-oophorectomy is enough in such cases. Malignancy in struma ovarii has good prognosis. Ten year survival rate of such patients is 80%. This tumor should be treated by hysterectomy and bilateral salpingo-oophorectomy along with radioactive iodine therapy after thyroidectomy.

## Carcinoid

Ovarian carcinoid tumor represents less than 1% of ovarian teratoma and 1.7% of all carcinoid tumors of the body.[16]

*Clinical Features*

The tumor commonly occurs in peri- and postmenopausal patients. The patients commonly present with non-specific symptoms that include abdominal pain, swelling, vaginal bleeding and menstrual irregularities. Only 25% patients with carcinoids present with typical carcinoid syndrome such as flushing, diarrhea, bronchospasm and hypertension. The majority of such patients show insular type of carcinoid tumor.

### Gross

Carcinoid tumor of ovary is unilateral and occasionally contralateral ovary is involved by mature teratoma, mucinous tumor or Brenner tumor. The tumor varies in size from microscopic size to several cm in diameter. Carcinoid is solid tumor and cut section shows yellowish to light brown in color (Figure 15.40).

### Histopathology (Figures 15.41 to 15.44)

Carcinoid tumor of ovary is morphologically classified as: (1) Insular, (2) Trabecular, (3) Mucinous, (4) Strumal carcinoid.

**Insular carcinoid (25–53%):** It resembles typical appearance of midgut carcinoid. The tumor is composed of multiple nests and acinar arrangement of cells. The individual cells are round with abundant amount of cytoplasm having round monomorphic nuclei. The cytoplasm often shows reddish brown granules. Mitotic activity is low.

**Trabecular pattern (29%):** The tumor simulates the foregut and hind gut carcinoid. The tumor is composed multiple anastomosing long ribbons, cords and trabecular cells. The cells are columnar with elongated nuclei. The long axis of the nuclei is parallel to each other. The individual cells have abundant cytoplasm with reddish granules.

**Mucinous pattern (1%):** Mucinous carcinoid resembles goblet cell carcinoma of the appendix. The tumor is composed of multiple small glands and acini within a loose edematous or dense fibrous stroma. The glands are lined by cuboidal to columnar cells having abundant mucin. The nuclei are small

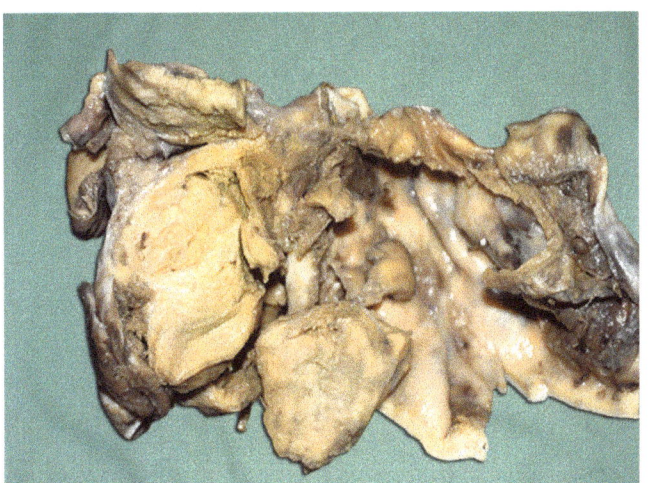

Figure 15.40: Carcinoid ovary: Solid gray white tumor

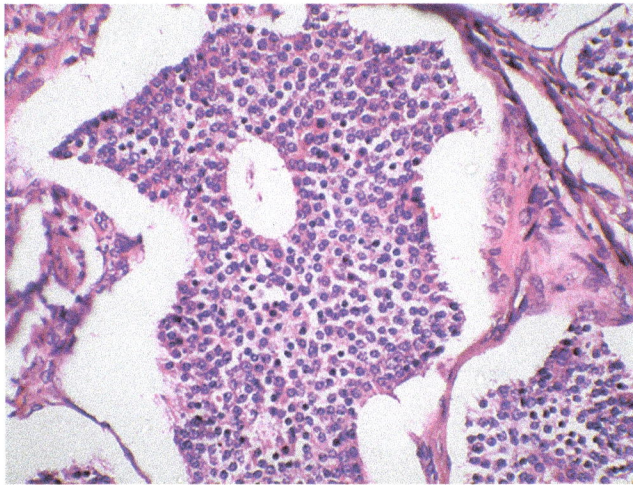

Figure 15.42: Carcinoid ovary: The tumor is composed of round cells with abundant amount of cytoplasm having round monomorphic nuclei

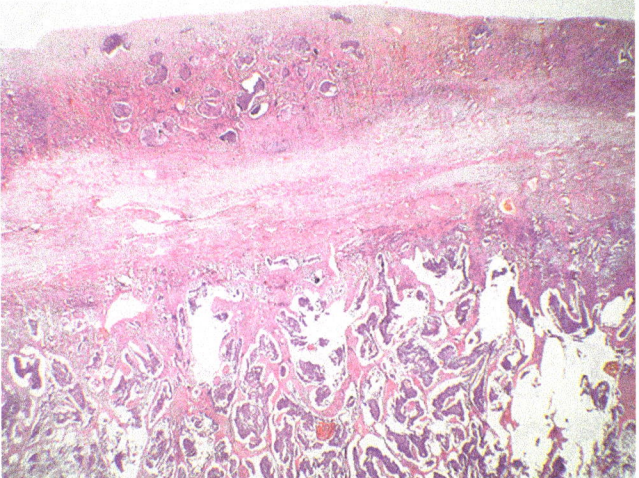

Figure 15.41: Carcinoid of ovary: Multiple nests of tumor cells

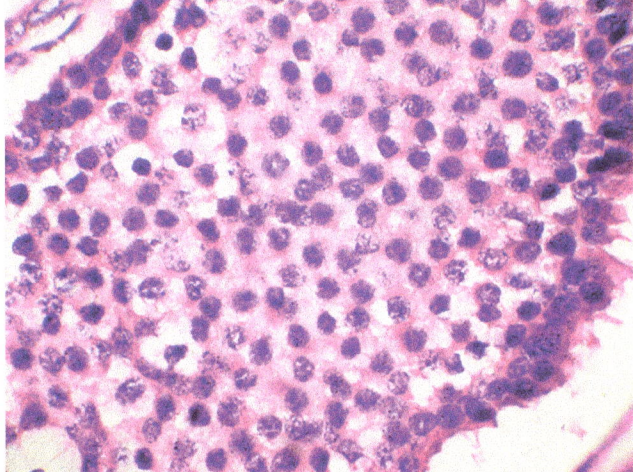

Figure 15.43: Carcinoid ovary: Higher magnification of the same

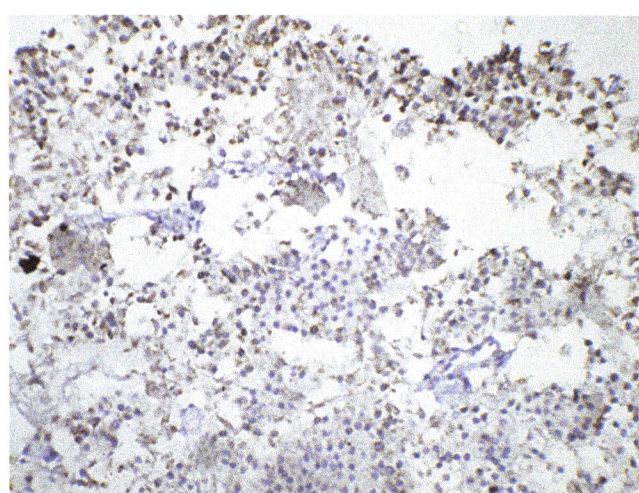

**Figure 15.44:** Carcinoid ovary: Strong chromogranin positive tumor cells

and round. The tumor cells may also contain neuroendocrine granules. There may be abundant mucin within the glands or in the stroma due to rupture of the mucin containing cells.

**Strumal carcinoid (26 to 44%):** Strumal carcinoid shows either contiguous or homogenous admixture of carcinoid and benign thyroid tissue. The tumor shows mostly trabecular pattern with long ribbons or cords of tumor cells in a dense fibrous stroma. The individual cells are columnar in shape with elongated hyperchromatic nuclei. The tumor cells invade the normal thyroid glands.

*Immunohistochemistry*

The carcinoid tumors are positive for chromogranin and synaptophysin. In addition, the trabecular and strumal carcinoids are positive for prostate specific acid phosphatase (PSAP). Carcinoid tumors are also variably positive for vasoactive intestinal polypeptide, serotonin, gastrin, insulin, glucagon, substance P, beta-endorphin and somatostatin.

*Differential Diagnosis*

a. Metastatic gastrointestinal carcinoid: The following features favors metastasis: (1) Bilateral involvement, (2) Multinodularity, (3) Absence of any other mature teratomatous component, (4) Clinical history.
b. Brenner tumor: Brenner tumor shows: (1) Characteristic urothelial cell nests, (2) Typical coffee bean appearance of nuclei.
c. Granulosa cell tumor: The characteristic differentiating features of granulosa cell tumor are: (1) Call-Exner bodies, (2) Grooved nuclei, (3) Hyperchromatic nuclei, (4) Positive inhibin and negative neuroendocrine markers.

*Treatment and Prognosis*

The ovarian carcinoids are low grade malignant tumor with very good prognosis. Simple salpingo-oophorectomy is adequate for young women. In postmenopausal patients the treatment of choice is hysterectomy with bilateral salpingo-oophorectomy. Five year survival of the patient is 95%.[17]

## Neuroectodermal Tumors

Neuroectodermal tumors are composed predominantly neuroectodermal tissues and they may resemble similar tumors of central nervous system.[18]

*Clinical Features*

The age of the patient varies widely from 6 to 69 years and the mean age is 28 years. The patient commonly presents with pelvic mass. Gross: The tumors are large and ranges from 4 to 20 cm in diameter. The tumor is solid or solid-cystic. Cut section shows pale yellowish appearance.

*Histopathology*

Kleinman GM et al.[18] classified this tumor in three groups:
1. Differentiated: Ependymoma,
2. Primitive: Medulloepithelioma, ependymoblastoma, neuroblastoma, and medulloblastoma, and
3. Anaplastic: Glioblastoma multiforme

Except ependymoma, the other neuroectodermal tumors are often associated with teratoma.

*Prognosis*

The patients of ependymoma has good prognosis whereas glioblastoma multiforme has poor outcome.

## MIXED MALIGNANT GERM CELL TUMORS

Mixed malignant germ cell tumors are composed of different germ cell elements in varying proportions and represent 5 to 15% of all malignant germ cell tumors.[19] The combination of benign mature teratoma with any other malignant germ cell element is not designated as mixed malignant germ cell tumors. The most common combination of mixed malignant germ cell tumor is dysgerminoma with EST. The patients are usually young child and the mean age of the patient is 16 years. They commonly present with abdominal pain, amenorrhea or precocious puberty. Majority of the patient behave mainly on the stage rather than the type of tumors.

## GONADOBLASTOMA

Gonadoblastoma is a rare tumor. It shows admixture of two elements: germ cells and sex cord stromal cells.[20] It is almost always associated with abnormal malformed gonads.

The patients are genotypically male with XY chromosome and phenotypically female due to virilization. Histopathology section of the tumor shows multiple nests and aggregates of cells containing central large germ cells encircled by smaller round cells resembling immature sertoli cells and granulosa cells. The cells are round with moderate amount of pale cytoplasm having central large nucleus with prominent nucleoli. The peripheral small sertoli cells are arranged in three different patterns: (1) The cells surround a central space with eosinophilic hyaline material resembling Call-Exner bodies, (2) The cells surround the individual germ cells, and (3) The cells lined the periphery of the nests of cells in a radiating fashion. The Leydig cells or luteinized stromal cells are seen in many cases that give rise to endocrine manifestation.

Three types of changes have been described within gonadoblastoma: (a) Calcification: The calcified bodies form concentric ring like structures and coalesce to form mulberry like structures. (b) Hyalinization: Hyaline plaques are formed within the epithelial nests. They coalesce and form large irregular network that replaces the tumor cells. (c) Dysgerminoma: Dysgerminoma occurs within the stroma outside the nests of the gonadoblastoma cells and may completely replace the gonadoblastoma.

## Prognosis and Treatment

Pure gonadoblastoma is a benign tumor and is treated by surgical excision. Gonadoblastoma with dysgerminoma also has good prognosis. Surgical removal of the tumor followed by combination chemotherapy is used in cases of gonadoblastoma with malignant tumors such as YST or embryonal carcinoma.

## REFERENCES

1. Kurman RJ, Carcangiu ML, Herrington S, Young RH. WHO classification of tumours of female genital reproductive organs. 4th Edition, International agency for research on Cancer, Lyon 2014.
2. Mueller CW, Topkins P, Lapp WA. Dysgerminoma of the ovary. An analysis of 427 cases. Am J Obstet Gynecol. 1950;60:153-9.
3. Cheng L, Roth LM, Zhang S, et al. KIT gene mutation and amplification in dysgerminoma of the ovary. Cancer. 2011;117:2096-103.
4. Gershenson DM. Update on malignant ovarian germ cell tumors. Cancer (Phila). 1993;71:1581-90.
5. Pedowitz P, Felmus LB, Grayzel DM. Dysgerminoma of the ovary. Prognosis and treatment. Am J Obstet Gynecol. 1955; 70:1284-97.
6. Bekaii-Saab T, Einhorn LH, Williams SD. Late relapse of ovarian dysgerminoma: case report and literature review. Gynecol Oncol. 1999;72(1):111-2.
7. Norgaard-Pedersen B, Albrechtsen R, Teilum G. Serum alpha-foetoprotein as a marker for endodermal sinus tumour (yolk sac tumour) or a vitelline component of "teratocarcinoma". Acta Pathol Microbiol Scand A. 1975;83(6):573-89.
8. Kurman RJ, Norris HJ. Cancer. Endodermal sinus tumor of the ovary: a clinical and pathologic analysis of 71 cases.1976; 38(6):2404-19.
9. Peccatori F, Bonazzi C, Chiari F, Landoni F, Colombo N, Mangioni C. Surgical management of malignant ovarian germ cell tumors: 10 years' experience with 129 patients. Obstet Gynecol. 1995;86(3):367-72.
10. Ueda G, Abe Y, Yoshida M, Fujiwara T. Embryonal carcinoma of the ovary: a six-year survival. Int J Gynaecol Obstet. 1990;31(3):287-92.
11. Beck JS, Fulmer HF, Lee ST. Solid malignant ovarian teratoma with "embryoid bodies" and trophoblastic differentiation. J Pathol. 1969;99:67-73.
12. Peccatori F, Bonazzi C, Chiari F, Landoni F, Colombo N, Mangioni C .Surgical management of malignant ovarian germ cell tumors: 10 years' experience with 129 patients. Obstet Gynecol. 1995;86(3):367-72.
13. Norris HJ, Zirkin HJ, Benson WL. Immature (malignant) teratoma of the ovary: a clinical and pathologic study of 58 cases. Cancer. 1976;37(5):2359-72.
14. Devaney K, Snyder R, Norris HJ, Tavassoli FA. Proliferative and histologically malignant struma ovarii: a clinicopathologic study of 54 cases. Int J Gynecol Pathol. 1993;12(4):333-43.
15. Garg K, Soslow RA, Rivera M, Tuttle MR, Ghossein RA. Histologically bland "extremely well differentiated" thyroid carcinomas arising in struma ovarii can recur and metastasize. Int J Gynecol Pathol. 2009;28:222-30.
16. Soga J, Osaka M, Yakuwa Y. Carcinoids of the ovary: an analysis of 329 reported cases. J Exp Clin Cancer Res. 2000;19(3):271-80.
17. Robboy SJ, Norris HJ, Scully RE. Insular carcinoid primary in the ovary: a clinicopathologic analysis of 48 cases. Cancer. 1975;36:404-18.
18. Kleinman GM, Young RH, Scully RE. Primary neuroectodermal tumors of the ovary. A report of 25 cases. Am J Surg Pathol. 1993;17:764.
19. Gershenson D M, del Junco G, Copeland LJ, et al. Mixed germ cell tumors of the ovary. Obstet Gynecol. 1984;64:200-7.
20. Scully RE. Gonadoblastoma: a review of 74 cases. Cancer. 1970;25:1340-56.

# Metastatic and Miscellaneous Tumors of Ovary

## METASTATIC TUMORS OF OVARY

Metastatic tumors of ovary represent 8% of all ovarian malignancy. The ovary may be involved from the adjacent organ by direct extension or by distant metastasis. The metastatic tumors in the ovary may masquerades as the primary ovarian tumor. However, certain features are helpful to suggest the metastatic origin of the tumor (Box 16.1).

**Box 16.1: Features suggestive of metastasis**
- Bilateral tumor
- Superficial small multiple nodules over surface
- Small tumor size
- Desmoplastic stroma
- Vascular invasion
- Extensive unusual metastasis
- Odd clinical history

### Common Primary Sites

The various primary sites are responsible for metastasis in ovary. The common primary sites are stomach, breast, large intestine and endometrium. The colonic carcinomas are responsible for 35% of metastatic carcinoma of ovary. Near about 28% of ovarian metastatic carcinomas are from breast. Recently, appendicular carcinomas are also considered as a rich source of metastatic carcinoma of ovary.

### Mode of Spread

The tumor spreads to ovary by the following routes: (a) Lymphatic and vascular route. (b) Transperitoneal. (c) Direct extension from the adjacent organs. (d) Transtubal spread via fallopian tube.

### Clinical Features

The metastatic ovarian tumor is detected mainly by:
1. During follow-up of the primary ovarian tumor,
2. Incidentally detected during a surgical procedure,
3. At the time of autopsy.

### Gross Features

In 70% cases, the ovarian metastatic tumors are bilateral. The size of the tumor varies from small microscopic to several cm in diameter. The tumor is usually solid and involves the superficial parenchyma of the normal sized ovary. Occasionally, the tumor is cystic.

### Intestinal Carcinoma

Majority of the metastatic intestinal carcinomas are from large intestine and they are the commonest primary site of origin. The rectosigmoid region is the commonest site of the primary tumor. In 50% cases, the tumor is bilateral. They are usually solid or cystic with soft and friable gray to red on cut section.

*Histopathology*

The features that are helpful to distinguish colonic carcinoma from the primary ovarian carcinomas are:[1] (1) Dirty necrosis: Eosinophilic necrotic debris within the glandular lumen. (2) Ring like distribution of the glands around the necrotic material. (3) Focal necrosis of the lining epithelium of the gland, (4) The presence of goblet cells. (5) Absence of any squamous metaplasia or adenofibromatous component, (6) Higher degree of nuclear atypia in colonic carcinoma. The metastatic tumor may occasionally show signet ring like cells (10% cases). The stroma is edematous and may show luteinized cells.

*Immunohistochemistry*

Colonic carcinomas are positive for CK 20 and CDX-2 and negative for CK7, whereas the endometrioid carcinomas are positive for CK7 and negative for CK 20 and CDX-2. In addition, colonic carcinomas are positive for nuclear stain of beta catenin.

## Metastasis from Stomach (Krukenberg's Tumor)

The metastatic carcinoma of signet ring like cells from the stomach is known as Krukenberg's tumor or signet ring cell carcinoma. Krukenberg's tumor may also be seen in from the metastatic tumor of breast, intestine, appendix, pancreas or biliary tract.[2] The average age of the patient is 45 years. The patient usually presents with non-specific symptoms such as pelvic pain, abdominal swelling, vaginal bleeding or virilization if the patient is pregnant.

### Gross

Krukenberg's tumor is bilateral in 85% cases. The tumor is solid, smooth with bosselated appearance. The cut section is firm or fleshy gelatinous in consistency with white or reddish brown in color (Figure 16.1).

### Histopathology (Figures 16.2 to 16.6)

The tumor shows alternate hyper- and hypocellular areas giving a pseudolobular arrangement in low power examination. The hypercellular areas are composed of numerous signet ring cells, glands or tubules. The tumor may also show diffuse sheets of tumor cells within the stroma.

The signet ring cells may be arranged diffusely, in small glands or as tubules. The number of such cells may be variable abundant to relatively less. The individual signet ring cells show abundant vacuolated cytoplasm with peripherally pushed nuclei. The cell may show targetoid cytoplasmic appearance characterized by central vacuole containing eosinophilic body.

### Differential Diagnosis

A. **Clear cell adenocarcinoma of ovary (CCA):** The occasional presence of signet ring type of cells in clear cell carcinoma of ovary may give rise to confusion. The following features help in the diagnosis of clear cell carcinoma: (1) The presence of hobnail cells, (2) Tubulocystic pattern, (3) Absence of targetoid cytoplasm, (4) Eosinophilic secretion.
B. **Sertoli-Leydig cell tumor (SLCT):** The absence of signet ring cell is important to distinguish SLCT from Krukenberg's tumor.
C. **Primary mucinous carcinoid:** Mucinous carcinoid may show signet ring cells. However, this tumor often shows other teratomatous component.
D. **Cellular fibroma:** Spindle cells stroma of Krukenberg's tumor may simulate fibroma. However, fibroma lacks the presence of signet ring cells.

## Tumors of Appendix

Metastatic appendicular carcinoma represents 1% of all metastatic carcinoma of ovary.

### Clinical Features

The patient is usually from 30 to 70 years with a mean age of 52 years. The patient commonly complains of pelvic mass.

### Gross

Tumor is mostly bilateral (80%) and large in size. Usually, the size of the metastatic tumor is much larger than the primary appendicular tumor. The tumor is solid and firm.

### Histopathology

The following types of appendicular tumors metastasize in the ovary:
1. Borderline appendicular tumor,
2. Mucinous carcinoid,
3. Signet-ring cell carcinomas,

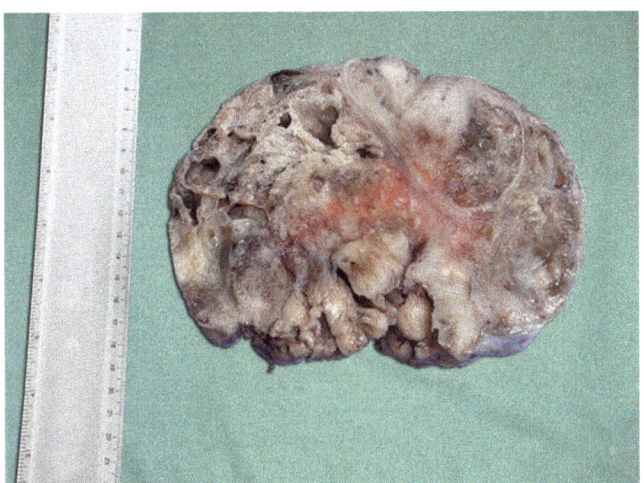

**Figure 16.1:** Krukenberg's tumor: Solid tumor with gray white color. Large areas of necrosis

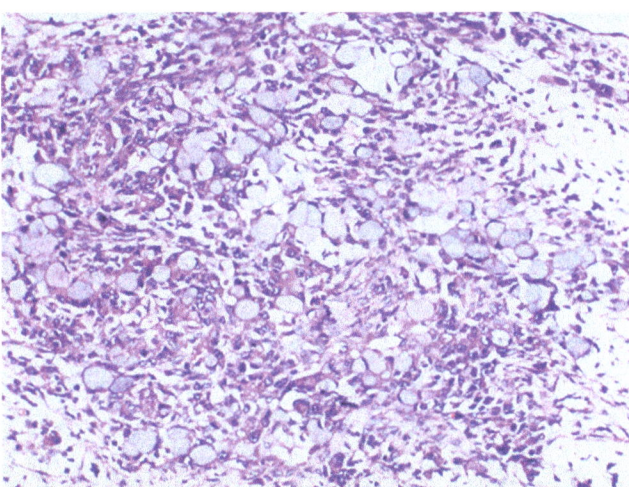

**Figure 16.2:** Krukenberg's tumor: Krukenberg's tumor: hypo- and hypercellular areas

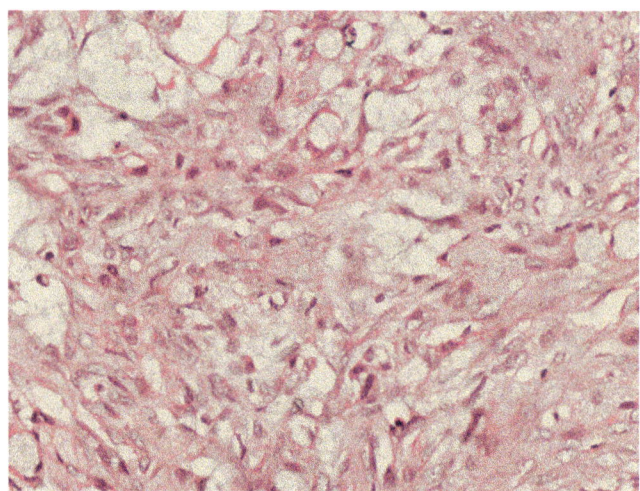

**Figure 16.3:** Krukenberg's tumor: Scattered signet ring cells in the stroma

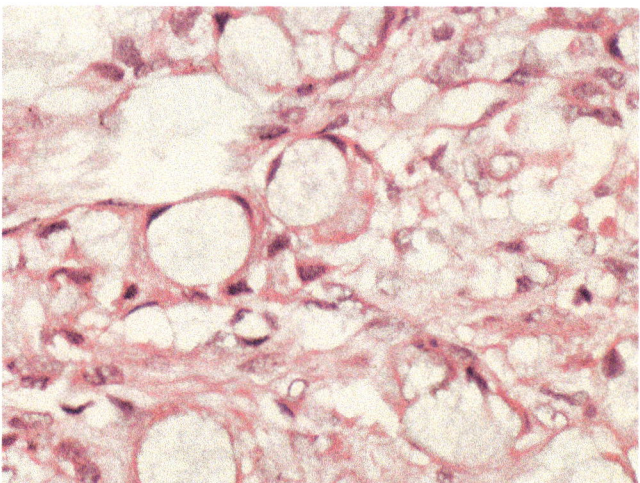

**Figure 16.5:** Krukenberg's tumor: The cells contain abundant mucinous material that pushes the nuclei in the periphery

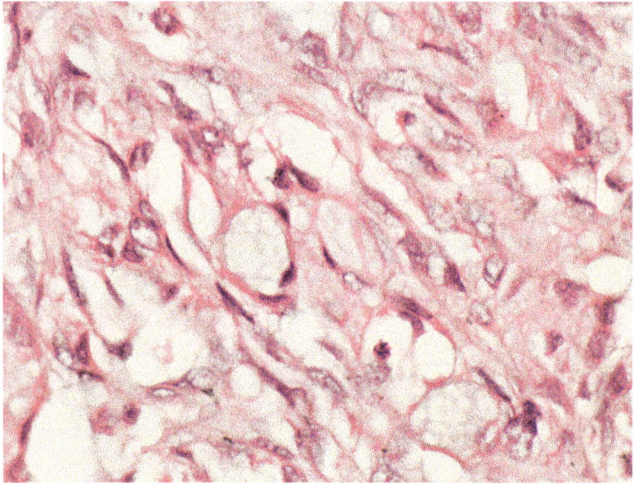

**Figure 16.4:** Krukenberg's tumor: Large cells with abundant cytoplasm having signet ring type of nuclei

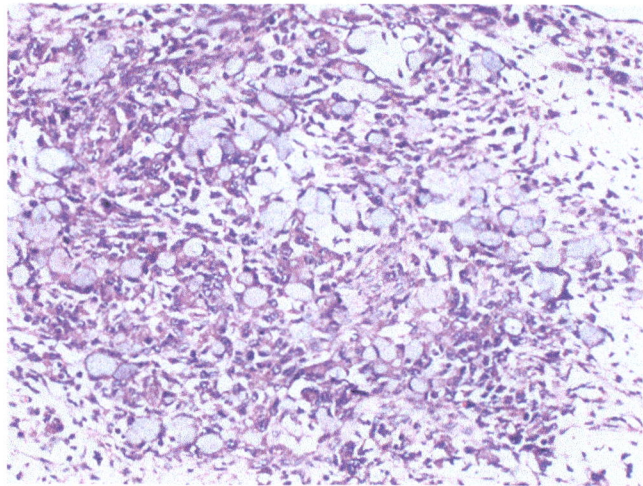

**Figure 16.6:** Krukenberg's tumor: Large number of signet ring cells

4. Rarely typical carcinoid. In pseudomyxomatous peritoneii the tumor may have both in appendix and ovary. The mucinous tumors of appendicular origin may be low grade mucinous type. Many times borderline tumor of ovary may also coexist. Clinical, immunohistological and molecular evidence confirm that the tumor in ovary is secondary to appendicular tumor.[3]

*Immunohistochemistry*

Appendicular carcinoma is typically positive for CK20 and may also show CK 7 positivity.

## Pancreatic, Biliary Tract and Liver Tumors

Metastatic tumors from the pancreas, biliary tract and liver tumors are rare. The pancreatic carcinoma are positive for CK 7 and MUC5AC and negative for CK 20. The pancreatic tumors are characteristically negative for dpc-4 (smad-4), whereas this stain is positive in mucinous adenocarcinoma of ovary.[4] Metastatic hepatocellular carcinoma in ovary is very rare and it should be differentiated from hepatoid yolk sac tumor.

## Breast Carcinoma

Metastatic breast carcinoma represents 1/3rd of ovarian metastatic carcinoma. Majority of metastatic breast carcinomas are usually incidentally detected particularly at the time of therapeutic oophorectomy.

*Gross*

Almost 80% of the tumor affects bilateral ovary. The tumor is solid firm, multinodular in appearance with firm and yellowish in color on cut section.

*Histopathology*

Metastatic lobular carcinoma is more frequent than ductal carcinoma. The ductal carcinoma may show diffuse sheets, glandular, tubular or cribriform appearance. The lobular carcinoma shows classical Indian file, trabecular and insular arrangement of cells. Discrete signet ring type cells are also noted.

## Immunostaining

The breast carcinoma cells are positive for ER/PR, EMA, and gross cystic disease fluid protein is a specific and sensitive marker of breast carcinoma.

## Metastatic Urothelial Carcinoma

The primary transitional cell carcinoma of ovary is positive for CK 7, and WT 1; and negative for CK 20 and thrombomodulin. Whereas transitional cell carcinoma of bladder shows positive CK 20 and thrombomodulin and negative for CK 7, and WT 1. PAX-8 is positive in primary transitional cell carcinoma of ovary and negative in the tumor of non-ovarian origin.

## Uterine Tumors

*Endometrial Carcinoma*

Ovarian metastasis from the endometrial carcinoma of uterus represents 15% of the metastatic tumors in ovary. In absence of any symptoms of primary endometrial carcinoma the ovarian mass may be mistaken as primary ovarian carcinoma. The metastatic carcinoma in the ovary is usually bilateral, less than 5 cm diameter and solid in appearance. The endometrioid and serous carcinoma of uterus mimic the primary ovarian carcinoma. The following features are suggestive of primary uterine carcinoma:
1. Deep myometrial invasion,
2. Vascular invasion,
3. Bilateral ovarian carcinoma,
4. Nodular surface involvement of ovary,
5. Absence of endometriosis in ovary. Endometrioid carcinomas are positive for ER/PR, and negative for p53. Serous carcinomas are strongly positive for p53 and weakly positive for WT1.

*Cervix*

Cervical squamous cell carcinoma metastasis in ovary is rare and represent only 1% of cases.[5] The primary ovarian squamous cell carcinomas develop mainly from mature teratoma. Therefore, the presence of other elements of teratoma indicates primary ovarian tumor rather than metastatic squamous cell carcinoma.

Metastasis from cervical adenocarcinoma is more common than cervical squamous cell carcinoma. The following features suggest metastatic adenocarcinoma from cervix: (1) Luminal cytoplasmic eosinophilia of the glandular epithelial cells, (2) Apical suspended mitosis, (3) High nuclear grade of the tumor cells, (4) Strong p16 positivity.

*Fallopian Tube Carcinoma*

Carcinomas of fallopian tube involves the ovary in 10 to 15% cases. The tumor usually extends directly from the fallopian tube. In case of extensive involvement of both ovary and tube, it may be difficult to decide the primary site of origin of the tumor. The recent evidences of molecular pathology suggest that most of the serous ovarian carcinomas are actually metastasis from the fallopian tube.[6]

## MISCELLANEOUS TUMORS OF OVARY

## Lymphoma and Leukemia

Approximately 25% of lymphomas involve ovary in autopsy study. Majority of ovarian lymphoma occurs as dissemination of lymphoma to the ovary. Lymphoma of the ovary represents less than 1.5% of all ovarian neoplasms.

*Clinical Features*

The age of the patients varies widely from 20 to 70 years with mean age is 43 years of age. The patients commonly present with pelvic mass, pain abdomen, fatigue, weakness and fever.

*Gross*

The tumor varies in size from microscopic foci to several cm. The mean size of the mass is 10–15 cm in diameter. Ovarian lymphomas are solid, firm in consistency with soft, rubbery and white to gray-pink in color on cut section.

*Histopathology*

The commonest lymphoma in the ovary is diffuse large B cell lymphoma (DLBCL). The other types of lymphomas include:
1. B-cell lymphoblastic lymphoma,
2. Burkitt lymphoma,
3. Peripheral T-cell lymphoma,
4. Follicular lymphoma.

*Differential Diagnosis*

## Dysgerminoma

Dysgerminoma may be mistaken as lymphoma. Immunohistochemistry shows positive placental alkaline phosphatase (PLAP) and negative CD45 in dysgerminoma cases.

## Leukemia

Ovary may rarely be involved by leukemia either by primary or secondary process. The secondary involvement of ovary by leukemia is more common. The primary ovarian granulocytic sarcoma may be noted in case of acute myeloid leukemia. The leukemic cells show diffuse involvement of ovary.

## Tumors of Soft Tissue and Bone

### Leiomyoma

This is an extremely rare tumor in ovary. Leiomyoma of ovary mainly occurs in between 30 to 65 years. The tumor is unilateral, solid and size varies from 1 to 15 cm in diameter. The cut section of the tumor is gray brown and shows whorled appearance. Microscopical appearance of leiomyoma of ovary is similar to that of uterine leiomyoma. This is a benign tumor and surgical removal of the tumor is the treatment of choice.

### Leiomyosarcoma (Figures 16.7 to 16.10)

This is an exceptionally uncommon neoplasm in ovary.[7] The mean age of the patient is 53 years. Leiomyosarcomas are usually more soft and fleshy and larger in size compared to leiomyoma of ovary. There is no definite criteria of diagnosis of leiomyosarcoma of ovary. Conventionally, the presence of any two of the following criteria indicate leiomyosarcoma:
1. Tumor cell necrosis,
2. Significant nuclear atypia,

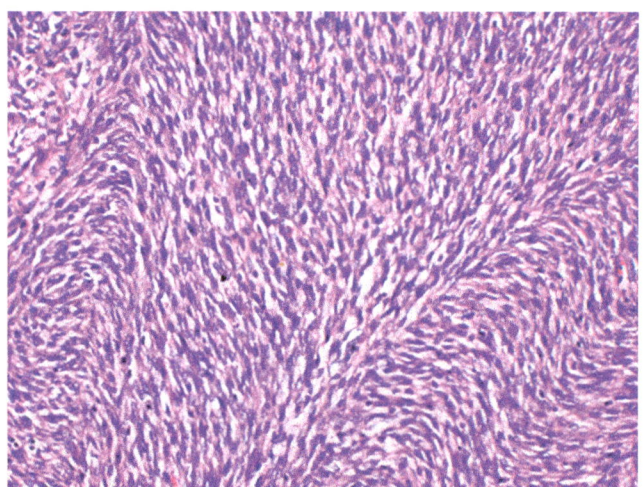

Figure 16.7: Leiomyosarcoma ovary: The oval to spindle cells arranged in fascicles

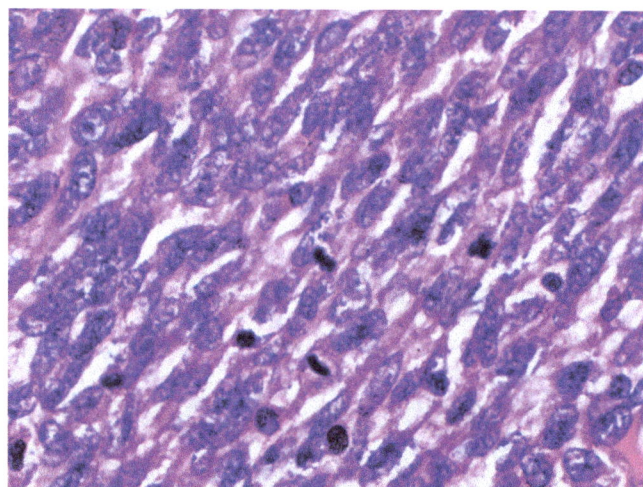

Figure 16.9: Leiomyosarcoma ovary: Frequent mitotic activities are seen

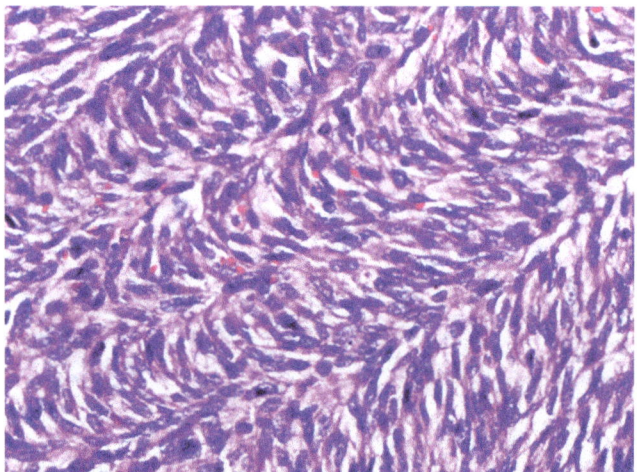

Figure 16.8: Leiomyosarcoma ovary: The cells are spindle-shaped with moderate nuclear atypia

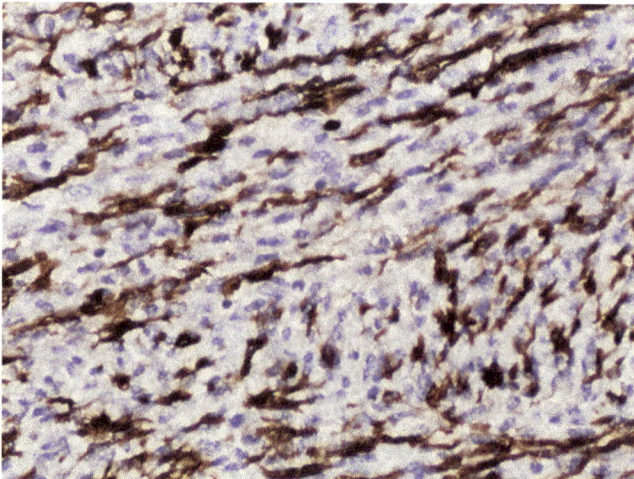

Figure 16.10: Leiomyosarcoma ovary: Desmin positive cells

3. ≤10 mitosis per 10 high-power fields. However, Lerwill MF et al.[7] suggested that even in the absence of any tumor cell necrosis the presence of more than ≤5 mitosis per 10 high-power fields along with nuclear atypia should be considered as leiomyosarcoma of ovary.

### Skeletal Muscle Tumor

**Rhabdomyosarcoma:** Primary rhabdomyosarcoma of ovary is very uncommon tumor. Rhabdomyosarcoma may often be associated with malignant mixed Müllerian tumor (MMMT) of ovary and therefore thorough sampling is needed before the diagnosis of primary rhabdomyosarcoma of ovary. The age of the patient varies widely from 2 to 84 years with a mean age 37 years.[8] The tumor is unilateral and varies in size from small to huge mass with smooth, solid and fleshy appearance on cut section. Histopathology the tumor may show embryonal, alveolar or pleomorphic type rhabdomyosarcoma. Ovarian rhabdomyosarcoma is an aggressive malignancy with very poor prognosis. Surgical removal of the tumor followed by combination chemotherapy is the treatment of choice.

### Tumors of Bone and Cartilaginous Tumor

Primary chondrosarcoma and osteosarcoma of ovary are extremely uncommon.[9,10] The exact histogenesis is unknown.

**Hemangioma of ovary:** Hemangioma of ovary is very uncommon. The tumor occurs in wide range of ages from few months to 63 years.[11] They are unilateral and of variable sized from few mm to several cm in diameter with spongy in appearance on cut section. Microscopically, the tumor shows multiple cavernous or cavernous-capillary patterns. Large vascular spaces are seen lined by endothelial cells.

**Angiosarcoma:** Angiosarcoma of ovary is an extremely uncommon tumors and only a few case reports have been recorded.[12] Angiosarcoma is usually large, soft, friable tumor. Histology section shows abundant varying sized vascular channels with intervening connective tissue stroma. The vascular channels are lined by endothelial cells that show marked nuclear enlargement, pleomorphism and increased mitotic activity. The tumor cells are positive for CD34, CD31 and von Willebrand factor. Angiosarcoma is an aggressive malignant tumor. The tumor may have favorable prognosis if it is confined within ovary at the time of diagnosis.

## REFERENCES

1. Lash RH, Hart WR. Intestinal adenocarcinomas metastatic to the ovaries. A clinicopathological evaluation of 22 cases. Am J Surg Pathol. 1987;11:114-21.
2. Saphir O. Signet-ring cell carcinoma. Mil Surg. 1951;109(4):360-9.
3. Szych C, Staebler A, Connolly DC, Wu R, Cho KR, Ronnett BM. Molecular genetic evidence supporting the clonality and appendiceal origin of Pseudomyxoma peritonei in women. Am J Pathol. 1999;154(6):1849-55.
4. Ji H, Isacson C, Seidman JD, Kurman RJ, Ronnett BM. Cytokeratins 7 and 20, Dpc4, and MUC5AC in the distinction of metastatic mucinous carcinomas in the ovary from primary ovarian mucinous tumors: Dpc4 assists in identifying metastatic pancreatic carcinomas. Int J Gynecol Pathol. 2002;21(4):391-400.
5. Young RH, Gersell DJ, Roth LM, Scully RE. Ovarian metastases from cervical carcinomas other than pure adenocarcinomas. A report of 12 cases. Cancer. 1993;71(2):407-18.
6. Levanon K, Crum C, Drapkin R. New insights into the pathogenesis of serous ovarian cancer and its clinical impact. J Clin Oncol. 2008;26(32):5284-93.
7. Lerwill MF, Sung R, Oliva E, et al. Smooth muscle tumors of the ovary: a clinicopathologic study of 54 cases emphasizing prognostic criteria, histologic variants, and differential diagnosis. Am J Surg Pathol. 2004;28:1436-51.
8. Sandison AT. Rhabdomyosarcoma of the ovary. J Pathol Bacteriol. 1955;70:433-8.
9. Talerman A, Auerbach WM, Van Meurs AJ. Primary chondrosarcoma of the ovary. Histopathology, 1981;5:319-24.
10. Fadare O, Bossuyt V, Martel M, et al . Primary osteosarcoma of the ovary: a case report and literature review. Int J Gynecol Pathol. 2007;26:21-25.
11. Talerman A. Hemangiomas of the ovary and the uterine cervix. Obstet Gynecol. 1967;30:108-13.
12. Nielsen GP, Young RH, Prat J et al. Primary angiosarcoma of the ovary. A report of seven cases and review of the literature. Int J Gynecol Pathol. 1997;16:378-82.

# Fallopian Tube 17

## WHO Classification of Fallopian Tube[1]

**Epithelial tumors and cysts**
- Hydatid cyst
- Benign epithelial tumors
  - Papilloma
  - Serous adenofibroma
- Epithelial precursor lesion
  - Serous tubal intraepithelial carcinoma
- Epithelial borderline tumor
  - Serous borderline tumor
- Malignant epithelial tumors
  - Low-grade serous carcinoma
  - High-grade serous carcinoma
  - Endometrioid carcinoma
  - Undifferentiated carcinoma
- Others
  - Mucinous carcinoma
  - Transitional cell carcinoma
  - Clear cell carcinoma

**Tumor-like lesions**
- Tubal hyperplasia
- Tubo-ovarian abscess
- Salpingitis isthmica nodosa
- Metaplastic papillary tumor
- Placental site nodule
- Mucinous metaplasia
- Endometriosis
- Endosalpingiosis

**Mixed epithelial-mesenchymal tumors**
- Adenosarcoma
- Carcinosarcoma

**Mesenchymal tumors**
- Leiomyoma
- Leiomyosarcoma
- Others

**Miscellaneous tumors**
- Adenomatoid tumor

**Germ cell tumors**
Teratoma
- Mature
- Immature

**Lymphoid and myeloid tumors**

## ANATOMY

Fallopian tube (FT) is joined to the upper part of uterus. It is located anterior to the ovary. Medially the tube ends in the uterine cavity and laterally it ends near the ovary in the peritoneal cavity. The total length of fallopian tube is 9–12 cm. FT is divided into four parts from medial to lateral: intramural, isthmic, ampullary and fimbrial.

1. **Intramural:** It is 1 cm long and 0.7 mm wide. This portion of FT lies within the uterine smooth muscle wall.
2. **Isthmic:** The length of isthmic part is 3 cm and width is 5 mm. It continues medially with intramural part and laterally with ampullary part of FT.
3. **Ampulla:** This is the widest part of the fallopian tube. The luminal diameter of ampulla is 1 cm. The ampullary part of FT is 5 cm long and is continuous with the infundibular part. Fertilization usually takes place in the ampullary part of FT.
4. **Fimbrial part:** The fimbrial part consists of 25 fingers like fimbrial projections. One of the fimbria is long and comes in direct contact with the tubal pole of ovary.

## HISTOLOGY

The fallopian tube is composed of three layers: Mucosal layer, muscularis layer and serosal layer.

a. **Mucosal layer:** The mucosa of FT consists of multiple longitudinal folds of epithelium which is made of single layer of cells that contains predominantly two types of cells:
   - Ciliated cells: These cells are more abundant in the lateral part of the FT. These are tall columnar

epithelial cells with eosinophilic cytoplasm having round regular nuclei. The cilia of the cells move only in one direction and helps propel the sperms towards the uterine cavity.
- Secretory cells: These cells are more abundant in the medial part of the FT. The cells are tall columnar with scanty eosinophilic cytoplasm and round regular hyperchromatic nuclei. These cells lack any cilia.

b. **Muscularis mucosa:** This consists of outer longitudinal and inner circular layer of muscle.
c. **Serosal layer:** The serosal layer consists of flattened mesothelial cells. Loose connective tissue and capillaries are seen underneath the mesothelial cell layer of serosa.

## BLOOD SUPPLY AND LYMPHATICS

Fallopian tube derives its vascular supply from the tributaries of the ovarian and uterine arteries. The lymphatic vessels of the FT drain into ovarian vessel and go to the para-aortic lymph node and uterine lymphatic system to the internal iliac lymph node.

## NON-NEOPLASTIC LESIONS OF FALLOPIAN TUBE

### Metaplasia of Fallopian Tube

The following metaplastic changes are seen:[2]
1. **Decidual metaplasia:** This is commonly seen during the peripartum tubal ligation. It shows focal collection of decidual cells within the lamina propria or sub-mesothelial location (Figures 17.1 and 17.2).
2. **Mucinous metaplasia:** Mucinous cells are tall columnar in appearance with basally located nuclei. There may be focal hyperplasia of the mucosal cells that may form cribriform appearance simulating carcinoma.
3. **Transitional cell metaplasia:** This metaplasia is common and does not bear any clinical significance (Figures 17.3 and 17.4).

### Walthard Cell Rest

Walthard cell rest appears as small 1 to 3 mm whitish nodule or cyst on the surface of the FT. It is composed of well-circumscribed nest of transitional epithelial cells (Figure 17.5). The cells show moderate amount of clear cytoplasm with centrally placed round nuclei having prominent longitudinal nuclear groove. It is a benign lesion and does not have any clinical significance.

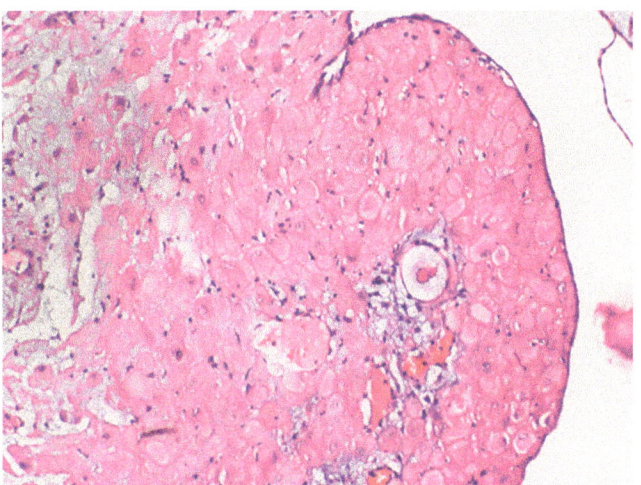

Figure 17.2: Decidual metaplasia: Higher magnification of the same

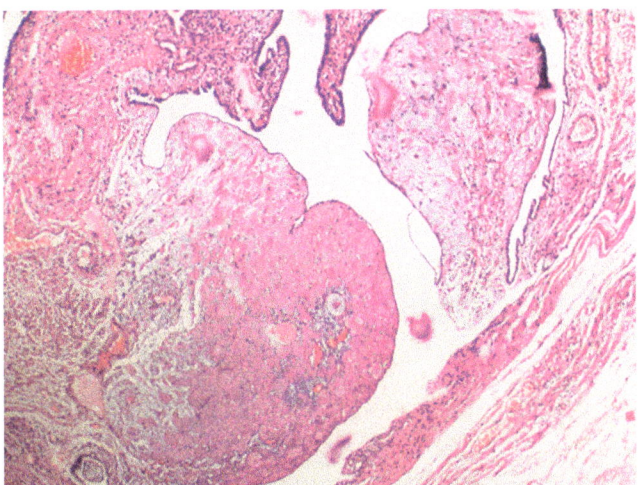

Figure 17.1: Decidual metaplasia: Foci of decidual metaplasia on the wall of the fallopian tube

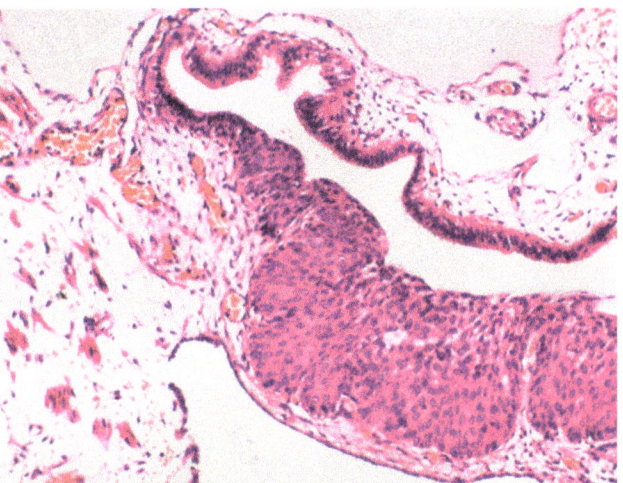

Figure 17.3: Transitional metaplasia of the fallopian tube: The tubal wall shows focal transitional metaplasia

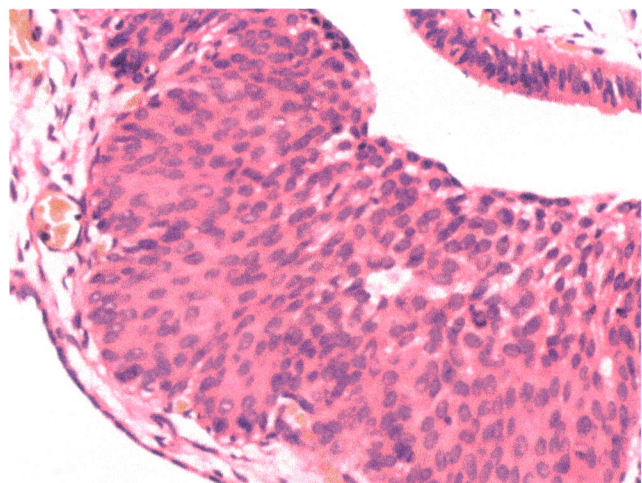

Figure 17.4: Transitional metaplasia: Higher magnification of the same

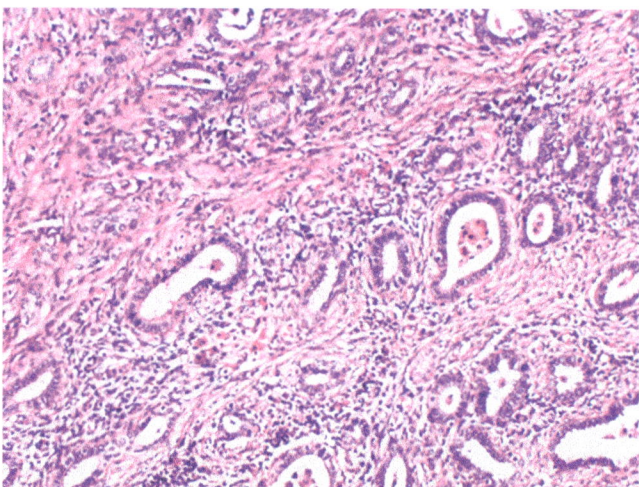

Figure 17.6: Salpingitis isthmica nodosa: Multiple irregular round to elongated glands within the muscular wall of the fallopian tube

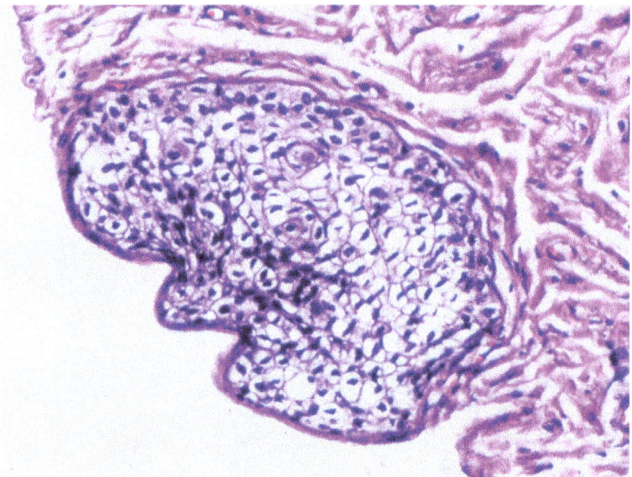

Figure 17.5: Walthard cell rest on the serosal aspect of the fallopian tube

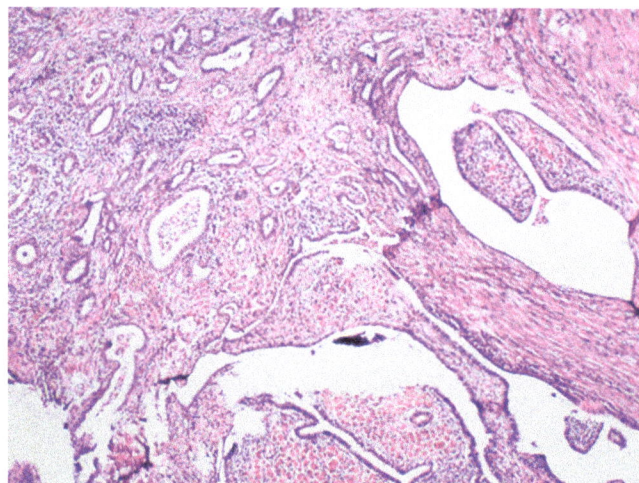

Figure 17.7: Salpingitis isthmica nodosa: The glands are of variable size and surrounded by muscle

## SALPINGITIS ISTHMICA NODOSA

Salpingitis isthmica nodosa (SIN) is also known as "adenomyosis" of the fallopian tube. The mean age of the patient is 30 years. SIN is seen in 0.6–11% female and is frequently seen with infertility and ectopic gestation.[3] SIN is usually bilateral and is seen as small one to multiple 1 to 2 cm yellowish nodules predominantly on the isthmic part of the fallopian tube.

### Histopathology (Figures 17.6 to 17.8)

Histopathology section shows multiple irregular round to elongated glands lined by bland looking fallopian tube epithelium. The glands are encased by proliferating disorganized hyperplastic muscle layer. Serial section often shows communication of the glandular lumen with the fallopian tube lumen.

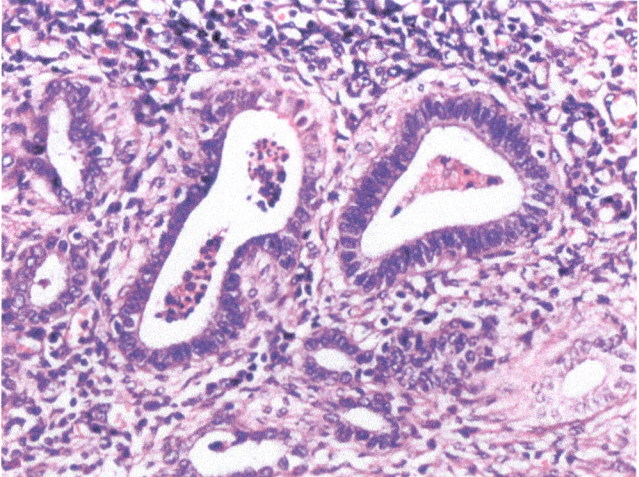

Figure 17.8: Salpingitis isthmica nodosa: The lining epithelium of the glands are made of bland looking fallopian tube epithelium

## Differential Diagnosis

a. **Follicular salpingitis**: The following features favor the diagnosis of follicular salpingitis: (1) the glandular structures are surrounded by fibrous tissue, (2) lymphocytic infiltration.
b. **Endometriosis**: The presence of endometrial stroma and endometrial glands are evident in closer inspection in case of endometriosis.

## Prognosis and Treatment

The most common sequel of SIN are infertility and ectopic pregnancy. Microsurgical removal of the affected segment is the treatment of choice.

## TUBAL PREGNANCY

Implantation of the blastocyst in the tubal lumen causes tubal pregnancy. Most of the ectopic pregnancy occurs in the fallopian tube. The other areas of ectopic pregnancy are in cervix, hepatic, diaphragmatic or splenic. The ectopic pregnancy occurs in 1-2% of all pregnancies. However due to frequent use of assisted reproductive technology the incidence of ectopic pregnancies is now increased.

## Risk Factors

The risk factors of tubal pregnancy include:[4]
1. Previous genital infection
2. History of induced abortion
3. Use of intrauterine device
4. Tubal pathology.

## Clinical Features

The main features of tubal pregnancy are:
1. Amenorrhea
2. Vaginal bleeding
3. Pain abdomen.
   The tubal rupture may cause intra-abdominal bleeding and produces the symptoms and signs of acute abdomen.

## Gross

The tube is grossly dilated with external congestion and hemorrhage. Cut section of FT shows blood clot, necrosis and friable fleshy tissue. Most of the time the products of gestation can be identified on the tubal wall. Placental tissue and parts of embryos may also be recognizable.

## Histopathology

Histopathological examination shows multiple chorionic villi, decidual tissue along with hemorrhage and necrosis in the tubal wall. The wall shows edema and inflammation.

## Treatment

Surgical removal of the affected tube (salpingectomy) is the treatment of choice. Treatment with methotrexate is an alternate management of tubal pregnancy.

## INFECTIONS

### Acute Salpingitis

The causative organisms of acute salpingitis are *Neisseria gonorrhoeae*, *Chlamydia trachomatis*, *Mycoplasma*, and anaerobic bacteria. This is predominantly seen in young female. The common risk factor of acute salpingitis include:
1. Early intercourse
2. History of sexual transmitted disease
3. Multiple sexual partners
4. Prior instrumentation
5. Application of intrauterine contraceptive device.

*Clinical Feature*

The patient commonly complaints of pelvic pain, fever, vomiting and menstrual irregularities. In chronic case the patient may have abscess formation or peritonitis.

*Gross*

The FT is enlarged, edematous with purulent exudates over the surface.

*Histopathology*

The mucosa of the FT shows focal denudation of the epithelial lining, edema, along with dense infiltration by polymorphs. The epithelium may be show proliferation and complex glandular branching.

*Therapy*

Acute salpingitis is treated by antibiotics, analgesics and rest.

### Chronic Salpingitis

Chronic salpingitis occurs due to repeated episode of acute salpingitis. The patient may have pelvic pain and infertility.

*Gross*

The tube is grossly dilated and adhered with the surrounding structures and ovary. Tubal wall is often thickened. The wall of the tube shows whitish scar. The cut section of the tube shows dilated lumen which is often filled with thin fluid or pus.

*Histopathology (Figures 17.9 and 17.10)*

The wall of the FT shows dense chronic inflammatory cells consisting of lymphocytes, plasma cells and histiocytes.

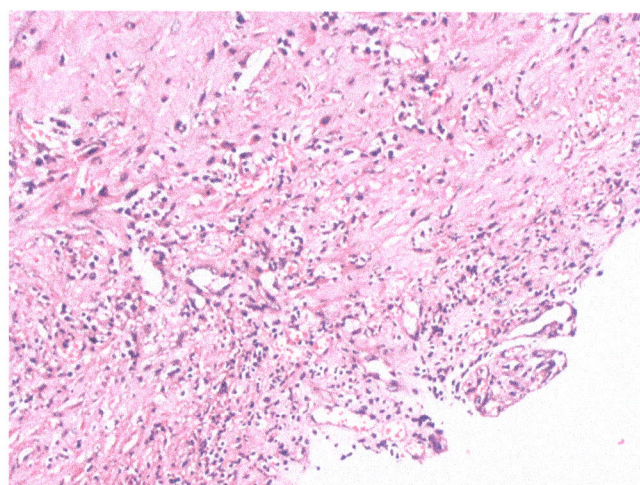

**Figure 17.9:** Chronic salpingitis: The wall of the fallopian tube shows chronic inflammatory cells

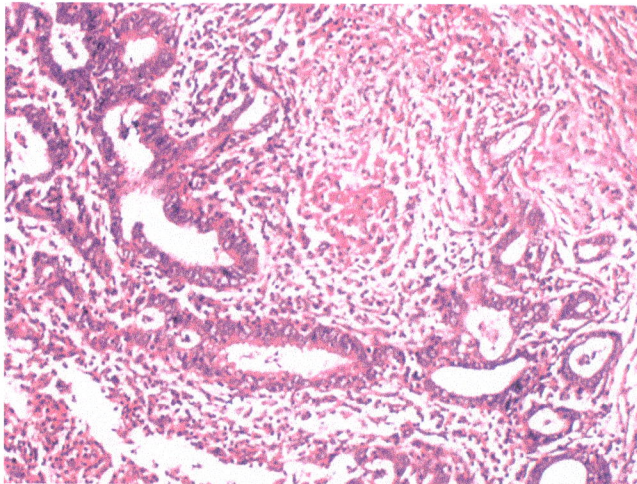

**Figure 17.11:** Tuberculous salpingitis: Epithelioid cell granuloma in the wall of the fallopian tube

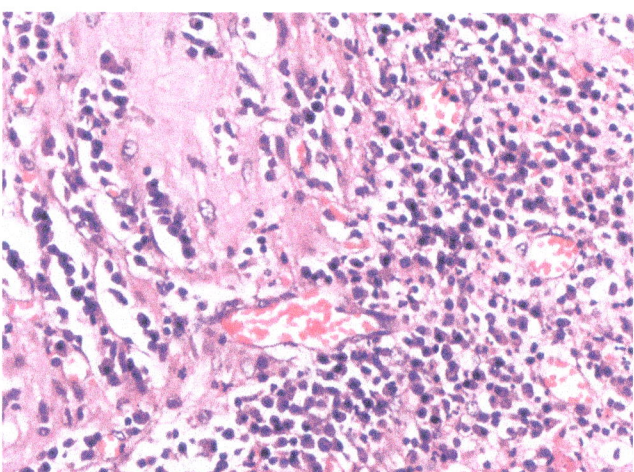

**Figure 17.10:** Chronic salpingitis: The inflammatory cells are composed of lymphocytes and plasma cells

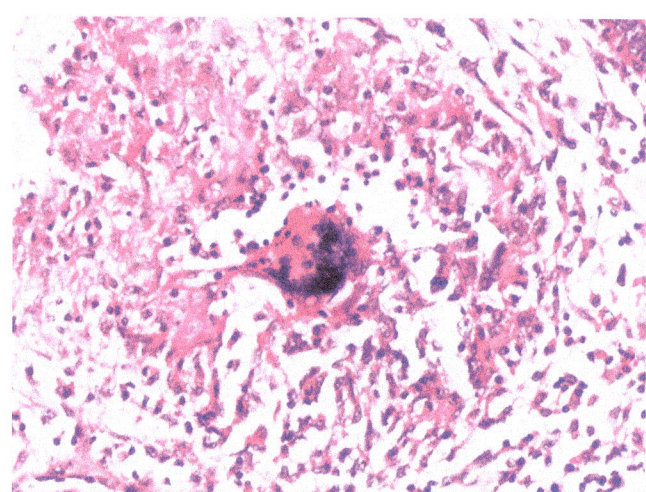

**Figure 17.12:** Tuberculous salpingitis: Caseous necrosis, epithelioid cells and Langhan's giant cells

The mucosa is often flattened. There may be fusion of the glandular space. The mucosal plicae of the FT often adhere with each other and form a cribriform-like appearance.

## Tubercular Salpingitis

Tuberculous salpingitis is caused by *Mycobacterium tuberculosis*. It may occur in any age group, but adolescent females are often involved by tuberculous salpingitis. The incidence of tuberculous salpingitis varies in different countries from 5 to 40% in infertile women.[5] The infection of FT commonly occurs by hematogenous spread from already infected lung and usually bilateral FTs are involved. In most of the cases, the infection is latent and remain silent for many years. The infection is detected at the time of investigations of infertility.

### Gross

Fallopian tube is usually enlarged, edematous with multiple small nodules over the surface. The tube may show adherence with the adjacent structures. The cut section of the lumen may show caseous necrosis.

### Histopathology (Figures 17.11 and 17.12)

The mucosal lining of the FT shows multiple caseating epithelioid cell granulomas. There may be focal hyperplasia of the mucosal lining. The muscularis mucosa shows dense lymphocytic infiltration. The mucosal granulomas may coalesce and rupture into the lumen of the FT along with caseous necrotic material. The FT may be dilated with thick wall and the epithelium may show proliferation with hyperplasia mimicking carcinoma. The presence of acid fast bacilli in Ziehl-Neelsen stain or bacterial culture is the definitive proof of tuberculosis.

*Differential Diagnosis*

a. **Lipoid salpingitis:** Lipoid salpingitis caused by contrast agent is characterized by variably sized, round to ovoid spaces containing lipid material.
b. **Parasitic infections:** Eosinophilic infiltration along with demonstrable parasitic ova are the diagnostic features of parasitic infections.
c. **Necrotic pseudoxanthomatous lesion:** This is the end stage of endometriosis and is characterized by necrotic center surrounded by palisading histiocytes.

*Treatment*

Antitubercular therapy including rifampicin, isoniazid, and ethambutol is the treatment of choice.

## TORSION

Isolated torsion of the FT is rare.[6] Torsion is usually associated with benign or malignant ovarian tumor. In addition the presence of hydrosalpinx or pyosalpinx may be related with the torsion of FT. The patients usually present with severe acute pain in lower abdomen that may mimic surgical emergency. Grossly, the FT may be mild to moderately enlarged, red and edematous. Microscopically, the FT shows edema, vascular congestion, hemorrhage and necrosis. Early diagnosis and surgical intervention may help to preserve the tube.

## TUMORS OF THE FALLOPIAN TUBE

WHO classified FT neoplasms in the main heading of: Epithelial, mesenchymal, metastatic and miscellaneous group.

## Adenomatoid Tumor

Adenomatoid tumor is the most common benign tumor in the FT. The tumor is of mesothelial cell origin.

*Clinical Feature*

This is usually seen incidentally in middle aged or elderly patient.

*Gross*

The adenomatoid tumor is mostly unilateral. Grossly, it appears as small well-circumscribed 1 to 2 cm diameter whitish nodule over the surface of the FT.

*Histopathology (Figures 17.13 and 17.14)*

Histopathological section shows multiple anastomosing pseudoglandular spaces with intervening band of connective tissue. The spaces may be slit-like, dilated or cribriform-like. The lumen may contain basophilic secretory material. The lining cells of the channels are cuboidal to flat with monomorphic round nuclei. Rarely signet ring-like cell is also seen. Mitosis is rare. Foci of chronic inflammatory cells may be present. Occasionally, the lymphoid aggregates are formed.

*Immunohistochemistry*

The tumor is positive for calretinin, low molecular weight cytokeratin and WT-1. And negative for EMA, Ber-EP4, and B72.3.

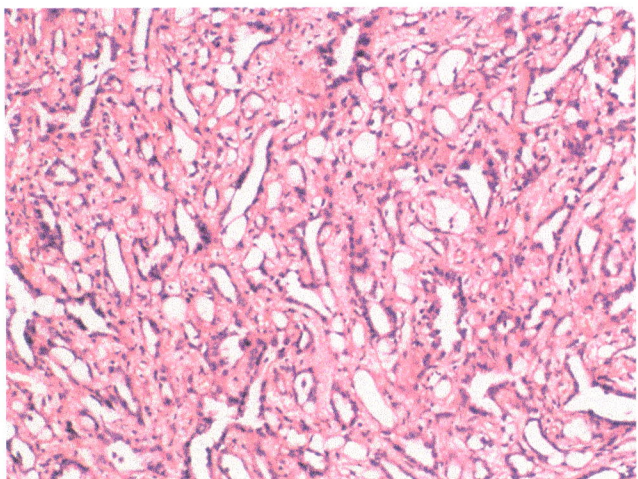

Figure 17.13: Adenomatoid tumor of fallopian tube: Multiple anastomosing pseudoglandular spaces with intervening band of connective tissue

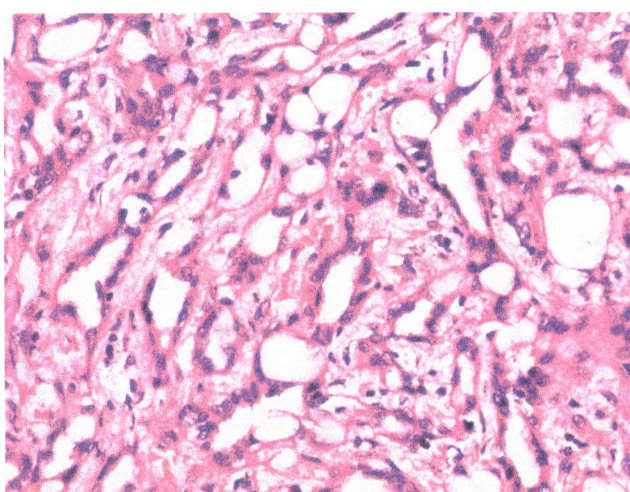

Figure 17.14: Adenomatoid tumor of fallopian tube: The lining cells of the channels are cuboidal to flat with monomorphic round nuclei

*Differential Diagnosis*

a. **Adenocarcinoma**: The following features support the diagnosis of adenomatoid tumor: (1) Well-circumscribed nodular appearance in gross, (2) No nuclear atypia, (3) No mitosis.
b. **Lymphangioma**: Lymphangiomas are positive for CD34 and negative for calretinin.
c. **Leiomyoma**: The leiomyoma is well-circumscribed and do not show infiltrative growth pattern.

## Epithelial Tumor

*Papilloma*

This is a rare tumor in fallopian tube.

**Clinical feature:** Papilloma is mainly detected incidentally in pregnant and postpartum patients.

**Pathology:** The tumor is seen as mass in the lumen of FT. Histological section shows multiple orderly branched papillae with fibrovascular core. The papillae are lined by single layer of columnar to cuboidal cells. The individual cells show abundant eosinophilic cytoplasm and bland nuclei. Mitotic activity is nil.

**Differential diagnosis:** (a) Borderline tumor: Unlike borderline tumor the papillae in papilloma are orderly arranged and individual cells are completely bland. (b) Metastatic papillary carcinoma: Clinical history is helpful.

## Carcinoma

Carcinoma of FT is uncommon and represents about 1% of all malignancies of female genital tract.[7] The diagnostic criteria of primary FT carcinomas are: (1) the tumor must be located within the FT and the tumor should show evidence of origin within the fallopian tube mucosa, (2) there should not be any coexisting endometrial adenocarcinoma of similar histology, (3) the parenchymal involvement of ovarian carcinoma should be less in volume than that of tube. Clinical features: The average age of the patient is 58 years. The three common complaints of the patient include: bleeding per vagina, pain in abdomen and abdominal mass. These symptoms are quite nonspecific and therefore patients are usually not diagnosed preoperatively. Fallopian tube carcinomas are associated with near about 30% cases of BRCA 1 and BRCA 2 mutation.[8]

*Gross*

The majority of the FT carcinomas are unilateral (97%). The tumor occurs mainly in the middle and lateral third of the tube. Gross appearance of the tumor resembles either hydrosalpinx or pyosalpinx. The fimbrial end of the fallopian tube is usually blocked by the tumor. The outer surface of the tube is smooth or in advanced case may show nodularity. The cut section of the tube shows necrotic material and gray white friable tissue.

*Histopathology*

Near about 80% of tubal carcinomas are serous adenocarcinomas followed by endometrioid, transitional and undifferentiated carcinomas.

**Serous adenocarcinoma (Figures 17.15 to 17.18):** It is the commonest carcinoma in the FT. The section shows multiple well-formed papillary structures with central fibrovascular core. The lining cells of the papillae are cuboidal to columnar cells with moderate amount of cytoplasm and mild nuclear atypia. The high-grade serous adenocarcinoma shows solid nests of cells with occasional papillary structures. The nuclei

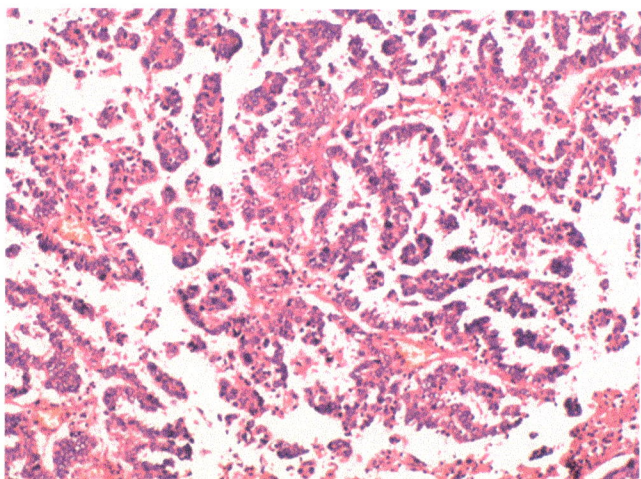

**Figure 17.15:** Serous carcinoma of fallopian tube: Multiple well-formed papillary structures

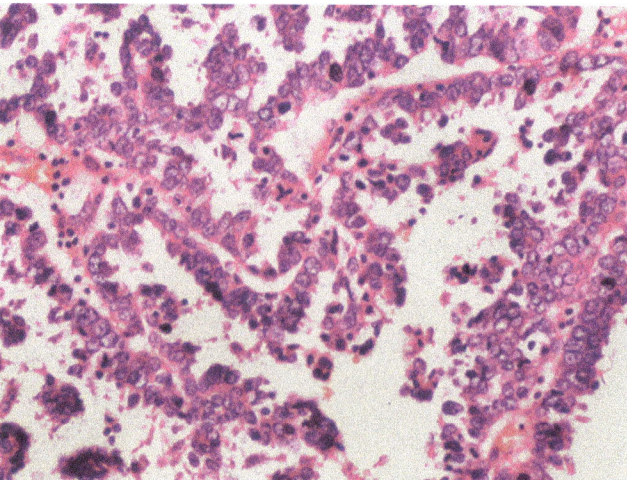

**Figure 17.16:** Serous carcinoma of fallopian tube: The papillae with central fibrovascular core

**258** Essentials of Gynecologic Pathology

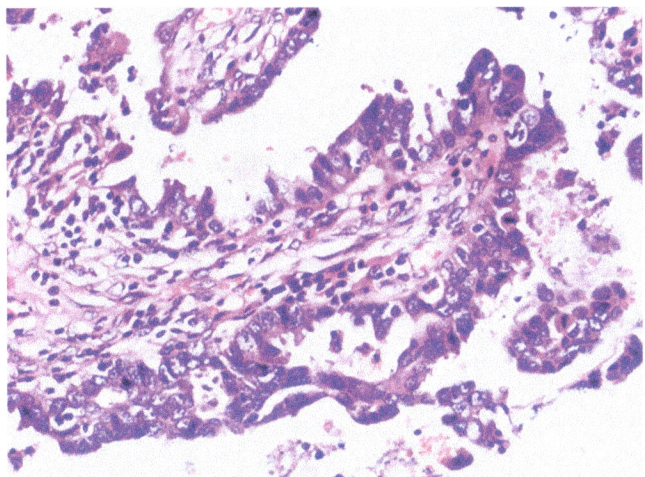

Figure 17.17: Serous carcinoma of fallopian tube: Higher magnification of the papillary structure

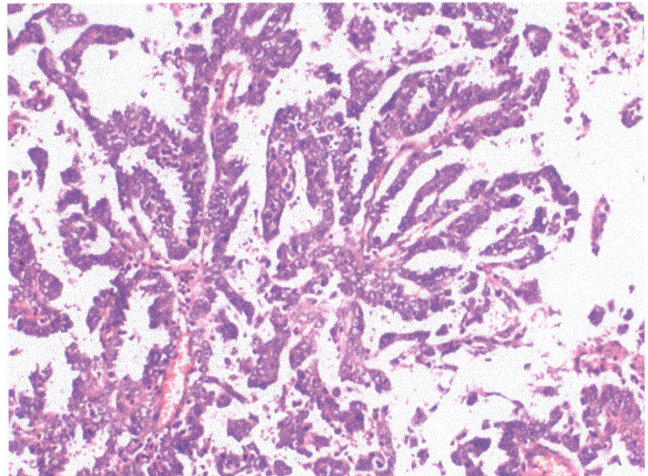

Figure 17.18: Serous carcinoma of fallopian tube: Thin and long papillae

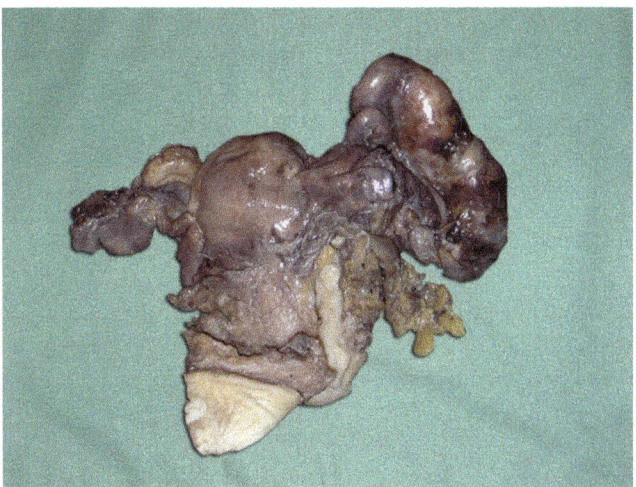

Figure 17.19: Transitional cell carcinoma of fallopian tube: Grossly enlarged left fallopian tube

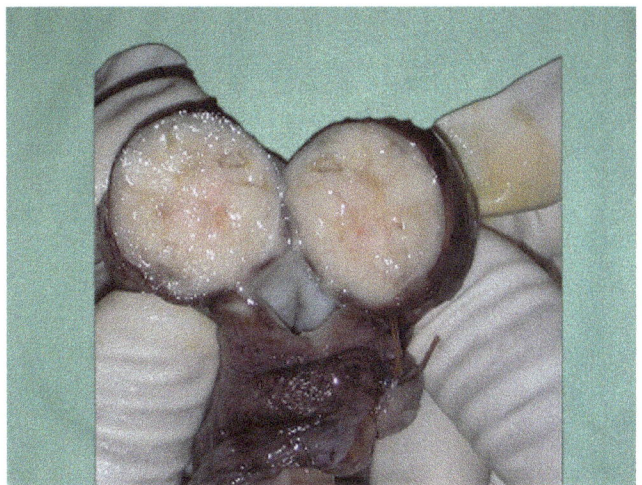

Figure 17.20: Transitional cell carcinoma of fallopian tube: Cut section shows gray white solid tumor

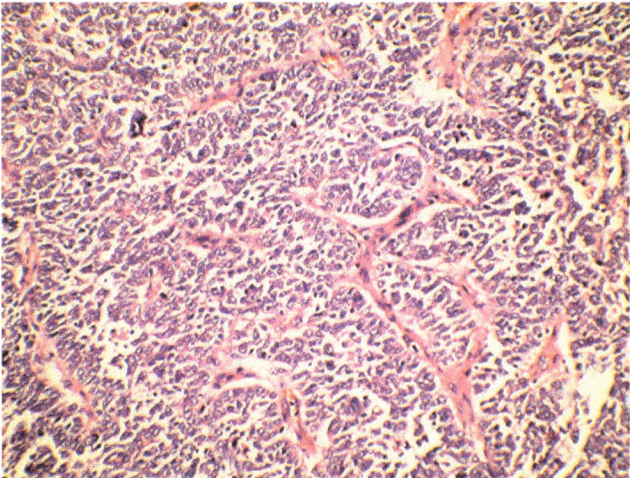

Figure 17.21: Transitional cell carcinoma of fallopian tube: The nests of tumor cells with moderately pleomorphic nuclei

of grade 3 carcinoma shows marked atypia. Majority of serous adenocarcinomas are grade 3. In addition, serous carcinoma of fallopian tube shows many multinucleated tumor giant cells and psammoma bodies.

**Endometrioid carcinoma:** It is usually confined within the mucosa and lamina propria of FT. The tumor simulates the morphology of endometrioid carcinoma of ovary and uterus. The tumor is made of dense collection of endometrioid-like glands with moderate nuclear pleomorphism of the lining epithelial cells. Squamoid differentiation or spindle cell type of epithelial cells are also seen. Endometrioid carcinoma often simulates the female adnexal tumor of probable Wolffian origin.[9]

**Transitional cell carcinoma (Figures 17.19 to 17.21):** This is an uncommon tumor of FT and is possibly developed from metaplastic transitional epithelial cells. The individual cells show scanty to moderate cytoplasm and moderately pleomorphic nuclei with prominent longitudinal nuclear groove.

**Mucinous carcinoma:** This is also an uncommon tumor of FT. The tumor is often associated with Peutz–Jeghers syndrome.

*Immunocytochemistry*

Tubal carcinomas show similar immunohistochemical pattern as that of ovarian tumor. The tumor cells show CK 7 positivity and CK20 negativity. In addition the nuclei of tumor cells are strongly positive for PAX 8.

*Staging*

International Federation of Gynecology and Obstetrics (FIGO) staging is applied for clinical staging of FT carcinoma (Box 17.1).

*Prognosis*

Carcinoma of FT has poor prognosis. Five year survival rate depends mainly on FIGO staging of the tumor. In addition the other prognostic factors are grade of the tumor and large volume of residual tumors. The overall five year survival rate of stage I, II, and stage III-IV are 80%, 16–58%, and 12–29% respectively.

**Box 17.1:** FIGO staging of fallopian tube carcinoma[10]

**Stage 0:** Carcinoma in situ

**Stage I:** Tumor confined to the fallopian tubes
- IA: Tumor confined to one tube, without involving the serosal surface and no ascites
- IB: Tumor confined to both tubes, without involving the serosal surface and no ascites
- IC: Tumor confined to one or both tubes with extension onto or through the serosa or with malignant cells in ascites or peritoneal washings

**Stage II:** Tumor involves one or both fallopian tubes with pelvic extension
- IIA: Infiltration or metastasis to the uterus or ovaries
- IIB: Infiltration to other pelvic structures
- IIC: Pelvic extension with malignant cells in ascites or peritoneal washings

**Stage III:** Tumor involves one or both fallopian tubes with peritoneal implants outside the pelvis
- IIIA: Microscopic peritoneal metastasis outside the pelvis
- IIIB: Macroscopic peritoneal metastasis outside the pelvis ≤2 cm or less in diameter
- IIIC: Peritoneal metastasis ≥2 cm in diameter

**Stage IV:** Distant metastasis

*Treatment*

The treatment of FT carcinoma is similar to that of ovarian carcinoma. Total abdominal hysterectomy with bilateral salpingo-oophorectomy is done. In advanced stage additional combination chemotherapy is administered.

### Tubal Intraepithelial Carcinoma

The tubal carcinoma was commonly related with serous carcinoma and was designated as "serous tubal intraepithelial carcinoma" (STIC). STIC lesion has been discussed in detail in Chapter 14.

### Metastatic Carcinoma

Metastatic carcinoma in the FT is far more common than the primary carcinoma of FT. Metastasis may occur from the adjacent ovary or endometrium by direct extension. Infrequently metastasis from the distant organ is seen.

## CYSTS

### Paraovarian Cyst

Paraovarian cysts represent 10% of all adnexal cysts. They are of three types: (1) Paramesonephric (Müllerian), (2) Mesonephric (Wolffian), (3) Mesothelial (Table 17.1). These cysts are usually asymptomatic. Large cysts may cause pressure effect and may produce symptoms such as abdominal pain. The cysts are few mm to several cm in diameter and mostly are unilocular filled with clear serous fluid.

**Table 17.1:** Comparison of different cysts in fallopian tube

| Features | Paramesonephric cyst | Mesothelial cyst | Mesoenephric cyst |
| --- | --- | --- | --- |
| Lining | Ciliated columnar epithelial cells similar to fallopian tube | Flattened mesothelial cells | Non-ciliated cuboidal epithelial cells |
| Wall | Smooth muscles | Fibrous stroma | Smooth muscles |

### Paramesonephric Cyst (Figures 17.22 and 17.23)

The cysts are lined by ciliated columnar epithelial cells. The wall of the cyst is formed by smooth muscles.

### Mesothelial Cyst (Figure 17.24)

The cyst wall is lined by mesothelial cells. The wall of is made of fibrous stroma.

### Mesonephric Cyst

The lining of the cyst shows non-ciliated cuboidal epithelial cells. The wall of the cyst contains smooth muscles.

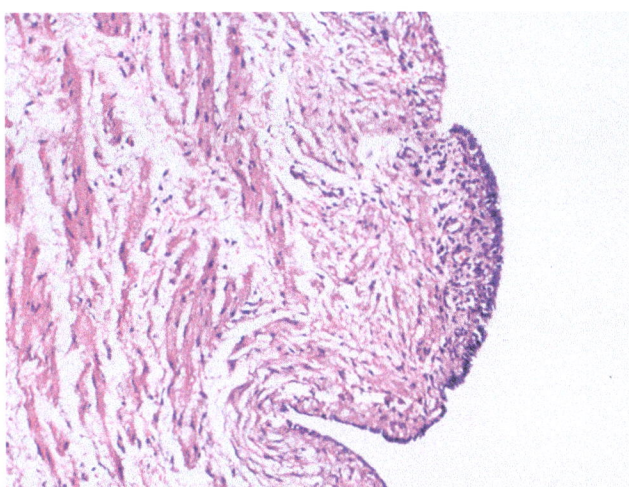

**Figure 17.22:** Paramesonephric cyst: The cyst wall is formed by muscle layer and the lining of the wall is formed by fallopian tube epithelium

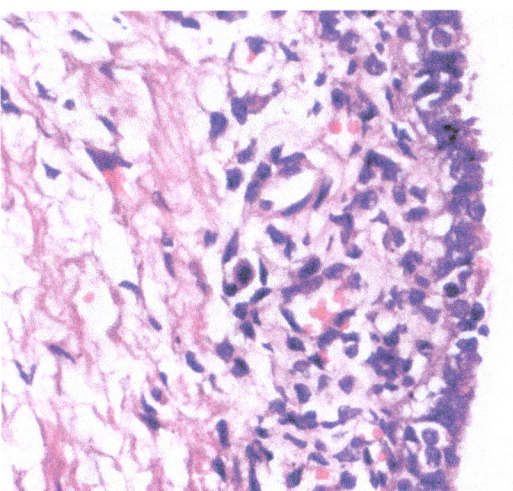

**Figure 17.23:** Paramesonephric cyst: Ciliated columnar lining

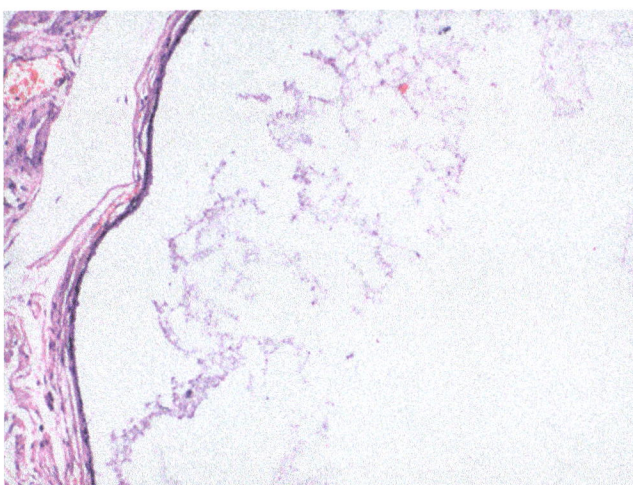

**Figure 17.24:** Mesothelial cyst: The cyst wall is lined by flattened mesothelial cells

### Differential Diagnosis

**Serous cystadenoma of ovary:** The serous cystadenoma does not have any smooth muscle wall. At times it is difficult to differentiate the paratubal cyst from a serous cystadenoma. In such difficult situation, the cyst should be labeled as simple cyst only.

## FEMALE ADNEXAL TUMOR OF PROBABLE WOLFFIAN ORIGIN

Female adnexal tumors of probable Wolffian origin (FATWO) is a distinctive group of tumor and are seen in broad ligament, mesosalpinx, hilum of ovary and also in the wall of the FT.[11] The tumor is probably developed from the remnants of the mesonephric duct (Wolffian).

### Clinical Feature

The mean age of the patient is 46 years. The tumor may be detected incidentally or the patients may have abdominal swelling and pain.

### Gross

The average size of the tumor is 8 cm. It is usually well-circumscribed and firm. The cut section of the tumor is homogenous and white to yellow.

### Histopathology

The tumor shows variable growth pattern such as tubular, trabecular, reticular and sieve like. There may be admixture of various patterns and one of the patterns may predominate. The individual cells are cuboidal, polygonal or spindle shaped. The cells contain pale eosinophilic cytoplasm and relatively monomorphic nuclei. Mitosis is minimal to nil. The features of malignancy in FATWO include high mitosis, nuclear atypia and vascular invasion.

### Immunohistochemistry

Female adnexal tumor of probable Wolffian origin is positive for CK7, CAM 5.2, calretinin, and CD 10 and negative for EMA.

### Differential Diagnosis

Female adnexal tumor of probable Wolffian origin may be confused with endometrioid carcinoma. However, endometrioid carcinoma shows true gland and often shows squamoid differentiation.

### Treatment

Female adnexal tumor of probable Wolffian origin is a benign tumor and simple surgical resection is adequate in this patient. Malignant FATWO should be treated by surgical resection followed by chemotherapy.

## REFERENCES

1. Kurman RJ, Carcangiu ML, Herrington S, Young RH. WHO classification of tumors of female genital reproductive organs. 4th Edition, International agency for research on Cancer, Lyon, 2014.
2. Rabban JT, Crawford B, Chen LM, et al. Transitional cell metaplasia of fallopian tube fimbriae: a potential mimic of early tubal carcinoma in risk reduction salpingo-oophorectomies from women with BRCA mutations. Am J Surg Pathol. 2009;33:111-9.
3. Jenkins CS, Williams SR, Schmidt GE. Salpingitis isthmica nodosa: a review of the literature, discussion of clinical significance, and consideration of patient management. Fertil Steril. 1993; 60(4):599-607.
4. Bouyer J, Coste J, Shojaei T, et al. Risk factors for ectopic pregnancy: a comprehensive analysis based on a large case-control, population-based study in France. Am J Epidemiol. 2003;157:185-94.
5. Parikh FR, Nadkarni SG, Kamat SA, et al. Genital tuberculosis – a major pelvic factor causing infertility in Indian women. Fertil Steril. 1997;67:497-500.
6. Batukan C, Ozgun MT, Turkyilmaz C, Tayyar M. Isolated torsion of the fallopian tube during pregnancy: a case report. J Reprod Med. 2007; 52(8):745-7.
7. Ajithkumar TV, Minimole AL, John MM, et al. 2005 Primary fallopian tube carcinoma. Obstet Gynecol Surv. 2005;60:247-52.
8. Zweemer RP, Van Diest PJ, Verheijen RH, et al. Molecular evidence linking primary cancer of the fallopian tube to BRCA1 germline mutations. Gynecol Oncol. 2000;76:45-50.
9. Daya D, Young RH, Scully RE. Endometrioid carcinoma of the fallopian tube resembling an adnexal tumor of probable Wolffian origin: a report of six cases. Int J Gynecol Pathol 1992;11:122-30.
10. Benedet JL, Bender H, Jones H III, et al. Staging Classification and Clinical Practice Guidelines of Gynaecologic Cancers by FIGO Committe on Gynecologic Oncology, 2000.
11. Devouassoux-Shisheboran M, Silver SA, Tavassoli FA. Wolffian adnexal tumor, so-called female adnexal tumor of probable Wolffian origin (FATWO): immunohistochemical evidence in support of a Wolffian origin. Hum Pathol. 1999; 30:856-63.

# Pathology of Placenta

Placenta is the important organ that separates the fetus from the endometrium of the uterus. It is also the main connecting link between the fetus and mother. Understanding the pathology of placenta may help us to know the cause of many fetal abnormalities.

## NORMAL DEVELOPMENT

Fertilization commonly occurs in the ampulla of the fallopian tube which is the widest part of the tubal canal. About 30 hours after the fertilization, the zygote undergoes mitotic division. The dividing cells form a morula that consists of 12 to 32 cells 3 days after fertilization. The spherical morula enters into the uterus in 3rd day of fertilization. Approximately 4th day after fertilization, a cavity appears within the morula and a fluid-filled cystic space develops, known as blastocyst cavity. The outer cell layer of the cavity is known as trophoblast. A group of cohesive cells is formed in one pole the morula which is known as inner cell mass. The fetus finally develops from this inner cell mass. The whole structure is known as blastocyst. The blastocyst freely floats within the uterine cavity for two to three days. Approximately 6th to 7th days after fertilization, the blastocyst implants on the endometrium (Figure 18.1). Usually, the attachment of the blastocyst occurs near the embryonic pole. Immediately after the attachment of the blastocyst, the trophoblast starts proliferation and slowly differentiates into two distinct layers: Cytotrophoblast (CT) and syncytiotrophoblast (ST). The ST rapidly proliferates and invades the uterine endometrial wall. The ST cells produce the human chorionic gonadotropin hormone (hCG) and maintain the activity of corpus luteum of the ovary. The blood-filled spaces develop in the uterine wall at the site of implantation (Figure 18.2). The multiple columns of cell with outer ST and inner CT layers appear. In 11th to 12th days, the ST erodes the maternal capillaries and many congested and dilated sinusoids form (Figure 18.3). The maternal blood now freely circulates within these blood filled sinusoids and uteroplacental circulation develops.

In the meantime, the extraembryonic mesenchyme develops from the wall of the yolk sac and invaginates within the core of these columns and chorionic villi develop. In the third week, the villi consist of only CT and ST cells and are known as primary villi. The secondary villi contain mesenchymal core within them. During the course of development, the mesenchymal tissue differentiates into blood vessels and tertiary villus develops. Intermediate trophoblast (IT) is seen in the anchoring columns and in the extravillous sites. IT cells are mixed with decidual cells and microscopically difficult to differentiate from the decidual cells. Initially, the chorionic villi encircle the entire chorionic sac but in course of time only the villi in relation to decidua basalis remain and proliferate to produce a disk-like structure known as chorionic plate that later on forms the definitive placenta. The blood is filled in the intervillous space in the placenta and is supplied by the eroded spiral artery. Multiple stem villi come out from the chorionic plate and undergo complex branching. Some villi connect from the fetal chorionic plate to the maternal basal plate. These villi are known as anchoring villi. Multiple wedge-shaped septa of decidua, known as placental septa, arise from the basal plate and are directed towards the chorionic plate. These placental septae

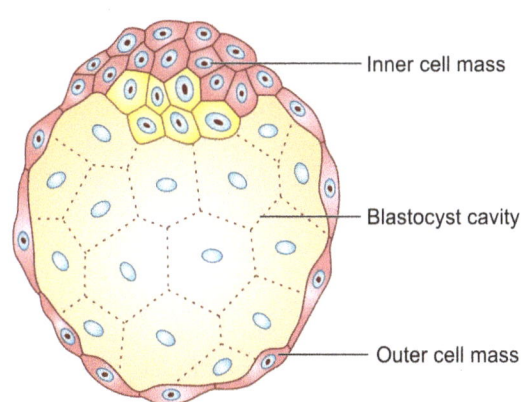

**Figure 18.1:** Placenta formation in 6th to 7th day after fertilization

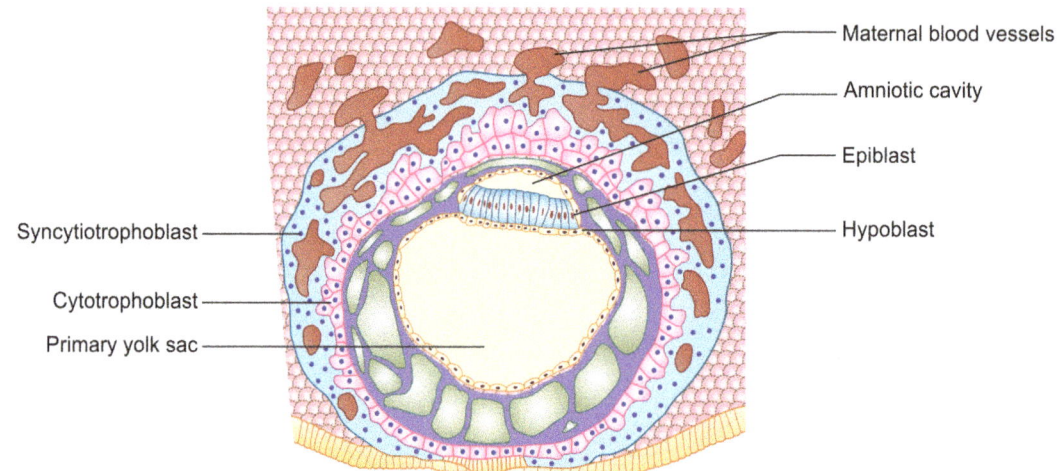

Figure 18.2: Placenta formation in 9th day after fertilization

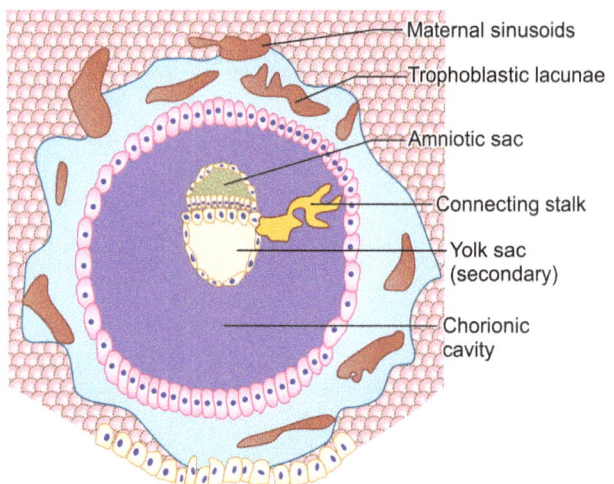

Figure 18.3: Placenta formation in 13th day after fertilization

separate the placenta into 10 to 40 compartments known as cotyledon. Each cotyledon contains one or two stem villi and their multiple branches. The cotyledon is the functional unit of the placenta and has its own blood supply. The fetus is attached with the trophoblast by a narrow connecting stalk known as umbilical cord. Umbilical cord contains two arteries and one vein. The arteries carry the deoxygenated blood and the vein carries the oxygenated blood to the fetus. Deoxygenated blood comes out from the fetus to the placenta by two umbilical arteries. These arteries divide multiple times before it reaches to the chorionic plate. The villi are bathed into the oxygenated maternal blood from the spiral arterioles of the endometrium. The gaseous and metabolic products are exchanged on the placental membrane. This membrane includes: (1) ST, (2) CT, (3) Basement membrane of the trophoblastic villous, (4) Mesenchymal tissue of the villi, (5) Endothelial cells of the fetal capillaries, (6) Basement membrane of the capillaries.

The oxygenated blood in the fetal capillaries of the chorionic villi ultimately comes to the vein and drains into the umbilical vein that carries the blood to the fetus.

## MICROSCOPY (FIGURE 18.4)

The placenta consists of multiple villi. The villi are lined by the CT and ST and the central core of the villi consists of blood capillaries containing blood.

### Cytotrophoblast

Cytotrophoblast is the mitotically active component of the trophoblast that ultimately gives rise to ST. The cells have well-defined border with clear cytoplasm. Nuclei are round and monomorphic. They cover the surface of the villi and merge with ST.

### Syncytiotrophoblast

Syncytiotrophoblast (ST) cell overlies the CT of the villi. The cells have indistinct border and contain abundant vacuolated cytoplasm with multiple small nuclei. These cells are differentiated and maintain many essential functions of the placenta that include hormone production, transport and protection.

### Intermediate Trophoblast

These cells may be seen as:
a. Villous Intermediate trophoblast (IT) that lines the trophoblastic column,
b. Implantation site IT that is seen in the implantation site. IT infiltrates in the endometrium and myometrium, and is intimately mixed with decidua.

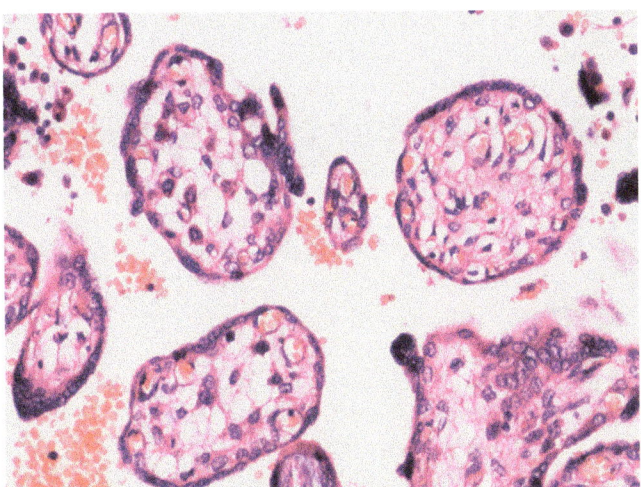

Figure 18.4: Chorionic villi: The villi are lined by both cyto and syncytiotrophoblastic cells

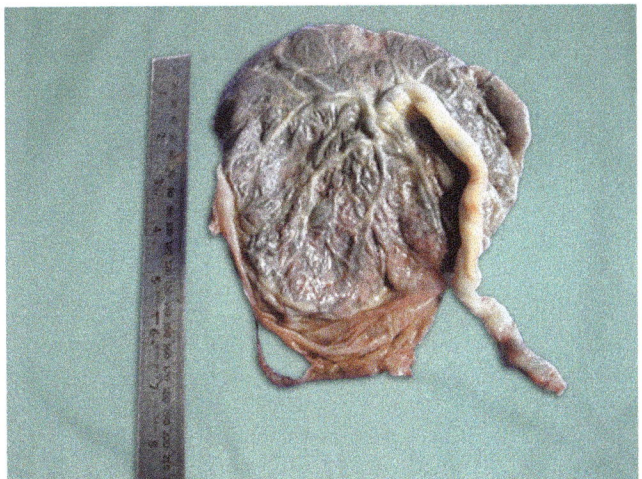

Figure 18.5: Placenta gross: Disk-shaped organ with attached umbilical cord

c. Chorionic type IT: These cells are present in the chorionic leave of the fetal membrane.

IT cells are positive for cytokeratin (CK) whereas the decidual cells are negative for CK.

## PLACENTA GROSS

Placenta is a discoid-shaped structure with 3 cm thickness and average diameter 15 to 25 cm. It weighs 500 to 600 g and is divided into 20 to 25 cotyledons (Figures 18.5 and 18.6).

## INDICATIONS OF PLACENTAL EXAMINATION

Indications of placental examination include maternal, fetal and placental causes (Box 18.1).

## ABNORMALITIES OF THE SHAPE OF PLACENTA

Normally, the placenta is a single disk-shaped structure. Following abnormalities may occur in shape (Table 18.1).

### Succenturiate Lobe

This is the commonest abnormality of the shape and occurs in 3% cases. In this condition, single or multiple small pieces of placenta is seen along with the main placental tissue. The umbilical cord is inserted into the dominant lobe. However, it may be inserted in other small lobe also. The succenturiate lobe may be retained within the uterus after the delivery. The small lobe is prone to infract. No histopathological changes are seen in succenturiate lobe.

### Bilobed

In case of bilobed placenta, the lobes are almost equal in size and are connected by the fetal membrane. Bilobed placenta is

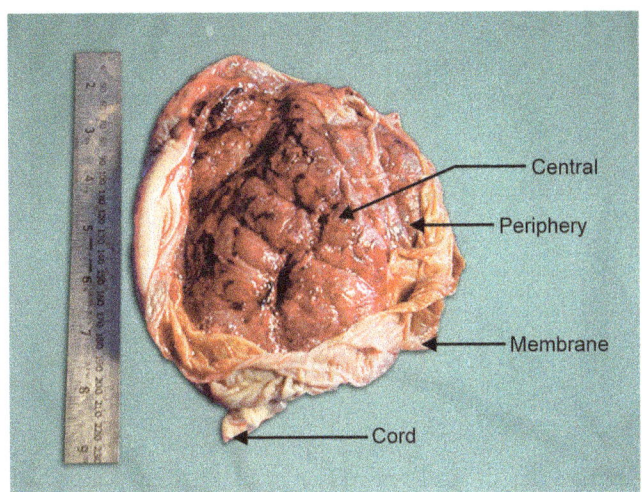

Figure 18.6: Placenta gross: Different parts of the placenta

**Box 18.1:** Indications of placental examinations

**Maternal**
- Preeclampsia
- Chronic hypertension
- Diabetes mellitus
- Oligohydramnios
- Polyhydramnios
- Abruptio placentae
- Preterm delivery
- Infection

**Fetal**
- Fetal malformations and intrauterine growth restriction
- Intrauterine or perinatal death
- Thick meconium
- Suspected infection
- Congenital anomalies

**Placental**
- Grossly abnormal placenta

Table 18.1: Abnormalities of shape of placenta

| Diagnosis | Altered shape | Clinical significance |
|---|---|---|
| Bilobed | Two equal size | • Higher incidence of first trimester<br>• Bleeding and placenta previa |
| Succenturiate | Two or multiple unequal lobe | • Small lobe is prone to infract |
| Placenta membranacea | Large and thin and multiple chorionic villi are seen along the whole gestational sac | • Extremely uncommon, high fetal mortality and pre term delivery |
| Fenestrate placenta | Focal absence of chorionic villi in the placenta | • No significance |
| Circumvallate | Membranous insertion is away from the margin of the placenta | • Moderate degree may cause intrauterine growth retardation, premature termination of pregnancy placental abruption, oligohydramnios and neurological impairment |

commonly associated with multiparity and advanced maternal age. There is higher incidence of first trimester bleeding and placenta previa in cases of bilobed placenta.

## Multilobated Placentas

In this condition, placenta contains multiple lobes defined by indentations.

## Placenta Membranacea

It is extremely uncommon in human. The placenta is large and thin and multiple chorionic villi are seen along the whole gestational sac. This is due to failure of atrophy of the chorionic leave. The placenta may not contain any proper thick disk and the whole placenta remains thin. These cases are associated with high fetal mortality and preterm delivery.

## Fenestrate Placenta

There is focal absence of chorionic villi in the placenta and the placenta is fenestrated.

## Extrachorial Placenta

In case of extrachorial placenta, the chorionic plate is smaller than the basal plate and does not come to cover the placental margin. Therefore, a thin rim of placental tissue remains at the periphery devoid of any chorionic tissue. Cause: Exact cause of extrachorial placenta is not known. Probably recurrent hemorrhage at the margin of placenta is responsible for the displacement of the membrane towards central part of the placenta. This recurrent marginal hemorrhage may occur due to chronic abruption placenta.

There are two types of extrachorial placenta: circumvallate and circummarginate.

## Circumvallate

It occurs in 1 to 5% of placenta. Circumvallate placenta is abnormal-shaped placenta characterized by folded fetal membranes at the periphery of the disk. There is marginal fold of the chorion and the membranes are rolled back and reflected centrally. In this type of placenta, the membranes are not attached at the edge of the placenta but within the inside part towards the umbilical cord. Fibrin and old blood clots are noted at the peripheral margin.

## Circumvaginate

In case of circumvaginate placenta, there is a flat transition from the chorionic plate to the membrane. There is no reflection of the membrane at the periphery and no fibrin or blood clot is seen.

### Significance

Minor circumvallate placenta has no clinical impact. However moderate or severe circumvallate placenta may be responsible for intrauterine growth retardation, premature termination of pregnancy placental abruption, oligohydramnios and neurological impairment.[1]

## ABNORMAL ADHERENCE OF PLACENTA

The placenta may be adhered to the uterine wall abnormally. Depending on the degree of adherence, this may be classified as: Placenta accreta, increta, and percreta.

**Placenta accreta:** Placenta is superficially adhered to the myometrium.

**Placenta increta:** Here the placental villi infiltrates within the deeper part of the myometrium.

**Placenta percreta:** Here the whole thickness of the myometrium up to the serosal layer is infiltrated by the chorionic villi.

## Etiology

The underlying pathology in all three conditions accreta, increta and percreta is same and there is only quantitative difference of invasion of the mole in deeper myometrium. In case of abnormal adherence of placenta, there is complete or partial absence of decidual tissue and lack of proper development of the Nitabuch's layer. Normally, the decidual cells prevent the deeper insertion of the chorionic villi and also help in the separation of the placenta from the myometrium at the time of delivery. However, in absence of decidual cells the chorionic villi infiltrate in the deeper myometrium. The patients with cesarian section and placenta previa have near about 40% risk of developing placenta accreta.[2] Other risk factors of placental adherence include uterine anomalies, cornual implantation, uterine instrumentation, infection, manual removal of placenta, submucosal leiomyoma, and placenta membranacea.

### Clinical Features

The incidence of placenta accreta is approximately 0.3 per thousand deliveries.[2] According to The American Congress of Obstetricians and Gynecologists (ACOG) Committee's opinion, the incidence of placenta accreta has increased 10-fold in last five decades.[2] The steady rise of incidence of placenta accreta is related with the increased rate of cesarian section delivery. Placenta increta and percreta are often diagnosed antepartum due to bleeding or even uterine perforation. USG of the uterus shows irregular hypoechoic areas in villous tissue due to abnormal disposition of the spiral arterioles.

### Complications

Abnormal adherence of placenta may cause severe bleeding resulting the death of fetus or mother. Placental percreta may cause uterine perforation and rupture. Therefore if this condition is diagnosed before delivery then the patient should be managed by cesarean section followed by hysterectomy.

### Gross (Figures 18.7 and 18.8)

In case of placenta accreta part of the placenta may be absent. However, the gross examination of placenta may not exclude the possibility of placenta accreta completely. In

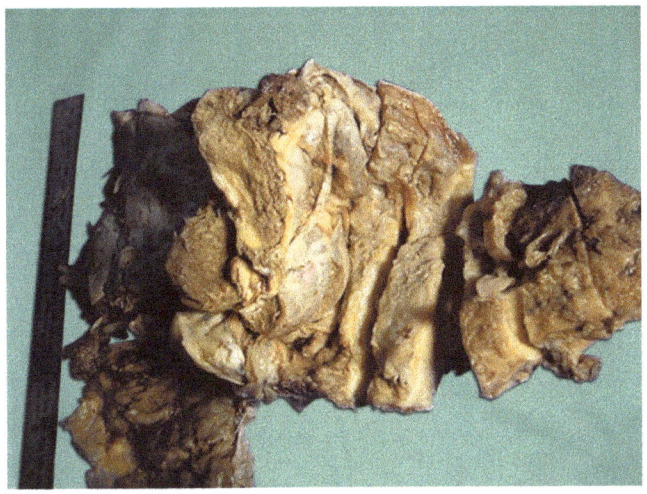

Figure 18.7: Placenta percreta: the placenta is deeply adhered in the uterine wall

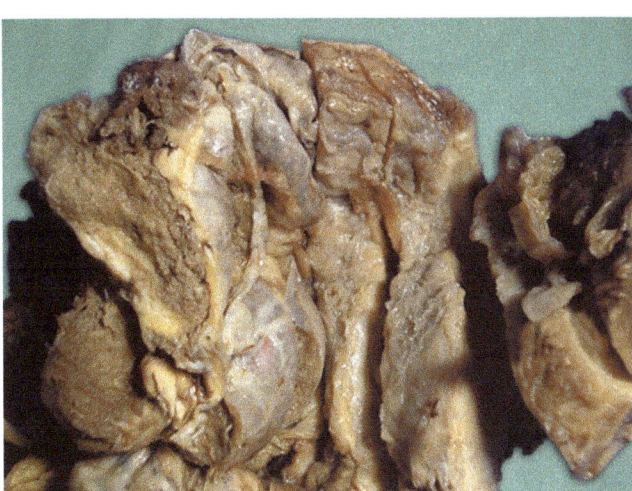

Figure 18.8: Placenta percreta: The placenta is reaching up to the serosa

small curetting, it is not possible to diagnose this condition. The placental adhesion is best judged in the hysterectomy specimen. Gross examination of the uterus shows thinned out myometrial tissue at the site of placental implant. The extension of villous tissue may also be recognized grossly. In placental percreta, the outer wall of uterus shows edema, hemorrhage and perforation.

### Histopathology (Figures 18.9 and 18.10)

Histology section of placenta accreta shows direct adherence of chorionic villi with the underlying myometrium without any intervening decidual cell layer. Lack of decidual cells in the interface between the villi and myometrium is the most important diagnostic feature of placenta accreta. The diagnostic criteria of placenta accreta is often used as direct contact of the villi on the myometrium. This may not be true as often extravillous trophoblast and fibrin may be present in the interface between the villi and myometrium. We must remember that the "lack of decidua" is the main diagnostic feature of placenta accreta.

In case of percreta and increta, the chorionic villi penetrate in the myometrium in varying depth.

## MULTIPLE GESTATIONS

Twin pregnancies are increasingly more common nowaday due to the increased application of assisted reproductive technologies. The examination of placenta is important to determine the zygosity and also to understand the mechanism of multiple gestations. Multiple gestations often contribute perinatal morbidity and mortality and also fetal malformation. Therefore, detailed placental examination is necessary in such cases.

**Zygosity:** Basically there are two types of zygosity:

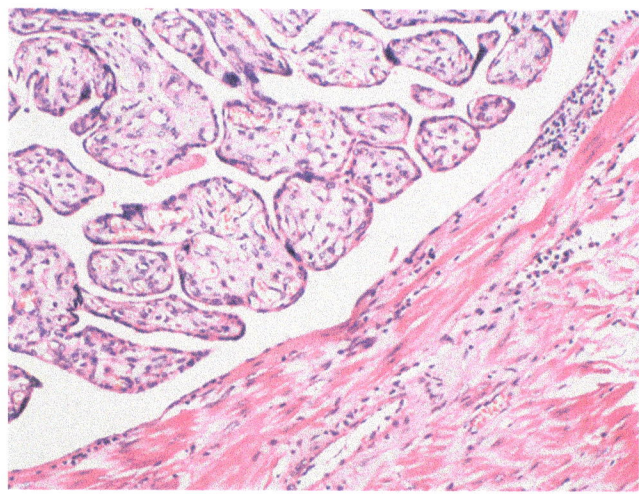

**Figure 18.9:** Placenta accreta: Villi directly on the muscle no decidua

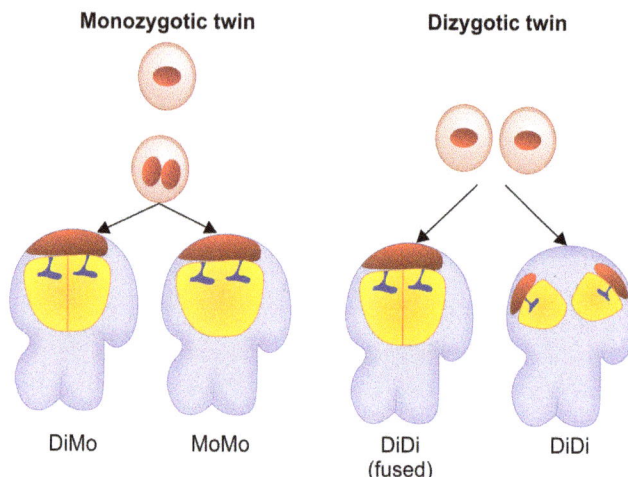

**Figure 18.11:** Twin pregnancy and zygosity

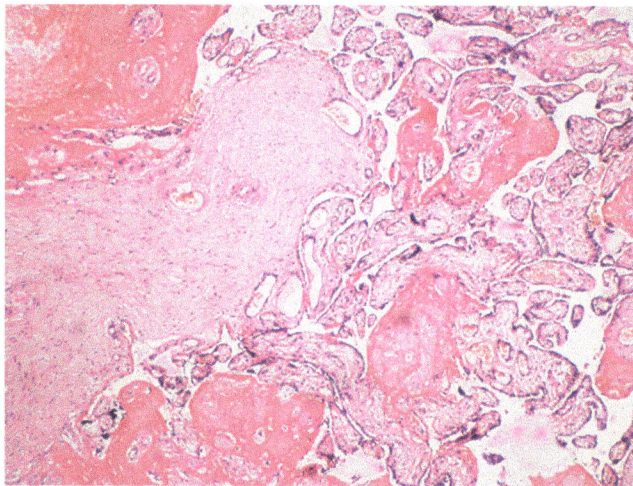

**Figure 18.10:** Placenta percreta: Chorionic villi invades deep in the myometrium up to serosal layer

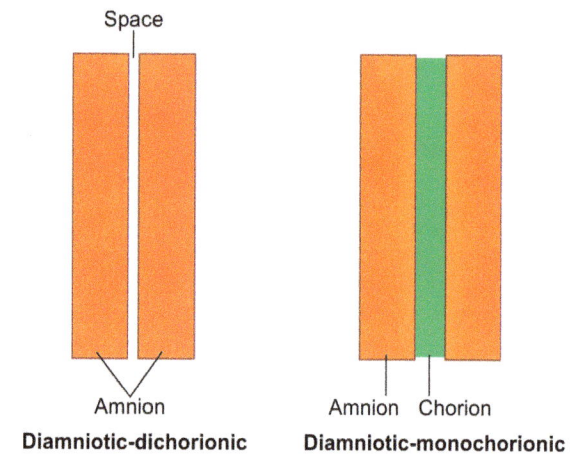

**Figure 18.12:** Placental membrane and chorion in twin pregnancy

### Monozygotic

One ovum is fertilized by one sperm only. The monozygotic (MZ) are identical genotypical and also phenotypically. They are usually of same sex.

### Dizygotic

In this process, two ova are fertilized separately by two sperms. The twins are genotypically different from each other.

The incidence of twin pregnancy is 1.25% of births.

### Placentation

The placentation of twin pregnancies are basically three types (Figures 18.11 and 18.12):
1. Diamniotic–dichorionic (DiDi): In DiDi placenta, there are two chorions and two separate amniotic cavities.
2. Diamniotic–monochorionic (DiMo): In DiMo cases, there is only one chorion and two amniotic cavities. DiMo placenta is always monozygotic.
3. Monoamniotic–monochorionic (MoMo): In MoMo placenta, there is only one chorion and amnion. MoMo placenta is always monozygotic.

*Monozygotic Twin*

In case of monozygotic twin, there is fertilization of one ovum by one sperm only. If the split occurs before the formation of the blastocyst (within 5 to 6 days after fertilization) then there will be two chorions and two amnions and the placentation will be DiDi. The dichorionic disks are always fused in such cases. If the split develops after the formation of chorions and before the development of the amnion then the placentation will have single chorion and two amnions (DiMo). In case of monoamniotic and monochorionic placentation (MoMo) the split occurs after the development of amnions.

### Dizygotic Twin

In dizygotic twin, the placentation is always DiDi. However, the chorionic disk may be closely spaced and fused.

**Pathogenesis:** The pathogenesis of dizygotic twin is different from the monozygotic twin. Dizygotic twin develops due to polyovulation. Polyovulation depends on ethnicity, race, maternal age and excessive stimulation by follicle stimulating hormone. The dizygosity is mostly familial or hereditary. The monozygotic twin is incidental and a sporadic event. There is no hereditary relation with monozygotic twin.

**Complication:** Congenital anomalies are more common in twin pregnancy than single pregnancy. Twin pregnancy is frequently associated with anencephaly, and visceral ischemic lesions. Twin pregnancy is also associated with various umbilical cord abnormalities such as defects in the insertion of umbilical cord or hypocoiled umbilical cord. Intrauterine growth retardation and premature delivery also occur in increased frequency in twin pregnancy.

**Gross examination:** Exact type of placentation can be determined by gross examination (Table 18.2). If the two placentas are completely separated from each other then they are clearly Diamniotic–dichorionic (DiDi). At times, the blastocyst may be closely spaced and fused and therefore appears to be a single chorion but the two chorions are separated distinctively by a membranous septum. The membranous septum is thick and the fetal blood vessels do not cross the membrane. It is important for the pathologist to distinguish monochorionic placenta from the fused dichorionic placenta. In fused dichorionic placenta, the septum is thick and opaque as they contain chorionic tissue whereas, in case of monochorionic placenta, the septum is thin, translucent and lacks any blood vessels. The septum lacks any chorionic tissue and is easily detachable.

Table 18.2: Differences between diamniotic dichorionic versus diamniotic monochorionic

| Features | Diamniotic dichorionic | Diamniotic monochorionic |
|---|---|---|
| Placental disk | Fused and appears single | Single |
| Dividing septum Thickness Color | Thick Opaque | Thin Translucent |
| Visible ridge on the fetal surface of the diving septum | Present | Absent |
| Abrupt termination of the surface vessels in the area of fusion | Present | Absent and vessels cross |

The study of the fetal blood vessels anastomosis in the chorionic plate is also very important to distinguish DiDi and DiMo placenta. In case of fused double chorion, the fetal blood vessels terminate at the septum and do not cross. Whereas, in DiMo placenta, the fetal circulation anastomoses in the septum and both the fetus share this portion.

## PLACENTAL INFLAMMATION AND INTRAUTERINE INFECTIONS

The infection of the placenta may be divided in:
a. Acute chorioamnionitis (ACA): Here, the inflammation is limited to the fetal membrane and umbilical cord. The infective organisms are mainly bacterial in ACA.
b. Villitis: Inflammation is mainly seen in the villous parenchymal tissue. This is mainly idiopathic.

### Clinical Features

ACA is seen in 10 to 15% cases of term delivery and two-thirds cases of preterm deliveries. Infections of the placenta may reach in several pathways:
1. Ascending pathway through vagina or cervix and infects the amnion. It is also known as "amniotic sac infection syndrome". It is often associated with rupture of membrane.
2. Hematogenous pathway through blood circulation.
3. By direct infection during amniocentesis.
4. By direct extension from endometrial infection. The diagnosis of clinical ACA is difficult as the patient may not show the clinical features of infection. However, clinically the patient may manifest as local or systemic symptoms or features such as fever, uterine tenderness, high leukocyte count and foul smelling vaginal discharge. In addition fetal tachycardia may also be seen. These clinical features may not coincide with the histopathology and therefore histopathological examination should be the ultimate gold standard of ACA.

### Pathology

Grossly, the fetal surface of the placenta loses it shiny appearance and it becomes white and opaque. In long standing infection, the fetal surface of the placenta becomes yellowish or greenish. The placenta may give malodorous smell. The placental membranes become more friable and focal areas of hemorrhage may be noted under the membranes. There is polymorphonuclear leukocytic (PMN) infiltration in the amniotic membrane and underlying chorion in ACA. The inflammatory exudates may also contain varying amount of macrophages and eosinophils in long standing cases. In case of subacute chorioamnionitis, the inflammatory exudates contain mixed cells consisting of lymphocytes and polymorphs both. In case of ACA, there may be maternal and fetal response to infection. Initial inflammatory response in ACA is maternal followed by fetal inflammatory response.

*Maternal Response (Figures 18.13 and 18.14)*

At first, the PMN migrates from the maternal vessels to intervillious space and decidual tissue under the membranes. Subsequently, the PMN accumulates into the connective tissue of the chorion and amnion. They traverse through the amniotic membrane to the amniotic cavity. The amniotic epithelial cells undergo necrotic changes and sledded within the amniotic fluid. The formation of abscess in the chorion is rarely seen. The maternal inflammatory response has been graded to assess the neonatal outcome (Table 18.3).[3] This grading system is not full proof and may not be reliable to predict the neonatal outcome.

Table: 18.3: Different stages of acute chorioamnionitis

| Stage | Terminology | Descriptions |
| --- | --- | --- |
| Early | Acute subchorionitis or chorionitis | Polymorphs in subchorionic area and membrane |
| Intermediate | Acute chorioamnionitis | Diffuse infiltration of Polymorphs in connective tissue of chorion and amnion |
| Late | Necrotizing chorioamnionitis | Necrosis of the amniotic cells and thickening of the basement membrane of amnion |

Grade: Mild or moderate: No special terminology, severe: Chorionic microabscess formation or severe confluent inflammation.

*Fetal Response (Figure 18.15)*

Fetal inflammatory response occurs only after 20th week of gestation. The inflammatory cells first involve the veins of the umbilical cord. PMN migrates through the venous wall and arterial muscular wall and then infiltrates in the Wharton's jelly. This is known as funiculitis. Focal areas of necrosis and abscess formation occur in the umbilical cord. The fetal inflammatory response is also staged as early, intermediate and advanced. The inflammatory response is graded as grade 1 (mild to moderate) and grade 2 (severe). In grade 1 infection, there is scattered PMN infiltration in the umbilical vessels and chorionic tissue. In grade 2, there is confluent collection of PMN in chorion and umbilical vessels (Table 18.4).

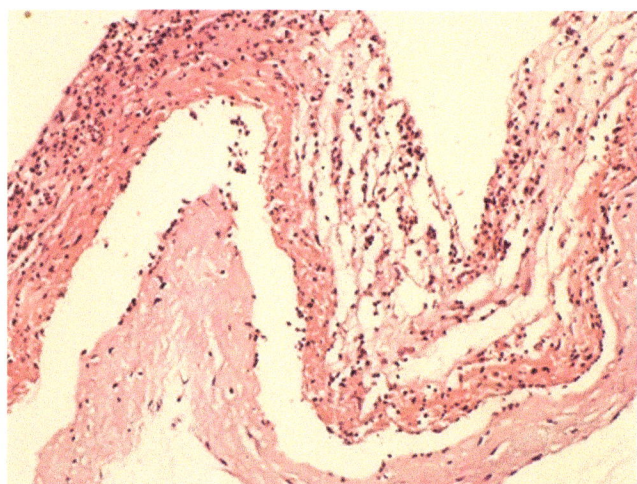

**Figure 18.13:** Acute chorioamnionitis: Polymorphonuclear leukocytic infiltration in the amniotic membrane and underlying chorion

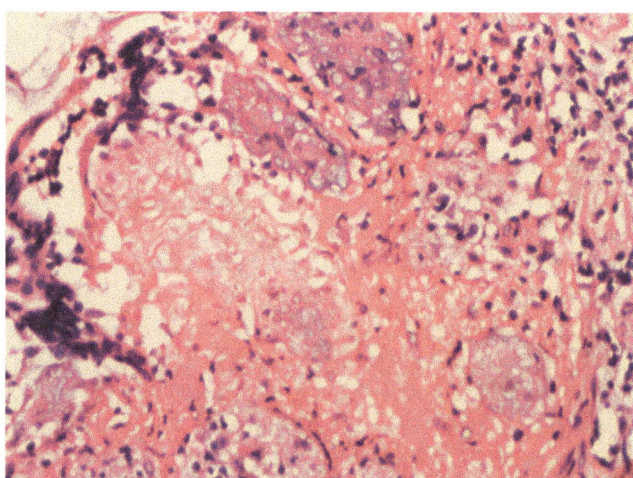

**Figure 18.14:** Acute chorioamnionitis: Diffuse infiltration of polymorphs in connective tissue of chorion and amnion along with necrosis

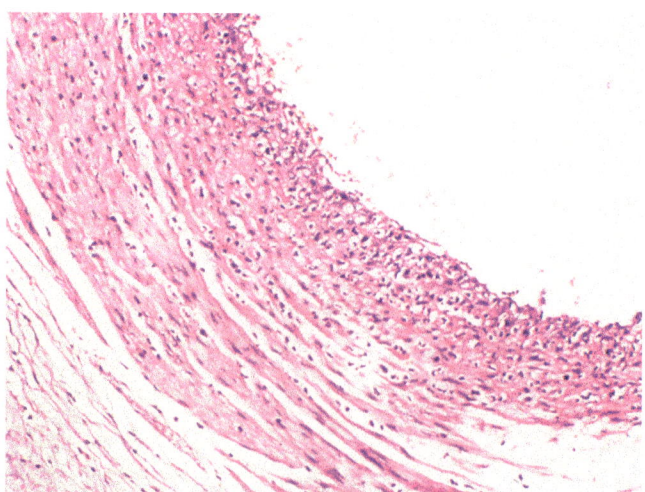

**Figure 18.15:** Fetal inflammatory response: Intramural PMN in umbilical artery

Table 18.4: Fetal inflammatory response

| Stage | Terminology |
|---|---|
| Early | With chorionic vasculitis or umbilical phlebitis |
| Intermediate | With umbilical vasculitis or umbilical panvasculitis (all vessels) |
| Late | Necrotizing funisitis or with concentric umbilical perivasculitis |

Grade 1 (mild to moderate): Scattered PMN infiltration in the umbilical vessels and chorionic tissue, Grade 2, there is confluent collection of PMN in chorion and umbilical vessels

### Clinical Impact

ACA is associated with various complications that include:
1. Spontaneous abortions,
2. Preterm birth,
3. Fetal death in utero, stillbirth,
4. Malformations,
5. Active infection,
6. Delayed sequelae: Chorioamnionitis may also lead to deafness and learning disabilities of the infant.

## Villitis

Chorionic villitis is characterized by chronic inflammatory cell infiltrates within the chorionic villi. The villitis may be due to infection or due to unknown etiology. Villitis due to infection is caused by usually viral infections that are transmitted from the mother to fetus.

### Pathology

The inflammatory infiltrate within the chorionic villi consists of lymphocytes, histiocytes, and plasma cells. Rarely, granulomatous inflammation may be noted. The inflammatory cells may be focal or diffuse in distribution. Necrosis and focal hemorrhage may also be seen. Depending on the severity of the inflammatory cells, the villitis is categorized from grade 1 to grade 4.[4]

Villitis of unknown etiology (VUE) constitutes the major component of villitis (more than 90%). The inflammatory cell infiltration is usually of mild degree and rarely the villitis may be severe. Morphologically, VUE is similar to that of villitis with specific etiology. Therefore, special stains should be done in all cases of villitis. Mild degree VUE is usually clinically silent and severe VUE may cause IUGR, mental impairment and cerebral palsy.

## Specific Infections

### Cytomegalovirus (CMV)

The CMV is a common infection and occurs in 0.2 to 2.5% of live birth. The infection is transmitted from mother to fetus in 20 to 50% of maternal infection by CMV. CMV infection of the fetus may have long standing side effects such as mental retardation, sensory hearing loss, blindness, learning disabilities, hydrocephaly and growth retardation.

**Pathology:** Histology section shows infiltration of plasma cells and histiocytes within the villi. Foci of hemorrhage and hemosiderin laden macrophages are also seen. The characteristic large eosinophilic intranuclear inclusion and small basophilic cytoplasmic inclusions are seen in the trophoblastic cells, Hofbauer cells and endothelial cells.

### Rubella

Currently, rubella infection is rare due to effective vaccination program. Rubella infection in the first trimester bears greatest risk for the fetus. The virus causes necrotizing villitis and vasculitis. Cord and membranes show mild chronic inflammation. The endothelial cells of blood vessels also show necrosis. The cytoplasm of these cells show eosinophilic inclusions.

### Herpes Simplex Virus

Herpes simplex virus (HSV) infection occurs mainly in the intrapartum by either ascending infection or by transplacental dissemination. Spontaneous abortion and congenital fetal malformation are more frequent in HSV infection. The virus causes necrosis of villous and also fibrinoid necrosis of blood vessels. HSV infection is also responsible for chorioamnionitis and funisitis. HSV inclusion may be demonstrated in amniotic cells.

### Toxoplasma

Toxoplasma infection mainly occurs due to primary infection from the mother at the time of pregnancy and almost half of the infected women transmit the infection to the fetus. The villi show lymphoplasmacytic infiltration, increased vascularity and increased Hofbauer cells. The inflammatory cells are seen in the decidua and umbilical vessels. The granulomatous inflammation with central necrosis and palisaded histiocytes are also seen within the chorionic villi. Toxoplasma cyst may be present in the subchorionic tissue, sub amniotic area or in umbilical cord. Usually, the cyst does not show any inflammation. However, the rupture cyst may show intense inflammatory reaction.

**Clinical significance:** Toxoplasma infection in the fetus is associated with hydrocephaly, hydrops, chorioretinitis, encephalitis and involvement of various other organs.

### Syphilis

Treponema pallidum infection may occur in any stage of gestational period. The infection is spread from the mother to fetus by hematogenous spread.

**Pathology:** The placenta is usually enlarged and overweight. The severity of the placental pathology largely depends on severity of the fetal infection. The chorionic villi are enlarged and immature. The endothelial cells of the fetal blood vessels show marked proliferation along with fibroblastic proliferation. There is infiltration of the plasma cells in the villi and decidua. In severe infection, abscess formation and necrosis of the villi are noted. Necrotizing funisitis may also be seen.

### Human Immunodeficiency Virus

Human immunodeficiency virus (HIV) infection causes chorioamnionitis, however no villitis is seen.

### Parvovirus B19

Parvovirus B19 infection is related with abortion in second trimester of pregnancy. The placenta is enlarged, edematous, pale and friable. The villi are relatively immature and edematous. The nucleated red blood cells of the villus blood show typical eosinophilic intranuclear inclusions. These infected cells look like Chinese lantern and so they are known as "lantern cells". In situ hybridization, immunohistochemistry, electron microscopy or PCR may be used as an additional help to detect such viral infected cells.

### Tuberculosis

Congenital infection of *Mycobacterium tuberculosis* may be seen occasionally. In this condition, the placenta may show white plaque. Microscopical examination shows typical epithelioid cell granulomas and necrosis (Figure 18.16). Ziehl-Neelsen stain may demonstrate the acid fast bacilli and confirm the diagnosis.

### Listeria

*Listeria monocytogenes* is an important cause of intrauterine infection. It is a gram positive rod like organism. *Listeria* infection in the placenta shows yellowish necrotic foci. The infection typically shows PMN infiltration within the villi and in the intervillous space. In addition, there may chorioamnionitis and funisitis.

### Others

Occasionally, placenta may show malarial pigment and trophozoites due to *plasmodium* infection (Figure 18.17 and 18.18). Rarely fungal infection may also be noted (Figure 18.19).

## CIRCULATORY DISORDERS OF PLACENTA: MATERNAL CIRCULATORY DISORDER

### Infarct

This is the area of ischemic necrosis of the placenta due to obstructed blood flow. Infraction is seen in 10 to 25%

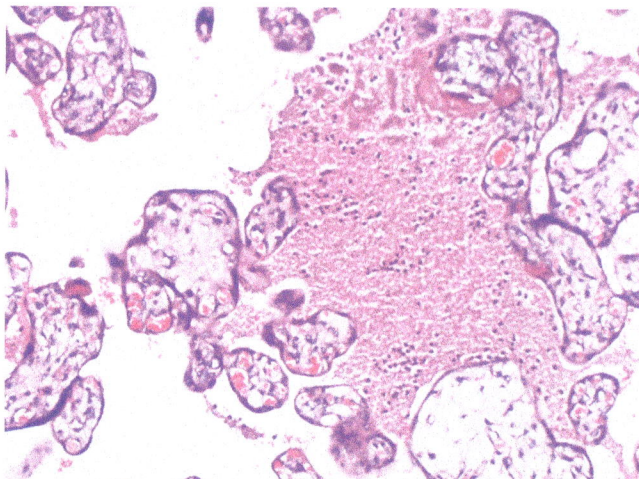
**Figure 18.16:** Placental tuberculosis: Necrosis and ill-formed granuloma in the villi

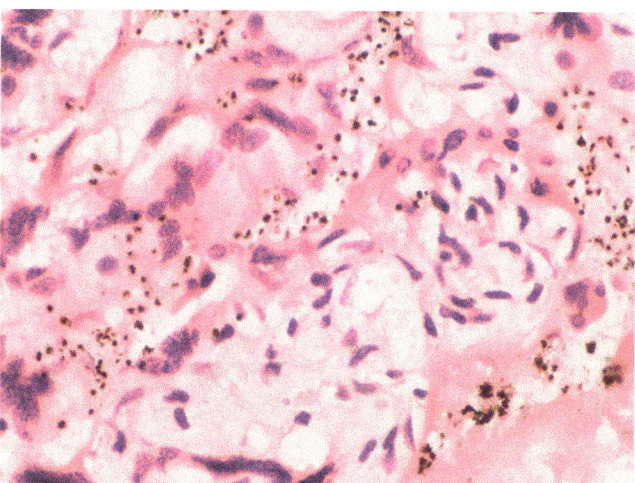
**Figure 18.17:** *Plasmodium* infection: Malarial pigment

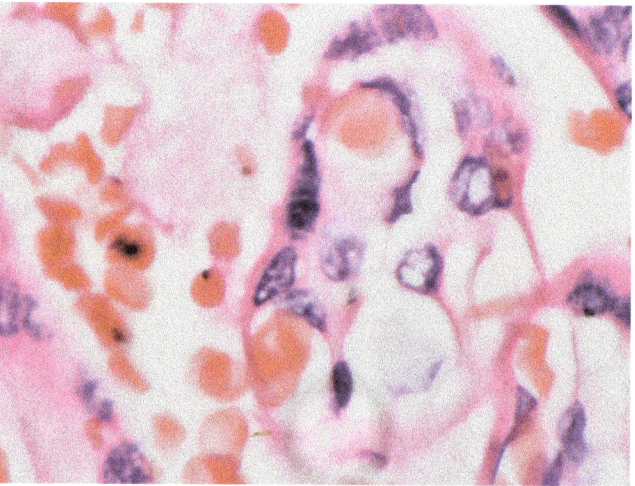
**Figure 18.18:** *Plasmodium* infection: Ring form of trophozoites of *Plasmodium vivax*

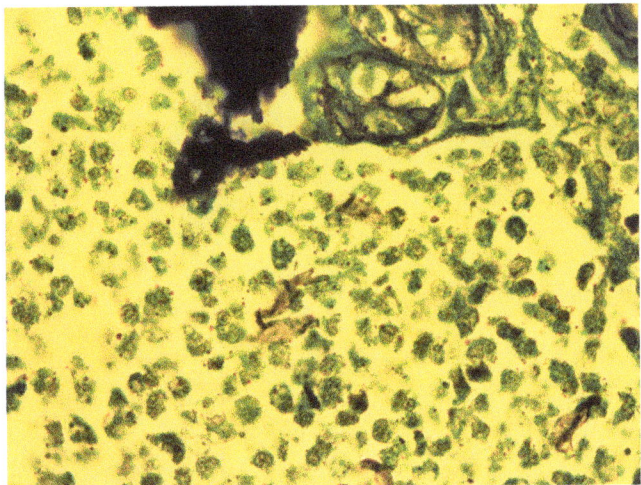

Figure 18.19: Mucormycosis in placenta: Broad fungal hyphae in the placenta (Grocot's stain)

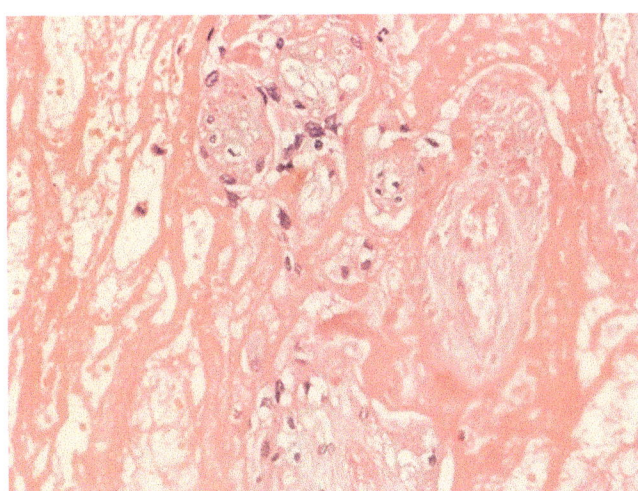

Figure 18.20: Necrosis: Only ghost-like margin of the villi

of termed placenta. The infraction is usually seen as small area in the periphery of the placenta. Infract is considered as significant if: (1) Multiple central location, (2) Larger than 3cm in diameter, (3) In first and second trimester of pregnancy.

*Pathology*

Infract is usually seen at the periphery of the placenta as wedge shaped area. Infracts are slightly different in color and mildly firm in consistency. On histology section the villi show necrosis and there is only ghost like outer margins are seen (Figure 18.20). The syncytiotrophoblast, blood vessels and stroma of the villi undergo necrosis. Later on the necrosed villi are replaced by fibrosis.

*Differential Diagnosis*

a. Perivillous fibrin deposition
b. Intervillous thrombohematoma: However, intervillous thrombohematoma does not contain any villi.

## Maternal Floor Infarct

Maternal floor infarct (MFI) is characterized by extensive fibrin deposition in the basal plate. The incidence of MFI is 0.09 to 0.5%.[5] In case of massive perivillous fibrin (MPF) deposition, the fibrin deposition is seen throughout the placenta rather than concentration in the basal plate region. Both MFI and MPF are similar in histology and they differ only in the distribution of fibrin deposition. They both share common pathophysiology.

*Etiology*

The exact etiology of MFI and MPF is unknown and various hypothesis have been proposed that include: (1) abnormal blood flow in the intervillious space, (2) cytotoxic effect of a pregnancy, related protein, (3) Final outcome of different insults to the placenta.[5]

*Pathology*

Grossly, the maternal surface of the placenta is thickened and firm with yellowish in appearance. Thick pale white material is extended on the surface to the interior of the placenta. Microscopically, the fibrinoid material is accumulated in the perivillous space (Figures 18.21 and 18.22). The entrapped chorionic villi loss the blood vessels and syncytiotrophoblast and become avascular leaving only the ghost outlines of the villi. These villi show extensive degeneration, however this is truly not an infraction. There are no strict criteria to the amount of area affected to qualify the term MFI. Fox et al. considered that at least 90% villi should be affected to label the case MFI.[4]

*Clinical Significance*

MFI is related with growth retardation, stillbirth and preterm delivery. The infants of MFI cases show increased incidence of central nervous system abnormalities.

## Marginal Hematoma

This hematoma occurs in the lateral margin of the placenta where the peripheral margins of the placenta join the fetal membrane.

*Etiology*

Marginal hematoma develops due to tear of the uteroplacental veins in the placentas that are situated in the lower part of the uterus.

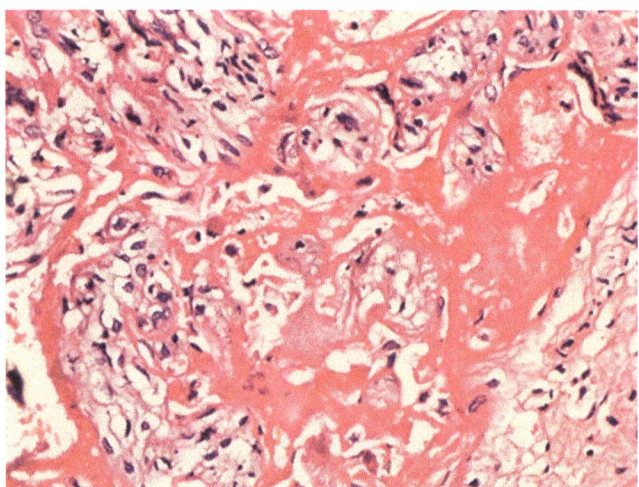

**Figure 18.21:** Maternal floor infract: Extensive fibrinoid material in the perivillous space

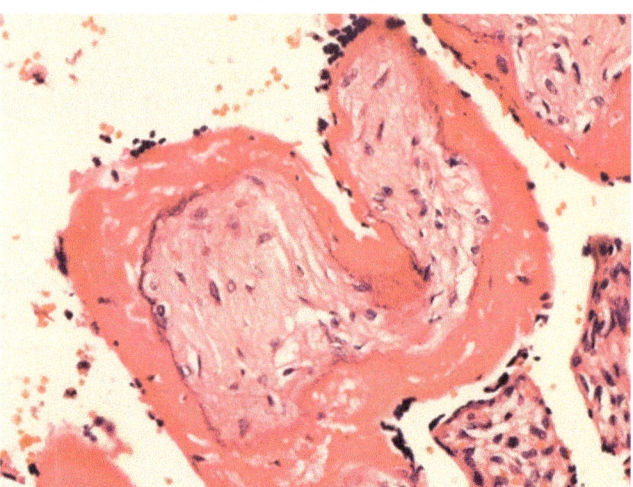

**Figure 18.22:** Maternal floor infract: Fibrinoid material is accumulated in the perivillous space

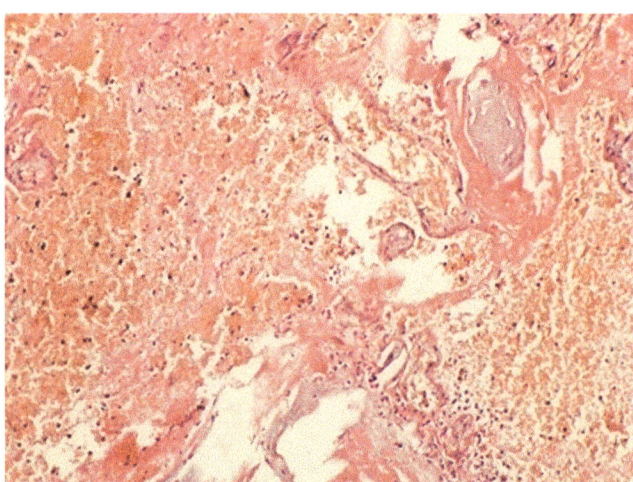

**Figure 18.23:** Retroplacental hematoma: Clot is located between basal plate of placenta and the myometrium

*Clinical Significance*

Marginal hematoma has usually no clinical significance.

*Pathology*

On gross examination, the placenta shows crescent-shaped clot at the peripheral margin. Microscopically, the clot is located outside the placental disk. In case of chronic marginal hematoma, there may be hemosiderin laden histiocytes around the clot.

### Retroplacental Hematoma

In case of retroplacental hematoma, the clot is located between basal plate of placenta and the myometrium (Figure 18.23). The incidence of retroplacental hematoma is near about 4.5% of the placenta.[4]

*Clinical Significance*

Clinical significance of retroplacental hematoma depends on the size, amount of infarction and the perfusion of placenta. Large clot may reduce the perfusion capacity of the placenta significantly and may cause abruption placenta, fetal hypoxia and even fetal death.

### Intervillous Hematoma

Intervillous hematoma is common and occurs in near about 48% of placenta. It is characterized by hematoma in the intervillous space due to bleeding. The intervillous hematoma is often associated with amniocentesis, injury or external torsion. Microscopically, the vessels show fibrin deposition and RBC. The peripheral villi adjacent to hematoma show infraction.

*Clinical Significance*

Small intervillous hematoma has little clinical significance. Large hematoma may cause fetal anemia and fetoplacental hydrops. Sudden severe hematoma may cause sudden death of the fetus.

### Fetal Vascular Thrombosis

Fetal vascular obstruction may occur due to obstruction at any level such as umbilical cord vessels, chorionic plate vessels or small vessels in villi. The clot is formed in the vessels and closes the fetal blood circulation. In case of fetal thrombotic vasculopathy (FTV), the stem vessels of villi undergo occlusion by thrombi.

*Etiology*

The etiological causes of thrombotic obstruction of the fetal vessels include:

a. Obstruction: The compression of the umbilical cord may cause thrombosis. The common causes of obstruction of the umbilical cord are long cord or hypercoiling.
b. Stasis: Vascular stasis occurs due to chorangioma or mesenchymal dysplasia.
c. Vascular wall injury: The damage of the vessel wall may be due to infection or irritation by meconium.

*Pathology*

The fresh thrombi show extravasation of RBCs and laminated fibrin layer. The endothelium of the vessel wall disappears followed by the muscle layer. Vessel wall shows calcification. The villi supplied by occluded vessels show karyorrhexis of the endothelial cells, and stromal cells of villi along with destruction of capillaries. The stroma shows increased mineralization. The overall process is known as villous stromal vascular karyorrhexis. The adjacent syncytiotrophoblast shows increased syncytial knots. In course of time the villus become fibrotic and hyalinized and is termed as fibrotic avascular villi.

*Clinical Significance*

It has been suggested that the term FTV should only be used if more than 15 chorionic villi are involved per slide.[6] FTV is related with increased risk of cerebral palsy, intrauterine fetal death and encephalopathy.

## Villous Edema

Villous edema is characterized by accumulation of fluid in the villous stroma. Villous edema is seen in infections by parvovirus B19, CMV, toxoplasmosis, and syphilis, etc., in Rh incompatibility and diabetes mellitus. Severe villous edema is seen in fetal hydrops. The exact etiology of villous edema is unknown. Possibly there is osmotic imbalance between the stroma and the maternal space. Fetal hypoproteinemia may be also the cause of villous edema. Villous edema is frequently seen in infant with neurologic impairment, cerebral palsy, premature delivery, neonatal hypoxia, and neonatal death.

## CHORANGIOSIS

Chorangiosis is characterized by hypervascular villi containing multiple capillaries. The diagnosis of chorangiosis can be done in examination of 10 X objective by following rule of 10. Ten or more terminal villi should contain ten or more capillaries in ten fields in 10 X objective examination in areas of non-ischemic placental tissue.[7] The prevalence of chorangioma is 5.5%.

## Pathogenesis

Chorangiosis is often associated with severe anemia of the mother, high altitude gestations, mothers who smoke, heart disease of the mother. This indicates that chorangiosis is an adaptive response to chronic hypoxia.

### Clinical Significance

Chorangiosis is associated with increased perinatal mortality. It is also more common in the infants having cerebral palsy or cord problems.

## PLACENTA IN MATERNAL AND FETAL DISORDERS

### Preeclampsia and Eclampsia

In case of preeclampsia, the placenta is usually small and occasional cases it may be large.

*Histopathology*

The placenta shows decidual vasculopathy, diminished growth of the villi, maldevelopment of the villi and infracts. Decidual vasculopathy is characterized by various changes in the decidual blood vessels including vasculitis, thrombosis, atherosis, fibrinoid necrosis and retention of the arteriolar smooth muscle. The cytotrophoblast shows proliferation. The villi become abnormally small with multiple syncytial knots.

### Essential Hypertension

Essential hypertension shows similar changes as that are seen in preeclampsia but in lesser extent and degree. The histopathology section shows thickening of the medial wall of the blood vessels and intimal hyperplasia resulting in narrowing of the lumen.

### Diabetes Mellitus

Diabetes mellitus shows large bulky heavy placenta. The chorionic villi are immature and edematous. The villi show marked capillary and cytotrophoblast proliferation. Basement membrane of the vessels show thickening and the decidual vessels show medial hypertrophy and fibrinoid necrosis.

### Sickle Cell Disease/Trait and other Hemoglobinopathies

Placenta is a good detector of sickle cells as the maternal RBCs show sickling in case of maternal sickle cell trait disease. Placenta in sickle cell disease is usually small due to repeated infraction. Sickle cell disease of mother shows increased fetal morbidity, mortality, intrauterine growth retardation and premature delivery.

### Rh Incompatibility

The destruction of fetal RBCs by maternal antibody is responsible for the development of hydrops fetalis that can also be labeled as erythroblastosis fetalis or immune hydrops. In most of the times, the maternal blood is sensitized by the fetal blood and Rh negative mother develops antibody against Rh antigen of the RBC of the fetus. The antibody against ABO blood group and Kell has also been noted rarely. The antibody passes through the placental barrier and destroys the fetal RBCs resulting in anemia of the fetus. The severity of the anemia depends on the severity of the condition. Due to chronic destruction of the RBCs, the fetus tries to compensate by releasing immature precursors of RBCs. Therefore, large numbers of nucleated RBCs come to the fetal circulation. Due to anemia, the heart undergoes more stress and develops congestive cardiac failure. In severe cases, the fetus shows severe anemia, ascites and generalized edema and ultimately develops hydrops fetalis.

*Pathology*

The placenta also develops placental hydrops and is characterized by large, pale bulky and edematous placenta. The histopathological features of placenta are nonspecific and the features are mainly due to severe hemolytic anemia and cardiac failure. The villi are large, immature and contain less number of capillaries. The vessels show large number of nucleated RBCs. Stroma of the villi shows edema and increased number of Hofbauer cells.

*Clinical Significance*

Hydrops fetalis can be diagnosed intranatally by radiological investigations and therefore should be treated by intranatal blood transfusion.

## PATHOLOGY OF MEMBRANES

### Squamous Metaplasia

This appears as multiple foci of mildly elevated pearly white macules with tiny to large plaques. On histology, the lesion shows squamous metaplastic cells. The lesions do not carry any clinical significance.

### Amnion Nodosum

Amnion nodosum is characterized by multiple small yellowish granular lesions on the amniotic surface. It is commonly associated with oligohydramnios and is also noted in prolonged rupture of the membrane or fetus with renal agenesis.

*Pathogenesis*

Amniotic membrane gets nutrition from the amniotic fluid and therefore in oligohydramnios the amniotic membrane does not get proper nutrition and dies. The vernix is deposited on the dead amniotic epithelium and forms small nodular lesion. The amniotic nodosum develops in the late fetal life because of insufficient vernix in the early fetal life.

*Histopathology*

Microscopically, the lesion shows acellular eosinophilic material, squames and hairs. Unlike squamous metaplasia the surface of the amniotic nodosum does not contain any metaplastic squamous cells.

### Amniotic Bands

The separation of amniotic membrane from the chorion causes small fragmented band like amniotic membrane. The membrane may entangle the fetal parts and prevents normal sequence of development of the fetal parts. The amniotic bands may encircle the fetal digits, limbs, neck or umbilical cord resulting in constriction or amputation of the fetal parts. Early formation of band causes multisystem defects. The later development of band causes amputation of the limbs or digits.

## NON-TROPHOBLASTIC TUMORS

### Hemangioma (Chorangioma)

Chorangioma is a benign vascular neoplasm and is characterized by the proliferation of capillaries within the villi, predominantly stem villi. The incidence of chorangioma is 0.1 to 1%. Chorangioma may be hamartomatous rather than a neoplastic one.

*Pathology*

The chorangiomas are usually well defined solitary nodule located more in the periphery of the placenta. They may be dark red like blood clot and also may be whitish firm area resembling infract. Microscopical examination shows numerous blood vessels within the villi with scanty connective tissue (Figure 18.24). The tumor may show necrosis, calcification and hyalinization. Chorangiomas are surrounded by proliferating trophoblasts.

*Clinical Significance*

Chorangiomas are related with fetal hydrops, intrauterine growth retardation, premature delivery, preeclampsia, still birth and heart diseases.

The other rare tumors of placenta include cholangio-carcinoma, leiomyoma, endometrial stromal sarcomas, teratoma and metastatic carcinoma.

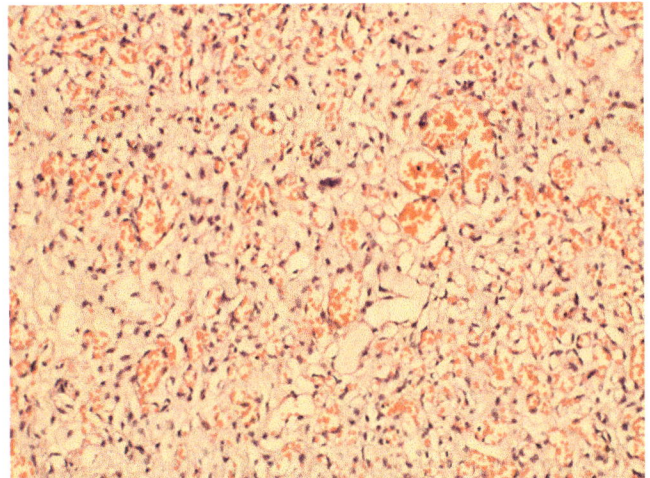

Figure 18.24: Chorangioma: Numerous blood vessels within the villi with scanty connective tissue

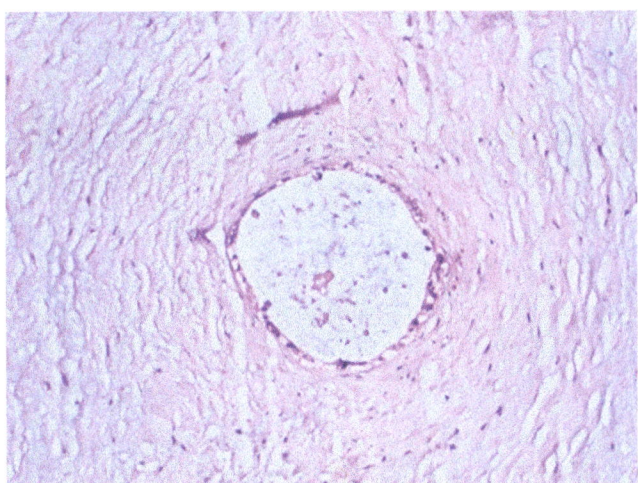

Figure 18.25: Allantoic duct: The duct in the umbilical cord lined by cuboidal epithelium

## UMBILICAL CORD PATHOLOGY

### Vestigial Remnants

*Omphalomesenteric Duct*

The persistence of the connection between the fetal ileum and the yolk sac gives rise to the formation of the omphalomesenteric duct. This duct is more frequent in the fetal end of the umbilical cord. Histologically, the duct is lined by columnar cells resembling intestinal epithelial cells. Occasionally, ganglion cells, pancreatic and hepatocytes are seen on the wall of the duct. Omphalomesenteric duct has no clinical significance.

*Allantoic Duct (Figure 18.25)*

The presence of allantoic duct is seen in 15% of the placenta. The presence of allantoic duct does not carry any clinical significance. The duct is more common in fetal side of the umbilical cord. The duct is present in between two umbilical arteries. The lining epithelium of the duct is transitional epithelial cells.

*Insertion of Umbilical Cord*

The following abnormalities are seen regarding abnormal insertion of placenta:

*Marginal (7%)*

The umbilical cord is inserted at the edge of the placenta. This condition is more common in twin pregnancies.

*Velamentous Insertion (1%)*

The umbilical cord is inserted into the membrane of the placenta. This type of insertion is more frequent in multiple pregnancies, single umbilical artery and higher maternal age.

**Clinical significance:** The blood vessels in the membrane in the velamentous insertion are prone to injury. Thrombosis is frequently seen in the velamentous insertion as the distensible vessels are prone to get compressed. Similarly, these vessels may undergo hemorrhage due to rupture of the wall. Severe fetal distress may occur due to hemorrhage and loss of blood during delivery.

### Cord Length

The normal umbilical cord is 55 cm long.

*Long Cord (4%)*

If the umbilical cord is more than 80 cm long then it is considered as long cord.[8]

**Clinical significance:** The long cord is associated with thrombotic vasculopathy due to vascular stasis, intrauterine growth retardation and fetal death.

*Short Cord (1%)*

Less than 35 cm long umbilical cord. Short cord is frequently associated with fetal distress, asphyxia, cord hemorrhage, cord hematoma, abruption, and uterine inversion.

*Thin Cord*

The average diameter of the cord is 1.2 to 2 cm.[9] Thin cord is associated with intrauterine fetal growth restriction.

### Torsion

Normally, the umbilical cord is coiled in a counterclockwise direction and average coil per cm is 0.2. More than 0.3 coil/cm of cord length is considered as hypercoiled umbilical cord. The incidence of hypercoiled umbilical cord is 10%. The hypercoiled umbilical cord is often associated with stasis of blood circulation and increased fetal death. The incidence of hypocoiled umbilical cord is 7.5%. The coiling of the umbilical cord is related with fetal activity. Therefore, hypocoiled umbilical cord is more often seen restricted fetal movement due to fetal malformation or anomalous uterus.

## Umbilical Knots

a. True knots (0.4%): The true knots are commonly associated with long umbilical cord, excessive amniotic fluid, multigravida and monoamniotic twins.

   Long standing true knot causes grooving of the umbilical cord. Wharton's jelly is lost at the site of true knot. True knots cause vascular stasis and increased thrombosis of the blood vessels. The knot becomes more tightened during the labor. This may cause fetal asphyxia and death. Intrauterine mortality rate in case of true knot is 10%.

b. False knots: False knots are characterized by focal accumulation of Wharton's jelly and focal excessive blood vessels. The false knot has no clinical significance.

## Single Umbilical Artery

The presence of single umbilical artery (SUA) in the umbilical cord is the most frequent congenital abnormality and its incidence rate is 2.5%. The presence of SUA should be judged a few cm (at least 3.5 cm) away from the placental insertion because the arteries may be fused together before the insertion.

### Etiology

SUA may be either aplasia of the umbilical artery or due to atrophy of the artery. Atrophy of one umbilical artery may be the more common cause of SUA.

### Pathology

The cross section of the umbilical cord does not show one umbilical artery. Occasionally remnants of the atrophic other artery may be present.

### Clinical Significance

SUA is frequently associated with antepartum bleeding, maternal diabetes, oligohydramnios and IUGR. Fetal malformation is also more common in SUA.

## REFERENCES

1. Redline RW, O' Riordan MA. Placental lesions associated with cerebral palsy and neurologic impairment following term birth. Arch Pathol Lab Med. 2000;124:1785-91.
2. ACOG Committee on Obstetric Practice. ACOG Committee opinion. Number 266, January 2002: placenta accreta. Obstet Gynecol. 2002;99(1):169-70.
3. Redline RW, Faye-Petersen O, et al. Amniotic infection syndrome: nosology and reproducibility of placental reaction patterns. Pediatr Dev Pathol. 2003;6:435-48.
4. Fox H, Sebire NJ. Pathology of the placenta, 3rd edn. 2007; Saunders, Philadelphia.
5. Naeye RL. Maternal floor infarction. Hum Pathol. 1985; 16:823-8.
6. Redline RW, Ariel IB, et al. Fetal vascular obstructive lesions: Nosology and reproducibility of placental reaction patterns. Pediatr Devel Pathol. 2004;7:443-52.
7. Altshuler G. Chorangiosis. An important placental sign of neonatal morbidity and mortality. Arch Pathol Lab Med. 1984;108:71-4.
8. Berg TG, Rayburn WF. Umbilical cord length and acid-base balance at delivery. J Reprod Med. 1995;40:1-12.
9. Silver RK, Dooley SL, et al. Umbilical cord size and amniotic fluid volume in prolonged pregnancy. Am J Obstet Gynecol. 1987;157:716-20.

# Gestational Trophoblastic Disease

Gestational trophoblastic disease (GTD) is a group of diseases with variable morphology, etiopathogenesis and prognosis. GTD develops from trophoblasts or extravillous trophoblasts related with pregnancy. World Health Organization (WHO) classifies this tumor into benign group and malignant group (Box 19.1). The benign group is comprised of hydatidiform mole, exaggerated placental site trophoblastic lesion and placental site nodule. The malignant group comprised of gestational choriocarcinoma and placental site trophoblastic tumor (PSTT).[1]

**Box 19.1:** Classification of trophoblastic disease

**Mole**
- Hydatidiform mole:
  - Complete
  - Partial
- Invasive mole

**Trophoblastic tumor**
- Placental site trophoblastic tumor
- Choriocarcinoma
- Epithelioid trophoblastic tumor

## HYDATIDIFORM MOLE

The complete hydatidiform mole (HM) has normal karyotyping (46XX). It develops from ovum with empty nucleus. In 85 to 95% cases the fertilization of the empty ovum is done by a haploid sperm (23X). In small number of cases (4–15%) the blighted ovum is fertilized by two sperm (23X). In case of partial mole the karyotyping is triploidy (69XXY, 69XXX or 69XYY). Here the ovum is fertilized by two haploid sperms. The incidence of hydatidiform mole varies widely. In North America the occurance of hydatidiform mole is 100 per 100000 pregnancies. The incidence rate is 10 times higher in Middle East and Asia.[2]

## Clinical Features

### Complete Hydatidiform Mole

More than 50% of the molar pregnancies are complete hydatidiform mole (CHM). The disease occurs more frequently before 20 years and after 40 years of age. The patients usually present in the 11th to 25th week of gestation. They commonly complain of vaginal bleeding, and occasionally passage of vesicles. The fetal heartbeat is missing. The patient has inappropriate enlargement of uterus related to gestational age. The urine and serum β hCG level is markedly increased. Ultrasound examination of uterus show typical snowstorm appearance. Nowadays HM is detected much earlier due to the routine use of ultrasound examination during pregnancy. Therefore, the signs and symptoms of HM may not be present and the patient may have only missed period. Preeclampsia occurs in 10–25% of CHM.

### Partial Hydatidiform Mole

The symptoms of partial hydatidiform mole (PHM) is almost similar to that of CHM. The patients also complain of vaginal bleeding at the end of first trimester. The uterus may be normal in size or shrunken relative to the age of gestation. The serum or urinary β hCG level may be normal or low. The toxemia of pregnancy may occur in PHM (42%), however it is usually seen in the later part of gestation.

## Gross

In case of CHM, multiple 1–2 cm diameter, transparent grape-like vesicles are seen. The vesicles replace the normal placenta and therefore no gestational sac, umbilical cord or fetus is identified.

In PHM, the amount of tissue is lesser in volume. Both grape-like vesicles and nonmolar placental tissue is seen. Fetus may also be identified in PHM.

## Histopathology

### Complete Hydatidiform Mole (Figures 19.1 to 19.4)

In cases of CHM the villi are dilated with cistern-like formation. The villous stroma becomes edematous and may contain the primitive thin walled vascular spaces. Fetal blood cells are typically absent in the villi. There is circumferential disorderly proliferation of cyto and syncytiotrophoblast over the surface of the villi. The proliferating trophoblasts may show nuclear atypia and high mitotic activity. Marked cytological atypia is also seen in the implantation site. Due to the early detection and evacuation of CHM, the above mentioned changes may not be evident in CHM. The CHM may show only subtle changes in early gestational period and is designated as "early complete mole". The characteristic features of complete mole include:[3]

1. Redundant polypoid club shaped terminal villi.
2. The villous stroma is hypercellular and contains stellate shaped cells.
3. Fluid filled canaliculi of the villous stroma form a labyrinthine network.
4. Cytotrophoblast and syncytiotrophoblast show focal hyperplasia on both villi and also under surface of the chorionic plate.
5. The trophoblastic cells in the implantation site are enlarged and hyperchromatic.

### Partial Hydatidiform Mole

Partial hydatidiform mole shows admixture of two types of chorionic villi:
1. Enlarged dilated villi.
2. Small villi with central fibrosis.

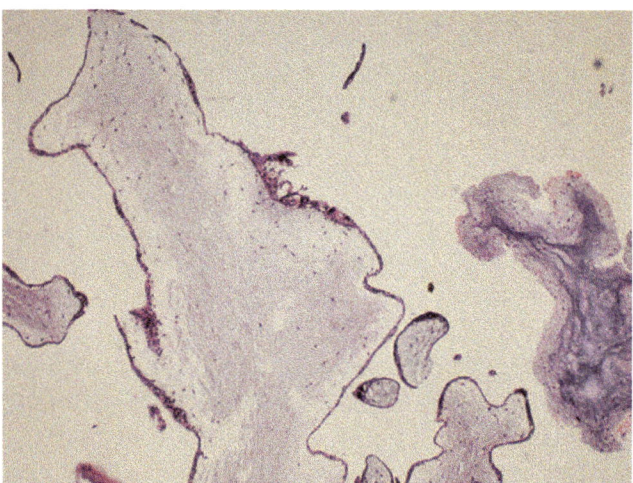

Figure 19.1: Hydatidiform mole: Large cystically dilated villous

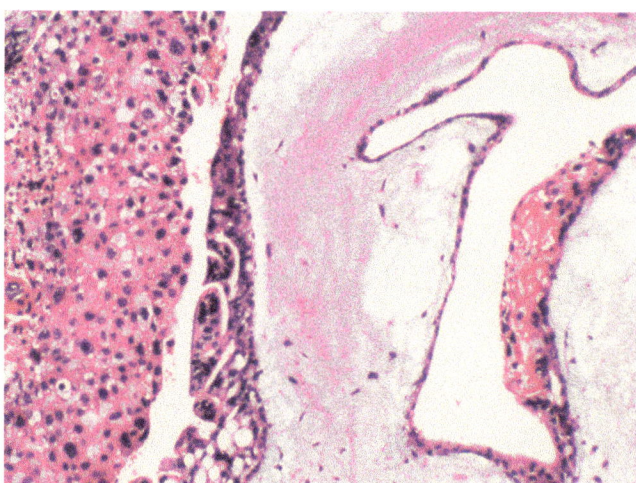

Figure 19.3: Hydatidiform mole: Marked trophoblastic proliferation

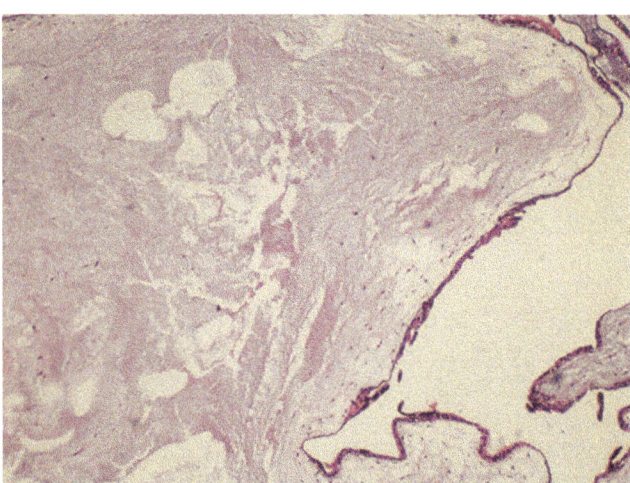

Figure 19.2: Hydatidiform mole: Villous with central degeneration

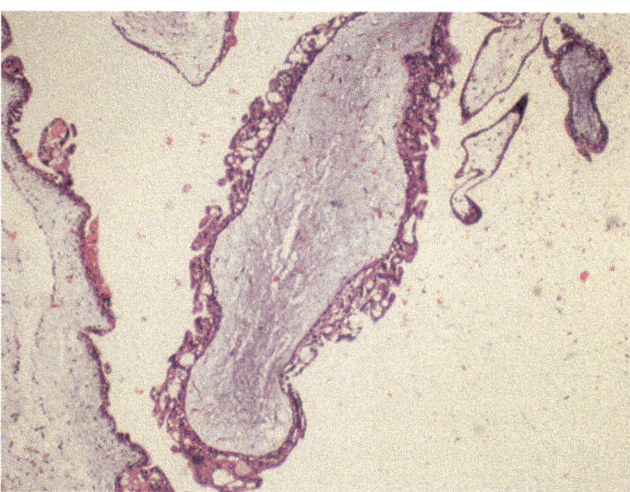

Figure 19.4: Hydatidiform mole: Circumferential trophoblastic proliferation

There are many enlarged cistern-like dilated villi. The stroma of the villi is acellular. The outer margin of the villi is scalloped with frequent invagination of the trophoblastic cells within the stroma. The cell proliferation is less marked in PHM. Stroma of the villi may often show fetal blood cells. There may be evidences of fetal development by the presence of fetal tissue, amnion or chorionic tissue in the section. The presence of fetal tissue should always raise the suspicion of PHM.

### Differential Diagnosis

a. **Hydropic abortus**: The villi in case of missed abortion may often show cistern formation and hydropic changes. However, the trophoblastic proliferation in such case is minimal to absent.
b. **Partial mole versus complete mole**: At times there may be difficulties in differentiating CHM versus PHM. However, PHM shows less proliferation of the trophoblastic cells, typical scalloped margin and presence of fetal parts[4] (Table 19.1).
c. **Choriocarcinoma**: Marked atypia in CHM without any evidence of villi may be confused with choriocarcinoma. However through sampling may help to detect villi. Destructive growth pattern is also absent in CHM.

Table 19.1: Complete versus partial mole

| Features | Complete hydatidiform mole | Partial hydatidiform mole |
| --- | --- | --- |
| Genetics | 46XX, 46 XY | 69 XXY, 69 XXX, 69 XYY |
| hCG level in serum and urine | High | Normal to low |
| Fetal parts in USG | Absent | Present |
| Types of villi | Only abnormal dilated villi | Both dilated and small sclerosed villi |
| Margin of villi | Regular, no trophoblastic invagination | Scalloped with frequent trophoblastic invagination |
| Trophoblastic proliferation | Relatively more and circumferential | Less and focal |
| Fetal parts | No evidence | Chorionic plate, amnion, cord and fetus |
| Chances of persistent GTD | More: One-fourth cases | Less: Less than 0.5–4% |

### Prognosis and Treatment

The occurrence of persistent gestational trophoblastic disease is the commonest complication of CHM. Persistent gestational trophoblastic disease is characterized by persistent elevation of β hCG level after evacuation of HM with or without any presence of extrauterine trophoblastic disease. Persistent gestational trophoblastic disease may occur in 20% cases of CHM and only rarely is seen in PHM (0.5 to 4%).[5,6] Histological representations of persistent gestational trophoblastic disease include persistent mole, invasive mole, and choriocarcinoma.

Complete evacuation of the mole is the treatment of choice in both CHM and PHM. The patient should be followed up by estimating serial β hCG level for one year until the level becomes completely normal. The level of β hCG level falls quickly after evacuation and usually becomes normal within 2–24 weeks. A chest radiograph should also be done before and after management to exclude any evidence of metastasis. In case of persistent gestational trophoblastic disease chemotherapy should be administered.

## INVASIVE HYDATIDIFORM MOLE

Invasive hydatidiform mole is characterized by the invasion of hydatidiform mole within the myometrium and/or blood vessels. Invasive mole is commonly seen as a sequel of either CHM or PHM. The uterus shows hemorrhagic and infiltrative lesion. Microscopically, there is infiltration of the hydatidiform villi along with trophoblastic proliferation within the myometrial wall. The villi are usually smaller in size than that of noninvasive HM. Occasionally, the villi may be seen in the extrauterine sites.

### Differential Diagnosis

The presence of chorionic villi is mandatory to exclude the possibility of choriocarcinoma on curetting. This may not be always possible in scanty curetting. A repeat endometrial curetting may be helpful in difficult situation. In case of difficulty the lesion should be designated as persistent gestational trophoblastic disease only.

### Prognosis and Treatment

The most common cause of persistent gestational trophoblastic disease is invasive mole. The prognosis of such patients is good and the patients survive even after distant metastasis. Chemotherapy is the treatment of choice of invasive mole.

## CHORIOCARCINOMA

Choriocarcinoma is an aggressive malignant tumor of trophoblastic cells. The incidence of choriocarcinoma is 1 in 160,000 pregnancies.[7] Gestational choriocarcinoma is noted after subsequent history of CHM (50%), abortion (25%), normal pregnancy (22.5%) and rarely after ectopic gestation (2.5%).[7]

### Clinical Feature

The patient commonly presents with abnormal vaginal bleeding. Occasionally, the patients may present first time with clinical feature of metastasis such as hemoptysis in lung secondary.

## Gross (Figures 19.5 and 19.6)

The uterus shows darkly reddish friable mass with areas of hemorrhage and necrosis. The mass may be soft and tan grayish color with less hemorrhagic. The size of the tumor may be small to large necrotic growth.

## Histopathology (Figures 19.7 to 19.12)

Choriocarcinoma shows characteristic bilaminar and dimorphic growth pattern. The tumor shows complete absence of any chronic villi. The tumor cells consist of mononuclear cytotrophoblast, intermediate trophoblast, and multinucleated syncytiotrophoblast. The small nests of central group of cytotrophoblasts are encircled by syncytiotrophoblast. The tumor does not show any intrinsic blood vessels and therefore it shows large areas of hemorrhage and necrosis. The tumor cells get nutrition from the invading blood vessels. Only peripheral thin rim of viable cells are present in choriocarcinoma. Extensive sampling of the tumor may be required to demonstrate the classical dimorphic pattern of the tumor.

## Immunohistochemistry

Syncytiotrophoblast of choriocarcinoma are strongly positive for β hCG and weakly positive for hPL. The tumor cells are also positive for CK18.

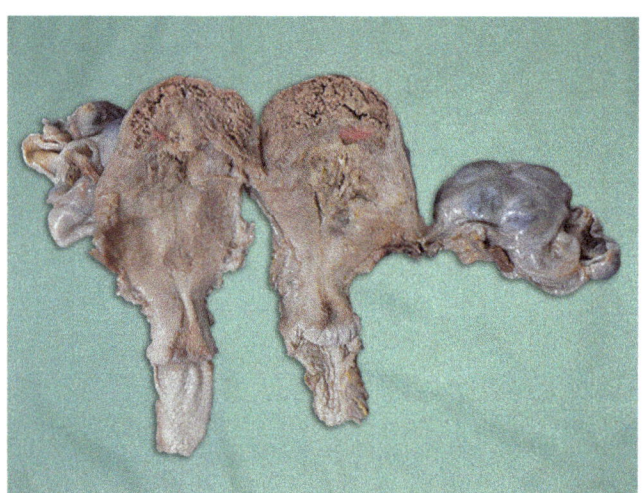

Figure 19.5: Choriocarcinoma: Hemorrhagic and necrotic mass in the fundus of uterus (Provided by Professor Uma Nahar Saikia)

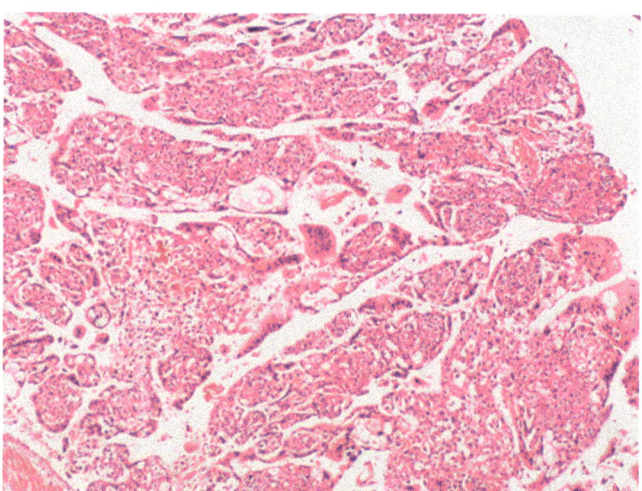

Figure 19.7: Choriocarcinoma: Nests of tumor cells consisting of both cyto and syncytiotrophoblast

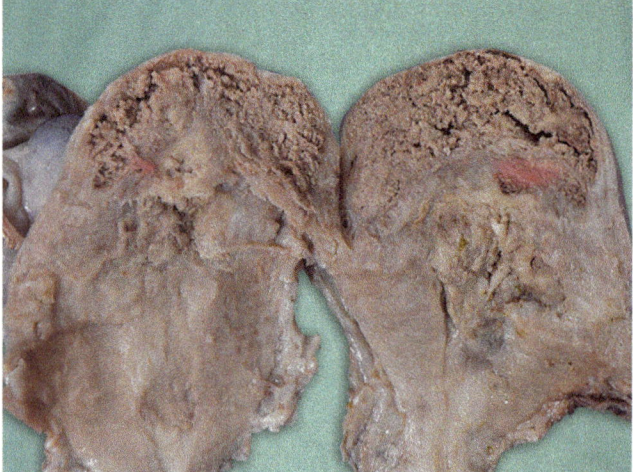

Figure 19.6: Choriocarcinoma: Close-up view of the mass

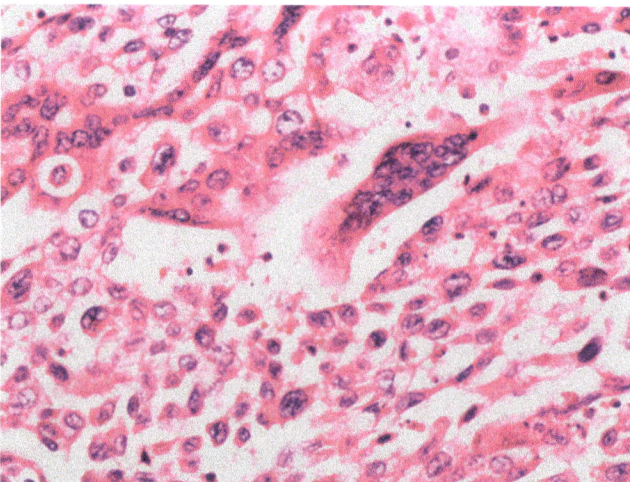

Figure 19.8: Choriocarcinoma: Characteristic bilaminar and dimorphic growth pattern. Both cyto and syncytiotrophoblast are seen

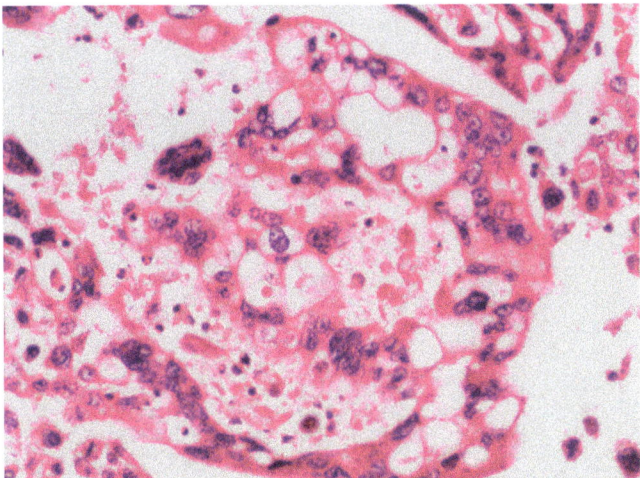

Figure 19.9: Choriocarcinoma: Cytotrophoblasts and scattered syncytiotrophoblast

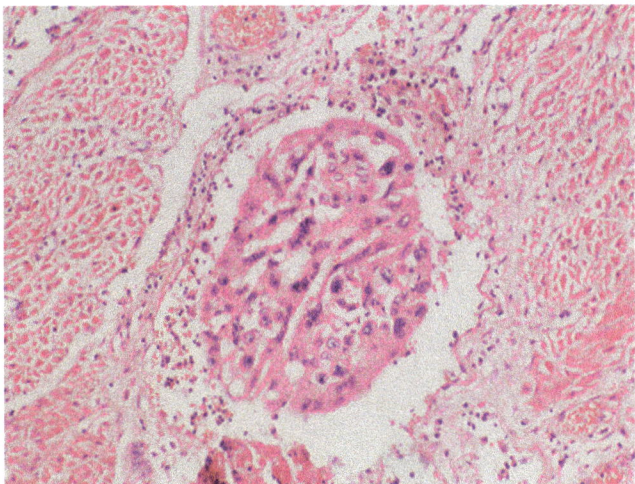

Figure 19.11: Choriocarcinoma: Vascular infiltration of the malignant cells

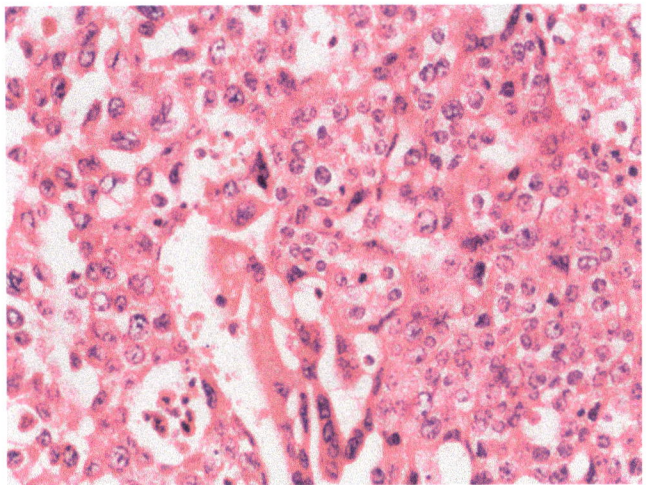

Figure 19.10: Choriocarcinoma: Round to oval cytotrophoblasts in sheet

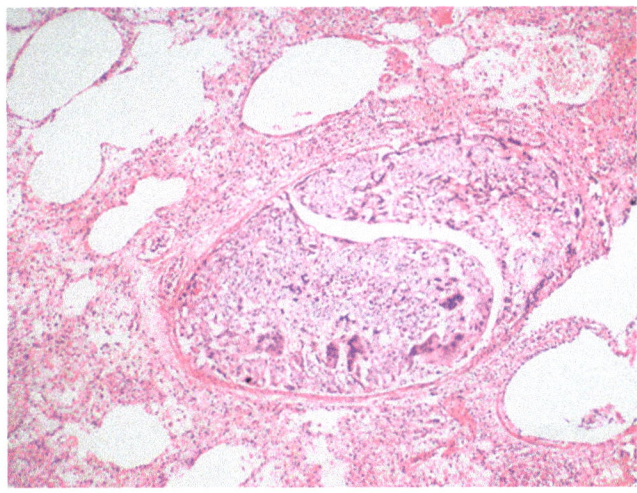

Figure 19.12: Choriocarcinoma: Lung emboli is seen in an autopsy section (Provided by Professor Uma Nahar Saikia)

## Differential Diagnosis

a. **Early normal pregnancy:** In case of early gestation there may not be any chorionic villi and the curetting may show only trophoblastic cells. However, lack of significant nuclear atypia of the trophoblastic cells and serial β hCG estimation help in the diagnosis of normal pregnancy.
b. **Poorly differentiated carcinoma:** In metastatic sites, choriocarcinoma may show only scanty syncytiotrophoblast and predominant cytotrophoblasts. In such cases differentiation from poorly differentiated carcinoma and choriocarcinoma may be problematic. In such case, β hCG level in serum or immunohistochemistry of β hCG may resolve the issue.
c. **Placental site trophoblastic tumor (PSTT):** Choriocarcinoma should be distinguished from PSTT. The following features favor the diagnosis of PSTT: (1) Monomorphic or single cell population, (2) Confluent sheets of cells with peripheral invasion, (3) Typical vascular invasion by tumor cells from the wall to lumen, (4) Relatively low β hCG level in serum, (5) Positive human placental lactogen (hPL).

## Prognosis and Therapy

Choriocarcinoma is a highly malignant tumor with frequent vascular invasion and distant metastasis. The common sites of metastasis are lung, liver and brain. The combination chemotherapy consisting of etoposide, methotrexate, actinomycin D, cyclophosphamide, and vincristine helps to achieve complete cure from this malignancy and 100% survival rate.[8]

## PLACENTAL SITE TROPHOBLASTIC TUMOR

Placental site trophoblastic tumor (PSTT) is an uncommon trophoblastic tumor that represents less than 3% of all gestational trophoblastic disease (GTD).[9] PSTT is mainly composed of intermediate trophoblasts originated from the placental site. The tumor mainly occurs after a normal pregnancy. However, it may also be seen after spontaneous abortion, or ectopic or molar pregnancy.

### Clinical Features

The mean age of the patient is 30 years. The patient typically presents with vaginal bleeding and amenorrhea. The uterus is mildly enlarged. The serum β hCG level of the patient is mildly elevated. Therefore, the presence of amenorrhea, mildly enlarged uterus and elevated serum β hCG level may wrongly be misinterpreted as normal pregnancy. The tumor mainly occurs after a normal pregnancy. However, it may also be seen after spontaneous abortion, termination of pregnancy, ectopic or molar pregnancy. A long latent period (even after 10 years) may occur from the development of PSST after normal pregnancy.

### Gross

Placental site trophoblastic tumor is a well-circumscribed solid lesion that often projects as polypoidal mass in the lumen of uterus (Figure 19.13). Occasionally, the tumor may be totally within the myometrium. The mean diameter of the tumor is 5 cm. The cut section of PSTT is soft tan with areas of hemorrhage and necrosis.

### Histopathology (Figures 19.14 to 19.19)

The tumor shows sheet or nests of single population of intermediate trophoblastic cells. Unlike dimorphic population

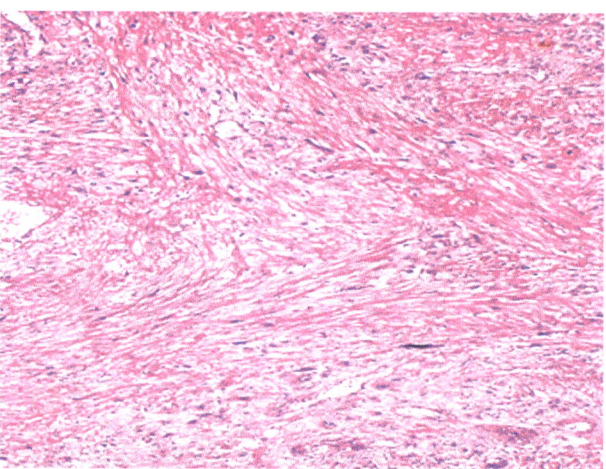

Figure 19.14: Placental site trophoblastic tumor: Infiltrating single population of intermediate trophoblastic cells

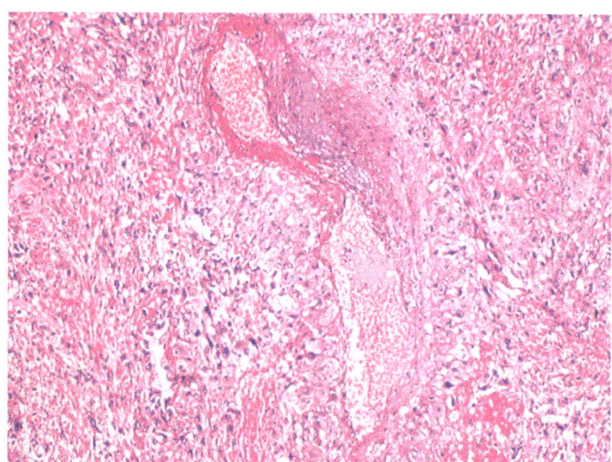

Figure 19.15: Placental site trophoblastic tumor: The trophoblastic cells around the blood vessels

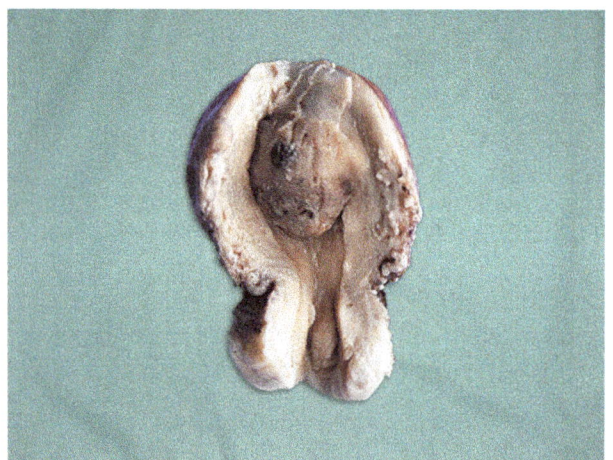

Figure 19.13: Placental site trophoblastic tumor: Polypoidal mass projecting in the lumen of uterus

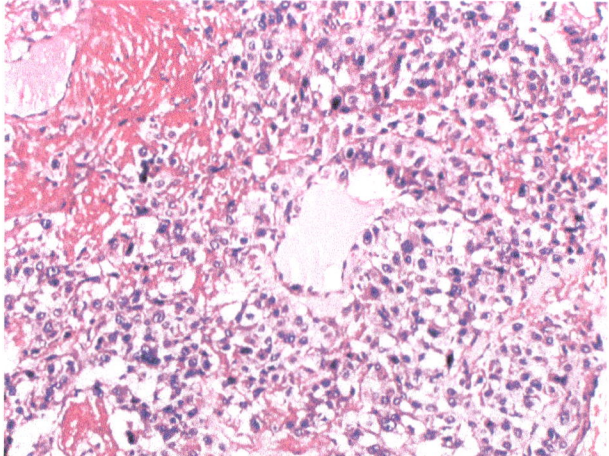

Figure 19.16: Placental site trophoblastic tumor: The individual intermediate cytotrophoblasts are large polygonal cells with abundant clear or eosinophilic cytoplasm

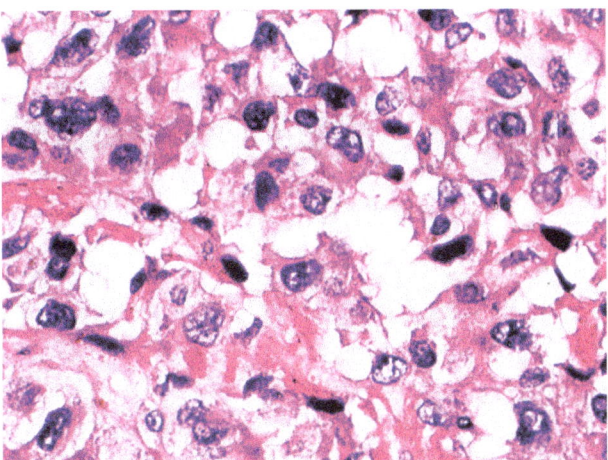

**Figure 19.17:** Placental site trophoblastic tumor: Moderate nuclear atypia in the tumor cells

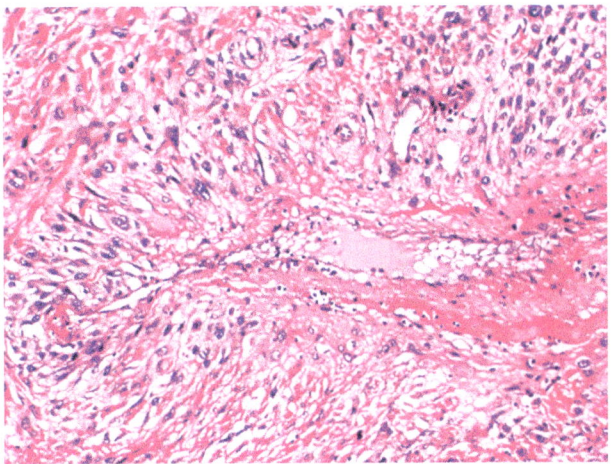

**Figure 19.18:** Placental site trophoblastic tumor: Fibrinoid necrosis in vessel wall and the tumor cells form lining of the vessel wall

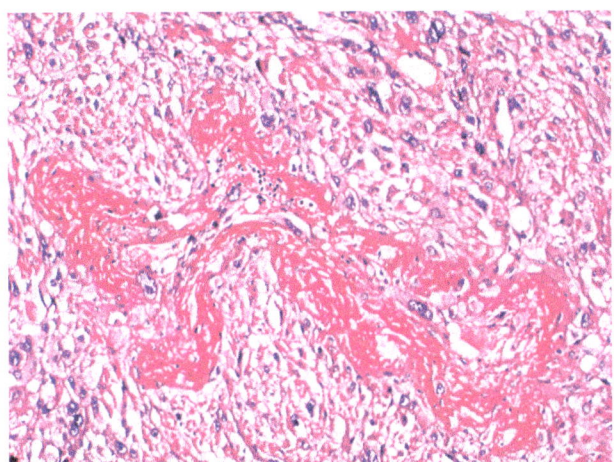

**Figure 19.19:** Placental site trophoblastic tumor: Fibrinoid necrosis in vessel wall

in choriocarcinoma, the cases of PSTT show monomorphic cell population. The individual intermediate cytotrophoblasts are large polygonal cells with abundant eosinophilic cytoplasm. The nuclei may be bland monotonous or may show moderate pleomorphism and hyperchromasia. The mitotic activity of the cells may be low to very high (30/10 HPFs).[10] PSTT characteristically presents unique vascular invasion. The wall of the blood vessels are infiltrated and replaced by the trophoblastic cells along with deposition of fibrinoid material. Occasionally, the tumor shows spindle shaped cells adjacent to the myometrium. The tumor often infiltrates the endomyometrium and may also show significant necrosis. In general, the tumor does not show any chorionic villi.

### Immunohistochemistry

The tumor is positive for hPL, CD146, CD10, and Mucin-4.[11] Less than 10% of tumor cells in PSTT are positive for hCG.[12]

### Differential Diagnosis

a. **Choriocarcinoma/gestational trophoblastic neoplasm (GTN):** Choriocarcinoma should always be distinguished from PSTT. The types of cell, pattern of growth and immunocytochemistry are helpful features to distinguish these two entities (Table 19.2).
b. **Exaggerated placental site reaction:** PSTT should be distinguished from exaggerated placental site trophoblastic reaction as both of them shared some common morphological similarities such as marked proliferation of intermediate trophoblastic cells and identical immunohistochemistry (Table 19.4). However, the following features favor the diagnosis of PSTT: (1) Mass-like lesion, (2) Destructive infiltrating pattern, (3) High mitosis, (4) Ki-67 index of PSTT is usually more than 10. However, this index is almost nil in exaggerated placental site trophoblastic reaction. (5) Relative lack of multinucleated giant cells in PSTT. (6) Lack of chorionic villi.
c. **Placental site nodule**
d. **Epithelioid type of leiomyosarcoma:** The distinctive vascular growth pattern and immunocytochemistry are helpful to differentiate PSTT from epithelioid type of leiomyosarcoma. The later tumor is positive for SMA and negative for hPL.

### Behavior and Treatment

Majority of PSTT behaves as a benign tumor. Simple hysterectomy cures the patient when the tumor is limited to uterus. PSTT is staged according to the FIGO staging of gestational trophoblastic disease. Only 10–15% PSTT are malignant. Metastasis may occur in lung, liver, central

Table 19.2: Placental site trophoblastic tumor versus choriocarcinoma

| Features | Placental site trophoblastic tumor | Choriocarcinoma |
| --- | --- | --- |
| Antecedent gestational history | Mostly normal pregnancy | Mostly molar pregnancy (50%) |
| Time interval from gestation to the disease | Long latent period months to many years | Short latent period, only few weeks to months |
| β hCG | Relatively low; less than 1,000 mIU/mL | Very high; more than 1,000000 mIU/mL |
| Pattern | Monomorphic cell population, only intermediate cytotrophoblast | Dimorphic cell population, both cytotrophoblast and syncytiotrophoblast |
| Vascular invasion | Typical vascular invasion and the wall of the vessels are formed by tumor cells | Vascular destruction |
| βhCG immunocytochemistry | Only 10% cells are positive | Majority of the cells are strongly positive |
| hPL | Strong and diffuse | Focal and weak |
| Ki-67 | 10–30% | More than 40% |
| Behavior | Usually benign | Highly malignant |
| Chemotherapy | Resistant | Highly sensitive |

Table 19.3: Placental site trophoblastic tumor versus exaggerated placental site trophoblastic reaction

| Features | Placental site trophoblastic tumor | Exaggerated placental site trophoblastic reaction |
| --- | --- | --- |
| Mass formation | Present | Absent |
| Chorionic villi | Absent | Present |
| Destructive infiltrating growth | Present | Absent |
| Multinucleated giant cells | Absent | Present, many |
| Mitosis | High | Low |
| Ki-67 index | More than 10 | 0 |

nervous system, etc. The following factors are related to bad prognosis:[13,14] (1) Higher FIGO staging of the tumor, (2) Metastasis at the time of first presentation, (3) High mitotic rate (more than 5 per 10 HPFs), (4) Longer interval from previous pregnancy to the disease (more than 2 years), (5) More than 35 years age. Malignant PSTT should be treated by multi-agent chemotherapy (etoposide, cisplatin/etoposide, methotrexate, and actinomycin D).[15]

## EPITHELIOID TROPHOBLASTIC TUMOR

Epithelioid trophoblastic tumor (ETT) is a very rare tumor and is distinct from PSTT or choriocarcinoma. The tumor is developed from cytotrophoblasts. ETT occurs in the patient of reproductive age period. The patient commonly presents with abnormal vaginal bleeding. Most of the reported cases of ETT have history of normal pregnancy, molar pregnancy or abortion.[16,17]

### Gross

The tumor presents as solid nodule from few mm to few cm in diameter in the endomyometrium. The cut section shows solid, tan to brown in appearance.

### Histopathology

The tumor shows of monomorphic small cytotrophoblasts arranged in small nest, cords and nodules. The tumor cells are small round with scanty cytoplasm. The nuclei of the cells are round and monomorphic. Mitosis activity is usually low and varies from 1 to 10 per 10 HPFs. The tumor often shows lymphocytic infiltration.

### Immunohistochemistry

The tumor cells are positive for E cadherin, CK18, epidermal growth factor receptor, inhibin and p63. ETT is focally positive for hPL.

### Differential Diagnosis

a. **Placental site trophoblastic tumor:** The characteristic nodular growth pattern, less pleomorphic cells and lack of typical vascular invasion seen in PSTT are helpful features to differentiate PSTT from ETT.
b. **Choriocarcinoma:** The dimorphic growth pattern, severe pleomorphic cells and large areas of hemorrhage and necrosis are diagnostic features of choriocarcinoma.
c. **Cervical squamous cell carcinoma:** Occasionally, ETT may be mistaken as cervical keratinizing squamous cell carcinoma in curetting sample. Immunohistochemistry positivity for cytokeratin 18 and inhibin may help to diagnose ETT.

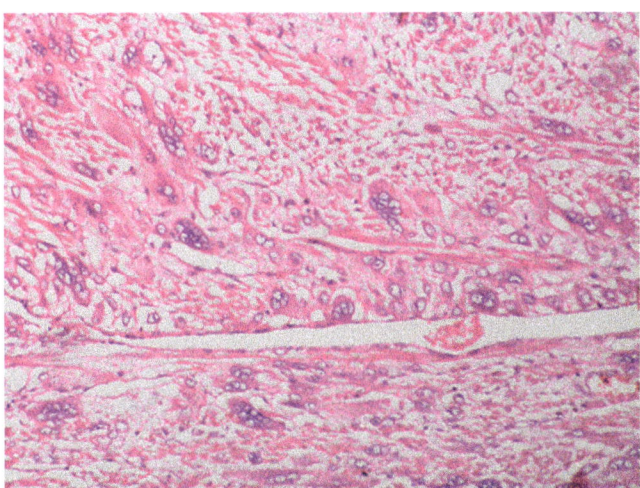

Figure 19.20: Exaggerated placental site reaction: Exuberant non-neoplastic proliferation of cytotrophoblast and syncytiotrophoblastic cells

## Behavior

ETT behaves as PSTT. No long-term follow-up data is still available in this relatively new entity.

## EXAGGERATED PLACENTAL SITE REACTION

Exaggerated placental site reaction characterized by exuberant non-neoplastic proliferation of cytotrophoblastic cells in the normal implantation site (Figure 19.20). In case of exaggerated proliferation the cytotrophoblastic cells diffusely infiltrate in the endometrium and myometrium. The orderly architectural arrangement of the tissue in the placental site is maintained. The cellular infiltration is usually around the spiral arterioles and glands of the endometrium. No necrosis is noted. The associated villi are normal.

## PLACENTAL SITE NODULE

Placental site nodule (PSN) is characterized by small well-circumscribed nodule in the placental site formed by the collection of cytotrophoblasts in a hyalinized stroma. The patients of PSN are mainly in the reproductive age period. PSN is an incidental finding and is detected in endometrial curetting, cervical biopsy, hysterectomy specimen for various causes.

## Gross

Placental site nodule is usually a small nodule and the lesion varies from microscopic size to 1 cm in diameter. The cut section of PSN is soft yellowish tan with foci of hemorrhage.

## Histopathology

Placental site nodule is composed of nodular collection of cytotrophoblasts. The nodules are made of isolated cytotrophoblasts embedded in dense hyalinized stromal material. The cells have abundant eosinophilic cytoplasm with central round monomorphic nuclei. Occasional cells show nuclear enlargement and pleomorphism. The nodules of cells are often surrounded by lymphocytes. Multinucleated giant cells are also seen.

### Immunohistochemistry

The cells of PSN are positive for cytokeratin 18, EMA, PLAP, and human leukocyte antigen. In addition, the cells are also positive for hPL, hCG, and CD146.

### Differential Diagnosis

Placental site nodule should be distinguished from PSTT and ETT. The small size of PSN with bland cells helps to distinguish PSN from the tumors.

### Prognosis and Treatment

This is a benign lesion and surgical removal of the lesion is optimum treatment.

## REFERENCES

1. Genest DR, Berkowitz RS, Fisher RA, et al. Gestational trophoblastic disease. In: Tavassoli F A, Derilee P (eds). World Health Organization Classification of Tumours: pathological genetics of tumours of the breast and female genital organs. IARC Press, Lyon, pp 250-4.
2. Altieri A, Franceschi S, Ferlay J, Smith J, La Vecchia C. Epidemiology and aetiology of gestational trophoblastic diseases. Lancet Oncol. 2003;4:670-8.
3. Keep D, Zaragoza MV, Hassold T, Redline RW. Very early complete hydatidiform mole. Hum Pathol. 1996;27:708-13.
4. Chew SH, Perlman EJ, Williams R, Kurman RJ, Ronnett BM. Morphology and DNA content analysis in the evaluation of first trimester placentas for partial hydatidiform mole (PHM). Hum Pathol. 2000;31:914-24.
5. Seckl MJ, Fisher RA, Salerno G, Rees H, Paradinas FJ, Foskett M. Choriocarcinoma and partial hydatidiform moles. Lancet. 2000;356:36-9.
6. Bagshawe KD, Lawler SD, Paradinas FJ, Dent J, Brown P, Boxer GM. Gestational trophoblastic tumours following initial diagnosis of partial hydatidiform mole. Lancet. 1990; 335:1074-6.
7. Hertig AT. Tumors of the female sex organs. Part 1. Hydatidifrom mole and choriocarcinoma. In: Atlas of tumor pathology, section 9, fascicle 33. 1956:Armed Forces Institute of Pathology, Washington DC.
8. Ilancheran A. Optimal treatment in gestational trophoblastic disease. Ann Acad Med Singapore. 1998;27(5):698-704.
9. Hassadia A, Gillespie A, Tidy J, Everard RGNJ, Wells M, Coleman R. Placental site trophoblastic tumour: clinical features and management. Gynecol Oncol. 2005;99:603-7.

10. Moore-Maxwell CA, Robbery SJ. Placental site trophoblastic tumor arising from antecedent molar pregnancy. Gynecol Oncol. 2004;92:708-12.
11. Lee Y, Kim KR, McKeon F, Yang A, Boyd TK, Crum CP, Parast MM. A unifying concept of trophoblastic differentiation and malignancy defined by biomarker expression. Hum Pathol. 2007;38:1003-13.
12. Kurman RJ. The morphology, biology and pathology of intermediate trophoblast, a look back into the present. Hum Pathol. 1991;22:847-55.
13. Papadopoulos AJ, Foskett M, Seckl MJ, McNeish I, Paradinas FJ, Rees H, et al. Twenty-five years' clinical experience with placental site trophoblastic tumors. J Reprod Med. 2002;47:460-64.
14. Hoekstra AV, Keh P, Lurain JR. Placental site trophoblastic tumor: a review of 7 cases and their implications for prognosis and treatment. J Reprod Med. 2004;49:447-52.
15. Newlands ES, Mulholland PJ, Holden L, Seckl MJ, Rustin GJ. Etoposide and cisplatin/etoposide, methotrexate, and actinomycin D (EMA) chemotherapy for patients with high-risk gestational trophoblastic tumors refractory to EMA/cyclophosphamide and vincristine chemotherapy and patients presenting with metastatic placental site trophoblastic tumors. J Clin Oncol. 2000;18:854-9.
16. Kuo KT, Chen MJ, Lin MC. Epithelioid trophoblastic tumor of the broad ligament. Am J Surg Pathol. 28:405-9.
17. Macdonald MC, Palmer JE, Hancock BW, Tidy JA. Diagnostic challenges in extrauterine epithelioid trophoblastic tumours: a report of two cases. Gynecol Oncol. 2008;108:452-54.

# Gross Examination of the Samples and Synoptic Reporting Format

# 20

Systemic examination of the specimen is a prerequisite for the correct diagnosis and management. Proper examination and sampling help to identify the lesion with its extent. It thereby reduces the turn overtime of reporting and also reduces the overall cost.

## ESSENTIAL THINGS REQUIRED BEFORE GROSSING

1. **Identification of the specimen and matching with the requisition form:** The information on the label on the container should be matched with the requisition form.
2. **Specimen preservative fluid:** The fixative should be identified and if the specimen is sent fresh then 10% buffered formalin should be added in the container.[1]
3. **Type of the operation:** The type of operation should be noted as it helps to examine the specimen accordingly.
4. **Essential clinical history:** The clinical history and diagnosis are mandatory information. The history of previous operation or history of previous therapy should be noted.

## GROSSING ROOM

The grossing room should be well-lighted, well-ventilated and should have adequate space. There should be continuous flow of water in the grossing station. The grossing station should be well-equipped with weighing machine, measuring tape and essential instruments such as sharp knife, forceps, petri dish, etc. The grossing station should have photographic facilities. The gross description of the specimen could be recorded in tape recorder and can be retrieved in future.

## INDIVIDUAL SPECIMEN

### Cervical Specimen

Cervical specimen can be discussed as follows:

*Endocervical Polypectomy*

The endocervical polyp is of variable in size from few mm to cm. The size, color, surface mucosa and stalk of the polyp should be described. Large polyp should be bisected through mucosa and embedded partially. Small polyp less than 1 cm should be bisected and embedded fully.

*Cervical Punch Biopsy*

Cervical punch biopsy is usually taken for the diagnosis of cervical intraepithelial lesion. The sample is usually colposcopic guided and only few mm in size. The whole tissue should be embedded.

*Cervical Wedge Biopsy*

The cervical wedge biopsy specimen is usually taken for confirmation of carcinoma before therapy. The biopsy is relatively larger than punch biopsy. The size of the sample should be described along with color. Any abnormality of the mucosal surface should be mentioned. The specimen should be bisected perpendicular to the mucosal surface and embedded totally.

*Manchester Repair*

Manchester repair is done in case of uterine prolapse and an amputated specimen of cervix is sent. The specimen has little significance and only two sections from anterior and posterior lip of cervix are enough.

*Cervical Cone Biopsy or Loop Electroexcision*

Cone biopsy is done in case of high grade squamous intraepithelial lesion to remove the affected area and also to treat Microinvasive carcinoma. The specimen is shaped as cone with a broad base representing ectocervix and tip pointing towards the uterine body (Box 20.1). Usually, the

**Box 20.1:** Cone biopsy grossing

**Description:**
- Length of the cone
- Diameter of ectocervix
- Mucosal surface
  - Color
  - Erosions
  - Lacerations
  - Any mass
  - Hemorrhage
- If fragmented record the number and size of the fragments

**Procedure:**
- Identify the suture at 12 o'clock
- Mark the surgical margins with India ink
- Open the specimen by a sharp scissor and the tissue is kept flat on a wax board by pin
- The entire cone specimen is cut by longitudinal strips of 2-3 mm interval
- The whole specimen is embedded

cone biopsy specimen is accompanied with a suture mark at 12 o'clock position. The length of the cone and diameter of ectocervix is measured in cm. The mucosal surface should be noted for its color, surface irregularities, erosions or any mass lesion.

**Procedure (Figures 20.1 and 20.2):** The suture mark indicating the position of the clock should be identified. The surgical margin should be marked by ink. The cone biopsy specimen should be opened by a sharp scissor and the tissue is kept flat on a wax board by pin. Now the entire cone specimen is cut by longitudinal strips of 2-3 mm interval. The sections should start from 12 o'clock to clockwise 11 o'clock position. In all such sections, the squamocolumnar junction should be present. The complete cone biopsy specimen should be submitted for the histopathological examination.[2]

### Endocervical Curetting

Endometrial curetting is done to exclude any neoplastic lesion in endocervical canal. Usually blood, mucus and small fragments of tissue are received. Color of the tissue, mucus, blood and total volume or dimension should be described. The specimen is wrapped in filter paper and processed as whole.

## Uterine Specimen

### Endometrial Curetting

Endometrial curetting is done predominantly (1) for work-up of infertility, (2) abnormal uterine bleeding and (2) in abortion.

The specimen is usually received as multiple fragmented tissue. The tissue is collected in filter paper or in cassette of fine mesh. The tissue is embedded in single to multiple cassettes depending on the amount. The following things should be noted:
- Total volume of tissue
- Color of tissue
- Any friable firm tissue: This is usually seen in carcinoma
- Fatty tissue: The presence of adipose tissue usually indicates uterine perforation

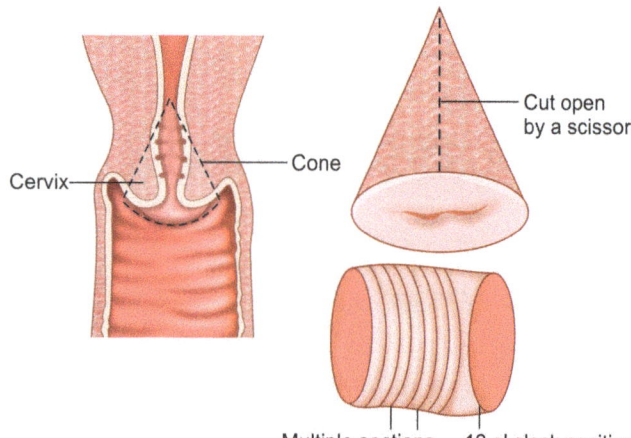

Figure 20.1: Cone biopsy of cervix: Schematic diagram of processing

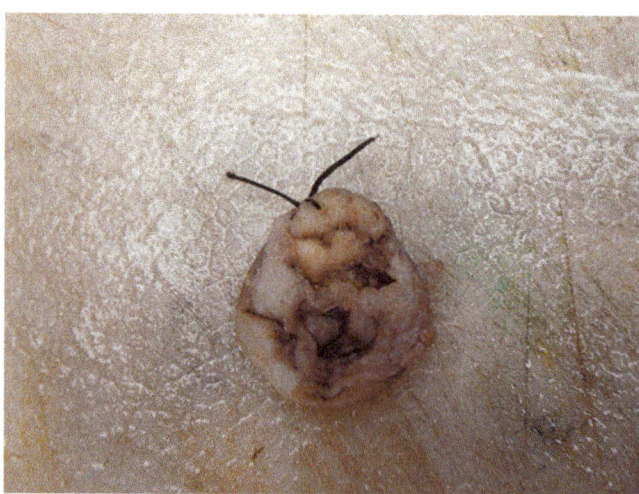

Figure 20.2: Cone biopsy specimen: Suture indicates 12 o'clock position

- In case of aborted material or product of conception: chorionic villi, fetal parts, gestational sac or grape-like vesicles (in molar pregnancy).

All the tissue fragments should be processed for endometrial curetting sent for histopathological examination of abnormal uterine bleeding.

### Myomectomy

Myometrial specimen is received for the confirmation of leiomyoma of uterus (Figure 20.3). The dimension and the weight of the specimen should be measured. The specimen is cut into maximum diameter and is processed for histopathological examination.

### Hysterectomy Specimen

The specimen of uterus may be received as:
- Only uterus
- Uterus with bilateral salpingo-oophorectomy
- Uterus with bilateral salpingo-oophorectomy and pelvic lymphadenectomy.

**Description:** Size of the uterus is measured and length from fundus to ectocervix, width from one to other corneal distance and diameter of cervix should be recorded. The weight of the uterus is also recorded. The anterior surface of uterus is less covered by peritoneum than the posterior surface. From anterior to posterior there are round ligament, fallopian tube and ovary are attached with uterus. The color of the surface and any abnormality of the outer surface is noted.

The uterus is cut through the lateral walls by a sharp knife or scissor from the cervix to the upper part of the fundus (Figures 20.4 to 20.7). The uterus is made of two halves: anterior and posterior uterus and is kept for proper fixation for several hours. Multiple parallel sections are cut

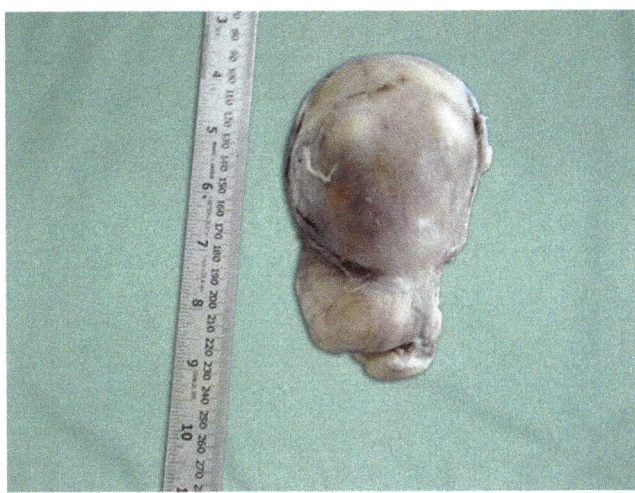

**Figure 20.4:** Simple hysterectomy

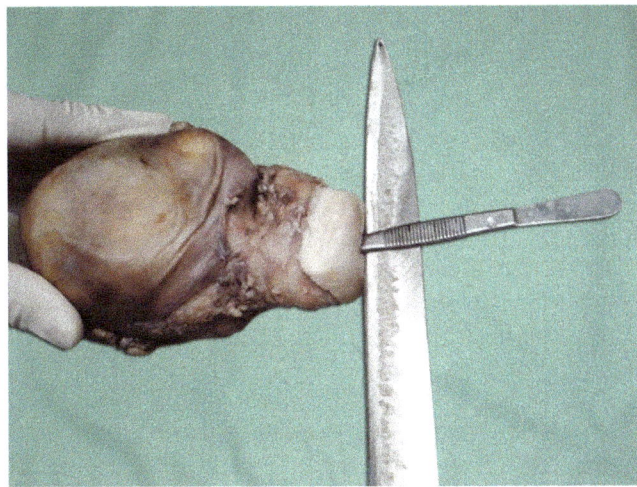

**Figure 20.5:** Specimen is cut through cervix to fundus

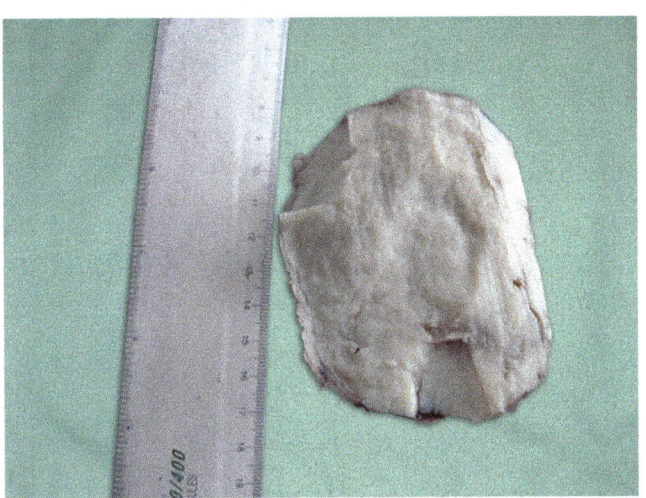

**Figure 20.3:** Myomectomy specimen

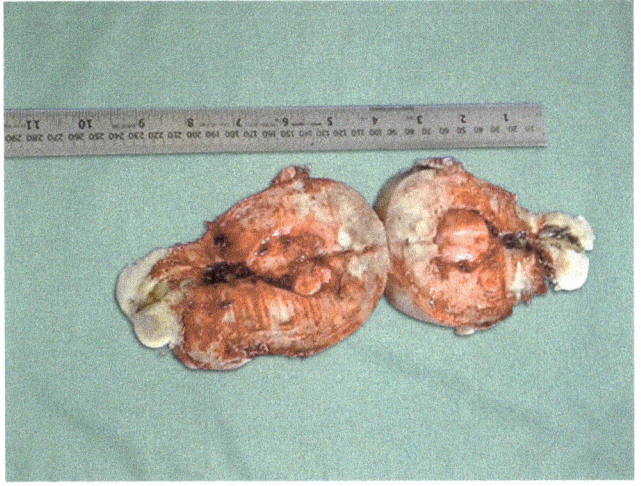

**Figure 20.6:** Two longitudinal halves of uterus, one anterior and other posterior half

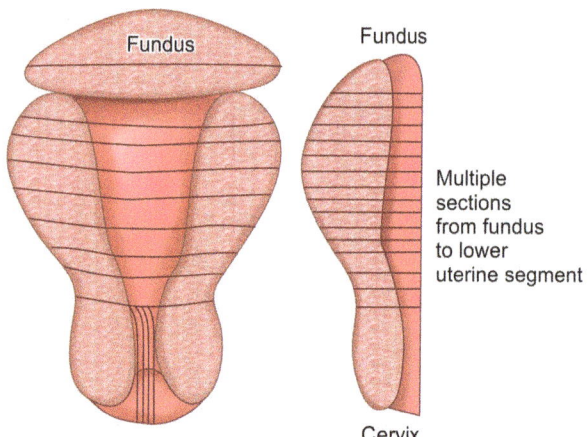

**Figure 20.7:** Grossing of uterus: Schematic diagram

about 1 cm apart from fundus to lower part of the body of uterus. The multiple longitudinal sections of cervix are cut. The following features should be noted:

- Any abnormality in serosa: adhesion, nodularity, change of color
- Length of uterine cavity
- Any lesion in the uterine cavity
- Thickness of endometrium
- Thickness of the myometrial wall
- Cervix:
  - Ectocervix: Size, color, mass lesion, ulceration, cyst, polyp
  - Endocervix: Length, color, mucosal surface, any polyp or cyst
- Any lesion in the myometrium such as leiomyoma. Total number of leiomyoma, site, size, etc. should be mentioned. Any hemorrhage or necrosis in leiomyoma should be described.
  - No macroscopic abnormality with no suspicion for malignancy: In this condition, two to four sections from the uterus are adequate.
    - The sections should be taken from the upper part of the body of uterus including endometrium and portion of the myometrium and if possible serosa should be included.
    - Two section from the cervix, one from anterior part and other from the posterior part of the cervix should be taken. Squamocolumnar junction should always be included in the block.
    - If vaginal part is included in the specimen then the section from the vagina should be taken.
    - The ovary should be cut through the hilum and section should be taken.
  - Benign condition:
    - Leiomyoma: In case of leiomyoma, multiple sections should be taken and blocks should be included from the myometrial and leiomyoma interface. The areas of hemorrhage and necrosis should be sampled adequately. In case of multiple leiomyomata at least three should be sampled and preference should be given to the large leiomyoma.
    - Adenomyoma: It may be present anywhere in the myometrial wall and multiple sections should be taken.
    - Endometrial polyp: The poly should be described properly such as stalk of the polyp, cut surface etc. The polyp should be sectioned from the larger axis and entire poly including the stalk should be embedded.
  - Malignant condition: In case of malignancy the following features should be noted:
    - Exact location of the tumor
    - Size
    - Color
    - Appearance: papillary, solid and circumscribed, cystic, ulcerated, etc.
    - Extent: Lateral extent of the tumor and downward extent in the cervix
    - Any evidence of tumor in the tube, ovary or serosa
    - Cut surface of ovary and tube
    - Vaginal cuff present or not
    - Gross description of lymph node: number, size, color, gross tumor in the node.

**Sections to be taken:** At first the whole serosa of the uterus should be inked preferable different color for anterior and posterior surface.

*Tumor:* The sections from the tumor along with myometrial and serosa should be taken. At least three sections should be taken and if possible the whole section should be embedded. If it is not possible to take the entire section then the tissue should be cut in two parts and embedded in two cassettes.

*Non-neoplastic endometrium:* Multiple sections from the fundus to lower part of the uterus should be taken. There is no need to take full section from the endometrium to serosa in such sections.

*Cervix:* The cervix should be cut longitudinally and two sections one each from the anterior and posterior lip should be taken.

*Parametrium:* Soft tissues from the left and right parametrium should be taken.

*Vaginal cuff:* The attached vaginal tissue should be taken in one or two cassettes.

*Ovary and fallopian tube:* Adequate sections should be taken from the left and right ovary and fallopian tube.

*Lymph nodes:* All the lymph nodes should be cut in their long axis and should be embedded. The following group of lymph nodes are received:
- Obturator
- External iliac
- Common iliac
- Internal iliac
- Para-aortic

**If no tumor is seen in naked eye:** If no visible tumor is present then the entire uterus should be cut 3 mm apart and sections should be taken from the fundus to the lower part of the body of uterus.

### Hysterectomy for Cervical Carcinoma

In cervical cancer, we usually receive radical hysterectomy specimen with lymphadenectomy specimen. An attached vaginal cuff and parametrial tissue are also included in the specimen.

**Description:** The following features should be noted:
- Size: The length of the cervix and diameter of the os should be mentioned.
- Mucosa: Color of the mucosa, any ulceration
- Growth:
  - Appearance: Solid, fungating, polypoidal, etc.
  - Necrosis or hemorrhage
  - Depth: The lateral and upwards extent of the tumor
  - Parametrium: Any macroscopic abnormality in the parametrium.
- Uterus: As instructed before
- Ovary, tube, lymph node: As instructed before.

**Sections:** The cervix should be amputated from the uterus and the uterus should be opened from the lateral wall as described before. The cervix is opened at the 12 o'clock position by a sharp scissor. The cervix is kept in formalin in several hours for fixation. Now the cervix is stretched and pinned in two sides. Multiple parallel longitudinal sections should be made and all the sections should be embedded. Precautions should be taken to include squamocolumnar junction and epithelial membrane in every section.

## VULVECTOMY SPECIMEN

The type of the vulvectomy should be identified:
- Hemi vulvectomy: Only one-half of the vulva that mean unilateral vulvectomy
- Partial vulvectomy: No deep fascia is included
- Total vulvectomy: Deep fascia included
- Radical vulvectomy: Lymph node also included (Figure 20.8).

## Description

- Size of the specimen: Two-dimension along with depth of the tissue
- Structures identification: Mention the structures included such as clitoris, labia majora, minora, deeper tissue, lymph node
- Tumor:
  - Location
  - Gross appearance: Verrucous, fungating solid, ulcerated
  - Size
  - Extent: invasion to the adjacent tissue and depth of invasion in the deeper tissue
- Non-neoplastic area: Appearance of the non-neoplastic area should be recorded.

## Procedure

At first the resection margins and the deep resection plane should be labelled with India ink. The following sections should be taken:[3]
- Multiple sections from the tumor proper
- Tumor with the deep resection plane
- All the resection margins
- Urethral margin
- Soft tissue and deep fascia near the tumor site in deep resection plane
- One or two sections also should be taken from the uninvolved structures in the specimen.

## SALPINGECTOMY SPECIMEN

Salpingectomy is done for the specific pathology of the fallopian tube or as a part of total abdominal hysterectomy.

The tube should be fixed properly. The tube is cut transversely in 5 mm interval and the following features should be noted:
- Length and diameter of the tube

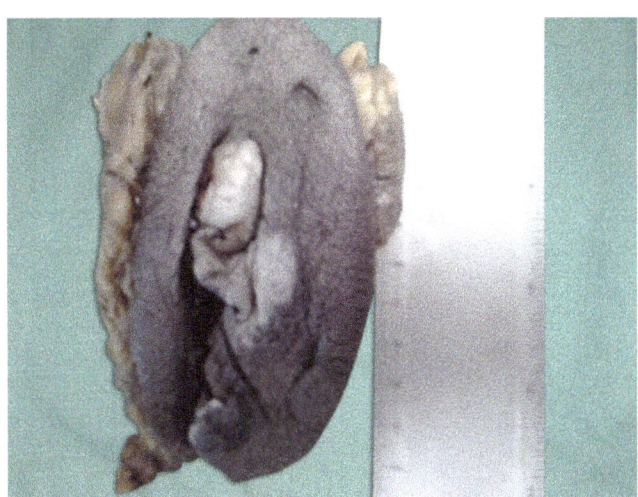

**Figure 20.8:** Radical vulvectomy specimen: Growth in the left side of vulva

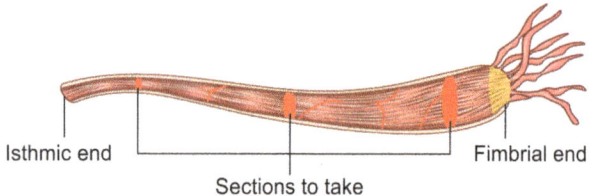

Figure 20.9: Salpingectomy specimen: Schematic diagram to take sections

- Any abnormality of the outer surface: Color, hemorrhage, nodularity, adhesion
- Lumen: The patency of the tubal lumen
- Lesion: If there is a mass lesion in the fallopian tube then the size of the tumor, color, cut surface and presence or absence of hemorrhage and necrosis should be noted.

## Sections (Figure 20.9)

- Normal appearing tube: Three cross sections from the fimbrial, ampullary and isthmic region of the tube are sufficient for normal appearing tube.
- Ectopic pregnancy: Multiple sections from the products of conceptions should be sampled. Fallopian tube from the adjacent site of the products of conception and rupture site should be sampled. In addition one should also take normal appearing fallopian tube.
- Tumor: Multiple sections from the tumor along with the fallopian tube wall should be sampled. In addition, at least 3 sections must be taken from the grossly normal area.

## OOPHORECTOMY

Oophorectomy may be alone or along with uterus and fallopian tube.
The following features should be noted:
- The dimension of the ovarian specimen is measured along with the measurement of the weight
- Ovarian shape and size
- Outer surface: Capsular breach, color, nodularity or any other abnormality
- Cut section
  - Appearance: Solid or cystic, any papillary projections, cystic spaces
  - Hemorrhage and necrosis
  - Calcification
  - Measurement of solid and cystic area
  - Color.

## Sections

- From the normal appearing ovary: One sagittal section of the ovary is enough
- Cyst: The cyst should cut open by sharp scissor and three to four sections from the cyst wall are sufficient. In case of papillary structures over the cyst wall one should take multiple sections from the cyst wall with papillae
- Tumor: The tumor should be cut transversely in multiple plane and from each cm of the tube one section should be taken.

## EXAMINATION OF THE PLACENTA

The placenta should be thoroughly examined to get various information (Figures 20.10 and 20.11).

### Fetal Membranes

*General*

- Color of the membrane:
  - Opaque color: Infection
  - Yellow-brown: Meconium stained
- Completeness: Whether the membrane is complete or torn and retained in the uterus

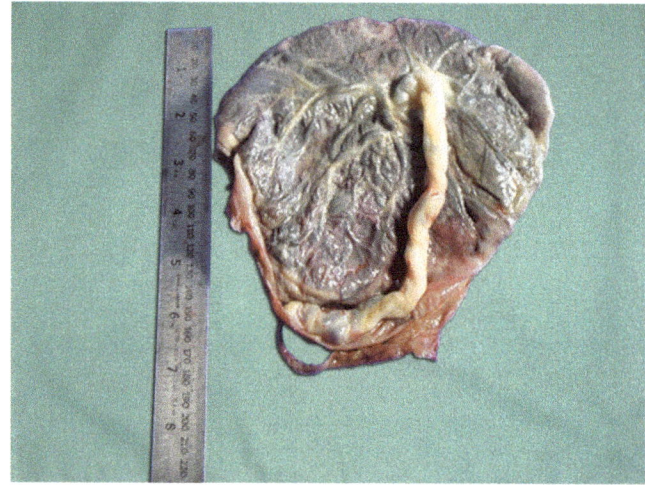

Figure 20.10: Placenta: Membrane and umbilical cord

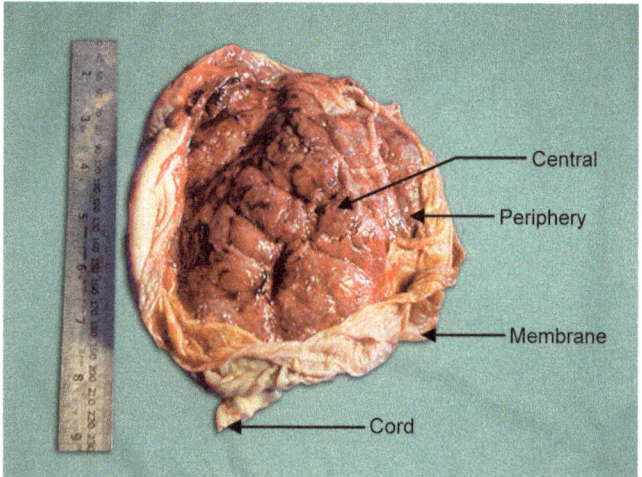

Figure 20.11: Placenta: Sections to be taken

- Insertion: Whether the membrane is properly attached with the placental margin.
- Hemorrhage: Any hemorrhage in the membrane or not.

## Umbilical Cord

- Length: Total length of the cord
- Diameter: Diameter of the cord
- Vessels: Number of the blood vessels
- Coiling: Hypercoiled or not
- Knots: Any true or false knot or not
- Insertion: The distance between the point of insertion and the closest margin of the placenta.

## Placenta

- Diameter: Exact diameter of the placenta
- Thickness: Measure the thickness
- Weight
- Shape
- Maternal surface: Any clot or tear and incomplete tissue that indicate the retained placental tissue within the uterus
- Fetal surface: Any abnormality present or not.

*Sections*

**Placenta:** At least three blocks should be taken from the central part, peripheral part and area of insertion of the umbilical cord. Multiple sections should be taken from the area of abnormality.

**Membrane:** Membrane should be rolled and embedded in one cassette.

**Umbilical cord:** The umbilical cord should be sectioned in proximal middle and distal part and the cross-sections of the three parts should be taken in one cassette.

## SYNOPTIC REPORTING OF GYNECOLOGICAL LESIONS

### Vulval Cancer

1. Number of primary tumor
2. Microscopic description of the tumor
3. Histological type: WHO typing of tumor is preferable
4. Degree of differentiation: Well/moderate/poor
5. Depth of invasion: Method of measurement should be mentioned
6. Resection margins and deep resection plane: Free/involved
7. The exact size of the microscopic tumor
8. Lymphovascular emboli: Present/absent
9. Any perineural invasion: Present/absent
10. Closest margin which is uninvolved: Distance
11. The presence of intraepithelial neoplasia: present/absent/VIN grade
12. Lymph nodes: Number of involved nodes/size
13. Ancillary tests:
    - Reports of immunohistochemistry
    - DNA ploidy
    - HPV type.

### Cervical Carcinoma

- Number: Usually single
- Description of tumor
- Histological type and subtype
- Grade:
    - Squamous cell carcinoma: Keratinizing/nonkeratinizing
    - Adenocarcinoma: Well-differentiated/moderately differentiated/poorly differentiated
- Size of tumor: The greatest microscopic size should be recorded in the transverse direction
- Depth of invasion by tumor: From the basement membrane to the deepest point of invasion
- Thickness of the cervical wall and the lateral extension of the tumor
- Any associated CIN or adenocarcinoma in situ: Present/absent
- Lymphovascular involvement: Present/absent
- Involvement of margins: Present/absent
- The distance of uninvolved margin
- Involvement of other organ:
    - Uterus: Present/absent: extent
    - Vagina: Present/absent: extent
    - Pelvic wall: Present/absent: Right/left
    - Bladder and rectum
- Lymph node: Number and location of the involved node
- Ancillary studies:
    - HPV type.

### Endometrial Carcinoma

1. Brief description
2. Histologic type
3. Histologic grade: FIGO grading is applicable to endometrioid carcinoma
   Grade1: The nonsquamous or nonmorular solid area is equal or less than 5%.
   Grade 2: The nonsquamous or nonmorular solid area is 6–50%.
   Grade 3: The nonsquamous or nonmorular solid area is more than 50%.
   The presence of significant nuclear atypia will increase the grade by 1.

Higher grade: Serous carcinoma, clear cell carcinoma also malignant mixed Müllerian tumor (carcinosarcoma)
4. Size of the tumor
5. The depth of myometrial invasion: The maximum depth of myometrial invasion should be mentioned along with thickness of the myometrial wall. The depth of tumor invasion is measured from the junction of endometrium and myometrium up to the maximum depth of tumor infiltration.
6. Lymphovascular invasion: Present/absent.
7. Cervical involvement: Cervical stroma or mucosa: present/absent.
8. Uninvolved endometrium: Atrophic/hyperplastic/intra-epithelial neoplasm.
9. Extrauterine involvement:
   - Parametrium
   - Vagina
   - Ovary
   - Fallopian tube
   - Omentum
   - Pouch of Douglas
10. Lymph node involvement: Sites, number
11. Ancillary tests:
    - Immunohistochemistry
    - Estrogen/progesterone receptors
    - DNA ploidy

## Ovarian Carcinoma

1. Brief description of tumor
2. Histological type
3. Histological grading:
   - Well-differentiated
   - Moderately differentiated
   - Poorly differentiated
   - Undifferentiated
4. Size of the tumor and its exact location
5. Capsular involvement: Rupture: present/absent
6. Lymphovascular involvement
7. Any other findings: Such as endometriosis
8. Contralateral ovary: No tumor/Involved by tumor of similar morphology/metastasis
9. Other organ involvement:
   - Uterus
   - Omentum
   - Pelvic peritoneum
   - Intestine
   - Liver
   - Vagina
10. Lymph node involvement: Location/number
11. Ancillary tests:
    - Immunocytochemistry
    - DNA ploidy
    - Electron microscopy
    - Tumor markers: CA 125, serum alpha-fetoprotein.

### REFERENCES

1. Hopwood D. Cell and tissue fixation. 1972-1982. Histochem J. 1985;17(4):389-442.
2. Heatley MK. How many histological levels should be examined from tissue blocks originating in cone biopsy and large loop excision of the transformation zone specimens of cervix? J Clin Pathol. 2001;54(8):650-1.
3. Wilkinson EJ. Protocol for the examination of specimens from patients with carcinomas and malignant melanomas of the vulva: a basis for checklists. Cancer Committee of the American College of Pathologists. Arch Pathol Lab Med. 2000;124(1):51-6.

# Index

Page numbers followed by *b* refer to box, *f* refer to figure, and *t* refer to table

## A

Acellular pinkish hyaline material 146*f*
Acid-fast bacilli 10
Actinomycosis 39, 39*f*, 55
   israelii infection 55
Adenocarcinoma 54, 61, 81, 257
   in situ 61, 78, 78*f*, 79*f*
   type of 83
Adenofibroma 93, 135, 138
Adenoid basal
   carcinoma 61
   cell carcinoma 88, 88*t*
Adenoid cystic carcinoma 34*f*, 35*f*, 87, 88*t*
   of cervix 87*f*
Adenomatoid tumor 153, 154*f*, 170, 251, 256
   of fallopian tube 256*f*
Adenomyoma 61, 94, 135, 154
Adenomyomatous polyp 110, 110*f*
Adenomyosis 154, 154*f*
Adenosarcoma 61, 135, 169, 197, 251
Adenosquamous carcinoma 61, 86
Adrenal cortical rest 167
Adult granulosa cell tumor 170, 209, 215*t*
Allantoic duct 276, 276*f*
Allergic contact dermatitis 16
Alveolar soft part sarcoma 61, 91
Amelanotic melanoma 30
Amenorrhea, primary 167
American Congress of Obstetricians and Gynecologists 266
Amnion nodosum 275
Amniotic bands 275
Ampulla 251
Ancillary tests 70, 295, 70*b*
Androgen abnormality 163
Androgen insensitivity, causes of 5*f*
Angiomyofibroblastoma 21, 22
Angiomyxoma
   aggressive 20, 21
   superficial 19, 21
Angiosarcoma 61, 250
Anovulatory cycle 117
Antepartum bleeding 277
Antral cavity 159*f*
Apoplectic leiomyoma 116
Appendix, tumor of 246
Arcuate uterus 6, 6*f*
Argentaffin cells 220
Arias-Stella reaction 53, 61, 103*f*, 125
Arterial supply 157
Asherman's syndrome 113
Atopic dermatitis 15
Atretic follicle 159
Atrophic endometrium 103*f*
Atypical hyperplasia, simple 118
Autoimmune oophoritis 164, 167

## B

B cell lymphoma 248
Bacterial
   infections 9, 56
   vaginosis 38, 38*f*
Bartholin cyst 18*f*, 42*f*
   cells in 18*f*
Bartholin duct cyst 17
Bartholin gland cysts 41
Basal cell carcinoma 30
Basaloid carcinoma 28
Basaloid squamous cell carcinoma 29*f*, 30, 74, 75*f*
Bicornuate uterus 6, 6*f*
Biliary tract tumor 247
Bizarre
   leiomyoma 147
   nuclei, large 147*f*
Blood supply 157, 252
Bone, tumor of 250
Breast carcinoma 247
Brenner tumor 169, 201*f*, 202*f*, 243
   benign 201
   borderline 169, 202
   malignant 169, 175, 202, 203*f*
Breslow's classification of melanoma invasion 34*t*
Bullous pemphigoid 16

## C

Canal, cysts of 18
Cancer cervix 71
*Candida albicans* 38
*Candida glabrata* 38
Candida infection 38
*Candida tropicalis* 38
Candidal hyphae 39*f*
Carcinoma, secretory 127, 133
Carcinomatous nodule 190
Carcinosarcoma 61, 86, 92, 135, 136*f*, 137*f*, 144, 169, 195, 251
Cartilaginous tumor 250
Caseous necrosis 255*f*
Cell
   crowding of 78
   layer
      intermediate 51
      superficial 51
   lymphoma, large 230
   malignant 150*f*
Cellular angiofibroma 21, 22

Cellular changes 172
Cellular fibroma 170, 246
Cellular leiomyoma 116, 141, 146, 147f
Cellular thecoma 214
Cervical
    adenocarcinoma, preneoplastic lesion of 78
    adenosarcoma 92
    cancer 71
    carcinoma 294
        hysterectomy for 292
        staging of 73t
    cysts 59
    intraepithelial
        neoplasia 25
        neoplasm 64, 65
    preneoplastic lesions 65t
    punch biopsy 288
    specimen 288
    squamous cell carcinoma 285
    wall, part of 83
    wedge biopsy 288
Cervicitis
    acute 55
    chronic 55, 55f
Cervix 50f, 248, 291
    adenomyoma of 92
    adenosarcoma of 92f, 93f
    adenosquamous carcinoma of 86f, 87f
    anomalies of 6
    atypical carcinoid of 89
    benign
        diseases of 50
            squamous lining of 51f
    carcinoma of 78, 83
    carcinosarcoma of 93f
    clear cell carcinoma of 85f
    endometrioid adenocarcinoma of 84f
    extension in 93
    fungal infection of 56
    hyperplasia of 56
    inflammation of 55
    inner wall of 58
    leiomyoma of 90
    leiomyosarcoma of 90f, 91f
    lymphoepithelioma of 76f
    lymphoid follicle in 52f
    lymphoma of 92
    metastatic carcinoma in 89
    microglandular hyperplasia of 104, 104f
    neoplastic lesions of 61
    neuroendocrine tumors of 88
    papillary serous carcinoma of 86f
    preneoplastic lesions of 61, 64
    small cell carcinoma of 88, 88f, 89f
    squamous cell carcinoma of 71, 133
    tuberculosis of 55
*Chlamydia trachomatis* 11, 56, 160, 254
Chorangioma 275, 274, 276f
Chorioamnionitis
    acute 268, 269f
    stages of acute 269t
Choriocarcinoma 235, 280, 281f, 282f, 284, 285

Chorionic villi 265
Cicatrical pemphigoid 16
Cilia, loss of 172
Ciliated carcinoma 128
Ciliated cells 193, 251
Clark's classification of melanoma 34t
Clear cell
    adenocarcinoma 45, 53, 131
    adenofibroma 169, 198
    borderline tumor 169
    carcinoma 46f, 56, 58, 61, 85, 86, 129, 129t, 131, 131t, 132f, 133f, 169, 195, 198, 199, 199f, 200f, 230, 234, 251
    cystadenoma 169
    metaplasia 112, 112f
    tumor 169, 179
        atypical proliferative 169
Clitoris 8
Clomiphene therapy 164
Coagulative necrosis, foci of 151
Colposcopy 66, 71
    of carcinoma 71b
Columnar epithelium 51
Condyloma accuminata 24, 61, 75
Cone biopsy
    grossing 289b
    specimen 289f
Congenital cyst 59
Corpus albicans 160, 160f
Corpus luteal
    cells 159f
    cyst 162, 163f, 170
Corpus luteum 159, 159f, 162f
    of pregnancy 160
Cortical granuloma 161
Cortical inclusion cyst 172
Cushing's syndrome 164
Cyclic endometrium 97
Cyclin dependent kinase 70
Cyst, surface inclusion 160, 180
Cystadenofibroma 179, 180f
    ovary 179f
Cystic atrophy 117
Cystic clear cell carcinomas 200
Cystic granulosa cell tumor 161
Cysts 59, 251, 259
    acquired 59
Cytogenetics 146
Cytokeratin 264
Cytomegalovirus 11, 270
Cytotrophoblast 262, 263

## D

Decidual metaplasia 252, 252f
Desquamative inflammatory vaginitis 40
Diabetes mellitus 274
Didelphus uterus 6f
Dissecting leiomyoma 116, 149
Dizygotic twin 268
DNA aneuploidy 70
Dysfunctional uterine bleeding 105
Dysplastic cells 73

## E

Eclampsia 274
Ectopic breast tissue 22
Ectopic decidua 166
Ectopic pregnancy 103
Edema, massive 170
Embryonal
   carcinoma 170, 230, 234, 234b
   rhabdomyosarcoma 46
   sarcoma 91
Emphysematous vaginitis 40
Endocervical
   adenocarcinoma 58, 61, 81, 82f, 125t
      type of 125
   adenomyoma 94
   crypt, blockage of 55
   curetting 289
   gland 53f, 83
      benign 52f
      deep 59
   glandular hyperplasia 58f
      diffuse laminar 58
   mucinous carcinoma 128
   polyp, atypical 92
   polypectomy 288
Endocervix 51f
Endodermal sinus 233
   tumor 230, 231f-233f
Endometrial biopsy 102, 103b
Endometrial cancer, molecular genetics of 121
Endometrial carcinoma 112, 116, 120, 120t, 121t, 124t, 134, 248, 294
Endometrial functional polyp 110f
Endometrial glands 97
   star-shaped 103f
Endometrial hyperplasia 117
   management of 119f
Endometrial hyperplastic polyp 110f
Endometrial intraepithelial neoplasia 119
Endometrial metaplasia, types of 111b
Endometrial metaplastic 111
Endometrial mucinous metaplasia 112
Endometrial nodule 140
Endometrial polyp 109, 117
Endometrial squamous metaplasia 111
Endometrial stromal
   cells 142f
   nodule 140, 141f
   sarcoma 90, 140, 214
      high-grade 116, 143, 169
      low-grade 116, 141, 142f, 143f, 169
   tumor 140, 146
      classification of 140t
      molecular genetics of 144
Endometrioid adenocarcinoma 57, 84
Endometrioid adenofibroma 94, 169
Endometrioid carcinoma 61, 116, 122, 123f, 124f, 125, 169, 175, 193, 194f, 195t, 214, 220, 225, 234, 251, 258
   of uterus, primary 85
Endometrioid cystadenoma 169

Endometrioid stromal sarcoma 115, 197
Endometrioid tumor 169, 179
   atypical proliferative 169
Endometriosis 22, 80, 113, 251, 254
Endometriotic cyst 169, 180
Endometritis 108
   chronic 108f, 117, 119
   nonspecific 108
Endometrium 97
   artifacts in 104
   changes in 106
   early secretory 100f
   non-neoplastic 291
   tuberculosis of 109f
Entamoeba histolytica 39
Enterobius vermicularis 40
Eosinophilic metaplasia 113, 113f
Epithelial cells, surface 171
Epithelial inclusion cyst 18, 42
Epithelial metaplasia 124
Epithelial ovarian carcinoma 172
Epithelial tumor 24, 37, 61, 116, 169, 257
   benign 61, 251
   malignant 251
   surface 215
Epithelial-mesenchymal tumors 37, 61, 169, 179, 204, 251
Epithelioid cell 255f
   granuloma 109f
Epithelioid leiomyoma 116, 148, 148f
Epithelioid leiomyosarcoma 116, 151, 152f
Epithelioid trophoblastic tumor 285
*Escherichia coli* 40
Estrogenic hormone 107
Exophytic condyloma 65
Extrachorial placenta 265
   cause of 265
   types of 265

## F

Fallopian tube 172, 251, 291
   carcinoma 248
   cysts in 259t
   metaplasia of 252
   non-neoplastic lesions of 252
   prolapse of 41
   serous carcinoma of 257f, 258f
   transitional metaplasia of 252f
   tuberculosis 55
   tumor of 256
Fascicles, focal areas of 144
Federation of Gynecologists and Obstetricians 176
Female adnexal tumor 260
Female genital tract development 1b
Fenestrate placenta 265
Fetal
   death in utero 270
   disorders, placenta in 274
   hydrops 275
   inflammatory response 269f, 270t
   membranes 293
   response 269
   thrombotic vasculopathy 273
   vascular thrombosis 273
Fever 254

Fibrin thrombi 106
Fibroepithelial
    mucosal polyp 25
    polyp 19f
    stromal polyp 19
Fibroma 170, 216, 217f
Fibromatous stroma 224
Fibrosarcoma 170, 217
Fibrotic stroma 109, 129
Follicle
    cyst 170
    early primary 158f
    tertiary 158
Follicular cyst 161, 162f, 214
Follicular salpingitis 254
Follicular stimulating hormone 97
Foreign body granuloma 161
Fungal infection 12, 56

## G

Gardnerella vaginalis 38, 40
Gartner's duct cyst 19f, 41, 41f
Genetic alteration 144b
Genital tract
    defects in female 1
    development, disorders of 4
Genitalia development, external 4
Genitalia, external 4f
Germ cell 171
    sex cord-stromal tumor 170
    tumor 61, 170, 171, 228t, 251
        mixed 170
Gestational trophoblastic disease 278, 283
Gestational trophoblastic neoplasm 284
Giant cells, multinucleated 30
Glands simulating crowding, collapsed 104
Glands, architectural abnormalities of 109
Glandular cell 79
Glandular tumors 37, 61
Glassy cell carcinoma 61, 86
Goblet cells 220
Gonadal abnormalities 4
Gonadal development 1
Gonadoblastoma 170, 243
Gonadotropin
    abnormality 163
    level, high 167
    releasing hormone 97, 107, 115
Graafian follicle 159f
Granulation tissue 41
Granuloma inguinale 9
Granulomatous infections 160
Granulosa cell 158f, 159f
    tumor 197, 209, 209f-213f, 241, 243
        diffuse 205
        type of 204
Gynandroblastoma 225
Gynecological lesions, synoptic reporting of 294

## H

*Haemophilus ducreyi* 9
Hemorrhage, large central 162f

Heart diseases 275
Hemangioma 275
Hematoma 272
Hematopoietic cells, foci of 145
Hemorrhage 294
Hemorrhagic cellular leiomyoma 147
Hemosiderin laden histiocytes 106
Hepatocellular carcinoma 234
Hepatoid pattern 233
Herpes simplex
    virus 9, 56, 270
    infection 11, 56
Heterozygosis, loss of 175
Hilus cell
    hyperplasia 165
    tumor 226
Hobnail metaplasia 112
Hormone-induced changes 107
Human
    chorionic gonadotropin hormone 262
    immunodeficiency virus 271
    papilloma
        viral infection 56
        virus 62
Hydatid cyst 251
Hydatidiform mole 278, 279f
    complete 278, 279
    partial 278, 279
Hydropic abortus 280
Hydropic leiomyoma 116
Hydrosalpinx 180
Hymen, imperforate 38
Hyperchromasia 172
Hyperinsulinemia 163, 164
Hyperplasia 57
    atypical 118, 119
    complex 117, 118t, 119
    nonatypical 117
    simple 117, 117f, 118t, 119
    without atypia, complex 118f
Hyperplastic polyp 109
Hyperreactio luteinalis 162, 170
Hypothalamic-pituitary disorders, primary 164

## I

Immature condyloma 66
Immature squamous metaplasia 54, 54f, 69, 69t
Immature teratoma 170, 236, 238f, 239f
    grading of 237b
Immunocytochemistry 19, 20, 22, 46, 47, 79, 83, 88, 89, 112, 137, 141, 142, 146, 200, 259
Immunofluorescence 13, 16, 17
Infection, specific 55, 270
Inflammatory cells, chronic 255f
Inflammatory disorders, infectious 38
Intervillous
    hematoma 273
    thrombohematoma 272
Intestinal carcinoma 245
Intraepithelial lesions, high grade 65

Intrauterine
    growth retardation 275
    infections 268
Intravenous
    leiomyoma 149f
    leiomyomatosis 116, 143
Invasive hydatidiform mole 280

## J

Juvenile granulosa cell tumor 170, 214, 215f, 215t

## K

Keratinizing squamous cell carcinoma 28, 71, 72f
Klebsiella granulomatis 9
Koilocytic cells 25f
Krukenberg's tumor 166, 200, 224, 246, 246f, 247

## L

Labia majora 8
Labia minora 8
Langhan's giant cells 255f
Leiomyoma 61, 90, 145, 146, 249, 251, 257
    atypical 147, 147f
    with lymphoid infiltrate 149
Leiomyosarcoma 47, 47f, 61, 90, 116, 144, 149, 150f, 249, 251
    diagnosis of 144
    ovary 249f
Leukemia 248, 249
Leydig cell
    hyperplasia 170
    tumor 170, 225, 226
Lichen planus 12, 14t
Lichen sclerosis 13, 14t, 27
    atrophicus 13, 14
Lichen simplex chronicus 14
Ligneous vaginitis 40
Lipoid salpingitis 256
Lipomatous leiomyoma 116
Listeria infection 271
Listeria monocytogenes 271
Liver tumor 247
Lobular endocervical glandular hyperplasia 58, 61, 83
Luteinized granulosa cell tumor 226
Luteinizing hormone 97
Lymph node 182, 292
    involvement 135, 295
Lymphangioma 257
Lymphatic drainage 8, 157
Lymphocytes, infiltration of 55
Lymphoepithelioma-like carcinomas 76
Lymphogranuloma venereum 11
Lymphoid tumor 37, 61, 170, 251
Lymphoma 248
    tumor 116
Lymphovascular invasion 134, 295

## M

Maternal
    circulatory disorder 271
    diabetes 277
    disorders, placenta in 274
    floor infarct 272, 273f
Mature squamous epithelium 53
Mature teratoma 170, 236, 236f, 237f
Mayer-Rokitansky-Küster-Hauser syndrome 6
Melanocytic tumors 24, 61
Melanoma 91
    cervix 91f, 92f
    superficial spreading 34
    vagina 47f, 48f
Menstrual
    cycle, changes in normal 53
    endometrium 102f
    phase 100
Merkel cell carcinoma 30
Mesenchymal tissue 19f
Mesenchymal tumors 37, 61, 90, 169, 251
    malignant 90
Mesodermal tumor, mixed 92
Mesonephric
    carcinoma 58, 61, 85
    cyst 41, 41f, 180, 259
    ducts 3f
    hyperplasia 57, 86
    remnants 57
Mesothelial cyst 259, 260f
Mesothelial tumors 170
Mesothelioma 170
Metaplastic
    cells, origin of 111
    papillary tumor 251
    theory 114
Metastasis from stomach 246
Metastasizing leiomyoma 116
    benign 149
Metastatic
    adenocarcinoma 115
    carcinoma 205, 259
    colonic carcinoma 195
    tumors 48
    urothelial carcinoma 248
Microcystic stromal tumor 170
Microglandular hyperplasia 56, 56f, 57f, 61, 85, 112
Microimmunofluorescence 11
Microinvasive adenocarcinoma 80, 81f, 82f
Microinvasive carcinoma 73, 73b
Micropapillary
    architecture 182
    serous carcinoma 174, 183
Mitogen activated protein kinase 174
Mitotically active
    cellular fibromas 217
    endocervical glands 80
    leiomyoma 116, 146
*Mobiluncus curtisii* 38
*Mobiluncus mulieris* 38
Molluscum contagiosum 11
Monodermal teratoma 170, 240
Monozygotic twin 267
Mons pubis 8
Morphea 14
Morules 111

Mucin core protein 32
Mucin rich cells 193
Mucin stain, positive 224
Mucinous adenocarcinoma 190
Mucinous adenofibroma 169
Mucinous adenoma 186
Mucinous borderline tumor 169, 187, 188f, 189f
    type of 187
Mucinous carcinoid, primary 246
Mucinous carcinoma 61, 116, 128, 128f, 129f, 129t, 130f, 133, 169, 191f, 192f, 194f, 251, 259
Mucinous cyst 18, 18f
Mucinous cystadenoma 169, 186f, 187f
Mucinous metaplasia 112, 251, 252
Mucinous tumor 169, 175, 179, 189
    atypical proliferative 169
      benign 186
      borderline 187
Müllerian adenosarcoma, low-grade 137
Müllerian cyst 41, 42f
Müllerian duct, development of 6
Mullerian tumor
    malignant mixed 111, 125, 135, 195, 196f, 197f, 224, 239, 250
    mixed 135
Multilayered granulosa cells 162f
Muscularis mucosa 252
Mycobacteria tuberculosis 255
Mycobacterium tubercle infection 108
*Mycobacterium tuberculosis* 271
Mycoplasma hominis 38, 160
Myeloid tumor 37, 61, 116, 170, 251
Myomectomy 290
Myometrial invasion 124, 134, 295
Myxoid
    leiomyoma 116
    leiomyosarcoma 116, 151f
    smooth muscle tumor 148
    variant 151

# N

Nabothian cyst 59f, 61
    formation of 55
Nasopharyngeal carcinoma 76
Necrobiotic granulomas 161
Necrotic pseudoxanthomatous lesion 256
*Neisseria gonorrhoeae* 56, 160, 254
Nerve sheath tumor 91
    malignant peripheral 61
Neuroectodermal tumors 24, 170, 243
Neuroendocrine
    carcinoma 61, 88, 205
      high grade 61
      large cell 61, 89, 116
    tumors 61
      low grade 61
Nodular melanoma 33
Non-gestational choriocarcinoma 170
Non-granulomatous infection 160
Noninfectious granulomas 161
Noninfectious inflammatory diseases 12, 40

Nonkeratinizing squamous cell carcinoma 28, 71, 89t
Non-trophoblastic tumors 275
Nuclear
    atypia 181
    moulding 172

# O

Omental deposit 176f
Omental implant 182
Omphalomesenteric duct 276
Oncocytic metaplasia 113
Oocyte, secondary 159f
Oophorectomy 293
Oral contraceptives 107
Original squamocolumnar junction 52f
Oropharynx 76
Ovarian
    cancer
      grading of 177t
      staging of 176b
    carcinoma 133, 295
    decidua 166
    dysgenesis 4
    endometriosis 114f
    hypoplasia 4
    stromal cells 171
    tumor 164, 169, 170b, 172
      classification of 169
Ovary 291
    absent 167
    anatomy of 157
    carcinoid 242f, 243f
    choriocarcinoma of 235f, 236f
    clear cell
      adenocarcinoma of 246
      carcinoma of 199f
      tumors of 198
    congenital lesions of 167
    contralateral 295
    cysts in 161
    endometrioid
      carcinoma of 192
      stromal sarcoma of 198f
    epithelial carcinoma of 179
    fibrosarcoma of 218f
    germ cell tumor of 228
    hemangioma of 250
    infections of 160
    metastatic tumors of 245
    mucinous tumor of 186
    neuroendocrine carcinoma of 205
    non-neoplastic lesions of 157
    serous
      adenocarcinoma of 184f
      borderline tumor of 180, 181f
      cystadenoma of 260
    sex cord tumor of 209
    squamous cell carcinoma of 205f
    tumors of 245, 248
Oxyphil cells 193
Oxyphilic endometrioid carcinoma 226

## P

Paget disease
  diagnosis of 32t
  of vulva 31
Paget's cells 32f
Pancreatic tumor 247
Papillary
  adenofibroma 84
  endocervicitis 84
  immature metaplasia 66
  serous carcinoma 113
  squamous cell carcinoma 75, 75f
  structures 129
  syncytial metaplasia 113
Papilloma 251, 257
Parabasal cell layer 50
Paramesonephric cyst 259, 260f
Paramesonephric duct 3f
Paraovarian cyst 259
Parasitic infection 56, 256
Parasitic vaginitis 39
Parvovirus B19 271
Pelvic
  examination 175
  pain 254
Pemphigus vulgaris 16, 16f
Periodic acid schiff 32
Peripheral basaloid cells 75f
Peritoneal cytology 134
Peritoneal implant 182
Peritoneal mucinous carcinomatosis 189
Perivascular epithelioid cell 143
  tumor 116, 153
Perivillous fibrin
  deposition 272
  massive 272
Persistent corpus luteum 107
Peutz-Jegher syndrome 225
Pithelial membrane antigen 32
Placenta 293, 293f, 294
  abnormal adherence of 265
  accreta 265
  circulatory disorders of 271
  increta 265
  membranacea 265
  mucormycosis in 272f
  multilobated 265
  pathology of 262
  percreta 265, 266f, 267f
  shape of 265t
Placental alkaline phosphatase, positive 248
Placental examination 264
Placental inflammation 268
Placental membrane 267f
Placental site trophoblastic tumor 283, 283, 283f, 284f, 285
Placental tuberculosis 271f
Plasma
  cells 55
  regain, rapid 9
Plasminogen 40
Plasmodium infection 271, 271f

Pleomorphic
  cells, moderate 82f
  leiomyoma 147
  rhabdomyosarcoma 137
Polycystic ovarian syndrome 163, 164b
Polyembryoma 235
Polyhedral cells 148f
Polymorphonuclear leukocytic infiltration 268
Polypoid adenomyoma, atypical 94, 110, 118, 119, 124
Postmenopausal endometrium 102
Preeclampsia 274, 275
Pregnancy
  early normal 282
  history of 125
  luteoma 166, 170, 225
Premature delivery 275
Preterm birth 270
Prevotella bivia 38
Primitive germ cells 2
Primordial follicle 157, 158f
Primordial germ cells 2, 4
Progesterone
  effect 107
  receptor 141
Progesterone-related disorder 106
Prostate specific acid phosphatase 243
Protein 63
Pseudohermaphrodite 5
Pseudomyxoma peritonei 189, 190f
Psoriasis 14, 15

## R

Radical vulvectomy specimen 292f
Resistant ovary syndrome 167
Rete ovarii
  adenoma of 170
  tumor of 170
Reticulin rich theca cell 214
Retiform SLCT 220
Retroplacental hematoma 273, 273f
Rh incompatibility 274
Rhabdomyoma 61
Rhabdomyosarcoma 61, 116, 144, 250
Rubella 270

## S

Salpingectomy specimen 292, 293
Salpingitis
  acute 254
  chronic 254, 255f
  isthmica nodosa 251, 253, 253f
Sarcoma botryoides 46, 91
Sarcomatous
  nodule 190
  overgrowth 138
Schistosoma haematobium infection 39
Schistosoma mansoni 39
Sclerosing stromal tumor 166, 170, 216, 218, 218f, 219f
Sebaceous
  adenoma 170
  carcinoma 170

Secretory carcinoma 127f, 128f
Secretory cell 193, 252
    outgrowth 173, 174b
Seminal fluid, reaction to 40
Septate uterus 6, 6f
Seromucinous
    borderline tumor 169
    carcinoma 169
    cystadenofibroma 169
    cystadenoma 169
    tumors 169
Serosa 97
Serosal layer 252
Serous
    adenocarcinoma 85, 257
    adenofibroma 169, 179, 251
    borderline tumor 169, 180, 182, 183, 183f, 251
    carcinoma 61, 116, 129, 130f, 131t, 133, 184, 186, 186b
        high-grade 169, 172, 175, 185, 186f, 251
        low-grade 169, 174, 184, 184f, 185f, 251
    cyst cystadenoma 179f
    cystadenoma 161, 169, 179, 180f
    endometrial intraepithelial carcinoma 131
    papillary adenocarcinoma 84
    surface papilloma 169
    tubal intraepithelial carcinoma 172, 172b, 173f, 251, 259
    tumor 169, 179
        atypical proliferative 169, 180
        benign 179
        borderline 174
Sertoli cell tumor 170, 224
Sertoli-Leydig cell tumor 170, 195t, 219, 220f-224f, 234, 241, 246
Sex chromosome 1f
Sex cord tumor 170
    pure 170
    with annular tubules 225
Sex cord-stromal tumors, mixed 170
Sex development, disorder of 5, 6, 6t
Sex differentiation, disorders of 5
Sickle cell disease 274
Signet ring
    carcinoma 83
    cell type 61
    stromal tumor 170, 219
Sinovaginal bulb fuses 3f
Skeletal muscle tumor 250
Slit-like glands 129
Small cell
    carcinoma 30, 89t, 133, 170, 205, 214
    type 207
Smooth muscle
    actin 22, 141
    cell 110f
    tumors 144
Society of Gynecologic Oncologists 73
Soft tissue, tumor of 24, 170, 249
Somatic genetics 200
Somatic type tumors 170
Spindle cell 193
    carcinoma 93

    fascicles of 90f
    nodule, postoperative 41
Spindle-shaped
    cells 145f
    nuclei 146f
Spontaneous abortions 270
Squamocolumnar junction 51, 52f
Squamoid cells 86f
Squamotransitional carcinoma 76
Squamotransitional cell carcinoma 45
Squamous cell 79
    carcinoma 30, 28, 28f, 44, 71, 73, 73f, 74, 75, 133, 170, 205
        prognosis of 76
    lesions, benign 61
    maturation to 54
    tumors 61, 179
Squamous epithelial cells 66
Squamous epithelium 50, 52f
Squamous hyperplasia 14, 27
Squamous intraepithelial lesion 54, 61
    high grade 61, 66
    low grade 61, 65
Squamous lining, benign 51f
Squamous metaplasia 53, 53f, 61, 111, 111f, 275
Squamous papilloma 61
Squamous tumors 24
*Staphylococcus aureus* 40
Stein Leventhal syndrome 117
Steroid cell tumor 170, 225, 226
Steroid tumor 165
Stic lesion 172
Stratum basalis 97
Stratum functional layer, glands of 99
Stratum functionalis 97
Stroma 51
Stromal
    breakdown 120
    collapse 106
    fibrosis in chronic bleeding 106
    hemorrhage 106
    hyperplasia 165, 170
    hyperthecosis 165
    invasion 185
    luteoma 225, 226
    metaplasia 113
    microinvasion in borderline tumor 182
    tumor, pure 170
Struma ovarii 224, 225, 240, 240f
    carcinomas in 240
    follicular carcinomas in 241f
Strumal carcinoid 170, 243
Subnuclear vacuoles 128
Succenturiate lobe 264
Symplastic leiomyoma 147
Syncytiotrophoblastic cells 235f, 236f
Syphilis 9, 270
    diagnostic tests of 9
    secondary 9
    serological test of 9
    tertiary 9
Systemic diseases 161

## T

Tamoxifen 108
Tampon ulcer 40
Telescoping gland 99f, 104
Testicular feminization 5
Testis determining factor 4
Theca cell tumor 214
Thecoma 216f
Thick-walled stromal blood vessels 109
Thyroglobulin positivity 224
Thyroid follicles 240f
Torsion 256, 276
Toxic shock syndrome 40
Toxoplasma 270
Transitional cell
    carcinoma 133, 175, 203, 251, 258
        of fallopian tube 258f
        of ovary 204f
    metaplasia 54, 252
    tumor 179, 201
Transitional epithelium 175
Transitional metaplasia 61, 253f
Transvaginal ultrasound 175
Transverse fusion of vagina, disorders of 7
Transverse vaginal septum 38
Traumatic injury 40
*Treponema pallidum* 9
*Trichomonas vaginalis* 39, 39f
Trichuris trichiura 40
Trophoblastic disease, classification of 278b
Tubal
    endometriosis 114f
    hyperplasia 251
    intraepithelial carcinoma 259
    metaplasia 54, 54f, 112f, 254
Tubercular salpingitis 255
Tuberculosis 55, 11, 108, 271
Tuberculous salpingitis 255f
Tubo-endometrioid metaplasia 80
Tubo-ovarian abscess 251
Tubular metaplasia 112
Tumor 155, 291
    benign 193
    bilateral 224
    borderline 180, 193
    carcinoid 61, 116, 224
    cell 129, 183
        cuboidal 232f
        discrete 152f
        necrosis 218
        proliferation 135
    invasion of 34, 138
    like lesions 37, 61, 170, 251
    of vulva, WHO classification of 2014 24
    secondary 61, 116, 171
    simulating endometrial glands 194f
    suppressor genes 135
    thickness 34
    unclassified 171
    unilateral 186

Twin pregnancy 267f
    chorion in 267f

## U

Umbilical
    artery 269f
    cord 294
        insertion of 276
        pathology 276
    knots 277
Unicornuate uterus 6, 6f
Uterine
    bleeding
        abnormal 105b
        causes of 105b
    carcinoma 133
    carcinosarcoma 93, 135
    cavity 97
    didelphys 6
    glands 109
    leiomyomatosis, diffuse 149
    leiomyomatous polyp 92
    segment, lower 102f, 104, 104f
    serous carcinoma 127, 129, 131t
    smooth muscle tumors 152
    specimen 289
    tumors 155, 248
    vascular supply 97f
Uterus 116
    anatomical parts of 97f
    anatomy of 96
    anomalies of 6
    endometrioid carcinoma of 85, 125
    grossing of 291f
    intravenous leiomyomatosis of 149
    mesenchymal tumor of 140
    normal 6f
    vascular supply of 96

## V

Vagina 40
    benign diseases of 37
    disorders of 37
    malignant diseases of 37
    melanoma of 47
    neoplasms of 44
    prolapse of 41
    staging of carcinoma of 45t
    upper part of 3f
Vaginal
    adenosis 42, 43f
    agenesis 7, 37
    cavity develops 3f
    cuff 291
    cysts 41
    development, anomalies of 7
    intraepithelial neoplasia 43, 43f
    squamous cell carcinoma 44f, 45f
Vascular leiomyoma 148
Vascular wall injury 274

Venous supply 157
Verrucous 61
   carcinoma 29, 29f, 30, 30f, 45
      diagnosis of 31t
   squamous cell carcinoma 75
Vestigial remnants 276
Villoglandular adenocarcinoma 83
Villoglandular carcinoma 61
Villoglandular endometrioid carcinoma 126f, 127f
Villous edema 274
Viral
   genome 62
   infections 11, 56
   life cycle 63
   protein interaction 62
Vulva 12, 28
   adnexal tumor of 19
   anatomy of 8f
   benign
      diseases of 17
      neoplastic lesions of 8
      squamous tumor of 19
   bullous lesions of 16
   conditions of 22
   cysts of 17t
   infections of 9t
   infectious diseases of 8
   malignant melanoma of 33
   malignant tumors of 24, 34
   melanoma of 33f
   mesenchymal lesions of 19
   metastatic tumors of 34
   mixed tumor of 22
   multinucleated atypia of 27
   premalignant tumors of 24
   squamous cell carcinoma of 27
   staging of carcinoma of 31t
Vulval
   cancer 294
   carcinoma 31f
   cyst 17
   intraepithelial neoplasia 25, 27t
      classification of 26t
      types of 27t
   lichen planus 12
Vulvectomy specimen 292
Vulvodynia 17

## W

Walthard cell 253f
Warty carcinoma 29, 75
Warty squamous cell carcinoma 75
Wolffian duct cyst 18
Wolffian tumors 170
World Health Organization 25, 171, 180, 278

## Y

Yolk sac tumor 133, 170, 200, 214, 224, 230, 230b

## Z

Zygosity 266, 267f